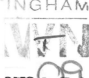
Design Concepts in Nutritional Epidemiology

DATE DUE FOR RETURN

The loan period may be shortened if the item is requested.

Design Concepts in Nutritional Epidemiology

Second Edition

Barrie M. Margetts
Wessex Institute for Health Research and Development

and

Michael Nelson
Department of Nutrition and Dietetics, King's College, London

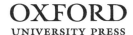

OXFORD

UNIVERSITY PRESS

OXFORD
UNIVERSITY PRESS

Great Clarendon Street, Oxford OX2 6DP

Oxford University Press is a department of the University of Oxford.
It furthers the University's objective of excellence in research, scholarship,
and education by publishing worldwide in

Oxford New York

Auckland Cape Town Dar es Salaam Hong Kong Karachi
Kuala Lumpur Madrid Melbourne Mexico City Nairobi
New Delhi Shanghai Taipei Toronto

With offices in

Argentina Austria Brazil Chile Czech Republic France Greece
Guatemala Hungary Italy Japan South Korea Poland Portugal
Singapore Switzerland Thailand Turkey Ukraine Vietnam

Oxford is a registered trade mark of Oxford University Press
in the UK and in certain other countries

Published in the United States
by Oxford University Press Inc., New York

© Barrie M. Margetts, Michael Nelson, and
the contributors listed on p. ix, 1997

A catalogue record for this book is available from the British Library

Library of Congress Cataloging in Publication Data
Design concepts in nutritional epidemiology / [edited by] Barrie M.
Margetts and Michael Nelson.—2nd ed.
Includes bibliographical references and index.
1. Nutritionally induced diseases–Epidemiology. I. Margetts,
Barrie M. II. Nelson, Michael.
RA645.N87D46 1997 616.3'9—dc20 96–43448

ISBN 978 0 19 262739 1

Printed in Great Britain
by
Biddles Ltd., King's Lynn, Norfolk

Preface

The need for this revised edition stems from the rapid rate of change in our understanding about the key issues in nutritional epidemiology. We are grateful to our many colleagues around the world who have been helpful in developing our appreciation of the influences in our understanding of epidemiological relationships that needed to be addressed in this new edition. We have added new chapters on qualitative and sociological measures (Chapter 9), anthropometric measures (Chapter 10), gene–nutrient interactions (Chapter 11), and cross-sectional studies (Chapter 13). In addition we have substantially revised the introductory section to bring a more practical focus to the theoretical concepts around study design, and all other chapters from the first edition have been revised to take into account recent developments. The material from two chapters from the first edition (use of existing nutritional data and measures of disease frequency and exposure effect) has been incorporated into relevant sections of other chapters.

We would like to acknowledge the continued support of our colleagues in the UK Nutritional Epidemiology Group whose work, comments, and discussion has helped to shape the contents of this revised edition. We would like to acknowledge the Department of Health, and particularly Martin Wiseman and Bob Wenlock, for their continued support of the Nutritional Epidemiology Group. By using the book as a course text for the European postgraduate summer course in public health nutritional epidemiology, we have had valuable feedback from both teachers and participants for which we are very grateful. We are also grateful to all the authors, and particularly new contributors whose work has so valuably extended the scope of the book, for making time to prepare their contributions to the book against a background of increasing pressures of other work.

Specifically, Barrie Margetts would like to acknowledge the support of colleagues in the Wessex Institute for Health Research and Development, particularly Rachel Thompson, Kip Pirie, and Julie Hickman. Michael Nelson would like to thank his colleagues in the Department of Nutrition and Dietetics, particularly Mary Atkinson and Charlotte Townsend for their hard work and continued support.

Southampton B.M.M.
London M.N.
September 1996

To Vanessa

Contents

Contents

Part C   The design of nutritional epidemiological studies

List of contributors

Anderson, Annie
School of Management and Consumer Studies, University of Dundee, Dundee

Bates, Chris J.
MRC Dunn Nutrition Centre, Cambridge

Bingham, Sheila A.
MRC Dunn Nutrition Centre, Cambridge

Burr, Michael L.
Centre for Applied Public Health Medicine, University of Wales, Cardiff

Cade, Janet E.
Nuffield Institute for Health, University of Leeds

Clayton, David
MRC Biostatistics Unit, Cambridge

Coggon, David
MRC Environmental Epidemiology Unit, University of Southampton, Southampton

Cole, Tim J.
MRC Dunn Nutrition Centre, Cambridge

DeMarini, David
Environmental Protection Agency, Triangle Park, North Carolina, USA

Gill, Caroline
MRC Biostatistics Unit, Cambridge

Hiller, Janet E.
Department of Community Medicine, University of Adelaide, South Australia

Inskip, Hazel
MRC Environmental Epidemiology Unit, University of Southampton, Southampton

Kohlmeier, Lenore
Departments of Nutrition and Epidemiology, University of North Carolina at Chapel Hill, NC, USA

Macintyre, Sally
MRC Medical Sociology Unit, Glasgow

Margetts, Barrie M.
Wessex Institute for Health Research and Development, University of Southampton, Southampton

McMichael, Anthony J.
Department of Epidemiology and Population Sciences, London School of Hygiene and Tropical Medicine, London

Nelson, Michael
Department of Nutrition and Dietetics, Kings College, London

Osmond, Clive
MRC Environmental Epidemiology Unit, University of Southampton, Southampton

Piegorsch, Walter
Department of Statistics, University of South Carolina, Columbia, SC, USA

Rouse, Ian L.
Department of Health, Perth, Western Australia

Thurnam, David I.
Human Nutrition Research Group, School of Biomedical Sciences, University of Ulster at Coleraine

Ulijaszek, Stanley J.
Department of Biological Anthropology, University of Cambridge, Cambridge and Department of Nutrition and Food Science, School of Public Health, Curtin University, Perth, Western Australia

van Staveren, Wija A.
Department of Human Nutrition, Wageningen Agricultural University, Wageningen, The Netherlands

West, Clive E.
Department of Human Nutrition, Wageningen Agricultural University, Wageningen, The Netherlands

Introduction

Barrie M. Margetts and Michael Nelson

After the supply of air and water, the supply of food is fundamental to human survival. The struggle to obtain enough food shapes the lives of all human beings, whether they grow their own food, or work to earn money to buy food from other people who produce it. At an individual level, whether it is explicit or only implicit, this struggle focuses on obtaining the right balance of foods to enable the body to function optimally. The way society maintains any coherence and order is also related to the capacity of the individuals within that society to meet these fundamental needs of water and food, as well as the capacity to meet with other people and form social networks (families, etc).

There are different social and biological imperatives which underlie how societies cope with an imbalance between the demands for foods and the ability of the society to supply them. A country or region (or town or village) may have health problems related to an excess of supply (e.g. obesity) as well as health problems related to an inadequate supply (anaemia, goitre, wasting, or stunting). The impact of the dietary excess or deficiency may be modulated by the effects of other factors, such as acute or chronic illness, clean water supplies, and medical services. The 'right' foods may be available, but not eaten for a wide variety of reasons.

It is our contention that whenever data are being collected which has anything to do with human nutrition and community health, then nutritional epidemiological principles need to be considered. Further, if a nutrition intervention programme is to be put in place, the effectiveness of that programme must be evaluated. This evaluation should be done following the principles of nutritional epidemiology. It is also important that the data are collected with a purpose in mind. Expressed another way, there should be a clear hypothesis that the activity/research addresses. This applies for nutritional surveillance or any other study. It is an important part of nutritional epidemiology to focus on the development of clear testable research questions. Another important part of a nutritional epidemiological approach is that the effects of other factors are also considered, and that both these other factors and the exposure and outcome of interest are measured with sufficient precision to enable a reliable estimate of the relationship of interest to be assessed.

Six years after the publication of the first edition, nutritional epidemiology has progressed dramatically. We now have a much better understanding of the characteristics of exposures that need to be measured in order to answer questions about diet-disease relationships. We now appreciate that risks are more likely to be associated with patterns of food consumption as well as the influence of individual components of foods. It is also becoming clear that the way foods are stored and prepared influences the impact they have on health; to date, few studies have measured the physical properties of food. This applies to what has traditionally been referred to as non-nutrients as well as nutrients.

We are also getting better at relating these improved measures of exposure to more specific aspects of outcome. For example, it is now becoming clearer that atheroma relates to a combination of levels of LDL and anti-oxidants, and that looking at either on their own is likely to be misleading. This ability to relate exposure to steps in the causal pathway more precisely, improves the value of the epidemiological findings in relation to public health recommendations.

We have also improved our understanding of both the sources, characteristics, and effects of errors in the measurement of dietary exposures. The ability to identify related aspects of exposure with independent errors has been helpful in understanding the limitations of the measures of diet which are currently used to assess exposure. While biomarkers may be able to be measured with greater technical precision, the relevance of these measures to understanding the underlying role of diet still needs further clarification. For many nutrients at present there are no biomarkers which reflect changes in dietary intakes with sufficient sensitivity for them to be useful proxies for dietary intake. The proxy function is often applied from one nutrient to another, for example, extrapolating the notion of the completeness of all aspects of diet (micronutrient levels) from only one measure, such as 24-hour urinary nitrogen excretion, may not be justified.

We can now derive estimates of measurement errors which can be used in the analysis and interpretation of studies to help us judge the likely impact of these errors on the estimates of risk. It is also possible to use statistical techniques to identify clusters or patterns of consumption (and behaviour) associated with risk, rather than focusing only on individual components of diet or related behaviour.

The use of biomarkers (e.g. energy and nitrogen, or energy intake/BMR ratios) to identify those respondents whose reported dietary intakes are unreliable has enabled us to be clearer about the generalizability of the results obtained from these studies. For example, energy intakes estimated from obese subjects are likely to have been under-estimated. This has helped us to appreciate that some of the recommendations that are made may apply only to specific subsets of the population; it may not be possible to make broad generalized statements because of the diversity of factors influencing diet, on the one hand, and disease risk on the other. Genetics and molecular biology may help us to identify susceptible individuals who may respond differently to other individuals at the same level of exposure; but this is likely to represent only a small proportion of the variation in sensitivity to exposure.

Public health nutrition

Nutritional epidemiology is the scientific basis upon which public health nutrition is built. Public health nutrition focuses on the promotion of good health through nutrition and the primary prevention of diet related illness in the population. The evidence upon which the promotion of good health, including the avoidance of illness and the maintenance of wellness, depends on research that is well done. In simple terms nutritional epidemiology provides the messages, and a function of many employed in public health nutrition is to take these messages and present them in the best possible way to promote optimal health.

Other skills are also required to function as a public health nutritionist. These include an understanding of the principles of nutritional sciences and the assessment of the nutritional status of individuals and populations; the principles of health promotion; skills in communication; and an understanding of the wider social, economic, and political context within which people live their lives and which influences their choices about diet.

Over the last six years since the first edition of this book, the understanding of the role of nutritional epidemiology in public health has increased. While many researchers undertaking nutritional epidemiological studies are not involved with public health and health promotion, the relevance of nutritional epidemiology to public health has become much clearer. There is now a better understanding of the need for skills from traditional academic research, through applied research aimed at evaluating nutrition health programmes, to the delivery of health programmes, all of which require training in nutritional epidemiology.

While it is not reasonable to expect academic research workers and those involved in health promotion to understand all aspects of each other's work, it is important that there is a dialogue between groups involved from the laboratory to the field.[1] This should be a two-way relationship: those working in research need to be addressing subjects of public health relevance, assessing the effects of dietary exposures that are of concern; while those involved in health promotion need to understand the strengths and limitations of the approaches which are used to gather the information about the role of diet in the aetiology of disease. Within the academic research community there is also a need to ensure that those involved in metabolic research and those involved in nutritional epidemiology can communicate in an effective way to ensure that the laboratory based work is exploring in detail the mechanistic basis for the associations revealed from epidemiological studies. Additionally, epidemiological researchers need to be aware of the characteristics of the biological measures used to inform the understanding of the mechanisms which underlie the reported associations. The use of biological measures to support interview/subject based data about food and nutrient intakes needs to be interpreted with some knowledge of the biological basis of the relationship between the dietary measure and the biological measure, as well as an understanding of the metabolic factors which control the biological measure used; concentrations in blood do not necessarily equate to levels of functional availability at the site of action.

Dietary guidelines to reduce the risks of chronic diseases have been prepared by many organizations in many countries; there is remarkable agreement between these guidelines, perhaps not surprisingly, because they are all based on a review and development of consensus from the same body of evidence. In the UK these guidelines have been promoted by the government, and as part of this promotion the government has set targets. While there is wide consensus on the desired changes required in diet to achieve these targets, what has been missing has been a clear way to measure progress toward these targets, even for something as seemingly straightforward as changes in the per cent energy from fat for the population. While national studies have been done to provide guidance about progress, all health authorities in the UK were charged with the responsibility for meeting the agreed targets; in order to do this the local health authorities required information at the local level. The question raised was how to measure diet accurately enough in groups of people in the population to know whether change is occurring in the right direction. The relevance of the questions being asked of nutritional epidemiological research about reducing measurement error and improving study design have become directly relevant to those who are involved in delivering the health service to the population. The skills traditionally linked only with academic nutritional epidemiological research are now also required for research aimed at evaluating the effectiveness of health promotion programmes aimed at achieving the dietary targets. The Health of the Nation diet and nutrition targets have therefore stimulated closer links between those involved in academic research and in the health service, as well as stimulating training centres to provide better, more relevantly trained, graduates.

The development of closer links between the requirements of research and monitoring the effectiveness of programmes stimulated in Europe was, in many ways, catching up with what had been occurring in the less economically developed countries, where nutritional surveillance has been part of routine monitoring of maternal and child health. This increasing emphasis on monitoring progress toward targets raised questions about how to measure these targets, and the level of accuracy required for these measures to allow a reliable assessment of the change in nutrition. We are becoming increasingly aware of the theoretical limitations of the measures being assessed, but the awareness of their limitations in applying these measures to address public health assessments of targets is less good. There is a need for the rigour applied in academic nutritional epidemiological research to be applied to public health as practised in the health service and health promotion.

Organization of the book

The book follows a progression from detailed definitions and clarification of concepts, through identification of the most appropriate methods for measuring exposures and outcomes, to a consideration of the study designs that are best suited to an exploration of hypotheses in nutritional epidemiological research.

Part A brings a practical focus to the scientific concepts underlying study design. Chapter 1 provides an overview of the principles of nutritional epidemiology. Chapter 2 considers the key elements in the design, planning, and evaluation of nutritional epidemiological studies. Chapter 3 reviews sampling, study size, and power; it provides guidelines on how to estimate the size of different study designs required to give appropriate power to these studies. Chapter 4 describes the effects of measurement error on study design and suggests some practical remedies.

Part B deals with the problems of the measurement and interpretation of a wide variety of variables relevant to nutritional epidemiology. Chapter 5 deals with the estimation of nutrient intakes from food consumption surveys using food composition tables. Chapter 6 describes the methods used to assess food consumption and nutrient intakes. Chapter 7 sets out the major techniques of assessing and evaluating biochemical markers of nutrient intake and nutritional status for use in nutritional epidemiological studies. Chapter 8 reviews the theoretical and practical issues of importance in the validation of dietary assessment. Chapter 9 provides a thought-provoking review of socio-demographic and psycho-social variables of relevance to nutritional epidemiology. Chapter 10 provides a review of anthropometric measures. Chapter 11 assesses the relevance and approaches to considering gene–nutrient interactions in nutritional epidemiological studies.

Part C addresses the principles of the design and interpretation of ecological studies (Chapter 12), cross-sectional studies (Chapter 13), cohort studies (Chapter 14), case-control studies (Chapter 15), and experimental studies (Chapter 16).

Reference

1. Margetts, B.M. (1994) Linking the field to the laboratory. *Proc. Nut. Soc.* **53**: 43–52.

Part A The scientific concepts underlying study design

1. Overview of the principles of nutritional epidemiology

Barrie M. Margetts and Michael Nelson

And the more I see – the more I know
The more I know – the less I understand
                          Paul Weller (1995) *Stanley Road*, CBS Records

The introduction discussed the wider context within which nutritional epidemiological research is conducted. This chapter sets out the basic principles of nutritional epidemiology as they apply to the study of relationships between nutrition and health outcomes.

1.1 Objective of nutritional epidemiological research

The main objective of nutritional epidemiological research is to provide the best possible scientific evidence to support an understanding of the role of nutrition in the causes and prevention of ill health.

Nutritional epidemiology is based on an understanding of the scientific principles of human nutrition and epidemiology. Epidemiology has been classically defined as having three aims:

(1) to describe the distribution and size of disease problems in human populations;
(2) to elucidate the aetiology of diseases;
(3) to provide the information necessary to manage and plan services for the prevention, control, and treatment of disease.[1]

Human nutrition describes the processes whereby cells, tissues, organs, and the body as a whole obtain and use the necessary substances to maintain their structural and functional integrity. Human nutrition is based on an understanding of the effects of the balance between the supply and demand of substrates and cofactors (e.g. nutrients) required to maintain optimal function (including growth, pregnancy, lactation, fighting infections, etc). Human nutrition seeks to understand the complexity of the effects of both social and biological factors on how individuals and populations seek to maintain optimal function. In nutritional epidemiological studies it is important to consider the factors that affect food supply (quality, quantity, balance) as well as those that affect what happens to the food once it has been eaten. Nutritional epidemiological research tries to take a wide view of the way in which diet affects/maintains health and well-being in individuals and populations.

The aim of nutritional epidemiological research is to ensure that the information upon which public health decisions are made is of the highest quality. To achieve this aim, clear research questions need to be addressed by well designed studies. This applies to basic as well as applied research. Poorly designed studies are a waste of time and money and in the widest sense they are unethical.

From a methodological perspective Riboli *et al.*[2] have recently highlighted four main limitations of nutritional epidemiology, particularly for cancer, but also for other disease endpoints:

(1) measurements of diet lack precision and specificity, particularly for estimates of food consumption;
(2) nutrient intakes are highly correlated, and attribution of causation to one nutrient considered to be acting on its own may be misleading;
(3) biological measures of nutrients in tissues may not accurately and reliably reflect dietary intake because the biological regulation of these measures is complex and may be influenced by levels of other nutrients;
(4) most studies undertaken to date have not considered the effects of the physical characteristics of food (e.g. an orange as a whole fruit or as juice, the way food is prepared) on the metabolic activity of the constituents of the food.

To assess the effect of dietary exposure it is necessary to measure dietary intakes; measuring intake is complex and inevitably the measure derived will not be a perfect representation of the true intake. The extent of this measurement error, the consistency across subjects in the study, and the effects these have on the statistical power and the interpretation of results is of prime concern in nutritional epidemiology.

Norrell[3] has suggested there are three steps in dealing with errors in epidemiological studies:

(1) identifying the principle sources of errors;
(2) exploring the impact of these errors on the results;
(3) designing studies which prevent or control these errors.

Even if it were possible to measure dietary intake with absolute accuracy, relating intake to the cause(s) of a disease requires an understanding of the steps by which what people eat leads to or protects against the occurrence of disease. It is not possible for an epidemiological approach to examine every step in the causal pathway, and here there is a need for close links with those involved in experimental work exploring metabolic processes. Because there will always be gaps in our knowledge of the exact causal pathways involved, we often have to infer causality from limited data when making suggestions about the likely role of a specific factor in causing or preventing the disease of interest. There are guidelines about how to draw causal inferences and these are explored later in this chapter.

Having a clear idea about the likely role of the nutritional factor of interest in the disease process of interest will help the researcher develop a research protocol which can test the role of that factor in the best possible way. The key issues involved in designing studies and the development of research protocols are covered in more detail in Chapter 2.

1.2 Types of epidemiological studies

Broadly, epidemiological studies can be divided into experimental and observational investigations (Table 1.1). The distinction between these types of study is that in experimental investigations exposures are assigned to subjects by the investigator, whereas in observational studies the investigator has no control over the way in which subjects are exposed. Practical and ethical issues may be important in determining which approach is used to address a particular question. In general, experimental studies provide the strongest evidence for the effect of an exposure on an outcome. However, it is not ethical (or permissible) to do experimental studies where the exposure is known to be harmful. Under these circumstances non-experimental study designs must be used.

In observational studies the investigator may be able to exploit 'natural experiments' where exposure is restricted in some groups in the community compared with other groups—for example, looking at groups of vegetarians who avoid meat and have other dietary differences compared with omnivores.

Among observational studies the main differences between study designs relate to the time when exposure and outcome are measured (Fig. 1.1). Cross-sectional studies measure both exposure and outcome in the present and at the same point in time; in case-control studies outcome is measured in the present and past exposure is ascertained; and in cohort studies exposure is measured in the present and outcome ascertained in the future. Experimental studies measure exposure in the present, modify the exposure, and then ascertain the effect of this change in exposure on outcome in the future. Generally cross-sectional studies sample from the population in such a way as to reflect the population characteristics for both exposure and outcome. Case-control studies sample from the population of people with the outcome of interest (with unknown levels of exposure) whereas cohort studies sample from groups of people with different levels of exposure (but unknown or unmeasured outcome). The sample for a cohort study is not always selected to represent the distribution within the whole

Table 1.1 Summary of study designs used in nutritional epidemiological research.

Study design	Study group	
	Populations	Individuals
Experimental	Community trials or community intervention studies	Clinical trials (therapeutic or secondary or tertiary prevention) Field trials (primary prevention) Field intervention studies
Observational	Ecological studies	Cross-sectional (prevalence) studies Case-control (referent) studies Cohort (longitudinal) studies

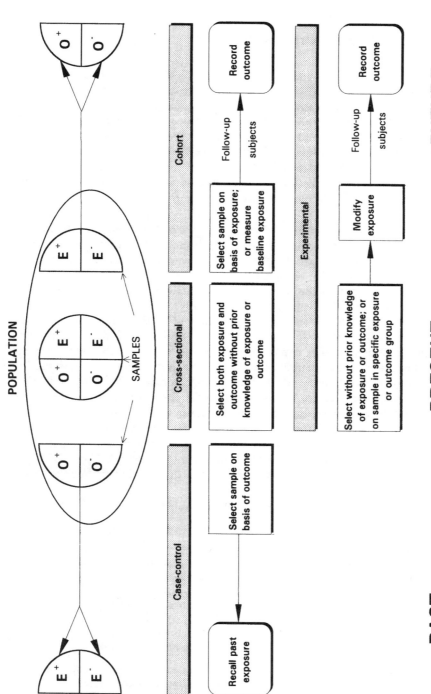

POPULATION

SAMPLES

O⁺ E⁺
O⁻ E⁻

E⁺
E⁻

O⁺
O⁻

E⁺
E⁻

O⁺
O⁻

Case-control

Select sample on basis of outcome

Recall past exposure

Cross-sectional

Select both exposure and outcome without prior knowledge of exposure or outcome

Cohort

Select sample on basis of exposure; or measure baseline exposure

Follow-up subjects

Record outcome

Experimental

Select without prior knowledge of exposure or outcome; or on sample in specific exposure or outcome group

Modify exposure

Follow-up subjects

Record outcome

PAST

PRESENT

FUTURE

NB: **O** = Outcome   **E** = Exposure

Figure 1.1   Summary of sampling and time order of study designs used in nutritional epidemiological studies.

population; it may be weighted to maximize heterogeneity of exposure. In a recent cohort study started in the UK we are recruiting all available vegetarian women, and equal numbers of women who eat fish and who are omnivores, despite the fact that in the general population only about 5% of women are vegetarians. This over-sampling of vegetarian and fish eaters enhances the dietary heterogeneity, but may affect the generalizability of the study. On balance generalizability from cohort studies is less of a concern than not having sufficient heterogeneity within the study sample. Experimental studies sometimes select representative samples of the whole population (community interventions), or sometimes samples of people from selected outcome groups (clinical trials). For both cohort and experimental studies the primary concern is to select a sample which is not going to be lost in the follow-up period. For example, a number of large cohort studies follow-up nurses or doctors who have to be registered to maintain their practice, and so can be traced through these registers. In some countries all the population is registered and therefore able to be traced.

Another way of classifying investigations is according to whether measurements of exposure and outcome are made on populations or individuals (see Table 1.1). It is possible to have population based experimental studies, such as community trials, and population based observational investigations, such as ecological studies. In ecological studies, measures of exposure routinely collected and aggregated at the household or national level are compared with outcome measures aggregated at either the local, district, regional, or national level. Ecological studies also compare differences between levels of exposure and outcome at an international level, as well as looking at changes over time within and between countries.

Both experimental and observational investigations can be conducted among individuals. Although population based studies consist of data collected from individuals (e.g. death certificate diagnosis or household food consumption data), exposure measures are only related to outcome measures at the group level. Information on the distribution of exposure within the group may or may not be known.

In an individual based study it is possible to relate exposure and outcome measures more directly. An advantage therefore of individual based studies over population based studies is that they allow the direct estimation of the risk of disease in relation to exposure. It is possible to assess, for example, whether individuals who eat more fat have higher rates of heart disease. With population based methods it might be shown that populations that have a higher exposure of fat intake also have a higher rate of heart disease, but it would not necessarily follow that the excess of heart disease was occurring in the higher consumers of fat.

It is also possible in individual based studies to measure, and take into account in the analysis, the effects that other factors may have on the relationship under investigation. In population based studies it is usually only possible to consider the effects of a limited number of other factors, and the possibility is greater that an association which is found could be due to the effects of other unmeasured factors.

The choice of a study method is often influenced by pragmatic issues such as cost and feasibility. This pragmatic approach should not, however, be the sole determinant of the study design. Optimally, the investigator should clarify the aim of the study, then decide the best way to do the study. At this stage the investigator usually has to make decisions about how far he or she is prepared to deviate from the ideal, before a study protocol is so compromised that it is no longer viable. If a study cannot address the research question adequately, then it may be better not to do the study.

Table 1.2 summarizes the design issues which are relevant for each type of study. For more details refer to Chapters 12–16 in this book and other texts.[4–9]

A primary factor in choosing between a case-control design and a cohort design is whether the exposure or outcome is rare; if the exposure is rare a cohort can be selected (as in the example of the vegetarian study) to over-sample the rare exposure; if the outcome is rare a case-control study would need a very large sample to have sufficient subjects with different levels of exposure. Cross-sectional studies are optimal where both the exposure and outcome are common. Because ecological studies are based on aggregated data usually collected from large groups of people (up to the whole country) they are good for exploring both rare and common exposures and outcomes.

The accuracy of the measurement of dietary exposure will generally be low unless special effort is taken to characterize the intakes of individuals; this is most commonly only the case in dietary clinical trials, although some cross-sectional and cohort studies do measure diet with greater precision using weighed records (although not all measures of diet obtained from a weighed record will be precise (see Chapter 6)). Ecological and community intervention studies particularly, but also case-control studies, measure diet less accurately. All studies, except very carefully controlled clinical trials, have a high potential for biased ascertainment of exposure. Where there is a long latent period between exposure and subsequent outcome, case-control and ecological studies are the best designs to use; cohort studies are optimal where there is a short latent period, unless pre-existing measures of exposure exist for a cohort which can be identified retrospectively.

Cohort studies are able to assess multiple outcomes (if the sample is large enough), but are restricted in the number of exposure measures that can be assessed (depending on the method of assessing diet); whereas case-control studies are restricted to assessing one outcome (or at the most subsets of related outcomes), but may be able to assess many different exposures (but also depending on the measure of diet used).

If an absolute measure of the effect of the exposure on the outcome (relative risk) is required, the only design which is appropriate is a cohort study, as ecological and cross-sectional designs can only measure prevalence, which relates to incidence but is affected by the duration of illness. For rare outcomes the odds ratio derived from a case-control study approximates a relative risk derived from a cohort study.

Cohort studies tend to be expensive and take a long time to complete, although not always, (for example, studies of maternal diet and birth outcome can be completed in nine months). Case-control studies are generally cheaper and finished more quickly.

1.3   Epidemiological measurements

The first critical stage in epidemiological research is to develop a clearly defined study aim. The investigator must have a sound knowledge of the literature already published. The aim must be specific (relating particular exposures to particular outcomes), feasible (it must be possible to measure exposure and outcome with sufficient accuracy), and relevant (the particular exposures to be measured must be clearly causally related to the outcomes, which are themselves appropriate markers of disease state or disease risk).

Table 1.2 Comparison of different study designs.

Design issues	Study design				Experimental	
	Ecological	Cross-sectional	Case-control	Cohort	Clinical trial, field trial	Community intervention
Exposure measures						
(1) Unit of measurement: populations/households/individuals	Populations	Households/individuals	Individuals	Individuals	Individuals	Populations/households
(2) Good for rare/common exposures	Rare	Common	Common	Rare	Rare/common	Common
(3) High/low accuracy of measurements	Low	High/low	Low	High/low	High	Low
(4) High/low potential bias of measurement, e.g. measure of exposure altered by outcome	High	High	High	Low	Low	High
(5) Good for long/short latent periods	Long	Short	Long	Short	Short	Long/short
Outcome measures						
(1) Unit of measurement: incidence/prevalence/mortality/absolute risk	Prevalence	Prevalence	Prevalence*	Incidence/mortality/absolute risk	Incidence†/absolute risk	Incidence/mortality/absolute risk
(2) Good for rare/common outcomes	Rare/common	Common	Rare	Common	Common, that can be changed	Common, that can be changed
(3) Able/not able to measure multiple outcomes	Able	Able	Not able	Able	Able†	Able‡
Cost						
Low/moderate/high	Low	Low	Low/moderate	High	Moderate/high	High
Duration to complete						
Short/medium/long	Short	Short	Short	Medium/long	Short/medium	Medium/long

* Some studies recruit incident cases.
† Disease, pre-endstage, or risk factor, e.g. blood pressure, serum cholesterol, body weight measured as a change from baseline.
‡ Most experimental studies have only one disease outcome, but they may measure different aspects of disease, and the potential exists to measure other outcomes after the trial is completed.

1.3.1   General issues in the measurement of exposure and outcome

Having defined the aim of the study the next step is to decide what to measure and how to measure it with required accuracy. In broad terms variables to be measured in a study can be defined as either measures of exposure or outcome. These measures can be defined in a variety of ways, and in different studies a measure may be either an exposure or an outcome, depending on the research question (Table 1.3). 'Exposure' is a generic term to describe factors (variables or measures) to which a person or group of people come into contact and that may be relevant to their health.[10, 11] This could include food and the constituents of food (nutrients and non-nutrients), smoking, alcohol, air pollution, noise, or dietary advice or health promotion via adverts etc., or the social environment; in other words any factor which has an impact on a person or group may be defined as an exposure. The way the exposure is measured will depend on the question being asked; exposure could be either a qualitative or quantitative measure. For example, the study may simply want to know whether a person eats carrots or not, or it may want to know how many carrots a person eats. The amount or dose of the exposure may be expressed as either the cumulative exposure over time (e.g. total lifetime calcium intake), the average exposure over time (e.g. amount of fat per day), or the peak exposure at a critical time (e.g. folate intake in first trimester of pregnancy).

Table 1.3   Measures of exposure and outcome.

Exposure measures	Outcome measures
Types of measures	*Types of measures*
Dietary habits	Dietary habits
– food patterns, meals, foods, nutrients	Anthropometry
– individuals, groups, populations	Biological
Anthropometry	Physiological
Biological	Disease/health status
Knowledge about food	– morbidity
Attitudes about food	– mortality
Expression of measures	*Expression of measures*
Continuous measure	Continuous measure
– total cumulative dose (e.g. lifetime intake)	or
– average dose (e.g. average amount per day)	Categorized into discrete measures:
– dose at critical times/induction period	– cut-off points of types of measures
– per cent of standard	e.g. blood pressure above a certain level = hypertension
Discrete measure	e.g. weight for age below a certain level = wasting
– eat a particular food item – yes/no	e.g. continuum of symptoms = disease/not disease
– divide distribution into thirds, fourths, etc. and express intakes in these groups	
– per cent above/below standard	

Exposure may be measured objectively or subjectively, on populations or individuals, in the present or in the past; the choice depends on the question and study design. A population estimate may give the available dose (e.g. estimated total fat available from food acquisition data), but it may not relate to the administered dose (the amount eaten by an individual), and the administered dose may not relate to the active or biologically effective dose at the site of action. Assumptions must be made about the relationship between these measures of exposure in different study designs (see Sections 1.3.2 and 4.7).

'Outcomes' is another generic term used to describe factors (measures/variables) which are being studied in relation to the effects of an exposure; often these outcome measures are disease states, but they may also be anthropometric or physiological measures. Depending on the study these outcome measures may be expressed as continuous or discrete variables. Often an outcome with a continuous distribution will be categorized and a measure of effect assessed across these categories. For example, blood pressure may be analysed as a continuous outcome measure or subjects may be categorized into those with or without hypertension on the basis of whether they fall above or below an agreed cut-off point. Even for nominally discrete outcome measures, such as disease state, it should be recognized that there is not a clear distinction between presence and absence of disease, that disease progresses, and at some point in that progression the disease may become diagnosed. Criteria need to be agreed for case definition for each outcome measure that is divided into diseased/not diseased. The point along the continuum at which a subject is diagnosed will differ in relation to, for example, when the subject complains about symptoms and seeks a medical opinion, and the level of sophistication of the health/diagnostic services for the disease.

Anthropometric measures may be defined in different studies as either an exposure or outcome measure, although, as pointed out in Chapter 10 by Ulijaszek, some caution needs to be exercised in using anthropometric measures as measures of nutritional exposure.

The selection of an appropriate method to measure exposure and outcome and the correct use of that method must be considered at the design stage in any study. The way in which information is obtained should be the same regardless of the level of exposure or outcome status. The level and variability of the exposure and outcome are important to consider when selecting a study population and research design. If all members of a community eat exactly the same diet, no matter how carefully diet is measured, the study will not show any effect of diet on outcome. The lack of variation in diet in many western countries has been suggested as the reason for weak and often statistically non-significant associations between diet and disease. Several recent studies have tried to address this problem by recruiting subjects from across many different countries with different dietary patterns.

Box 1.1 summarizes the measures commonly used to express the relationship between exposure and outcome. Association, expressed as a correlation (non-parametric = Spearman, or parametric = Pearson) gives an indication of the relationship between measures expressed as continuous variables; the association may be between exposure measures or between exposure and outcome measures. The correlation between two measures can be easily summarized into one number, with 95% confidence intervals and associated P-values (see Appendix, Chapter 8). It is also informative to have a

Box 1.1   Measures commonly used to express the relationship between exposure and outcome.

Average level of group outcome in discrete categories of exposure (e.g. blood pressure levels by thirds of fat intake)

Regression (change in outcome per unit change in exposure, adjusting for other factors)

Standardized morbidity or mortality ratios

Absolute risk or absolute risk reduction (incidence or prevalence/ change from baseline of an outcome at different levels of exposure)

Relative risk (the ratio of the rates of appearance of outcomes in different categories of exposure)

Attributable risk percent (the proportion of cases in the exposed population that can be attributed to the risk factor)

Number needed to treat (at a given level of exposure–outcome risk, the number of subjects in whom the exposure needs to be altered in order to save one person from getting the outcome)

scatterplot of the relationship summarized by a correlation coefficient, as the two dimensional plot can show any outliers or can give a more intuitive impression of the relationship across the range of values.

In some studies it may be helpful to assess the average level of group outcome in discrete categories of exposure (e.g. average blood pressure levels by thirds of fat intake); the statistical significance can be assessed using one way analysis of variance (specific differences assessed by least significance difference test). It may also be helpful to assess average differences in average levels of exposure broken down by levels of discrete variables (e.g. average fat by age group or gender). It is informative to assess average levels of a continuous measure against categories of another measure.

Once a set of key variables has been identified which the investigator believes may be related to the outcome of interest, regression analysis may be used to explore the relationship between the dependent variable and these key variables of interest, while taking into account the interaction of effects between the measures. Regression analysis is a powerful technique, which should be used with caution; there are important assumptions which must be met before the method is used.

Outcome can be measured in simple terms such as rates of death in groups with different levels of exposure; but often the measures used are combined to give an estimate of the risk difference between different groups in the study. The standardized mortality or morbidity ratio gives an indication of the level of morbidity or mortality in the study population compared to that of a standard population. When the study seeks to assess the public health impact of the exposure–outcome relationship, the attributable risk or number needed to treat are often used. The attributable risk gives an indication of the effect that eliminating the exposure as a risk factor would have on rates of the outcome measure. The number needed to treat gives an indication of the number of people that would need to be treated, given the relative risk estimate of the disease, to avoid one outcome (e.g. save one life, or prevent one case of disease).

Specific issues for measuring exposure

Considerable effort has been directed toward improving measures of food consumption from which levels of nutrient intakes have been derived, but relatively little effort has been directed toward developing valid measures of individual foods or food patterns. The issues around using different measures of dietary intake are covered more fully in Chapter 6. For large studies the choice of method to assess dietary intake will be dictated by practical constraints of time and money; the effects of these constraints on the quality of data have been widely debated, particularly with respect to the relative validity of questionnaire methods compared with weighed records (see Chapter 8).

Unlike nutrient intakes, there have been few studies which have sought to validate measures of food intake. The interest in food as the exposure of interest has largely arisen from interest in understanding the role of fruit and vegetable consumption in reducing the risk of cancer, and the fact that studies picking out key nutrients from these foods have not given results that are in total agreement with results for the whole food, suggesting that there may be other components (or combinations of components) of fruits and vegetables which are important in influencing risk.

In a number of recent multi-centre cohort studies greater emphasis has been placed on collecting biological samples. Concentrations of the nutrients of interest are measured in blood samples, for example, and these biological measures are then used as the measure of dietary exposure. Several reviews have been published recently which provide some important lessons about the assumptions that need to be made to infer that a biological sample is a good proxy for dietary exposure (see Chapter 7). The key issues to summarize here are the assumption that the biological measure is a relevant measure of the exposure of interest, and this relates to the question the study seeks to address. If the aim is to understand food patterns in order to change these food patterns, then the food pattern is the relevant exposure. If the aim of the study is to understand the causal mechanisms involved, then the relevant exposure is the amount of the nutrient of interest at the level of action in the cell. Concentration in blood may not reflect the level available to the cell if circulating levels are tightly regulated (for example, serum ionized calcium or iron); a high concentration may reflect high tissue stores, or it may reflect the lack of availability of factors required to remove the nutrient from the blood to the site of action. Ideally what is required is a dynamic measure which reflects the state of flux, and takes account of all the sources of the substance being measured, both external and internal. For example, the nitrogen pool in the body is a product of dietary intake plus that which is salvaged from the colon.[12] Measuring dietary intake of protein without taking this colonic salvage into account will lead to an underestimate of the available nitrogen, and particularly in vegetarians where there is greater salvage in the colon than in omnivores.[12]

Figure 1.2 summarizes the balance between supply and demand which operates from the individual to the international level. The factors which affect this balance may also be broadly grouped as basic factors (economic, social, political structures); underlying factors (level of education, sanitation, water supplies, food security); intermediate (operating at the household level); or immediate (availability of sufficient food, health status). These basic and underlying factors operate at the international and national level to influence household supply, and factors within the household influence levels of

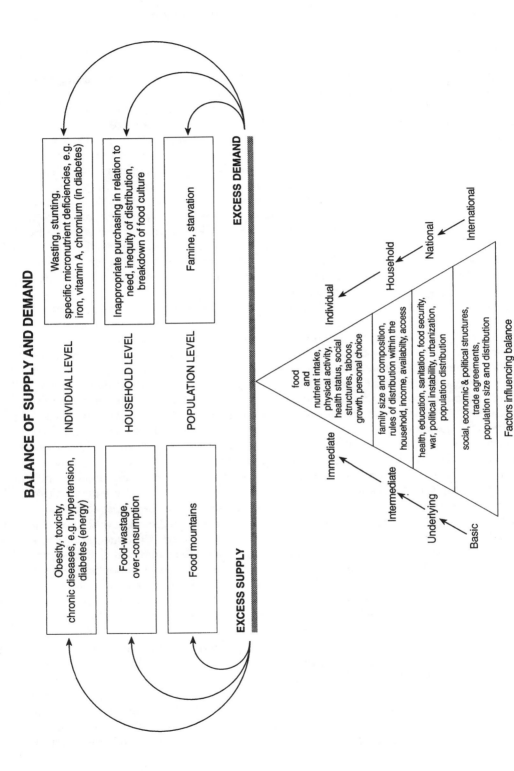

Fig. 1.2 Conceptual framework for understanding human nutrition and defining exposure

individual consumption. These factors all interact to affect the balance between supply and demand and the consequences of any imbalance will be different depending on the level of observation. At the population level, if supply exceeds demand there will be food mountains, whereas if demand exceeds supply there will be famine and starvation. At the household level an imbalance will either lead to food wastage and over consumption, or inappropriate purchasing in relation to need, and breakdown of the traditional patterns of eating and food gathering and distribution. At the individual level excess supply will lead to, for example, obesity (energy intake) or chronic diseases linked with excess (diabetes, high blood pressure, and high blood lipid levels), or toxicity if the excess element cannot be eliminated. Where supply is inadequate to meet the demand at the individual level wasting or stunting will occur (energy), or there may be specific micronutrient deficiencies (iron, iodine, or vitamin A), with related clinical signs and symptoms; the deficiency may be in trace elements which affect chronic diseases (e.g. in diabetes where chromium deficiency is suspected).

Depending on the level at which the research is aimed, the relevant measures of exposure and outcome will differ. The relevant exposure is a measure of the real available supply at the exposure level of interest (e.g. community, individual, cell); the balance between supply and demand will vary depending on the factors affecting both supply and demand. For example, the energy demands of a child with an infection will be increased, and an energy supply which is constant may be adequate for the child without an infection but inadequate for the child with an infection. At a national level, the adequacy of the food supply will depend on the demographic and health characteristics of the population, as well as the way in which the national crop production plus imports are made available to the population, or are affected by wastage due to pests or spoilage. The consequences of the imbalance between supply and demand will be manifested in different rates of outcome measures. The requirements for measuring this balance are different for international and individual studies, and where supply is excessive or deficient.

It is not usually possible to measure exposure at the critical time when, if the exposure is going to cause the outcome, the effect is occurring. Often exposure is measured after the effect has occurred, and it is assumed that the measure at this later point is related to the exposure which caused the effect. For example, in embryological development the neural tube is closed by about the twelfth week of pregnancy, so any measure of dietary intake taken after this time will not cover the relevant time frame. For a measure taken at a later time to be a relevant proxy for the true exposure, there must be a known and consistent relationship between the level of the measure which is used and the true level which is the relevant measure.

Other issues are discussed in a recent review.[13]

Specific issues for measuring outcome

Errors in measuring outcomes are as serious as errors associated with measuring exposure. Classifying someone as not diseased when they are diseased will distort the estimates of risk. It is therefore essential in the planning stage to determine whether an outcome can be measured with sufficient validity (sensitivity and specificity).

Many studies rely on death certificates for the ascertainment of outcome. For common diseases it may be reasonable to expect that the cause of death will be included on the death certificate. If this is the case the death certificate may provide a sensitive measure of outcome. Where the cause of death under study may not be routinely recorded on the death certificate, using death certificates for estimating the outcome may be misleading. In several studies that have compared death certificate diagnosis with autopsy diagnosis there has not always been good agreement between the two measures.[14] Death certificates will probably be of little use in identifying subjects where the disease of interest is not related to the immediate or underlying cause of death, such as, for example, hip fractures.[15]

If routinely collected data, like death certificates, hospital activity analysis, or mother and child health clinic attendances are used to measure an outcome, some estimate needs to be made of the likely completeness of case ascertainment. If the aim of the study is to derive a sample of the whole population, using clinic attenders may give a biased sample. For example, in The Gambia rates of diarrhoea in children attending a clinic in the village may be quite different from rates obtained from a census of all the children living in the village. If the factors determining attendance at the clinic are related to the exposure of interest, a biased exposure–outcome relationship may occur.

If outcome is measured by the observer there is the potential for biased ascertainment of outcome. An observer interviewing a subject may lead the subject into answers which the subject feels the observer wants to hear. A medical examination by a doctor in a white coat may evoke different responses from examination by a nurse who is perceived to be more friendly and approachable.

It may be difficult to check the accuracy and completeness of information obtained using a self-administered questionnaire, although the accuracy can be improved by careful questionnaire design (see Chapter 2). Response rates to questionnaires sent by post are generally lower than where the information is obtained by an interviewer. Those who respond are likely to be different in some ways from those who do not reply and it is therefore possible that the measured outcome (and exposure) does not reflect the distribution seen in the whole population.

For outcome measures like blood pressure, the observer can have a considerable effect on the level of measurement. This effect may alter over time as a subject becomes more familiar with the procedure. This error is in addition to any errors introduced in the way the observer measures the blood pressure.

1.3.2   The assessment of validity, relative validity, calibration, and reproducibility

Validity

A study is considered to be valid if the findings can be taken as being a reasonable representation of the true situation. For this to apply the study must measure diet at the relevant time, in the relevant population, and using a measure of diet which measures the true relevant exposure, and that there is no misclassification of outcome. It assumes that there are no errors in the way the data are collected, analysed, and interpreted. This broad definition of validity implies that the measures used in the study give valid measures of exposure and the relationships between exposure and outcome derived from the study give valid measures of effect. The assessment of the validity of the measures used in the study and the conduct of the study are often referred to as the internal validity, and the generalizability of the findings referred to as the external validity. To be externally valid a study must be internally valid, but a study may be internally valid, but not externally valid because the subjects studied may not reflect the population from which they came. To be internally valid there must be no bias in the way the data are collected, analysed, and interpreted. Judging whether a study is externally valid involves some judgement about the relevant characteristics of the study which affect the external validity; these characteristics are rarely able to be measured.

Validity of measures of exposure   From the above it is clear that the validity of the measure of exposure is only part of what constitutes an internally valid study. With respect to measuring nutritional exposure, a measure is valid if it measures what it purports to measure. This implies that there is a true measure of the variable against which the new or alternative measure (test) is compared. In most situations it is not possible to have an absolute measure of the true exposure, and the new or test measure of exposure is usually compared with another measure which is considered from previous research to be more accurate (the reference measure) than the new measure. A study which compares these measures is a validation study, but should be referred to as a study of the relative validity (sometimes called concurrent validity) of the test compared with the reference measure. To be a proper validation study the whole process of study design should be considered. Recently it has become popular to refer to studies which assess the relative validity of a test measure as calibration studies. Calibration studies do not estimate all sources of measurement errors; they are designed to assess those parameters which are needed to correct measures of association for measurement error for given increments of intake. Kaaks *et al.*[16], Plummer and Clayton[17, 18], and Chapters 4 and 8, discuss this further. These authors have characterized a measurement error model where the measured intake is related to the true intake multiplied by a proportional scaling factor PLUS systematic error PLUS random individual measurement error. These models must always be extended to include the occurrence of bias (see Section 1.4.2).

   If the new measure of the exposure gives the same results as the reference measure, then the new method is said to provide a valid measure of the true exposure. It is common to assess the association between the test and reference measure using a correlation coefficient. It is then assumed that if the correlation coefficient is statistically significant the test measure is a suitable proxy for the reference measure. However, there may be poor agreement (mean, slope, etc.) even though the correlation may be high. Other approaches to describing the agreement between test and reference measures are available and include the per cent difference between means of measures; Bland-Altman plots of the difference between the reference and test measure plotted against the average of the two measures[19]; the proportion of subjects grossly misclassified into opposite thirds, fourths, or fifths of the distribution, assuming the reference measure is correct. It is also becoming more common to include a third measure of exposure, usually a biological measure, and to compare the relationships between the three measures (see for example,[20]) (see Chapter 8).

   If the new method consistently records higher or lower than the reference measure of intake it may not affect the measure of association between exposure and outcome. For example, if a food frequency questionnaire estimate of fat intake differs on average from a 14-day weighed record estimate of fat intake, but it ranks subjects in the distribution of fat intake in exactly the same way, then the measure of effect (e.g. relative risk) across rankings will be the same. It is possible to use measures of absolute intake to correct for this scaling effect.[21] These issues are explored further in Chapter 4.

Measures of sensitivity and specificity relate to the validity of a measure. To be valid a measure should be both specific and sensitive. Sensitivity measures the proportion of truly exposed or diseased subjects who are correctly classified as such. Specificity measures the proportion of truly unexposed or non-diseased subjects who are correctly classified as such. Positive predictive value is the proportion of subjects measured to be exposed who are truly exposed. Negative predictive value is the proportion of subjects measured to be unexposed who are truly not exposed (Table 1.4).

In studies estimating the prevalence of an outcome the proportion classified as diseased will be a function of the prevalence of the disease as well as the sensitivity and specificity of the measures used. Unless a measure is 100% sensitive and specific, the measure of prevalence of the disease (or outcome) will be affected. If sensitivity and specificity are known it is possible to correct the prevalence measure. Any loss of validity in measuring either exposure or outcome will reduce the ability to determine risk accurately.

Reproducibility

Reproducibility refers to the process of assessing the repeatability of a measure. The repeatability is often referred to as precision or reliability and refers to the consistency

Table 1.4 Definition of sensitivity, specificity, and predictive value.

| | | True status | | |
		Diseased	Not diseased	Total
Measured	Positive	a	b	a+b
status	Negative	c	d	c+d
Total		a+c	b+d	a+b+c+d

Sensitivity = $\dfrac{a}{a+c}$

Specificity = $\dfrac{d}{b+d}$

Predictive value (positive) $\dfrac{a}{a+b}$

Predictive value (negative) $\dfrac{d}{c+d}$

The above are appropriate where there is a dichotomous variable.

with which a measure of exposure measures that exposure. A study of the reproducibility takes into account the circumstances in which the measure of repeatability is performed. Differences between repeat measures may be due either to true subject variation for that measure or to the effect of observer (measurement) error, or differences in other characteristics of the subjects. Subject variation may be either random or systematic. It is, however, difficult to distinguish between the true subject variation and the effects of the repeated observation of that subject by an observer because it is difficult to have exactly the same conditions for the initial and repeat measures. This is particularly true in repeat measures of diet where learning effects may exert a powerful influence. It may therefore be difficult to assess the reproducibility of a measure.

Lack of reproducibility in a measure indicates that it is not valid and reduces the possibility of correctly identifying a causal relationship.

1.4   Interpretation of epidemiological research: the role of chance, bias, and consideration of the effects of other variables

Having collected and analysed the data, the last step is to try to work out what the results means. There are several questions which need to be asked before it is reasonable to assume that the association can be interpreted as showing a cause–effect relationship. How likely is it that the finding did not occur by chance, or was not due to some bias, or was the result of some other factor which was not considered in the analysis? In this section these issues will be discussed, followed by a discussion of causality.

1.4.1   The role of chance

In assessing the findings of a study the investigator needs to know whether the results obtained could have occurred by chance alone. This can be assessed by hypothesis testing (significance testing and P-values) or by estimation and confidence intervals.

Hypothesis testing
This requires a clear statement of the hypothesis being tested and the formulation of an appropriate null hypothesis. The null hypothesis usually states that there is no relationship between exposure and outcome; the alternate hypothesis states that there is an association present. In a case-control or cohort study for example, the null hypothesis might be that the odds ratio (case-control study) or relative risk (cohort study) is equal to one (i.e. that there is not effect); the alternative hypothesis is that the effect is either greater or smaller than one. This hypothesis can then be addressed using an appropriate test of statistical significance. The principle of these tests of statistical significance is usually that there is a difference between groups (or observed and expected values) that can be measured and that the variance of the estimate of the difference can be estimated. The general form of the test (although this is not always the case) is the observed minus the expected divided by the square root of the variance. For a given variance, the bigger the difference between groups (or observed and expected) the more likely that the observed outcome has not occurred just by chance alone and

can be described as a statistically significant result (see Chapter 3). For a given difference, the variance of the estimate will also affect the level of significance, the smaller the variance the more statistically significant the recorded difference. The standard error of the estimate is a function of the sample size. The larger the sample the smaller the standard error and therefore the greater the ability to detect a statistically significant result (if one exists).

It is customary to express the level of statistical significance in terms of how likely it is that the result would have occurred by chance if there really were no association (i.e. if the null hypothesis were true). The larger the value of the test of statistical significance (either positive or negative) the smaller the P-value, or the less likely that such a result would occur by chance alone. If the P-value is 0.05 it means that there is only a one in 20 chance that a result as extreme as that observed would have occurred by chance alone, if the null hypothesis were true. If this is the case it is conventional to reject the null hypothesis and accept the alternative hypothesis that there is an association between exposure and outcome. If the P-value is greater than 0.05 it is customary to conclude that the result could have occurred by chance alone and that it is therefore not possible to reject the null hypothesis. If the null hypothesis is rejected, it is possible that this decision is incorrect. This type of error (incorrectly rejecting a null hypothesis) is called a type I or alpha error. On the other hand if the null hypothesis is false and is not rejected, this is referred to as a type II or beta error (Table 1.5, and see Chapter 3).

The P-value chosen as representing statistical significance is arbitrary and should only be used as a guide. For example, it does not make any sense to reject a P-value of 0.06, which is only just considered not statistically significant, if there is a clear notion as to how the exposure and outcome variables are related. This result may sensibly lead to another study being conducted which more specifically addresses that association.

In reporting P-values it is always preferable to present the exact P-value rather than to simply say that it was greater or less than 0.05. This enables readers to make their own judgements about whether a P-value of 0.06 or 0.10 (for example) is a useful guide to a potentially important observation.

Table 1.5 Summmary of type I and type II errors in hyopthesis testing*

The true situation	The decision	
	Accept H_0	Reject H_0
H_0 is true	*Correct decision*: Probability $= 1-\alpha$	Type I error: Probability $= \alpha$ (Level of significance; P-value)
H_0 is false	Type II error: Probability $= \beta$	*Correct decision*: Probability $= 1-\beta$ POWER (%) $= (1-\beta) \times 100$

* H_0 is the null hypothesis.
Modified from Conover[41].

Unless there is a clear hypothesis as to the direction of the effect expected, it is better to use (where possible) a two-sided or two-tailed test of statistical significance. If a two-sided test is used there is no assumption made as to the direction of the effect. A one-sided test of statistical significance assumes that the effect is in a particular direction. The two-tailed test is more conservative statistically and less likely therefore to lead the researcher into assuming there is a relationship present when in fact one does not exist. The level of statistical significance should not, however, be the sole arbiter of the importance of the results.

In some situations data are available on a whole range of variables which may have been included with no specific question in mind. If an investigator inspects the data and finds some comparisons which reach statistical significance, but before the analysis began the investigator had no idea that this comparison was important, care should be taken in the interpretation of the findings (this is referred to as *post-hoc* analysis). If these variables are examined and some happen to be statistically significant, it should be born in mind that even if no real associations exist, on average, one in 20 such associations will be statistically significant by chance alone. Some would argue that it is not acceptable to do *post-hoc* analyses, but if interpreted with caution they can often lead to new insights which can then be tested more formally in further research.

The major problem in using hypothesis testing is that it gives no direct indication of the size of the effect. For example, in a study assessing the effect of a change in diet on blood pressure, a P-value of 0.05 for the change in blood pressure gives no indication of the absolute change. If the sample size is very large small differences will be statistically significant, but these differences may not have any biological importance. It may not be reasonable to equate statistical significance with the importance of the effect.

Estimation and confidence intervals

Another way of quantifying the possible contribution of chance to observed results is to derive confidence intervals. A confidence interval expresses a summary of the data in the original units of measurement, as opposed to the dimensionless probability scale of significance testing.[22] This summary of the data is more intuitive than a P-value; the confidence interval represents the range within which the variable (risk, prevalence, etc.) that is being estimated is likely to lie. The width of a confidence interval based on a sample statistic, such as the mean, depends on the standard deviation and the sample size.[22] The standard error, which is used to determine the confidence interval, is calculated from the sample size and standard deviation and represents the estimate of the uncertainty of the sample statistic. The larger the sample size, for a given mean and standard deviation, the smaller the standard error and therefore the narrower the confidence interval. The confidence interval also depends on the degree of confidence required for the interval. Separate formulae are available for calculating confidence intervals for means, proportions, and their differences. These formulae usually depend on the assumption that the data are normally distributed, but there are techniques for estimating a confidence interval about a median, for instance. The common underlying principle is the addition and subtraction of a multiple of the standard error to the sample statistic.

It is most common to see a 95% confidence interval, but this is arbitrary and it is possible to use other intervals (e.g. 90 or 99% interval as required). The effect of a vegetarian diet on blood pressure was assessed in a sample of mildly hypertensive subjects.[23] When subjects were on the vegetarian diet systolic blood pressure fell by, on average 3.5 mm Hg. The 95% confidence interval for this test statistic was −7.0 to −0.1 mm Hg. If the study were repeated on many different samples from the same population and the 95% confidence interval was calculated for each study, 95% of these would include the population difference between means. It would be reasonable to assume from the above results that the effect of a vegetarian diet on blood pressure is therefore compatible with an effect as small as −0.1 mm Hg and as great as −7.0 mm Hg, although the best estimate is −3.5 mm Hg, the difference between the sample means.

Wide confidence intervals, even if the result is statistically significant, indicate that the estimate is not very precise. That is, the data are compatible with a wide range of potential effects.

There is a relationship between the two-sided hypothesis test and confidence interval. For example, the 95% confidence interval corresponds roughly to the 5% level of statistical significance under the null hypothesis as assessed using an appropriate test of statistical significance. In the above cited study of the effects of a vegetarian diet on blood pressure, a zero difference in blood pressure between vegetarians and non-vegetarians corresponds to the null hypothesis. The results showed that zero was not included within the 95% confidence interval and therefore the study could be considered statistically significant at the 5% level. Had the zero value fallen within the 95% confidence interval, this would have indicated a non-significant result, that is the probability of finding the mean difference obtained given a true null hypothesis would have been greater than 5%.

Where possible both the P-value and confidence interval should be presented, although the latter is likely to be more useful in interpreting the results of the study. The confidence interval provides an indication of the likely magnitude of effect, which the P-value derived from a test of statistical significance does not.[22] Relying on tests of statistical significance incorrectly implies that the purpose of a study is to obtain 'statistical significance'. Walter[24] has recently expressed the opinion that editorial policies of journals with respect to the way results are presented should remain flexible; he notes that the *American Journal of Epidemiology* reports results using both significance testing (*P*-values) and estimation (95% confidence intervals), whereas the *British Medical Journal*, *Lancet*, and *Annals of Internal Medicine* recommend 95% confidence intervals.

Where no statistically significant association has been found (i.e. P is greater than 0.05, or the 95% CI includes the value which was expected if the null hypothesis were true) it is important to consider the possible reasons why this may be so. It is important to look at the design and conduct of the study before assuming that the results obtained are a reliable reflection of the true situation. It could be that the study was too small, or there was an unusually large random sampling variation in the particular study sample, and that if the study were repeated in a larger or different sample, a statistically significant result might be obtained. Irrespective of the width of the confidence interval or level of statistical significance obtained, it is important to consider the effects that bias and confounding may have on the results obtained. These will be considered in the next two sections of this chapter.

1.4.2 Bias

Bias may be defined as: 'Deviation of results or inferences from the truth, or processes leading to such deviation. Any trend in the collection, analysis, interpretation, publication, or review of data that can lead to conclusions that are systematically different from the truth' (p. 15).[11] This wide definition suggests that bias can occur at any stage from developing the initial idea to writing up the completed study. Many different types of bias have been defined[25], but there are two main types of bias that can affect the validity of a study. These are selection bias and information bias. The effect these biases might have on the results of the study must be assessed before the study can be properly interpreted. Bias may be inherent at the design stage if the variables selected for measurement do not properly address the hypothesis to be tested.

Poor response rate may introduce bias in general, but especially if the response rate is different, for example, between cases and controls. Cases, having recently been diagnosed, may be more likely to participate because they may feel that they have a vested interest in finding out more about what caused their disease. Controls, on the other hand, may not have the same concern, and those who participate may be more health conscious or behave differently from the population they are meant to represent.

Selection bias

Most epidemiological studies are concerned with comparing and contrasting two or more groups in some measure of their exposure or outcome. The objective of drawing a sample from a population is to obtain a measure of effect such that the measure obtained in the sample is a reasonable reflection of the true effect in the population. A bias occurs if the relationship between exposure and effect is different for those who participate compared with those who are eligible to participate but do not (response bias). Therefore, any factors that affect the inclusion of subjects at the beginning of a study might introduce bias. It is then a matter of judgement as to how important this bias might be in interpreting the results of the study. In the design of the study some strategy should be considered as to how information could be obtained on those people who refuse to participate or subsequently drop out. Even if this information is only age, gender, and occupation it will allow an estimate of whether those who participate in the study reflect the population from which they are drawn. A non-representative sample may not, however, affect the internal validity of the study, especially in clinical or field trials, in which potentially causal pathways are being tested and in which the external validity may also be protected.

A number of specific types of selection bias are listed below.

1. Self-selection bias: In a retrospective cohort study of, for example, the relationship between infant feeding patterns and childhood diarrhoea, some subjects might be traced through health visitor records and some might be obtained through subjects contacting the investigators themselves; it is likely that the latter group might be different from the group obtained from the records. This may be termed self-selection bias.[4]

2. Referral bias: Referral bias may occur in, for example, case-control studies where cases are referred to a hospital which is a regional centre of excellence, but the controls are recruited only from subjects within the usual catchment area of the hospital. The

control group may not then reflect the population from which cases were drawn. In case-control studies where cases are recruited as they present at hospital, consideration needs to be given to the selection of appropriate control groups to represent the exposure in the dynamic population from which the cases are drawn.

3. Diagnostic bias: Subjects might be selected as cases in a case-control study using different diagnostic criteria in different centres. This may be a problem in multi-centre studies, but should be minimized by careful standardization prior to the commencement of the study.

Information bias

Information bias occurs when there are either random or systematic differences in the way exposure and outcome are measured in the study groups. There is a distinction between *differential* and *non-differential* bias: in the former, the information that is obtained is systematically different between different groups in the study; in the latter the bias is the same in different groups. Differential misclassification may lead either to over- or under-estimation of an effect. Non-differential misclassification biases towards the null. As with selection bias, the probable effects of information bias on the inter-pretation of the study findings is a matter of judgement, and is influenced by whether the bias is likely to be different for cases and controls.

There are many potential sources of information bias, but there are three common ones.

1. Social desirability bias: This sort of bias occurs when the individual wishes to convey a desirable image, or to convey an image in keeping with social norms (summarized in [26]). This sort of bias may occur in overweight men and women or among those on special diets, or even among nutritionists(!) who have a lot of interest in food and have a good idea of which foods may be considered 'better' or 'worse'. Scales have been developed to assess the extent of this sort of bias; for example, the Marlowe-Crowne Social Desirability Scale (MCSD)[27] or the Martin-Larsen Social Approval Scale (MLSA).[28] The study by Herbert *et al.*[26] was the first to use these scales to adjust the data collected; these scales may also be used in validation studies.

2. Recall bias: Any studies attempting to obtain information from subjects about events in the past may be subject to recall bias.[29] Recall bias can be affected by:

- the time interval since exposure;
- the degree of detail about the exposure that is required;
- personal characteristics of the subjects (e.g. memory);
- the perceived social desirability of the exposure under investigation;
- current public knowledge about the dietary component in the disease under study;
- the significance of the events under study.

In designing the study the aim should be to minimize any differences in recall biases which may occur between different groups of subjects in the study.

There are several factors which might contribute to differential recall between cases and controls. The motivation to participate may be greater in cases than controls, where the former might be seeking an answer as to why they have got the disease. They might reflect on past exposures, or have been asked about the exposure under investigation by physicians responsible for their care, and they might therefore recall past exposure differently from controls who, before being recruited into the study, had not thought about the exposure under investigation. In a case-control study of, for example, folate and neural tube defects, the mothers of the cases may be more likely to think back over events that occurred during their pregnancy to try to explain why their child has developed the defect. They may, therefore, recall exposures differently from mothers of controls who have not had the same incentive to think about exposures during their pregnancy. This effect may be reduced by the selection of appropriate controls, as, for example, another group of congenital malformations with an aetiology unrelated to neural tube defects.

In case-control studies where a measure of dietary exposure is required for some point in the distant past, it has generally been shown that the recalled exposure tends to be more like the current exposure (see Section 6.12). If current diet has changed from that consumed in the past a bias may occur. This bias may lead to either differential or non-differential misclassification depending on whether it differs between cases and controls.

3. Interviewer bias: Interviewer bias may occur when there is any difference in the way information is obtained, recorded, processed, and interpreted in different groups in the study by the interviewer. If interviewers assess exposure in case-control studies and they know whether the subject is a case or a control, they may solicit the information differently. This is less likely to be a problem in a prospective cohort study where outcome is not known at the time of obtaining the exposure information, but other biases (e.g. regarding occupational or ethnic groups) may influence interviewer behaviour and data quality. There will also be biases which may occur between interviewers. Interviewers should be blinded as to the nature of the question under investigation and they should be carefully trained so that they collect information in a standardized way throughout. The potential effects of observer bias need to be assessed and minimized before the study begins.

Bias: general issues

In a cohort or experimental study, the way in which subjects are followed or the completeness of information obtained during follow-up may also introduce a bias. If a distinct subset of subjects (the less healthy or poorer, or those with high or low exposure status) are lost to follow-up, a biased result may occur. In a cohort or experimental study it may be better to select a group of subjects that can be followed up over a long period of time even though they may not represent the general population. For example, in the classic study of Doll and Hill on smoking[30] they chose doctors as their cohort because they knew that they were an easy group to define and follow up. It is possible that the results from this study were not generalizable (although they probably were), but it was considered more important to have an internally valid study that provided information that could be reliably interpreted.

A major consideration in epidemiological research is to reduce bias. The potential effect that bias has on the measurement of a cause–effect relationship needs to be assessed wherever possible in all studies. In practice it is difficult. It is optimal to anticipate the likely sources of bias in a study at the design stage, and to consider how to collect information in a way that is likely to reduce that bias to an acceptable level. Consideration needs to be given as to how the study population, methods of data collection, and sources of information on exposure and outcome may be selected to reduce bias.

1.4.3 External validity

As already mentioned there are two components of validity: one relating to the information obtained from the subjects in the study (internal validity) and the other relating to how the information obtained relates to people outside the study sample (external validity or generalizability).

In discussing generalizability, it is important to consider which characteristics of the sample may affect the generalizability of the findings. This requires an understanding of the likely mechanism whereby such characteristics may affect the outcome. In some situations it may be reasonable to generalize, say, from a study of men to women, but in others it may not (for example, where female sex hormones are believed to play a key role in the causal process).

There are two broad views about the importance of external validity or generalizability. One view takes the position that the study sample should be representative of the population from which it was drawn and that it is, therefore, important to assess how the study sample differs from the population from which it was drawn. Thus for example, data on age, gender, and other socio–economic data would be compared between the sample and the population from which the sample was drawn. If they are similar it would be considered reasonable to generalize from the sample to the population. It may be, however, that the variables for which comparable information have been obtained, or are available, are irrelevant to the causal process under investigation. Generalizing from middle-aged people to children, for example, may not always be appropriate.

The other point of view argues that the generalizability of a study is not assessed by such simple comparisons between the study sample and the population from which it was drawn. This view argues that generalization is from the experience of the actual study to the abstract and is founded on judgement rather than statistical sampling and technical sample-to-population inference. Studies which are assessing the effects of metabolic processes, such as clinical trials, may not recruit subjects that are representative of any general population, but it is assumed that the metabolic processes under investigation will apply in all subjects in the same way. If this is true the phenomena described in these clinical trials of unrepresentative samples may be generalizable.

In reality, both views are similar in that they rely on the investigator making a sensible judgement about whether the results obtained in the present study are likely to be the same in a repetition of the study carried out using a different sample. The objective of the research should be to increase understanding about a particular process. This understanding requires going from the information that is available to the abstract formulation of a particular theory that can subsequently be tested and redefined. In terms of trying to understand the causal process, a non-representative sample from which good quality data are obtained may be more helpful than a representative sample from which biased data are obtained. In interpreting the results of the study the researcher needs to consider the potential biases in the sample studied and then consider whether the processes identified or results obtained may be likely to apply in other groups of the population not included in the present study.

1.4.4   Assessing the effects of other factors: effect modification, confounding, and interaction

The third major issue to consider in interpreting epidemiological research is the possibility that variables other than the exposure of interest have influenced the outcome. These factors may alter the estimate of the effect of the exposure on outcome. They are of three types which are defined below, and their influence is illustrated in Figs 1.3 and 1.4.

Outcome modifiers have an effect on the outcome variable but are independent of the exposure of interest. They do not lie in the causal pathway of interest, but can influence the population estimate of absolute risk of an outcome based on a given level of exposure. They do not change the relationship between the exposure of interest and the outcome (they do not change the slope of the line defining change in risk in relation to change in exposure).

Confounders are associated with both exposure and outcome. They can provide a true explanation for an apparent association (or lack of association) between the exposure of interest and the outcome, and typically include age, gender, and social class. For a variable to be a confounder:

• it must be associated with, but not causally dependent upon the exposure of interest;
• it must be a risk factor for disease, independent of its association with the exposure of interest;
• these must apply *within* the population under study.

Effect modifiers help to account for differences in the relationship between the exposure of interest and the outcome according to the level of the effect modifier. Such an effect is referred to as an *interaction*. An effect modifier will lie in the causal pathway which relates the exposure of interest to the outcome. A confounder cannot lie in the causal pathway.

In any study design, therefore, the most important likely outcome modifiers, confounders, and effect modifiers must be identified and included for measurement. This may be more difficult than it at first appears, simply because in many studies the important modifiers and confounders may not be known. It is therefore essential at this early design stage to have read the literature carefully both in relation to the epidemiology of the disease in question (in order to avoid carrying out unnecessary repetition of previous studies) and in relation to likely causal mechanisms (in order to be aware of factors which have already been described as being associated with the disease). It then requires judicious thought to identify those additional variables (modifiers and confounders) which need to be included amongst the study measurements.

Failure to measure a confounder will result in an apparent but spurious association between the exposure of interest and outcome, or it may obscure a relationship that would otherwise be apparent. It is never possible to eliminate the effects of all potential confounders, and it is therefore important to measure known or suspected confounders so that they can be considered in the analysis. Where variables are known to be confounders, the investigator can control for them either in the design (by randomization, restriction, or matching) or in the analysis (by stratification and/or multiple regression), provided sufficient valid information is available on the confounding factor. A poorly measured confounding factor may not give a correct estimate of the true effect of that confounder on the relationship under study. It will not be possible to control for the confounder if it has not been measured. Confounders mask the true effect, whereas effect modification and interaction offer important insights into underlying causation. Considering all other factors as confounders may be misleading. If a factor is in the causal pathway and is considered a confounder, the true effect of the exposure on the outcome will be underestimated. Measurement of variables which are neither modifiers nor confounders will waste resources.

Figure 1.3 illustrates what might result if an outcome modifier or confounder were not measured. Consider a study in which the aim is to determine the effect of fruit consumption on risk of coronary heart disease (CHD). Smoking would be an *outcome modifier* if it were associated with an increase in heart disease risk but not with fruit consumption (graphs (c) and (d)). The effect being measured is the risk of CHD at a given level of fruit consumption. Failure to measure smoking in graph (c) would result in the association being depicted by the dotted line, which would vary in position according to the proportion of smokers and non-smokers in the sample, and would affect the estimate of absolute risk of CHD in the population. In (d), failure to measure smoking would be more serious, because the proportion of smokers in the sample might influence the estimate of the threshold of fruit consumption that was believed to be protective, although it would not influence the estimated *change* in risk of CHD in relation to change in fruit consumption (the slope of the line would be unaltered). In (d), smoking is an independent cause of the outcome but not a confounder (because it is not associated with the exposure of interest). In graphs (a) and (b), where smoking is associated with neither CHD risk nor fruit consumption, it has no effect on the observed relationship between exposure and outcome and to measure it would be a waste of resources.

Smoking would be a *confounder* if people who smoke buy less fruit and smoking increases risk of CHD, as in graphs (g) and (h). Again, the dotted line depicts what would be observed if smoking were not measured. In (g), fruit would be assumed to be protective (when in fact it was not) because smokers (who have higher risk of CHD) buy less fruit than non-smokers. Similarly in (h), the apparent protective effect of fruit would be heavily exaggerated. The apparent relationship between fruit consumption and CHD risk (not corrected for confounding) is the same in both graphs (g) and (h), whereas the true relationship is different in the two examples. In graphs (e) and (f), where smoking is assumed not to be associated with CHD risk, the proportion of smokers in the sample would affect the estimate of mean fruit consumption and, in (f), the absolute estimate of CHD risk, but failure to measure smoking would not affect the

If smoking *IS NOT* associated with fruit consumption:

Smoking associated   **Fruit consumption protective:**
with CHD risk:

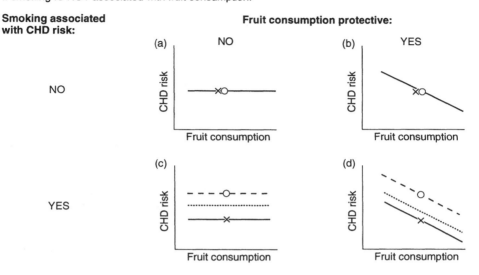

If smoking *IS* associated with fruit consumption:

Smoking associated   **Fruit consumption protective:**
with CHD risk:

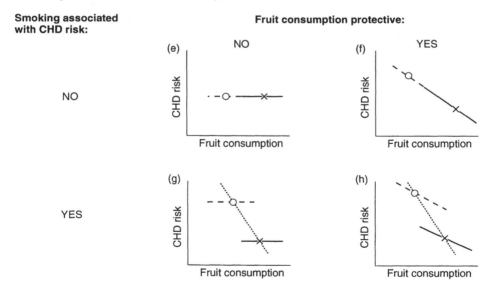

Non-smokers (———, ✕ = mean intake), smokers (– – –, O = mean intake). Dotted and short dashed lines indicate apparent relationship if smoking is not measured.

Fig. 1.3   Effects on CHD risk of smoking when assessing the influence of fruit consumption: outcome modifying and confounding.

determination of the slope of the line indicating rate of change in CHD risk in relation to change in fruit consumption.

The most complex situations exist where smoking is an effect modifier and there is some form of interaction between smoking, fruit consumption, and CHD risk. For example, assume that smoking increases CHD risk, that eating more fruit reduces risk, and that smokers eat less fruit. In the first type of interaction, depicted in Fig. 1.4(a), assume that smoking makes fruit less effective as a protective factor. Hence, the decrease in CHD risk with increasing fruit consumption is not as great in smokers as in non-smokers. (This contrasts with the situation depicted in Fig. 1.3(h), where the effects were additive (independent) and there was no interaction: the lines are parallel, and the change in CHD risk is the same in smokers as in non-smokers for a given change in fruit consumption.) Failure to measure smoking would again (as in Fig. 1.3(h)) result in the relationship depicted by the dotted line, heavily exaggerating the apparent protective effect of fruit consumption. Moreover, the interaction would be undetected. In the second type of interaction, assume that heavy smokers buy less fruit than light smokers. The two types of interaction are depicted together in Fig. 1.4(b), where the mean fruit consumption for heavy smokers is less than for light smokers, and the slope of the line is more shallow (i.e. fruit is less protective for heavy smokers than light smokers). The slope of the line depicting relative risk of CHD in relation to fruit consumption in studies in which smoking had not been measured would thus vary between the dotted and short dashed lines according to the proportions of light smokers and heavy smokers in the sample. The higher the proportion of heavy smokers, the greater the exaggeration in the apparent protective effect of fruit. Again, as in (a), the interaction would remain undetected. These graphs all depict a linear relationship between risk and fruit consumption. If the relationship were not linear (i.e. there was an upper threshold of the effectiveness of fruit consumption in protecting against CHD), the same basic

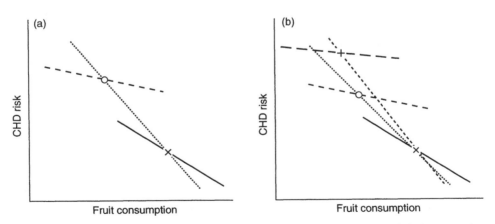

Non-smokers (——— , ✕ = mean intake), light smokers (– – – , ○ = mean intake), heavy smokers (— — , + = mean intake). Dotted and short dashed lines indicate apparent relationship if smoking is not measured.

Fig. 1.4 Effect on CHD risk of smoking when assessing the influence of fruit consumption: interaction.

principles would apply but the ability to detect relationships might be reduced at the extremes of the range of fruit consumption.

This problem may become even more difficult to control for when dietary variables are themselves the modifying or confounding variables. It is known that certain nutrients operate differently at different levels of other nutrients. It is also clear that people eat diets which consist of many different food items which contain many different nutrients and other factors. People who eat certain foods also tend to eat other foods. For example, in the Diet and Nutritional Survey of British Adults, a principal components analysis revealed that people who ate wholemeal bread were more likely to drink low fat milk and eat more fruit and vegetables, and those people who ate more white bread were more likely to drink more whole fat milk and to eat more fried foods and less fruit and vegetables.[31] It is virtually impossible to disentangle the effects of these foods and their related nutrients when trying to assess single nutrient exposure–outcome relationships. Adjusting for energy, which is now common (see Section 6.10), may not always eliminate the effect of energy intake, particularly if there is differential measurement error of energy intake in different subjects in the study. It may not always be appropriate to adjust for energy intake. This complexity highlights the need for careful consideration of the biologically plausible mechanisms involved, and consideration of the ways in which different aspects of diet may either interact or modify the effect of the dietary component of interest on the outcome of interest. It also suggests that for many nutrients it is desirable to have both a dietary and a biochemical measure if possible, in order to understand the causal pathway associated with a particular dietary exposure.

The complexity of dietary interaction can be illustrated using the example relating risk of CHD to fruit consumption. Assume that iron intake is a confounding variable (higher tissue iron stores increasing risk of CHD) and vitamin C intake is the protective factor of interest. Increasing amounts of vitamin C increase iron absorption. If vitamin C intake is protective, but there is an interaction between higher vitamin C intake and higher iron stores, it may be impossible to observe a protective effect of vitamin C unless iron storage in tissues (e.g. ferritin levels) is controlled for in the analysis. This illustrates the extraordinary care in thought required to disentangle potential dietary confounding and interactions which take place at different levels within the causal chain (e.g. iron intake versus tissue stores).

1.4.5 Interpretation

Once the researcher has considered the effects of chance, bias, and confounding, the final step is the interpretation of the results. After having considered everything that went wrong with the execution of the study, and the effect these problems had on the results, it is important to consider what weaknesses still remain in the study findings. Investigators must be as sceptical about their own results as they are about those of others. The results of the current study must be compared with those done previously in order to judge whether the current paradigm within which the research is operating still holds.

Criteria have been put forward to provide some guidance as to how to judge whether the results support the notion that the exposure under investigation caused the outcome. This judgement is usually made within the current consensus or paradigm about the relationship under study. According to the view of Popper it is possible to progress ideas only by falsification.[32] This philosophy suggests that you cannot prove anything and that the only way to conduct research is by trying to disprove hypotheses. However, to make some order of the world we live in requires accepting generalities that cannot be proved as a best guess estimate of the 'truth'. This current notion of 'truth' should be accepted only until such time as better generality of the real truth can replace it. Research should be seeking this underlying truth, not trying to re-enforce the existing notion of that truth.

In public health terms what is required is some way of judging what is the best guess estimate of what should be recommended for action, based on an objective review of the evidence. The elimination of the major causes of illness is of prime concern. Defining what is a cause is complex and relies on drawing causal inferences from the existing evidence. Criteria have been established to help judge whether the evidence supports drawing causal inferences.[4,33,34] There is disagreement about the need to satisfy all these criteria before suggesting that a factor may be causal. The only criteria that is absolutely agreed and essential is that the exposure/cause must occur before the outcome.

Rothman has proposed a terminology for causation.[4] The onset of disease is equivalent to the completion of a sufficient cause. A sufficient cause is made up of component causes; if a component cause must be present for the completion of a sufficient cause then it is defined as a necessary cause. For some complex diseases there may be more than one sufficient cause, and by implication therefore there may be different combinations of component causes which may lead to the presence of disease in different settings. Only if a component cause is necessary, will elimination of that cause eliminate the occurrence of that disease. The disease will still occur if other sufficient causes exist. The strength of any measured association may not give a true indication of the importance of a factor in causation of disease. It is also possible that if there are more than one sufficient causes of a disease, that adding together all the estimates of the size of the effect of various exposures on outcome (for example, per cent variance accounted for in a regression model), may total more than 100%.

Relevant time frame

In the interpretation of the results (and more importantly before the study begins!) it is important to consider whether the measure(s) of exposure covers the relevant time frame. What is required is a measure of the exposure at the time when it is believed that the exposure contributes to the causation or prevention of the outcome. This is illustrated in Fig. 1.5 for a number of different dietary or nutritional exposures. The figure shows the theoretical likelihood of developing or being diagnosed with a disease or disorder at various stages throughout the lifespan.

Some disorders may have a clearly defined window of time (period of critical exposure (PCE)) in which inadequate exposure may prevent normal development being established. For example, neural tube defects (NTD) are strongly related to maternal intake of folic acid in weeks 6–12 of the first trimester of pregnancy. A foetus growing in a mother with poor preconceptual folic acid status will have an increased risk of developing NTD even at the moment of conception. The NTD may be diagnosed prior

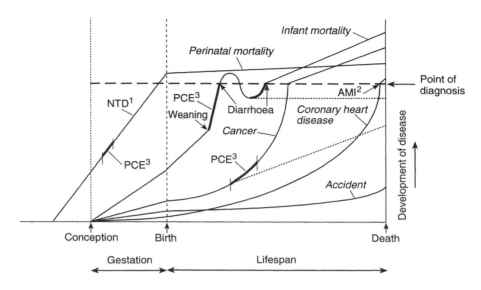

Fig. 1.5   Association of disease induction and progression with diagnosis, morbidity, and mortality.

to birth (e.g. using ultrasound). If the defect is severe, it is likely that death will follow rapidly and contribute to perinatal mortality (lifespan is short). Relevant exposures of folic acid in relation to risk of NTD would therefore be in all young women of child-bearing age (in relation to population risk of NTD) or in pregnant women in the first trimester (in relation to individual risk). Similarly, iodine intake during the 12th–15th week of gestation will influence the development of thyroid function in the foetus, and it would therefore be relevant to measure maternal iodine status during this period (not shown in the figure).

There may be important interactions with the nutritional exposure of interest. For example, under-nutrition in relation to infant mortality may be especially important at weaning and the switch to bottle feeding with the added dangers of diarrhoea due to use of contaminated water supplies. The critical period of exposure may therefore be during the initial period of weaning (determination of nutritional status before or after weaning may not help to explain the relationship between nutritional status and infant mortality). Diarrhoea may be episodic, in which case there may be several periods of critical exposure. The dotted line continuing horizontally following the second episode illustrated in the figure illustrates the outcome (e.g. no further diagnosis of diarrhoea and infant survival through a longer lifespan) if a clean water supply were introduced.

For chronic diseases such as cancer, there may be a critical point in time when the disease process began, but the exact period of critical exposure may not be easy to establish. In biological terms this may be considered as the point when normal cell turnover is altered such that the supply of substrates and co-factors is not sufficient to maintain function; this could be because the demand has increased, or the supply of essential factors has decreased. There may be some initial breakdown of the regulation of cell turnover; this slight defect of turnover may continue for some time without causing any obvious loss of cellular function, and then the rate of growth of the cancer speeds up under the influence of some promoting factor(s). For nutritional epidemiological studies it is likely that the exposure that is being considered is that which promotes the disease. Exactly when this promotion begins (PCE for cancer in Figure 1.5), and therefore when to measure dietary exposure is not clear. Conventional wisdom says that diet at least 10 years before diagnosis is likely to be nearer the relevant exposure.

Once the initial disease process has begun, it will not be diagnosed immediately (latent period) and the rate of progression of the disease to the point where it can be diagnosed may be affected by exposure to other factors which speed up (promotion) or slow down (inhibition) the rate of progress. The line relating to cancer shows that factors affecting the phenotypic expression of the genetic potential of an individual are likely to occur from the moment of conception. The dotted line which continues from the initial segment of the PCE shows that the disease may progress but not to the extent that it is diagnosed, and that death may be from other causes.

For heart disease the clarification of the relevant exposure may be more complex because of the more complex nature of the development of the disease. For an AMI to occur it is likely that there is both atheroma (narrowing of the vessel) and increased viscosity of cells in the blood (platelet aggregation) such that the flow of blood through a narrow lumen is restricted, oxygen supply to the heart is then interrupted, and the acute event occurs. Both atheroma and increased blood viscosity take some time to develop. Recent evidence suggests that the atheroma begins with some endothelial damage related to an imbalance of the level of LDL and antioxidant intake, making the LDL more likely to stick to the endothelium and the consequent formation of foam cells. The relevant dietary exposure is (at least) the combination of factors related to the levels of serum cholesterol (type and amount of fat in the diet), the balance of lipo-proteins (HDL, LDL), and the balance of free radical production (affected by smoking and infection) and antioxidant defences which affects the stability of the lipoprotein membrane around the LDL and the likelihood of this modified LDL sticking to the endothelium. There may not therefore be a single period of critical exposure, and the cumulative lifetime effects of a number of factors may need to be measured in order to understand the full range of dietary effects. Figure 1.5 illustrates for heart disease that the appearance of disease may be diagnosed only immediately preceding the time of death.

For many outcomes the effect of a given level of exposure as an adult may result in different levels of risk because of the effects of sub-optimal nutrition (where supply of essential factors has limited the development of certain cellular function) during early life. The exposures of interest are both the early life and adult exposures. This appears to be the case for diabetes and heart disease.[35] Another example (not shown in Figure 1.5) relates to calcium intake and risk of osteoporosis and hip fracture. There may be at least two relevant exposures, the total amount of calcium during pubertal growth affecting peak bone mass, and the amount of calcium later in adult life which may slow down the rate of loss of bone. Measuring either on its own may give misleading results.

The distance/time between diagnosis and death will depend on the stage at which the disease is diagnosed and the extent to which the health services can treat the disease once diagnosed. At the point of death a person may have several different diagnoses and the attribution of the cause of death may be a matter of judgment of the person writing the death certificate. In terms of trying to understand the meaning of epidemiological research the effects of competing causes of death may be important. Also the progression of one disease may be increased by other related diseases, or changes to, for example, host defence mechanisms, as may be the case with AIDS.

The line relating to accidents (e.g. car accident) illustrates that there may be some instances in which the cause of death is unrelated to nutrition, but that there have been a progression of nutrition related diseases that remain undiagnosed at death. (This does not deny the possibility that accidents may be more likely to occur if the driver has been drinking or may be hungry and have their attention diverted.)

In summary, failure to consider the model of disease progression and the relevant time period in which to measure exposure may mean that the wrong exposure is measured at an irrelevant time. In terms of drawing causal inferences, such information may be misleading.

1.5 Systematic reviews and the role of meta-analysis

When drawing causal inferences, results from different study designs should not be considered as offering information of equal weight, and the estimates of effect should not be pooled across study designs without careful consideration of the implications (Table 1.6). The strongest evidence comes from well conducted experimental studies, provided the study outcome measure is relevant, which may not be the case for some studies of pre-end stage markers of cancer.

The findings of any single study need to be placed in the context of findings from other studies. A systematic approach is required to review the literature objectively,

Table 1.6 Strength of causal inference in different study designs.

Study design	Strength of causal inferences which can be drawn
Ecological studies	Very weak
Cross-sectional studies	Weak
Case-control studies	Less weak
Cohort studies	Stronger
Experimental – community intervention studies	Stronger
Experimental – clinical or field trials	Strongest

particularly when the review will guide public action and health policy. There are now several texts and reviews of the procedures required to undertake a systematic review. The most critical aspect is the thoroughness and completeness of the review of the literature.[36,37] Once the literature has been compiled, the next key issue is to develop a systematic and objective approach to judging the scientific quality of the papers. We have recently undertaken such an exercise as part of the UK Nutritional Epidemiology Group review of the literature on diet and cancer,[38] and others have developed similar approaches for other outcomes.[39,40]

A pooled analysis of the results from a systematic review is often presented to give an overall estimate of effect. This pooled analysis is often called a meta-analysis. Unless the meta-analysis is based on a systematic review of all the available literature the summary estimate may be misleading. Before pooling risk estimates from different studies the researcher should assess whether it is appropriate to do this; it must be assumed that studies are sufficiently comparable in terms of their design, conduct, and presentation of data. There should be a test of the heterogeneity of the data before pooling. Often the pooled estimate, with more subjects, will have smaller confidence intervals and may give a statistically significant effect.

The value of the mathematical summary of the data included in the review, such as an overall estimate of risk, is critically dependent on the studies included in the review, and confidence about the comparability of the data from these studies. Caution is therefore required in assuming that the results of a meta-analysis will provide the best and most accurate measure of effect. However, without systematic reviews the decisions about what should be recommended will be based on hearsay and personal opinion. There is now a major international initiative, the Cochrane Collaboration, to bring together the scientific evidence on randomized controlled trials in order to facilitate a more objective, evidence based approach to decisions about optimal approaches to the delivery of health care. (The Cochrane Database of Systematic Reviews is available on disc and CD-ROM from BMJ Publishing Group, BMA House; fax 0171 383 6662.) More details about the Cochrane Collaboration can be obtained on the World Wide Web (http://www.ncl.ac.uk/~nphcare/GPUK/a_herd/research.htm).

1.6   Summary

The purpose of this chapter has been to outline the basic principles in the design and interpretation of nutritional epidemiological research. The aim has been to delineate the major problems and where appropriate offer some guidance as to how to avoid or handle the problems. Several key points should be restated.

1. Clear research objectives are essential to the development of good research.
2. Although nutrition is a complex exposure to measure, it is possible to obtain useful information, provided the right measures are used correctly.
3. Measurement error will always be present and some assessment is essential as to the likely effect of this error on the interpretation of the results.
4. When it comes to analysing the study, the effects that chance, bias, and confounding may have on the exposure–outcome relationship of interest should be carefully assessed.

References

1. Alderson, M. (1983) *An introduction to epidemiology*. 2nd edn. Macmillan, London.
2. Riboli, E., Slimani, N. and Kaaks, R. (1996) Identifiability of food components for cancer chemo-prevention. In: Stewart, B. W., McGregor, D. and Kleihues, P. (eds.) *Principles of chemoprevention*. IARC Sci. Publ. No. 139. IARC, Lyon, pp. 23–32.
3. Norell, S. E. (1995) *Workbook of epidemiology*. Oxford University Press, New York.
4. Rothman, K. J. (1986) *Modern epidemiology*. Little, Brown and Co., Boston.
5. Hennekens, C. H. and Burring, J. E. (1987) *Epidemiology in medicine*. Little, Brown and Co., Boston.
6. Kelsey, J. L., Thompson, W. D. and Evans, A. S. (1986) *Methods in observational epidemiology*. Oxford University Press, New York.
7. Mienert, C. L. (1986) *Clinical trials: design, conduct, and analysis*. Oxford University Press, New York.
8. Schlesselman, J. J. (1982) *Case-control studies: design, conduct, analysis*. Oxford University Press, New York.
9. Breslow, N. E. and Day, N. E. (1987) *Statistical methods in cancer research. Volume II. The design and analysis of cohort studies*. IARC Scientific Publications No. 82. International Agency for Research on Cancer, Lyon.
10. Armstrong, B. K., White, E. and Saracci, R. (1992) *Principles of exposure measurement in epidemiology*. Oxford University Press, Oxford.
11. Last, J. M. (ed.) (1995) *A dictionary of epidemiology*. 3rd Edn. Oxford University Press, New York.
12. Jackson, A. A. (1995) Salvage of urea-nitrogen and protein requirements. *Proc. Nut. Soc.* **54**: 535–47.
13. Margetts, B. M. and Nelson, M. (1995) Measuring dietary exposure in nutritional epidemiological studies. *Nutrition Research Reviews*. **8**: 165–78.
14. Barker, D. J. P. and Rose, G. (1984) *Epidemiology in medical practice*. 3rd Edn. Churchill Livingstone, Edinburgh.
15. Wickham, C. A. C., Walsh, K., Cooper, C., *et al.* (1989) Dietary calcium, physical activity and risk of hip fracture: a prospective study. *Br. Med. J.* **299**: 889–92.
16. Kaaks, R., Riboli, E. and van Staveren, W. A. (1995) Calibration of dietary intake measurements in prospective cohort studies.. *Am. J. Epid.* **12**: 548–56.
17. Plummer, M. and Clayton, D. (1993) Measurement error in dietary assessment: an investigation using covariance structure models. Part I. *Stat. Med.* **12**: 925–35.
18. Plummer, M. and Clayton, D. (1993) Measurement error in dietary asessment: an investigation using covariance structure models. Part II. *Stat. Med.* **12**: 937–48.
19. Bland, J. M. and Altman, D. G. (1995) Comparing two methods of clinical measurement: a personal history. *Int. J. Epid.* **24**: S7–S14.
20. Ocke, M. and Kaaks, R. (1997) Biomarkers as additional measurement in dietary validity studies: experience with data from the EPIC study. *Am. J. Clin. Nutr.* (In press.)
21. Kaaks, R. (1997) Validation and calibration of dietary intake measurements in the EPIC study: methodological considerations. *Int. J. Epid.* (In press.)
22. Gardner, M. J. and Altman, D. G. (1986) Confidence interval rather than P-values: estimation rather than hypothesis testing. *Br. Med. J.* **292**: 746–50.
23. Margetts, B. M., Beilin, L. J., Vandongen, R. and Armstrong, B.K. (1986) Vegetarian diet in mild hypertension: a randomised controlled trial. *Br. Med. J.* **293**: 1468–71.
24. Walter, D. (1995) Methods of reporting statistical results from medical research studies. *Am. J. Epid.* **141**: 896–906.

25. Sacket, D. L. (1979) Bias in analytic research. *J. Chron. Dis.* **32**: 51–63.
26. Herbert, J. R., Clemow, L., Pbert, L., Ockene, I. S. and Ockene, J. K. (1995) Social desirability bias in dietary self-report may compromise the validity of dietary intake measures. *Int. J. Epid.* **24**: 389–98.
27. Marlowe, D. and Crowne, D. (1961) Social desirability and responses to perceived situational demands. *J. Consult Clin. Psychol.* **25**: 109–15.
28. Martin, H. A. (1984) A revised measure of approved motivation and its relationship to social desirability. *J. Pers. Assess.* **48**: 508–16.
29. Coughlan, S. S. (1990) Recall bias in epidemiological studies. *J. Clin. Epid.* **43**: 87–91.
30. Doll, R. and Hill, A. B. (1950) Smoking and carcinoma of the lung: preliminary report. *Br. Med. J.* **3**: 739–48.
31. Gregory, J., Foster, K., Tyler, H. and Wiseman, M. (1990) *The dietary and nutritional survey of British adults*. HMSO, London.
32. Popper, K. R. (1983) *The logic of scientific discovery*. Hutchinson & Co., London.
33. Bradford-Hill, A. (1971) *Principles of medical statistics*. 9th Edn. The Lancet, London.
34. Susser, M. (1991) What is a cause and how do we know one? A grammar for pragmatic epidemiology. *Am. J. Epid.* **133**: 635–48.
35. Barker, D. J. P. (1994) *Mothers, babies, and disease in later life*. BMJ Publishing Group, London.
36. Oakes, M. (1993) The logic and role of meta-analysis in clinical research. *Statistical Methods in Medical Research*. **2**: 147–60.
37. Petiti, D. B. (1994) *Meta-analysis, decision analysis, and cost-effectiveness*. Oxford University Press, New York.
38. Margetts, B. M., Thompson, R. L., Key, T., Duffy, S., Nelson, M., Bingham, S., *et al.* (1995) Development of a scoring system to judge the scientific quality of information from case-control and cohort studies of nutrition and disease. *Nutr. Cancer*. **24**: 231–39.
39. Friedenreich, C., Brant, R. F. and Riboli, E. (1994) Influence of methodologic factors in a pooled analysis of 13 case-control studies of colorectal cancer and dietary fiber. *Epidemiology*. **5**: 56–79.
40. Doll, R. (1994) The use of meta-analysis in epidemiology. Diet and cancers of the breast and colon. *Nutr. Rev.* **52**: 233–7.
41. Conover, W. J. (1980) *Practical Nonparametric Statistics*. 2nd Edn. John Wiley, New York.

2. Design, planning, and evaluation of nutritional epidemiological studies

Michael Nelson and Barrie M. Margetts

2.1 Introduction

Nutritional epidemiological studies should not be undertaken lightly. They require meticulous design, planning, and interpretation which is best achieved through collaboration and teamwork. Measurements of exposures and outcomes invariably have errors which must be carefully ascertained and described; the number of factors which may need to be taken into account requires statistical analysis which, though sometimes complex, must be intelligible both to the researcher and the readership; and the interpretation of the results requires a fertile and incisive imagination[1] which must draw upon a deep knowledge of the relevant literature. The purpose of this chapter is to outline the key stages in the design and interpretation of nutritional epidemiological studies; consider some of the pitfalls likely to be met; review the ways in which new techniques may be of benefit; and to present a scheme for the systematic evaluation of study designs and published papers.

2.2 The design and planning of nutritional epidemiological studies

The many stages of design (see Fig. 2.1) need careful consideration before embarking on a study. Each stage requires clear statements regarding theoretical models (e.g. the hypothesis, determination of sample size, proposed methods of biochemical and statistical analysis, etc.) or practical steps (e.g. field work, data entry and validation, etc.). Where issues have been discussed elsewhere in the book, references are given to the relevant chapter or section.

2.2.1 Design

Study aims

Every study needs a clear and concise statement of the research question to be investigated (the hypothesis: H_1). The investigator must ensure that the question is one which can be answered within a reasonable time-scale and cost, and that the measurements which will be needed to answer the question can be obtained. The

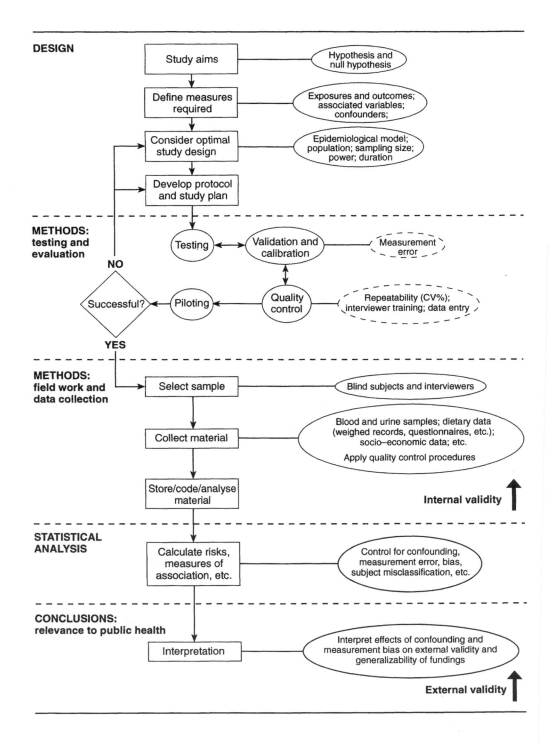

Fig. 2.1 Stages in the design of a nutritional epidemiological study.

hypothesis will have a greater chance of being proven if the exposures and outcomes to be measured are clearly specified (e.g. identification of intakes of individual caroten-oids; measurement of body fatness on a continuous scale [BMI] rather than an ordinal scale [lean, normal, overweight, obese]). Consideration of time, cost, and the ability to obtain measurements may result in appropriate modification of the hypothesis. If the modified hypothesis becomes so limited in its scope (e.g. precise measurements can be obtained only in a small subsection of the population) as to fail to address the original research question, then the study may have to be abandoned. Equally important is the formulation of the null hypothesis (H_0). Most statistical tests are based upon mathematical models which assume that there are no associations between variables, or that the difference between group means or medians is zero. If the observed outcome is very different from that which the model predicts (e.g. $P < 0.05$), then the null hypothesis can be rejected. A precise specification of the null hypothesis will in part dictate the nature of the statistical tests to be used.

Defining the measures required

The choice of appropriate measures for exposure and outcome is one of the primary themes of this book and others.[2,3] In terms of study design, measures must:

(1) address the questions posed in the hypothesis;
(2) be available within the resources of the study;
(3) be unbiased;
(4) be independent of confounders.

In order for the study to achieve its stated aims, it is essential that the measurements are appropriate to test the hypothesis. For example, if the hypothesis stated that neural tube defect (NTD) in newborns was related to the folic acid status of the mother, it would be necessary to specify the time period in which maternal levels of folic acid (in the diet or in serum) would be relevant (around the 12th week of gestation). A specific hypothesis would test the relationship between the occurrence of NTD and levels of folic acid before or at week 12. Measurement of folic acid after pregnancy in those women who had given birth to NTD infants would be less likely to show a relationship. Similarly, if a long history of exposure is needed (e.g. the assessment of lifetime intakes of calcium in relation to risk of osteoporotic fracture), then current measures may be of little value, and an estimate of past intake which might relate to dietary habits such as milk drinking in childhood and adolescence[4] may be appropriate. Exposures of nutrient intake may need to include dietary supplements.[5]

Outcome measures must also be relevant. Mortality is a poor measure to use with a disease which has a high morbidity but good prognosis (e.g. osteoporotic fracture in subjects under 75 years of age; non-insulin dependent diabetes in 45–74 year-olds). Measurements must also be available within the resources of the study. For example, an investigator may wish to test the hypothesis that intake of quercetin and related non-nutrient anti-oxidants reduces risks of large bowel cancer. If a case-control study is chosen as the appropriate study design, it may be that food composition data on the non-nutritive anti-oxidants in food are not adequate for an accurate calculation of intake. While it may be possible to collect duplicate diets to measure the anti-oxidant content of the diet directly, the disease process in the cases may have resulted in dietary modification, so that the present diet is no longer a reflection of the diet that may have been relevant to disease induction and progression. The resources available for the study may not permit the use of a cohort design (where duplicate diets could be collected at baseline, or dietary data could be collected at baseline and the necessary food analyses carried out during the follow-up period). Until such time as better food composition data or more resources were to be made available, it may not be possible to test this hypothesis using these kinds of observational models. Further problems relating to non-nutrient intakes are discussed by Petersen *et al.*[6]

In some studies, the primary source may not be available or appropriate, and it may seem desirable to use surrogate sources of data (e.g. a husband reporting wife's food consumption, or vice versa). For example, gastric cancer has a profound influence on dietary intake, and it may be felt to be more appropriate to ask a spouse about their partner's previous eating habits than to ask the subject directly. Also, mortality among gastric cancer patients is high, and subjects may have died before they can be interviewed. However, the reported quality of surrogate dietary data is poor.[7]

The measurements should be unbiased. It is rare, however, that unbiased measures are available. It is almost always necessary, therefore, to undertake validation, calibration, and reproducibility studies to measure the biases which exist, and to allow the biases to be taken into account during analysis and interpretation. Chapters 4 and 8 deal specifically with problems of measurement error, validation, and calibration. Chapters 5–7 and 9–11 describe in detail the types of biases which are likely to exist in relation to exposure measurements of different types, and Chapters 12–16 describe the types of errors characteristic of many outcome variables.

The effect of exposure on outcome should ultimately be expressed independently of confounders and effect modifiers (see Chapter 1 for definitions and discussion). The implication is that these additional factors must also be measured accurately. Biases associated with their measurement will lead to misinterpretation of both their influence and that of the exposure of interest. For example, risk of oesophageal cancer is related to smoking, but the effect of smoking is greatest in people who also have a high alcohol consumption. Heavy smoking and high alcohol consumption are positively correlated. If alcohol consumption were underestimated (as tends to occur in most surveys of alcohol consumption) not only would the influence of alcohol on risk be underestimated, but the effect of smoking on disease risk would be overestimated.

Effect modifiers alter the relationship between the exposure and the outcome. Such variables may or may not be independent of the exposure of interest, but they must lie in the causal pathway. For example, risk of kidney stones is positively related to vitamin C intake due to the metabolism of vitamin C to oxalic acid and the precipitation of calcium oxalate in concentrated urine in the kidney. Subjects with higher intakes of water have a reduced risk of disease because of the dilution effects. Water is thus an effect modifier because the association between vitamin C intake and disease risk is different at different levels of water intake. It is not a confounder, however, because water intake and vitamin C intake are not related. Failure to measure water intake would reduce the apparent effect of high vitamin C on disease risk. To take the influence of water intake properly into account, some form of stratified analysis according to level of water intake would be appropriate.

Finally, decisions need to be taken concerning the types of variables to be measured. In nutritional terms, this may mean choices between methods of dietary assessment (see Chapter 6) or the use of biochemical markers (see Chapter 7). It may require careful consideration of sociological and qualitative measures (Chapter 9), anthropometric variables (Chapter 10), or genetic markers of risk or nutrient interaction (Chapter 11). Each variable type requires a specific approach to its measurement and validation, and the help of experts should be sought.

Creating an optimal study design

Having generated a clear hypothesis and decided on the variables to be measured, it is necessary to create a study design which optimizes the chances of describing statistically significant risks (should they exist). The principal components will be:

1. The *epidemiological model*. The types of designs available have been outlined in Chapter 1 and are detailed in Chapters 12–16. To some extent, the type of design chosen will dictate the variables which are appropriate to measure: e.g. ecological studies require population based data, case-control studies require individually derived data, clinical trials demand very tight control of variability in the exposure of interest.

2. *Population*. The population from which the study sample is to be drawn must be clearly defined. Clever selection of populations with characteristics which are different from the general population in one or more aspects of lifestyle (e.g. vegetarians, nuns, Seventh-Day Adventists) or who have a unique history (e.g. women born during the Dutch famine 1944–45[8]) may help to achieve study aims by controlling for or determining exposures which are thought to influence the outcome measures. This applies particularly in relation to studies in which past diet is to be assessed and its validation will need to take place in a group of subjects for whom reliable dietary data were collected at the time in the past believed to be relevant to the dietary causation.[9]

It is also important to ensure that the exposure variables of interest vary sufficiently between study groups to make an estimate of risk feasible. The recently designed EPIC study maximizes variation of exposure by studying populations in a number of European countries[10], but this raises important problems concerning standardization of measurement which must be addressed. The same careful consideration must be given to the measurement of effect modifiers or confounding variables.

3. *Sampling*. Issues concerning the representativeness of samples in relation to populations have been discussed in Chapter 1, and techniques for sampling described in Chapter 3. Samples do not always have to be representative of the populations from which they are drawn to allow valid conclusions to be derived from a study (e.g. in field trials), but they must be representative of the aspect of the relationship between exposure and outcome that the study aims to address (e.g. a physiological mechanism). In certain types of study, however, (e.g. case-control studies) failure to obtain representative samples (selection bias) can undermine valid interpretation and generalizability of the results.

Sampling also relates to the timing of collection of repeat observations (i.e. the sampling of all possible repeat observations within the experimental unit). While considerable work has gone into estimating the *number* of repeat observations which may be needed to characterize a particular variable (e.g. blood pressure, 'usual' diet), the spacing and selection of observations have not been so carefully considered except insofar as they may have an impact on estimates of variables for which there is an obvious periodic element (e.g. day of week, season of year). The choice of observations will have an effect on the estimate of variance[11,12] which in turn will influence the extent to which subjects are believed to be correctly classified in the extremes of intake (see Chapter 4).

4. *Study size*. Study size must be a judicious choice between obtaining a sufficient number of observations to achieve a reasonable chance of demonstrating a statistically significant finding (should one exist), and obtaining sufficiently accurate and detailed information from each unit of observation (individual subject, household, country) to be able to test the hypothesis. A study size which is too large is clearly wasteful of resources. Equally, a study size which is too small is also wasteful if the study aims cannot be achieved. Optimal study size is discussed in Chapter 3, Section 3.3.

5. *Power*. Power is the ability of a study to demonstrate statistically significant associations, if they exist (see Figure 1.2). Its calculation for different types of study is described in Chapter 3, Section 3.3.3.

6. *Duration, dosage, lag times*. The duration of a cohort study depends on the number of cases expected within a given period, and the length of time over which the exposure of interest may be expected to have its effects. In case-control studies, the induction period and lag time will determine the point in time at which previous exposure should be estimated. In ecological studies, the lag time between exposure and outcome will dictate the collection of measurements relating to particular points in time. There may be a period of time over which a cumulative exposure needs to be measured. Each of these relate in effect to dosage, and a specific choice regarding dosage or degree of exposure (e.g. to nutrition education) needs to be made in clinical and field trials on the basis of previous estimates of dose-response or dose-risk.

Develop protocol/study plan

Once decisions about optimal design and measurements have been made, it is possible to start drawing up a protocol. This will contain the broad outlines of the study design, the population and sampling procedures, and the methods to be used to measure each variable and ensure its validity.

2.2.2   *Method testing and evaluation*

This stage involves deciding upon and writing into the protocol the detailed procedures that will be followed when carrying out the study. The first and often very time-consuming steps involve the standardization of instruments. They will typically include:

1. *Testing*. This concept applies to both laboratory and field measurements. It ensures that the procedures which are to be followed are consistent, and are in keeping with the meaning of the measurement which the investigator wishes to determine and convey to his or her audience. In relation to questionnaires, the interpretation or understanding of questions by the respondent must correspond with the meaning which the investigator intends to convey. A summary of the steps in the development of a questionnaire is given in Appendix I, and a more full procedure relating to questionnaire design is given

by Armstrong *et al.*[2] McKinney[13] and Gittlesohn *et al.*[14] have suggested that training subjects in the use of portion size estimation has a beneficial effect on quality of data.
2. *Validation and calibration.* This stage is vital to every nutritional epidemiological study, and two chapters in this book (4 and 8) are devoted to this issue. No measurement is perfect, and in nutritional studies especially, the errors may be very large. A knowledge of the size of the measurement errors is essential to an intelligent interpretation of the findings of the study. For example, the relationship between measures of nutrient intake assessed by questionnaire and by weighed inventory and a biochemical measure of that nutrient in blood which is sensitive to differences in nutrient intake will help to elucidate the true relationship between dietary intake and disease risk. Identification of differential misclassification is an important part of this process. In the absence of these measurements, it will not be possible to take into account the effects of bias, the sources of which are described in Chapters 1, 4, and 8.

A second important stage in the development of the methods is the need to ensure that procedures are appropriate and are being followed as described in the protocol.

3. *Quality control.* It is essential at all stages of data collection and entry and biochemical analysis to ensure that procedures are being followed correctly. This affects the precision (repeatability) of measurements. It is necessary to apply the same standards of quality control to information retrieved from subjects using questionnaires, diet records, etc., as to biochemical measurements in the laboratory. The problem is one of separating the 'noise' in the measurement from the true underlying variation.

Errors in replicate biochemical analyses can be used to determine which measurements are regarded as acceptable and which may need to be repeated. Errors in data entry must be trapped[15,16] either by having some form of range-checking (if a value entered for a particular variable falls outside the expected range, the computer queries the entry and offers an opportunity for the value to be re-entered) or a repeat entry system whereby values which are entered a second time which do not agree with the original entry are queried. In addition, it may be necessary to check the integrity of data in food composition tables used to estimate nutrient intakes (see Chapter 5) and ensure that apparent differences between centres, for example, are not due to differences between databases used to calculate nutrient intakes.[17] Interviewers must be trained to follow standard procedures and *not* use their initiative when responding to problems in the field: variations in interviewer technique will be likely to bias the estimates of risk towards the null.

4. *Piloting.* Piloting involves having a practice run of all the procedures that are to be carried out in the main study. It is usually carried out on a small subsample of the main sample, and its purpose is to discover those aspects of collecting, coding, and entering data which are likely to cause problems and which may need modification.

2.2.3 *Fieldwork and data collection and entry*

Only when the four steps above have been completed should data collection in the main study begin. Failure to ensure robust procedures in data collection and data management will result in undescribed errors being incorporated into the data. The likely effect is to undermine the ability to describe statistically significant associations between diet and disease (bias toward the null), although inaccurate data which is unevenly biased throughout the sample may result in differential misclassification and the observation of spurious associations.

Throughout the period of fieldwork and data collection and entry, the quality control procedures adopted should be rigorously applied. If there has been a major error in the choice of method or procedure, the study should be halted until the problem can be resolved. Changes of procedure midway in a study may make comparisons over the whole of the data set invalid, and delays in rectifying a problem may waste resources.

2.2.4 Statistical analysis

The choice of methods for statistical analyses is an important part of the development of the design of a study. It should be known at the outset exactly which statistical tests are to be used to describe the data and to test for associations between variables. This can be determined in part by deciding exactly what conclusions are to be drawn based on the hypothesis, and by thinking about the tables and figures which will be used to convey information about the results (e.g. 2×2 tables, scattergrams, estimates of relative risk). This process can save time both in relation to data collection and final statistical analyses, but it is necessary to remain aware of the problems that measurement error may introduce (e.g. differential misclassification) and how it is to be dealt with in the analyses. Clarification of the analyses to be used will help to define the characteristics of the variables to be measured (e.g. continuous or discrete) and will help to avoid problems where there is a mismatch between types of data needed for particular analyses (e.g. recording serum glucose levels rather than the presence or absence of diabetes in order to facilitate multiple regression analyses of energy, carbohydrate, and chromium intake as predictors of disease severity).

Decisions about inclusion or exclusion of data have important implications for statistical analysis. If dietary supplements are to be included in estimates of nutrient intake, this will have a profound effect on the distribution of intakes and hence the appropriateness of both the methods of analyses and the interpretation of the findings.[5] At every stage of analysis it is vitally important that the techniques used and reported are within the competence of the researcher to understand and describe. Modern statistical software packages such as SPSS[18] offer a range of very sophisticated analyses, but they should not be used if the researcher is not familiar with their application and interpretation. Techniques such as cluster analysis[19,20] offer new ways in which to assess the characteristics of exposure of diet, but should not be attempted without expert guidance. Detailed suggestions for appropriate analyses for different types of studies and variables are given throughout the book, particularly in Chapters 4 and 8 and the Appendix to Chapter 14 on cohort studies.

2.2.5 Interpretation

Sound interpretation of nutritional epidemiological findings is achieved through an accurate knowledge of the effects of chance, bias, and confounding on the measures of association between exposure and outcome, and on a thorough awareness of the likely mechanisms that may link the two. Reviewing the stages in Figure 2.1 and ensuring that correct procedures have been followed at each stage will improve overall interpretation. Interpretation will be enhanced especially by the ability to:

(1) distinguish the effects of confounding from effects which may lie in the causal pathway;
(2) recognize the influence of measurement bias and differential misclassification (knowledge derived from calibration and validation studies) – these are the issues around internal validity;
(3) consider whether the results have external validity and consider bias in relation to the study population.

Statistical analysis is the key transition between (2) and (3) above. In addition, there are many factors which may have influenced the choice of study design, variables, and methods which need to be considered again when interpreting the results. Their influence on external validity is a key issue.

A common dilemma is the need to choose between excluding from the analyses those subjects whose results are believed to be biased, and retaining subjects in the analyses in order to be able to generalize the findings. The former choice may lead to a clearer expression of a diet–disease relationship, but if the subjects who are excluded from the analyses differ from those retained in relation to the exposures of interest, then the strength of the diet–disease association may be mis-represented in terms of the general population. For example, if risk of osteoporotic fracture was being related to intakes of calcium, body weight, and levels of physical activity, and heavier subjects were excluded because they tended to under-report their dietary intakes, then the loss of information relating to bodyweight may lead to an overstatement of the importance of calcium and activity in relation to prevention of fracture. If the overweight subjects were retained, however, the conclusions may understate the importance of calcium as a protective factor. Correction of under-reported intakes in relation to energy intake may partly address the problem (see Chapter 6, Section 6.10) only if the biases in reporting are similar for different nutrients. Recent reports by Haraldsdóttir[21], Pryer et al.[22], Bellach and Kohlmeier[23], and Price et al.[12] suggest that energy adjustments may not adequately address these problems of dietary distortions which result in altered nutrient densities in under-reporters. Any conclusions would need to make explicit the population groups to which the results were believed to apply.

2.3 Other aspects of study design

In addition to the broad issues discussed in the previous section, there are other factors to be considered at the design stage that will have an influence on the outcome of a study.

Cognitive aspects. It has long been recognized that certain groups of subjects (e.g. young children, or even adolescents[24], who have an inadequately developed sense of frequency, type, or amount of food consumed; older subjects with memory loss[25]) may not be able to provide the information which is required to test a hypothesis. More recently, workers have been addressing the extent to which cognitive function may be related to differential biases. Abusabha and Smiciklas-Wright[26] were unable to show in a cross-section of women aged 60 years and over that factors such as memory and organizational abilities influenced outcome. Wirfält et al.[27] identified triggers to recall such as location of eating which were associated with improved recording. When comparing obese with normal weight subjects, Kretsch and Fong[28] showed that psychological factors were better discriminators of under-reporting in obese subjects, whereas adiposity was more strongly related in normal weight subjects. Price et al.[12] have also suggested that 'restrained' eating characteristics (restraint followed by bingeing) is more likely to be associated with under-reporting, although Lissner et al.[29] claim to have overcome some of the problems of under-reporting in relation to obese subjects. Birkett and Boulet[30] have used factor analysis to characterize the psychometric properties of responses from a food habits questionnaire to assess the internal consistency of responses as a way to identify weaknesses in design. Smith[31] has discussed general issues around information retrieval which may be important in relation to questionnaire design, and Domel and co-workers[32] have examined this specifically in relation to children. Further application of psychological profiling may help to identify the cognitive and personality characteristics associated with poor diet reporting.

Cultural factors. Studies which are aimed at a particular cultural subgroup within a population or which include a diversity of cultural or language groups require special care in their design. These relate particularly to aspects of comprehension[33], cultural taboos[34], portion size[35,36] and the diversity of food patterns.[10,37] The limitations of a tool for cross-cultural comparisons need to be evaluated before it is applied.[38,39,40,41]

Follow-up, compliance, and measurements of change. When planning cohort and experimental studies, decisions must be made at the outset concerning the ways in which continuity and compliance will be measured. Subjects who fail to continue in a cohort study (due to death, migration, or lost contact), or whose compliance in an experimental study is poor, may differ in their dietary habits from those who are retained or show good compliance.[42] Compliance can be maximized by securing and publicizing the support of the leadership of the social structure (school, factory, general practice, community), and through practical steps such as use of appointment reminder cards and thank-you letters.

If repeat dietary measures are to be used to assess change or compliance, the effect of the repetition of the measurements on the validity of the measures and the extent to which repetition may cause people to alter their dietary habits need to be assessed during the course of the study. In a cohort study, for example, repeat measurements may result in a dietary drift in the cohort away from mainstream dietary habits in the population. This may have the effect of reducing the generalizability of the results. If repeat dietary measures are used in a clinical trial to boost compliance, and subsequent analysis is based on those with good compliance rather than on an 'intention to treat' basis (see Chapter 16), then it will be important to include as part of the study design an assessment of the relationship between the characteristic of diet at baseline and subsequent compliance. Changes in the quality of dietary reporting during the course of intervention studies also need careful evaluation.[43] All plans relating to the analyses of the effect of follow-up on compliance must be included in the original study design.

2.4 New issues in study design and use of computers

The same general approaches to eliciting information from individuals about their eating habits have persisted since the 1930s: dietary records[44], 24-hour recall[45], and diet history.[46] Elaborations have included food frequency and amount questionnaires and the introduction of new technology. There are still major gaps in our ability to assess diet accurately, however, and some suggestions for improvements are outlined in this section.

Buzzard and Sievert[47] have identified several areas for improvement. These include:

1. *Better understanding of the cognitive and communication processes as they relate to food intake assessment.* These include sensitivity to cultural factors, age, styles of communication, and cognitive abilities. Kohlmeier[48], for example, has examined differences in response according to whether questions are list-based or meal-based, illustrating that differences may relate to the strategies that individuals have for recalling information.

2. *The need to minimize bias and other sources of error.* Substantial progress is being made in the development of new techniques to assess the impact of bias and measurement error on the interpretation of nutritional epidemiological studies. Of particular importance is the need to understand when it is appropriate to adjust for energy intake and which technique is best to use. Non-response bias also needs to be addressed.

3. *Improved estimation of portion size.* Recall of diet and some forms of record keeping require assessment of portion size without the use of scales. The finding that inclusion of portion size data does little to improve classification based questionnaire data[49] is counter-intuitive (more information should, in theory, give better classification). It may be that the reference measures against which the results utilizing portion size data are being compared are themselves too far from the truth, and that the true extent of improvement is thereby being underestimated. Carefully designed studies by Nelson et al.[50,51] and others[52,53] all suggest that photographs improve estimates of consumption.

4. *More rapid and cost-effective methods for collection and analysis of food intake data.* Innovative assessment methods based in part on the use of new technology will improve the accuracy and speed with which dietary data are reported. Use of tape recorders and hand-held computers linked to electronic digital food weighing machines and optical mark readers has already begun to reduce the number of errors inherent in transferring data from one format to another, and will help to overcome problems of coding errors.[15,16] Further development of computer-assisted data entry[54], portion size databases, and imaging (e.g. use of laser video to enable subjects to indicate portion size on screen) will facilitate this process. Analytical software for questionnaires is available.[55] The development of questionnaires especially must address differences in reporting by age, ethnicity, and culture, as well as keep up with the changes in food diversity and composition.[49]

5. *Development of food composition databases.* This is discussed extensively in Chapter 5. The main problems relate to ensuring that databases are sufficiently comprehensive to reflect the breadth of food consumption within a population, and that the analytical

data are accurate and complete, and reflect changing research interests (e.g. non-nutrient anti-oxidants).

6. *Development of tools for evaluating dietary change.* Problems concerning learning and compliance in studies where subjects are asked to make repeat measures of diet may undermine accurate measures of dietary change. Such efforts may be confounded by changes in databases or methods of chemical analysis over time.

7. *Development of improved methods for international comparisons.* This relates to measures collected at both the individual[10] and national[56] level and embraces the notion of calibration studies (see Chapters 4 and 8). The problems relating particularly to the consistency and continuity of data, such as the development of a single European food coding system, are discussed by Pietinen and Ovaskainen.[57]

8. *Improved use of biochemical, anthropometric, and whole body functional measurements.* The development of improved biochemical markers is discussed in Chapter 7, and the use of anthropometric measures is described in Chapter 10. Functional measures relate to the consequences of imbalanced nutrition (e.g. measures of psychological development in infants suffering from protein–energy malnutrition). It is important to obtain repeat measurements within individuals in order to have within-subject estimates of variability. Habitch and Pelletier[58] discuss the extent to which nutritional indicators are likely to reflect either the risks in the population or the benefits which accrue from intervention. The measure used, 'responsiveness', relates the difference of the observed measures from the situation in which there are no nutritional risks (d) to the standard deviation of the measures in the population (SD), that is, d/SD. This is a useful theoretical measure to help with decisions about which variables to include in a study and relates to both study size and power.

2.5 Evaluation of study design

There are two stages when it is important to evaluate the quality of study designs: when planning a study, and when reading the literature. In the former, the aim is to ensure that the most effective and robust design can be devised with the given resources. In the latter, the aim is to decide whether previous reported work is robust, whether it needs to be repeated, and if the conclusions can be used to inform the development of a new study.

Several sets of guidelines have been published to help researchers appreciate the type of information which needs to be included in a description of study designs.[59,60,61] By implication, the design of a study must be sufficiently detailed and comprehensive to allow that information to be reported. The elements of study design outlined in this chapter must be translated into specific items such as number of subjects, techniques of measurement, etc. In addition, the appropriateness of the methods and analyses relevant to the choice of design (e.g. case-control study) must also be described. Appendix II provides a set of guidelines which researchers can follow in order to ensure that their study designs are well described, relevant to their study hypothesis, and consistent with the literature.

When reading the literature, it is clear that some studies are better than others in their design and analysis. A difficulty therefore arises when comparing studies, or combining data from several studies in order to increase the power of an analysis. The UK Nutritional Epidemiology Group undertook a review of papers on diet and cancer[62] with a view to clarifying current opinions on diet–disease relationships. In order to facilitate this process, a scoring system was developed to enable the quality of the data presented to be evaluated in a systematic way. The scoring system was itself assessed.[63] Points were awarded in relation to relevance of study design and choice of variables in relation to the study hypothesis, sample choice and size, and analytical techniques. A scoring system of this type is not foolproof. It does, however, offer an objective measure of quality. This is an improvement on subjective evaluations, and at the very least allows for the weakest studies to be excluded from consideration. It should encourage researchers who are developing new studies to be more rigorous in their designs. In addition, it should encourage those who are writing papers to provide the level of detail which will enable their results to be properly evaluated.

Appendix I: Preparing a questionnaire

Questionnaires are used in all forms of epidemiological studies to measure exposures both to possible causal agents (e.g. nutrient intake) and to interacting or confounding variables (e.g. age and gender). They may also be used to measure outcomes (such as disease status) in cross-sectional studies.

A1.1   Objectives of questionnaire design

1. Valid measurements of the variables under study.
2. Ease of completion by the interviewer and/or subject.
3. Ease of processing and analysis.

A1.2   Principles of questionnaire design

1. *Content*. The questionnaire should be designed to ask the minimum amount about a subject's experiences which will provide sufficient information to investigate the research question. The questionnaire should be as brief as possible, with every question justified in terms of the objectives of the study.
2. *Types of question*.
   (a) Open: these allow respondents to answer in their own terms (verbatim).
   (b) Closed: these specify in detail the possible answers.
   Epidemiological questionnaires usually contain a majority of closed questions to reduce the possibility of interview, response, interpretation and/or coding bias, and to facilitate processing. The following points should be considered:
   (a) Open questions should be used for non-categorical data (e.g. age, date of birth).
   (b) In closed questions, where only one out of a selection of responses is allowed (e.g. 'Tick one box only'), the final option should always be 'Other, please specify', unless the investigator believes all possible responses have been offered.
   (c) In closed questions, where multiple responses are allowed (e.g. 'Tick one or more boxes'), each response should be coded as a separate variable.
   (d) When using mainly closed questions, respondents should be invited to make comments either in writing or to the interviewer.
3. *Wording of questions*. Questions must be written in simple, non-technical language, avoiding the use of jargon. Wording should avoid any suggestion that a particular answer is preferred, that is, 'leading' or 'loaded' questions should be avoided. Each question should contain only one idea.
4. *Question sequence*. Questions should follow a logical sequence resembling, as far as possible, the sequence that the respondents might expect to follow (this information can be derived from appropriate pre-testing of the questionnaire – see below). On each subject, questions should proceed from the general to the particular. When a

response to a general question makes further responses on that subject irrelevant or unnecessary (e.g. a lifetime non-drinker need not answer questions about present and past drinking), a branching of the question sequence may be introduced. This should be as simple as possible.

5. *Questionnaire layout.* This is important for both interviewer- and self-administered questionnaires, to arouse and maintain interest and ensure correct completion. An introduction, explanatory notes, and instructions and examples of how to complete particular questions should be brief. They should occupy pages which are separate from the first question, except where instructions and examples may immediately precede a new type of question. Different typefaces may be used for different components of each question, and to distinguish examples from actual responses.

6. *Method of administration.* Questionnaires can be self-administered or interviewer-administered. The advantages of self-administered questionnaires are their lower cost and absence of interviewer bias, but their disadvantages include a tendency to partial completion, unresolved or unidentified problems of question interpretation, and the need for literacy skills. Interviewer-administered questionnaires have the advantages of ensuring completion, use of complex question structures and sequences, clarification of meaning (although this may introduce bias), and support which facilitates cooperation. The main disadvantages are in terms of cost, time, and interviewer bias. Computer-administered questionnaires combine the advantages of self- and interviewer-administered questionnaires while minimizing the disadvantages. They have the advantages of 'intelligent' question sequencing (e.g. skipping irrelevant questions) which allows for complex question structures or sequences, confirmation of responses (e.g. it is not possible to continue until an answer has been provided, and unusual answers can be queried in a systematic way), and help with clarification of meaning which will be consistent across subjects. At the same time they are cheap to administer and avoid interviewer bias. They do of course require literacy and minimal computer skills (e.g. ability to use a keyboard).

7. *Recording of responses.* The relevant objective is to obtain clear and unambiguous answers to each question which are both easy to provide and easy to process. Self-coded questions, optical mark readers, and computer administration all reduce errors relating to data entry of responses. It is vital to ensure that when using closed questions all the possible responses are included in the list of options provided: failure to do so will result in biased responses which do not reflect the true range of behaviours in the sample, and will frustrate subjects' attempts to provide appropriate answers, thereby reducing care in completion and cooperation.

8. *Coding.* It is important at the outset to decide on the coding scheme to be used for each variable. This often highlights problems with question design, and helps to ensure that appropriate variables are being collected for analysis. Most responses are best coded and entered into the computer as numbers rather than letters, with the exception of obvious variables such as name or country of birth. A coding guide should be constructed which provides the key to the meaning of numerical responses (e.g. 1 = 'Yes', 2 = 'No'), and this can be used to clarify output in analysis programs such as SPSS (Statistical Package for the Social Sciences) which allows for the specification of 'value labels'.

A1.3 Evaluation of questionnaires

Questionnaires should be subject to two forms of evaluation:

1. *Pretesting and piloting.* This is an essential part of the development of any questionnaire. Pretesting involves administration of drafts of the questionnaire to samples of subjects similar to those to be studied. Its purpose is to identify questions which are poorly understood, ambiguous, or which evoke hostile or other undesirable responses. Multiple pretests are usually required. Pretests should ultimately lead to a formal pilot test, in which the questionnaire is administered in exactly the way in which it will finally be administered in the main study. At each stage the questionnaire will need modification until the researcher is satisfied that for every question the response corresponds to the understanding by the subject which the researcher intended to convey, and that the response is a true response insofar as the subject is able to provide it.

2. *Assessment of validity.* The main concern will usually be with the validity of questionnaire estimates of dietary variables, but other information (e.g. regarding lifestyle, smoking) may also require validation. This will require administration of another measuring instrument to obtain reference measures to which the question- naire responses can be compared. Validation is time-consuming, difficult, ex- pensive, and absolutely vital to the success of a study. Sometimes it may be impossible (e.g. validation of dietary intakes in the distant past), in which case researchers need to provide a description of a model which underlies the assumptions regarding the validity of the question responses. See Chapter 8 for a full description of the validation process.

A1.4 Use of standard questionnaires

Where a standard questionnaire exists for measurement of a particular exposure, it will be desirable to use it for the following reasons:

(1) It will usually have been used extensively and proved satisfactory in use;
(2) It may have been independently validated (although validity in one population does not ensure validity in another);
(3) It will facilitate comparison of results from your study with data collected by other workers;
(4) It will expedite questionnaire design.

Any change of format of standard questionnaires may affect the nature of response to them and therefore their validity and comparability. A modification can, of course, be tested for validity against the original questionnaire and, ideally, against an independent reference measure.

Appendix II: Guidelines for describing nutritional epidemiological study designs and methods

It is essential that studies are fully described in published papers. This relates to the rationale for the hypothesis and choice of methods, the description of the methods themselves, and the nature of the analyses to be undertaken. Especially important is the need to describe dietary assessment methods fully and accurately, as a method given the same name by different investigators may have the same broad approach but may differ in detail. See Chapter 6 for further descriptions.

A2.1 Design characteristics

1. Study design (e.g. cohort, case-control, intervention)
   * Rationale for choice of design
   * Rationale for choice of variables
2. Sample recruitment (includes cases, controls, other units of measure, e.g. country, GP practice)
   * How were subjects recruited?
   * What was the population or sampling frame?
   * Response rate: numbers contacted, recruited, and completing study
   * Reasons for non-compliance or non-completion
   * Use of incentives
3. Sample characteristics
   * Age, gender
   * Height, weight, other anthropometry
   * Social class, other demographic information
   * Clinical information, nature and confirmation of diagnosis
   * Whether sample represents the population studied
   * Geographic coverage
4. Other information relevant to response or interpretation of results
   * Power of study
   * Timing of study in relation to:
     – disease processes
     – interventions
     – season
   * Length to follow up (cohort or experimental studies) and rationale

A2.2 Methods of assessment

In any report, the methods should be described in sufficient detail to enable other workers to carry out the same study using the same techniques. While this is generally accepted in relation to biochemical techniques, it is rarely applied to dietary techniques.

A2.2.1 Information required for all dietary methods

1. Method of dietary assessment
   See Section A2.3 below for definitions

2. Validity of the method
   - Rationale for choice of method
   - Whether instruments used have been pre-tested on a similar population
   - Whether the method has been validated against another dietary method or external markers of intake
   - Whether the reproducibility has been assessed
3. Method used for quantifying portions
   See Section A2.3 below for definitions
   - Specify source of 'average' portions
   - Give details of aids used to help quantify portions
   - Give specifications of scales used for weighing
   - Describe method for quantifying unweighed foods in weighed records
4. Food composition database used for the analysis
   - Which database was used?
   - How were foods dealt with which were not in the database?
   - Describe supplementary analytical work
   - Describe any modifications of the database
5. Interviewers or field workers
   - Whether qualified (dietitians/nutritionists)
   - Training given to unqualified fieldworkers
   - Whether the same workers both collected and coded the data
6. Data collection procedures and method of administration
   - Where and how data were collected (home/clinic/by interview – face to face or telephone/self-completed – by post or by computer)
   - Number of interviews per subject
   - Duration of interviews
   - Level of detail of data collection (e.g. fat trimmed from meat, use of salt)
   - Nature of probes to elicit information
   - Nature of follow-up regarding queries
   - Who provided information(e.g. subject, relative, friend)?
7. Checking procedures (quality control)
   - When and how often records were checked with respondents
   - Checks for coding errors
   - Checks on the consistency of field workers

A2.2.2 Information required specific to different dietary methods

For all dietary methods, the question of weighting of results is important wherever there are differences in diet relating to the timing of the assessment. These may apply to days of the week (weekday/weekend differences), weeks of the year (e.g. Ramadan), season (affecting availability of specific foods), etc. Results should be presented in the way which best serves the study design, and not necessarily weighted if the comparison with disease or outcome does not warrant it.

1. Recall method
   - How many and which days recalled

- Were all days of the week included?
- If not, were results weighted?

2. Diet history
   - Attempted time-scale (current/recent past/distant past/season/whole year)
   - Open-ended questions or fully structured interview
   - Structure of interview
     - Did it start with a 24-hour recall;
     - Did it take each meal or each day of the week in turn to build up a picture of the diet?
     - Did it include any cross-checks for types or frequency of foods consumed?
     - If so, what?
   - Were the subjects given any prompt lists? If so, describe

3. Food frequency (and amount) questionnaires
   - Whether interviewer-administered or self-completed
   - Rationale for the choice of foods
   - Whether instrument was pre-tested in a similar population
   - Foods covered and options for frequency
   - Number of foods listed
   - Time taken to complete

4. Study-specific questionnaires
   - Whether interviewer-administered or self-completed
   - Rationale for the form of the questionnaire
   - Whether the instrument was pre-tested in a similar population
   - Include the questionnaire as an appendix (see note below)

5. All record methods
   - How many and which days were studied
   - Were all days of the week included?
   - If not, whether any adjustment or weighting was used
   - How food eaten away from home was quantified
   - What instructions and equipment were given to the respondent

General note on questionnaires. It is desirable for the questionnaire to be included as an appendix even if much reduced in size. This best describes the methods since it shows the questions asked and the foods and frequencies chosen. For the instrument to be 'available from the authors' is unsatisfactory since it does not permit immediate evaluation of the study and in later years is unobtainable. At the very least a copy of the questionnaire must be made available for review purposes.

A2.3 Definitions of dietary assessment methods

Dietary questionnaire: This phrase has no precise meaning. It is not an adequate description.

1. **Diet recall:** The respondent is asked to recall the actual food and drink consumed on specified days, usually the immediate past 24 hours (24-hour recall) but sometimes for longer periods.

2. **Diet history:** The respondent is questioned about 'typical' or 'usual' food intake in a one to two hour interview. The aim is to construct a typical seven days' eating pattern. The interview may discuss each meal and inter-meal period in turn or each day of the week in turn. Questions are usually open-ended, although a fully structured interview may be used. The diet history may be preceded by a 24-hour recall and/or supplemented with a checklist of foods usually consumed.

3. **Food frequency (and amount) questionnaires (FFQ or FAQ):** The respondent is presented with a list of foods and is required to say how often each is eaten in broad terms such as x times per day/per week/per month, etc. Foods listed are usually chosen for the specific purposes of a study and may not assess total diet. The FFQ may be interviewer-administered or self-completed. Assessment of the quantities of food consumed on each eating occasion/day may also be included.

4. **Study-specific dietary questionnaire:** A term covering all dietary assessments using a set of pre-determined questions but not conforming to any of the classic techniques defined above. *The method is defined only by the questionnaire itself.* The question-naire may be interviewer-administered or self-completed.

A2.3.1   Record techniques

Diet record: A blanket term for all record methods. In American literature the term is often used without qualification but with 'quantified in household measures' under-stood. Since there are other forms of record, it is an inadequate description. A **record** is of actual food and drink consumed on specified days after the first contact by the investigator. The number of days recorded classically is seven but may be fewer or more.

1. **Menu record or food frequency record:** The first term is preferable to avoid confusion with food frequency questionnaires. Record obtained without quantifying the portions, analysed in terms of frequencies or 'average' weights.

2. **Checklist:** Printed list of foods on which subjects check off each day which foods were eaten[64]. Portion size may be indicated, and space left to report consumption of unlisted items.

3. **Estimated record:** A record with portions described in household measures (cups, spoons, etc.) with/without the aid of diagrams or photographs. This method aims to estimate the actual quantity eaten.

4. **Weighed record (weighed inventory technique):** Record with weights of portions as served and the plate waste. (Weighed records are rarely fully weighed; estimated portions are usual for food eaten away from home.)

5. **Precise weighed record:** A record kept by the respondent of all ingredients used in the preparation of meals, also inedible waste, total cooked weight of meal items, cooked weight of individual portions, any plate waste.

6. **Cardiff photographic record:** Method of Elwood and Bird.[65] Respondents photo-graph food on the plate at the time of consumption. Portions are quantified by comparison with reference photographs of portions known weight projected along-side the survey photographs.

7. **Semi-weighed method for measuring family food intake:** Method of Nelson and Nettleton.[66] Total quantity of food served to a family is weighed and quantities served to individuals are given in household measures. The term is sometimes mistakenly used for a weighed diet record where the authors acknowledge that not all food is in fact weighed.

A2.3.2 Techniques of direct analysis

1. **Duplicate diets:** Respondents keep a weighed record and also weigh out and put aside a duplicate portion of each food as consumed for later analysis by the investigator.
2. **Aliquot sampling technique:** Respondent keeps a weighed record and puts aside aliquot samples of food as consumed for later analysis.
3. **Equivalent composite technique:** Respondent keeps a weighted record. Subsequently a combined sample of raw foods, equivalent to the mean daily amount of foods eaten, is made up by the investigator for analysis.

A2.3.3 Computer assessment

The phrase 'computer assessment' does not define a method. Assessments conducted by computer should be described in the terms defined above.

Computer conducted assessments differ from person conducted assessments in the mechanics used. The computer may substitute for the paper and pencil of a self-completion questionnaire or it may substitute for the interview in a diet history by fully-structured interview.

Computerized interviewing may be combined with nutrient analysis to provide 'instant' information on nutrient intake. Here the assumptions necessary to code foods and quantify portions are built into the programme. The computer substitutes for the investigator in performing the post-interview coding tasks.

A.2.4 Definitions: quantifying portions

1. **Qualitative (or unquantified) assessment:** An assessment made only in terms of foods eaten, usually by counting frequency of consumption.
2. **Quantitative assessment:** A dietary assessment that quantifies the portions of foods eaten in order to calculate nutrient consumption.
3. **Average portions:** Investigator assigns 'average' portion weights derived from previous studies or experience. 'Small', 'medium', or 'large' may also be used to indicate portion size in relation to the 'average'.
4. **Household measures:** Respondent describes portions in terms of household measures, e.g. cups, spoons, etc. 'Standard' weights are assigned to the descriptions.
5. **Photographic measures:** Respondent is shown photographs of portions of known weight and asked how their own portion relates to the pictured portion. (Not to be confused with the Cardiff photographic record; see above.)
6. **Food models/replicas:** Respondent is shown three-dimensional models representing foods and asked how their own portion relates to the models. Models may be realistic replica foods or a variety of neutral shapes and sizes.
7. **Weighed:** The subject weighs and records each food item as it is consumed.

A2.5 Analysis

There are no fixed rules regarding the types of analyses to be undertaken, simply because of the diversity of types of study. A few basic points should be considered:

1. Has basic information been provided (e.g. mean age, nutrient intake)?
2. Where other factors have been measured, have they been:
   - assessed properly?
   - taken into account using appropriate analyses?
   - where appropriate, has due regard for matching been observed?
3. Where relative risks or odds ratios have been calculated, are the categories of grouping sensible?
4. Where adjustment for other variables has been used, are both the unadjusted and adjusted results presented? If adjustment has been made for energy, is this appropriate;
5. In cohort studies:
   - have incident cases in the first year (or other appropriate interval) been excluded?
   - have baseline exposures been presented?
   - are there repeat measures, and have they been used appropriately in the analysis?
6. Have calibration techniques been used appropriately to allow combining of results from multi-centre studies?
7. If there are both dietary and biochemical measures of nutritional status, have the data been used together to strengthen the analysis?

References

1. Ashton, J. (1994) *The epidemiological imagination: a reader*. Open University, Buckingham.
2. Armstrong, B. K., White, E. and Saracci, R. (1992) *Principles of exposure measurement in epidemiology*. Oxford University Press, Oxford.
3. Dunn, G. (1989) *Design and analysis of reliability studies*. Edward Arnold, London.
4. Sandler, R. B., Slemenda, C. W., LaPorte, R. E., Cawley, J. A., Schramm, M. M.,Barresi, M. L., *et al.* (1985) Postmenopausal bone density and milk consumption in childhood and adolescence. *Am. J. Clin. Nutr.* **42**: 270–4.
5. Block, G., Sinha, R. and Gridley, G. (1994) Collection of dietary supplement data and implications for analysis. *Am. J. Clin. Nutr.* **59**(Suppl): 232S–9S.
6. Petersen, B. J., Chaisson, C. F. and Douglass, J. S. (1994) Use of food-intake surveys to estimate exposures to non-nutrients. *Am. J. Clin. Nutr.* **59**(Suppl): 240S–3S.
7. Metzner, H. L., Lamphiear, D. E., Thompson, F. E., Oh, M. S. and Hawthorn, V. M. (1989) Comparison of surrogate and subject reports of dietary practices, smoking habits, and weight among married couples in the Tecumseh Diet Methodology Study. *J. Clin. Epid.* **42**: 367–75.
8. Lumey, L. H., Ravelli, A. C., Wiessing, L. G., Koppe, J. G., Treffers, P. E. and Stein, Z. A. (1993) The Dutch famine birth cohort study: design, validation of exposure, and selected characteristics of subjects after 43 years follow-up. *Paed. Perinat. Epid.* **7**: 354–67.
9. Sobell, J., Block, G., Koslowe, P., Tobin, J. and Andres, R. (1989) Validation of a retro-spective questionnaire assessing diet 10–15 years ago. *Am. J. Epid.* **130**: 173–87.
10. Kaaks, R. (1997) Validation and calibration of dietary intake measurements in the EPIC study: methodological considerations. *Int. J. Epid.* **26**(Suppl). (In press.)
11. Hartman, A. M., Brown, C. C., Palmgren, J., Pietinen, P., Verkasalo, M., Myer, D., *et al.*

(1990) Variability in nutrient and food intakes among older middle-aged men. Implications for design of epidemiologic and validation studies using food recording. *Am. J. Epid.* **132**: 999–1012.

12. Price, G. M., Paul, A. A., Cole,. T. J. and Wadsworth, M. E. J. (1997) Characteristics of the low energy reporters in a longitudinal national dietary survey. *Br. J. Nutr.* (In press).

13. McKinney, S. (1995) Impact of intensive food portion size training on the accuracy of visual assessment of food portions and recall of quantity of food consumed. [abstract]. Second International Conference on Dietary Assessment Methods, Harvard.

14. Gittelsohn, J., Shankar, A. V., Pokhrel, R. P. and West, K. P. (1994) Accuracy of estimating food intake by observation. *J. Am. Diet. Assoc.* **94**: 1273–7.

15. Black, A. E. (1982) The logistics of dietary surveys. *Hum. Nutr. Appl. Nutr.* **36A**: 85–94.

16. Meltzer, S. T. and Lambert, M. (1995) The variability among dietitians in coding and analyzing reported food intake. [abstract]. Second International Conference on Dietary Assessment Methods, Harvard.

17. Guilland, J. C., Aubert, R., Lhuissier, M., Peres, G., Montagnon, B., Fuchs, F., *et al.* (1993) Computerized analysis of food records: role of coding and food composition database. *Eur. J. Clin. Nutr.* **47**: 445–53.

18. SPSS. (1988) Statistical Package for the Social Sciences. SPSS, Chicago.

19. Pryer, J. A., Elliott, P., Diamond, H. and Nichols, R. (1995) Dietary patterns among a national random sample of British men. [abstract]. Second International Conference on Dietary Assessment Methods, Harvard.

20. Wirfält, A. K. E. and Jeffrey, R. W. (1995) Differences in population characteristics across food pattern clusters. [abstract]. Second International Conference on Dietary Assessment Methods, Harvard.

21. Haraldsdóttir, J. (1995) Dietary composition among subjects reporting implausibly low energy intake. [abstract]. Second International Conference on Dietary Assessment Methods, Harvard.

22. Pryer, J. A., Vrijheid, M., Nichols, R. and Elliott, P. (1995) Who are the 'low energy reporters' in the dietary and nutritional survey of British adults? [abstract]. Second International Conference on Dietary Assessment Methods, Harvard.

23. Bellach, B. and Kohlmeier, L. (1995) Energy adjustment and exposure assessment error. [abstract]. Second International Conference on Dietary Assessment Methods, Harvard.

24. Feunekes, G. I. J., Burema, J. and van Staveren, W. A. (1995) Relative validity of a food frequency questionnaire to assess fat intake for adolescents, adults, and elderly. [abstract]. Second International Conference on Dietary Assessment Methods, Harvard.

25. Van Staveren, W. A., de Groot, L. C. P. G. M., Blauw, Y. H. and van der Wielen, R. P. J. (1994) Assessing diets of elderly people: problems and approaches. *Am. J. Clin. Nutr.* **59**(Suppl): 221S–3S.

26. Abusabha, R. and Smiciklas-Wright, H. (1995) Food frequency questionnaire reproducibility: diet and cognition. [abstract]. Second International Conference on Dietary Assessment Methods, Harvard.

27. Wirfält, A. K. E., Krinke, U. B. and Elmer, P. J. (1995) Recall strategies of usual diet – an exploratory study. [abstract]. Second International Conference on Dietary Assessment Methods, Harvard.

28. Kretsch, M. J. and Fong, A. K. H. (1995) Correlates of over- and under-reporting of energy intake in healthy normal-weight and obese women using estimated food records. [abstract]. Second International Conference on Dietary Assessment Methods, Harvard.

29. Lissner, L., Lindroos, A-K. and Sjöström, L. (1995) A dietary questionnaire developed for Swedish obese subjects (SOS). [abstract]. Second International Conference on Dietary Assessment Methods, Harvard.

30. Birkett, N. J. and Boulet, J. (1995) Validation of a food habits questionnaire: poor performance in male manual laborers. *J. Am. Diet. Assoc.* **95**: 558–63.

31 Smith, A. F. (1993) Cognitive psychological issues of relevance to the validity of dietary reports. *Eur. J. Clin. Nutr.* **47**(Suppl 2): S6–S18.

32. Domel, S. B., Thompson, W. O., Baranowski, T. and Smith, A. F. (1994) How children remember what they have eaten. *J. Am. Diet. Assoc.* **94**: 1267–72.

33. Murphy, S. P. and Ikeda, J. P. (1995) Evaluation of a dietary profile method of assessing usual nutrient intake. [abstract]. Second International Conference on Dietary Assessment Methods, Harvard.

34. Benavente, J. C. and Pobocik, R. S. (1995) Culture-specific dietary assessment interview techniques for Pacific islander and Filipino populations. [abstract]. Second Internaitonal Conference on Dietary Assessment Methods, Harvard.

35. Sharma, S., Cade, J. and Cruickshank, J. K. (1995) Developing and using a food frequency questionnaire in a British Afro–Caribbean population. [abstract]. Second International Conference on Dietary Assessment Methods, Harvard.

36. Taren, D. L., de Toabar, M., Ritenbaugh, C., Teufel, N. and Aickin, M. (1995) Portion size differences between NCI's FFQ and the Mexican–American portion of NHANES: implications for the development of FFQs. [abstract]. Second International Conference on Dietary Assessment Methods, Harvard.

37. Campbell, M. and Polhamus, B. (1995) Culturally sensitive dietary assessment for a rural African–American population. [abstract]. Second International Conference on Dietary Assessment Methods, Harvard.

38. Newell, G. R., Borrud, L. G., McPherson, R. S., Nichaman, M. Z. and Pillow, P. C. (1988) Nutrient intakes of whites, blacks, and Mexican Americans in southeast Texas. *Prev. Med.* **17**: 622–33.

39. Hankin, J. H. and Wilkens, L. R. (1994) Development and validation of dietary assessment methods for culturally diverse populations. *Am. J. Clin. Nutr.* **59**(Suppl 1): 198S–200S.

40. Forsythe, H. E. and Gage, B. (1994) Use of a multicultural food-frequency questionnaire with pregnant and lactating women. *Am. J. Clin. Nutr.* **59**(Suppl): 203S–206S.

41. Coates, R. J., Serdula, M. K., Byers, T., Mokdad, A., Jewell, S., Leonard, S. B., *et al.* (1995) A brief telephone-administered food frequency questionnaire can be useful for surveillance of dietary fat intakes. *J. Nutr.* **125**: 1473–83.

42. Buzzard, I. M., Jeffrey, R., McBane, L., McGovern, P. and Baxter, J. (1995) Estimating compliance bias and other sources of error in assessing dietary intake in a low fat diet intervention study. [abstract]. Second International Conference on Dietary Assessment Methods, Harvard.

43. Johansson, G., Callmer, E. and Gustafsson, J. A. (1992) Validity of repeated dietary measurements in a dietary intervention study. *Eur. J. Clin. Nutr.* **46**: 717–28.

44. Widdowson, E. M. (1936) A study of English diets by the individual method. Part I: Men. *J. Hyg.* **36**: 269–92.

45. Wiehl, D. G. (1942) Diets of a group of aircraft workers in Southern California. *Millbank Memorial Fund Quarterly.* **20**: 329–66.

46. Burke, B. S. (1947) The diet history as a tool in research. *J. Am. Diet. Assoc.* **23**: 1041–6.

47. Buzzard, I. M. and Sievert, Y. A. (1994) Research priorities and recommendations for dietary assessment methodology. *Am. J. Clin. Nutr.* **59**(Suppl 1): 275S–80S.

48. Kohlmeier, L. (1994) Gaps in dietary assessment methodology: meal- vs list-based methods. *Am. J. Clin. Nutr.* **59**(Suppl 1): 175S–9S.

49. Willett, W. C. (1994) Future directions in the development of food-frequency questionnaires. *Am. J. Clin. Nutr.* **59**(Suppl): 171S–4S.

50. Nelson, M., Atkinson, M. and Darbyshire, S. (1994) Food photography 1. The perception of food portion size from photographs. *Br. J. Nutr.* **72**: 649–63.

51. Nelson, M., Atkinson, M. and Darbyshire, S. (1996) Food photography 2. Use of food photographs for estimating portion size and the nutrient content of meals. *Br. J. Nutr.* **76**: 31–49.

52. Faggiano, F., Vineis, P., Cravanzola, D., Pisani, P., Xompero, G., Riboli, E., *et al.* (1992) Validation of a method for the estimation of food portion size. *Epidemiology.* **3**: 379–82.

53. Robinson, F., Morritz, W., McGuinness, P. and Hackett, A. (1996) A study of the use of a photographic food atlas to estimate served and self-served portion sizes. *J. Hum. Nutr. Diet.* (In press.)

54. Kretsch, M. J. and Fong, A. K. H. (1990) Validation of a new computerized technique for quantitating individual dietary intake: the Nutrition Evaluation Scale System (NESSy) vs the weighed food record. *Am. J. Clin. Nutr.* **51**: 477–84.

55. Block, G., Coyle, L. M., Hartman, A. M. and Scoppa, S. M. (1994) Revision of dietary analysis software for the Health Habits and History Questionnaire. *Am. J. Epid.* **139**: 1190–6.

56. Vassilakou, T. and Trichopoulou, A. (1992) Overview of household budget surveys in 18 European countries. *Eur. J. Clin. Nutr.* **46**(Suppl 5): 137S–53S.

57. Pietinen, P. and Ovaskainen, M-L. (1994) Gaps in dietary-survey methodology in Western Europe. *Am. J. Clin. Nutr.* **59**(Suppl): 161S–3S.

58. Habitch, J-P. and Pelletier, D. L. (1990) The importance of context in choosing nutritional indicators. *J. Nutr.* **120**: 1519–24.

59. Margetts, B. M. (1991) Basic issues in designing and interpreting epidemiological research. In: Margetts, B. M. and Nelson, M. *Design concepts in nutritional epidemiology.* 1st edn. Oxford University Press, Oxford. pp. 13–52.

60. Nelson, M., Margetts, B. M. and Black, A. E. (1993) Editorial guidelines for the methods section of dietary investigations. *Br. J. Nutr.* **69**: 935–40.

61. Wheeler, M. L. and Buzzard, I. M. (1994) How to report dietary assessment data. *J. Am. Diet Assoc.* **94**: 1255–6.

62. UK Nutritional Epidemiology Group. (1993) *Diet and cancer: a review of the epidemiological literature.* The Nutrition Society, London.

63. Margetts, B. M., Thompson, R. L., Key, T., Duffy, S., Nelson, M., Bingham, S., *et al.* (1995) Development of a scoring system to judge the scientific quality of information from case-control and cohort studies of nutrition and disease. *Nutr. Cancer.* **24**: 231–9.

64. Bingham, S. A., Cassidy, A., Cole, T., Welch, A., Runswick, S., Black, A. E., *et al.* (1995) Validation of weighed records and other methods of dietary assessment using the 24 h urine technique and other biological markers. *Br. J. Nutr.* **73**: 531–50.

65. Elwood, P. C. and Bird, G. (1983) A photographic method of diet evaluation. *Hum. Nutr.: Appl. Nutr.* **37A**: 474–7.

66. Nelson, M. and Nettleton, P. A. (1980) Dietary survey methods. I. A semi-weighed technique for measuring dietary intake within families. *J. Hum. Nutr.* **34**: 325–48.

3. Sampling, study size, and power

Tim J. Cole

3.1 Sampling

3.1.1 *Populations*

After deciding on the research question to be investigated, the next most important decision to make concerns the population to be studied. There are many possible populations of individuals identifiable by their place of residence or occupation and personal characteristics, for example inner-city families, vegans, hospital patients, or nuns. Imaginative choice of population can make the difference between a dull study which just reiterates known facts and an interesting study providing a useful extension to knowledge.[1]

The choice of population inevitably depends to a large extent on the nature of the research question. However, it is important that the results found can be extrapolated confidently to the broader population of which the study population is a part. There is no point in studying, say, hospital patients with a peptic ulcer and presuming that the results will automatically apply to people with the condition in the community. The very fact of their being in hospital makes them different from those in the community, and care should be taken to be aware of and avoid biases in interpretation due to selection.

It is important then to specify very precisely what the population is, where it comes from, and how the sampling frame is constructed. This will then make clear to which population the conclusions of the study refer. For example, a population might be defined as 'pregnant mothers recruited in the district maternity hospital during the last trimester of pregnancy, and living within five miles of the hospital'. This population might then be further qualified in terms of race, parity, or recent morbidity, allowing almost unlimited scope for defining different sub-populations of the broader population of urban pregnant women. The more clearly the population is defined at the outset, the easier subsequent recruitment, data collection, and writing up will be.

In case-control studies (Chapter 15) it is necessary to define two populations, the cases and the controls. Here the population of controls should match the population of cases with respect to major potential confounders such as gender and age, the principle being that the controls and cases should have equal chances of being exposed to the agent being investigated. When the cases ascertained are in-patients in a general (as opposed to a specialized) hospital, it is common practice to obtain as controls in-patients from other departments of the same hospital, where their condition is unrelated to the exposure. This increases the likelihood that the cases and controls come from the same catchment area (that of the hospital), which matches roughly for social and occupational conditions as they might affect exposure.

An alternative to hospital controls is a control group obtained from the community. This usually involves some form of sampling from population registers, but it can be much simpler, being based on friends or neighbours of the cases. Community controls tend to be more expensive to obtain than hospital controls, as the sampling and visiting is more extensive, so that hospital controls are very commonly used.

3.1.2 Sampling

The target population, once defined, is usually too large to investigate in its entirety. To produce a workable number of subjects, some form of sampling procedure is necessary. In the simplest case, for example subjects presenting to hospital or their GP clinic, all suitable cases identified between two points in time are sampled. The sampling period is assumed not to be atypical, so that any conclusions drawn apply to patients presenting to the hospital or clinic at other times. This assumption may actually be invalid; if there is an infectious epidemic, say flu, current at the time, this would obviously influence the pattern of cases seen, and might make the conclusions relevant only to cases seen during flu epidemics.

In cross-sectional or prospective studies, the sample is likely to be obtained from the target population by selection based on criteria other than time. It has already been stressed that the results obtained from the sample must be applicable to the target population. This will not be the case if the sample is not representative of the population, i.e. if any selection effects operate. The correct way to avoid selection in the drawing up of the sample is to make use of randomization. This device ensures that no biases, conscious or unconscious, on the part of the researchers, influence the choice of subjects. The other major benefit of randomization is that standard statistical methods can be applied to the sample data to obtain population estimates, and the estimates can be given confidence intervals. This latter point is crucial. It may be much easier and cheaper to go out into the street and recruit the first 100 people that pass by, but there is no way of knowing how closely their results reflect those of the target population (unless, of course, the target population happens to be people in that particular street at that particular time).

There are a variety of different forms of random sampling, of increasing complexity. The purpose of having different forms is to provide a trade-off between the precision of the population estimate (i.e. the width of its confidence interval) and the complexity of the sampling design. It is possible to shrink the confidence interval substantially while keeping the total cost of sampling fixed, by choosing a sampling design which exploits the structure of the population appropriately.

Formulae to derive estimates of the population mean and standard deviation for many of the simpler sampling designs are given by Kelsey, Thompson, and Evans.[2]

Sampling units and sampling frames

The items that are to be sampled are called *sampling units*. Sampling units are usually subjects, but in more complex multi-stage designs they may be GP clinics in a town, or schools in a county, or counties in a country.

All forms of sampling require a *sampling frame*, a real or imaginary list of the sampling units eligible to be sampled. In some cases the list actually exists, e.g. electoral registers or school registers; in others it exists only notionally, e.g. the filing cabinets of case notes in a GP surgery; in others still it does not exist at all, e.g. the patients attending a hospital clinic – here the actual sampling frame can only be known retrospectively, although the rule for its construction must of course be defined at the outset of the sampling procedure.

Simple random sampling

Simple random sampling requires a pre-existing sampling frame, where the sampling units are numbered sequentially. Random numbers (from random number tables or computer generated) are then drawn to identify the sampling units to be sampled according to their position in the sampling frame. This ensures that every unit in the frame has an equal probability of being sampled, and this probability is known as the *sampling fraction*. For example it might be a 1 in 10 sample, with a sampling fraction of 0.1.

The disadvantage of simple random sampling is the requirement for an existing and numbered sampling frame. Even where the sampling frame actually exists it is often unnumbered, so that a form of sampling which avoids these two requirements is of more practical value.

Systematic sampling

Systematic sampling is a version of simple random sampling which avoids the need for a sampling frame at the outset, and so simplifies the randomization procedure. Like simple random sampling, it ensures the same sampling fraction for each sampling unit, but in practice only the first unit sampled is randomly selected. If the required sampling fraction is say 1 in k, then the first unit is randomly selected from the first k in the sampling frame, and thereafter every kth unit is drawn.

It is clear that if the first k units have an equal chance of being drawn, then the same applies to all subsequent units. On this basis, systematic sampling is equivalent to simple random sampling, and the same formulae apply. The one occasion in which the two are not equivalent is when there is some form of cyclical pattern within the sampling frame, with a wavelength close to a simple multiple of k. Examples of this would be school classes, or households, where the individuals are clustered into groups.

Stratified sampling

The measurement made in each sampling unit may differ substantially in magnitude from one subgroup (or stratum) to another within the sampling frame. Obvious examples are weight, or other measures of body size, in children of different ages or in men versus women. If each stratum is sampled separately, and the results are combined appropriately, then this gives a population estimate with a tighter confidence interval than simple random sampling.

Another advantage is that separate estimates are available for each stratum, ensuring that each is adequately sampled. The results for the different strata can be combined using suitable weighting coefficients, thus adjusting for the distribution of units between strata within the population.

Cluster sampling

Stratified sampling splits the sampling frame into more homogeneous groups (strata). Cluster sampling by contrast splits it into groups that are, in general, less homogeneous (clusters) but which are administratively linked in some way. All the units within each cluster are then sampled.

Households are an example of clusters. Although they are more heterogeneous than the population at large, they are very cheap to sample. Thus for a given total cost more clusters can be sampled, and the population estimate is more precise than the equivalent under simple random sampling.

Multi-stage sampling

It is quite possible to combine the different forms of sampling, so as to work from larger to progressively smaller sampling frames. The sampling units at one level then provide the sampling frame for the next level down. This is a form of extended cluster sampling where the clusters are sampled rather than included in their entirety.

The British National Food Survey, discussed in Chapter 6, provides a good example of a multi-stage sample.

3.1.3 Non-response

All surveys have a degree of non-response. Subjects refuse to take part, or do only some of the questions or tests they are supposed to complete. It has been widely observed that non-responders as a group are different from responders, so that the effect of non-response is to make the sample unrepresentative of the sampling frame and the target population.

The level of non-response varies widely, according to the amount of commitment required of the subjects taking part. In nutritional studies involving the measurement of food intake over several days, the degree of non-response can be 30% or more. In simpler studies the figure ought to be less. This is a perennial problem with nutritional surveys, as it seriously weakens the value of the study. Indeed the high level of non-response is often implicitly recognized by workers who restrict studies to volunteers, where the drop-out rate is, by definition, much smaller. Unfortunately, in most epidemiological studies, the results for a survey of volunteers cannot be extrapolated to any larger population, and the study may be of less value for that reason. An exception is certain types of intervention study where the end point is a measure of metabolic change within individuals; here the use of volunteers, if well described, may be acceptable.

To minimize the effects of non-response, it is important first of all to encourage all the subjects to take part in the study, and to keep on encouraging them as it progresses. Secondly, as much information as possible should be obtained from a sample of the non-responders, for example, age, gender, and occupation as a minimum. This provides the opportunity to adjust the results to take account of the non-responders, and to come up with a less biased result.

Another effect of non-response is that the final sample size is smaller than originally planned. It is important to include a scaling-up factor in the calculation of sample size to cover this. So if the final sample size required is calculated to be 100, but the response rate is expected to be only 70%, then 100/0.7 or 143 is the number to be sampled initially.

3.2 Variability

Designing an epidemiological study requires an understanding of the nature of variability, the different sources of variability, and how they can be controlled for. Central to the concept of variability is the idea that measurements come from a hypothetical population of such measurements, whose mean needs to be estimated. This population is effectively the same as the target population discussed in the previous section, except that in this context it is usually assumed to be infinitely large.

The quantity to be measured may be a continuous variable (like weight or energy intake) or it may be grouped (like blood group or gender). An important special case of grouped data is where the quantity is either present or absent. This is particularly relevant for studies of disease where the cases have the disease and the controls do not, and some of the subjects are exposed to the agent of interest while others are not.

For continuous variables, the population mean and variance are estimated from the sample mean and variance. For binary and categorical variables, the population proportions in each category are estimated from the sample proportions. If σ^2 is the variance for a continuous variable, then the standard error of the mean based on a sample of size n is given by $\sigma/\sqrt{n}$, and the variance of the mean is σ^2/n.

The variance of a proportion derived from a binary variable differs from that for a continuous variable in that it can be estimated directly from the proportion. If the proportion is p, based on a sample size n, then the variance of p is given by $p(1-p)/n$. This shows that proportions near to zero or unity have a small variance, and the largest variance, $1/4n$, occurs when $p=0.5$.

There are two particular aspects of the process of data collection which can adversely affect the quality of the data. The first of these is *bias*, which is the name given to a consistent discrepancy between the sample mean and the population mean. It is inevitable that the two means will not be exactly the same, but in theory, with large enough sample size, the difference between the two should be very small. In situations where this does not happen, bias is said to be present. The other aspect of the data that reflects the quality of data collection is its *variance*. All data are by their nature variable, but the variance can be increased by the way the data are measured.

3.2.1 Bias

Bias is a very real problem in dietary intake studies, but one which nutritionists have in the past tended to ignore. Two particular factors have conspired in this, one being the plethora of different methods that are available to measure dietary intake, the other the absence of a 'gold standard' or accurate and unbiased estimate of dietary intake against which other methods can be validated. Nutritionists have felt that if one method of intake assessment is similar to another, then this provides the validation, when in fact both methods may be equally biased.

The precise mechanism for bias in dietary intake assessment depends on the particular method used (Chapter 8). Many of the methods have an inbuilt tendency to be biased downwards, in that subjects are more likely to forget a food they ate than to invent a food they did not eat. Diary or weighed intake methods, where the eating and the recording of food eaten occur largely concurrently, ought to be less prone to this than recall methods. However, there is ample opportunity, by any method, for subjects to consciously or subconsciously distort their apparent eating pattern to better suit their self-image. This distortion has been shown to generate under-reporting of up to 30% in the energy intakes of obese women.[3,4]

Biochemical methods of estimating nutrient intake (see Chapter 7) provide the opportunity to validate some aspects of dietary assessment. Even so, they are unlikely to remove the possibility of bias in existing methods, rather they quantify and perhaps reduce the bias. Nutritionists need to be aware of the importance of bias, and its ability to devalue otherwise well-designed studies. That said, bias is not always a problem. There are situations where the bias may cancel itself out, for example, a sample surveyed on two separate occasions or a correlation study. If the bias in the method is uniform throughout the sample, and tends to reduce the estimate of intake for every observation by some fixed amount, say 10 per cent, then the comparison in the two examples, i.e. the change in intake between surveys or the size of the correlation, is likely to be relatively unaffected. However, the situation where bias is very serious is when it affects only a subset of the sample, so that relationships between intake and other health measures become distorted. In this situation genuine relationships can be hidden and spurious relationships generated. An obvious example is the one cited above where obese subjects under-recorded their energy intake, so disguising the strong association between obesity and raised energy intake. Normal controls in the same study did not show a bias, so that there was no apparent difference in intake between them and the cases.

3.2.2 Variance

There are many different factors which contribute to the variance of a quantity. Three factors in particular can be identified, and these can be subdivided in a variety of ways.

The first and perhaps most important source of variability is between-subject or inter-individual variance, denoted by σ_b^2. This assumes that each individual in the population has some fixed but unknown constant value for the measurement which is appropriate to them. In terms of nutrient intake, for example, this might be called their usual or habitual intake. The between-subject variance is then the population variance of these true means. As a quantity it cannot be measured directly, since the true means cannot be measured without error, but it can be obtained by calculation.

The second source of variation is within-subject or intra-individual variance, denoted by σ_w^2. This represents the variation of individuals around their true mean value when measured repeatedly by a valid measurement instrument.

The third category of variability is measurement error. This is the difference between the observed value and the corresponding true but unknown value, for a particular observation. It is also called reproducibility. The term measurement error is confusing, as it implies that an error has occurred in taking the measurement. Errors of measurement do occur, e.g. writing down the wrong figure or failing to calibrate the instrument properly; however if the error is large enough it can be identified as an outlier from the main body of data. So, gross errors like these are assumed to have been identified and dealt with, and measurement error as used here describes the combined variability of all the factors influencing the measurements.

In some circumstances the measurement error is included with the within-subject error, where the two cannot easily be separated. Nutrient intake provides an example; the variance of daily intake as obtained by weighed inventory in a single individual combines the day-to-day variability about the true mean and the measurement error of the weighed inventory method.

The magnitude of the within-subject variance may depend on how frequently the measurements are made. The weight of a child measured every few minutes has a relatively small variance, whereas the variance of daily or weekly measurements is progressively larger. The minute-to-minute variance represents measurement error, because it is known from physiological considerations that true weight does not change on this time-scale. However daily and weekly variances are larger because they include within-subject variance, and also because the true weights of individuals themselves change. When quantifying within-subject variance it is useful to define the frequency with which measurements are taken, so as to standardize for the time component in the variance.

Of the three sources of variation – between-subject, within-subject, and measurement variance – the first is the most important in the calculation of sample size and power. The other two are nuisance variables which by their presence weaken associations and obscure differences. For this reason it is important to minimize their impact on the power calculations.

Measurement error, unlike within-subject variance, is affected by the quality of the data collection. It is often a good idea to design a pilot study specifically to investigate the size of the measurement error, and to split it up into its component parts. What the components are will depend on the measurements being made; height, for example, is influenced by the observer, the time of day and the type of measuring scale used. The relative contributions of the separate factors to the reproducibility of the measurement can be obtained by analysis of variance from a suitably designed study. For details of the design and analysis of such studies see, e.g., Snedecor and Cochran.[5] The results of such a pilot study can then be used to reduce the measurement error, e.g. by retraining outlying observers or by recalibrating aberrant instruments.

Minimizing the impact of within-subject variance on the power calculations is less easy, as the variance cannot be manipulated by the observer. It is a property of the individuals being studied and is a fixed quantity. However, one way of keeping it small is to study subjects whose within-subject variance is likely to be relatively small. The usual assumption in epidemiological studies is that subjects all have the same within-subject variance, but in practice it may be possible to identify in advance subjects whose variability is greater or less than average. Nurses or students are likely as a group to be more variable than housewives or nuns in their eating habits, so that a given dietary study would need to be slightly larger if based on nurses than if nuns were used.

A second and more important strategy for dealing with within-subject variation is to take several measurements for each subject, and to work with the mean. If the within-subject variance for a single measurement is σ_w^2 and k measurements are averaged, then the variance of the mean is σ_w^2/k. In principle, if k is large enough, the effect of the within-subject variance can be reduced almost to zero. In practice though, there is no sense in making k too large, as beyond a certain point the cost of each extra measurement outweighs its benefit.

There is a substantial literature addressed to the question of the number of days of dietary intake required to distinguish adequately between individuals. Consider a particular nutrient, energy or vitamin C say, and assume that the between-subject variance is σ_b^2. If the intake is measured over k days, then the within-subject variance is σ_w^2/k. The total variance for an individual sampled at random from the population is therefore $\sigma_b^2 + \sigma_w^2/k$, obtained by adding the two variances together, and the standard error is $\sqrt{\sigma_b^2 + \sigma_w^2/k}$.

Extending this to a sample of n individuals from the population, the variance of the mean intake for the sample is $(\sigma_b^2 + \sigma_w^2/k)/n$ or $\sigma_b^2/n + \sigma_w^2/kn$, and the standard error is $\sqrt{\sigma_b^2/n + \sigma_w^2/kn}$. The standard error of the sample mean in the absence of within-subject variance would be $\sigma_b/\sqrt{n}$, so the ratio of standard errors is:

$$\frac{\sigma_b/\sqrt{n}}{\sqrt{\sigma_b^2/n + \sigma_w^2/kn}} \qquad \text{or} \qquad 1/\sqrt{1 + \sigma_w^2/k\sigma_b^2} \qquad (3.1)$$

This, or more correctly its square, is a measure of the *efficiency* of the estimate of the mean, a statistical term indicating how much the variance of the estimate is increased because of within-subject variance. Note that the efficiency factor depends on k, the number of days of measurement, but not on the sample size n.

The presence of within-subject error also means that individual means are measured with error, so that there is an imperfect correlation between the true intakes of individuals and their intakes as measured. This correlation is given by $\sigma_b/\sqrt{\sigma_b^2 + \sigma_w^2/k}$, which is the same as eqn (3.1) above. This term (3.1) can be referred to as the *coefficient of attenuation*. As well as being the correlation of the true versus the observed intake, it also measures the extent to which the correlation of the intake with other factors is reduced (i.e. attenuated). The factor might be some disease marker, e.g. serum cholesterol or blood pressure.[6,7]

If the number of days k is sufficiently large, then the coefficient can be made very close to unity. However, the crucial issue is the ratio of σ_w^2 to σ_b^2, the within- to between-subject variance. If this is small, i.e. subjects in the population are widely spaced relative to the standard errors of individual means, then the attenuation is not too important. Conversely if the ratio is large, so that subject means are relatively close together, then the effect of within-subject error can be large and serious. As well as weakening correlations, it also leads to gross misclassification when the population is split into groups, e.g. thirds or fifths, on the basis of intake. Gross misclassification means that individuals with true intakes in the lowest group are classified into the highest, and vice versa. So a comparison of high versus low intake groups is weakened due to a fraction of the individuals being allocated to the wrong group.

For the special case of weighed intakes, many studies have documented the ratio σ_w^2/σ_b^2 for different nutrients in a variety of populations (see Nelson *et al.*[8]). The results show that for the coefficient of attenuation to be 0.9 or greater, less than 7 days of weighed intake are adequate for many nutrients, but that for certain vitamins and minerals, several weeks of intake need to be measured (Chapter 6). It is clear that for the latter class of nutrients, the detection of a correlation or a difference between groups requires a much increased sample size, to compensate for the attenuation due to the large σ_w^2/σ_b^2 ratio. This topic is discussed in more detail in later sections.

3.3 Sample size

3.3.1 Null hypothesis

The calculation of sample size and power is closely tied up with the concept of the *significance test*. A significance test involves a *test statistic*, that is, a statistical quantity with known distribution whose value is to be tested, and a *null hypothesis*, which states that the test statistic is equal to some predefined value. The test statistic is commonly the difference between two sample means, and the null hypothesis is that this difference is zero.

The purpose of the significance test is to decide whether to accept or reject the null hypothesis. The wrong decision can be reached in either of two ways – rejecting the hypothesis when it is true, and accepting it when it is false. The former risk, rejecting the hypothesis when true, is controlled by the significance test, which works to a preset error rate. The error rate is called the Type I error, or α, or the significance level. The latter risk, of accepting the hypothesis when false, is discussed in the next section.

Figure 3.1 illustrates the distribution of a test statistic, the difference between two sample means, which is to be tested for significance, and the null hypothesis is that the mean of the distribution is 0 (in other words that the two group means are equal). The axis of the distribution indicates a range of values that the test statistic can take, and the height of the bell-shaped Normal curve above the axis shows the probability of each particular value occurring. Thus values near 0 are relatively likely, while extreme values in the tails of the distribution are unlikely. The uncertainty about the mean, i.e. its standard error, is represented by the area under the distribution. The total area sums to unity, so that the statistic has a probability 1 (i.e. certainty) of taking a value some-where along the axis. The width of the curve is inversely related to the number of observations.

The distribution shows that, even when the true difference is zero, the *observed* difference between the groups may lie anywhere over a wide range of values. In particular, there is a small probability that it will fall beyond one or other of the two cut-offs marked d_- and d_+. These cut-offs define areas in each tail of the distribution of size $\alpha/2$ (marked I_- and I_+ in Fig. 3.1), a total area (or probability) of α.

The basis of the significance test is that if the null hypothesis is true, the observed value ought to be near 0. Conversely, if the null hypothesis is false, the value ought not to be near 0. Thus the further away from 0 the value is, the less likely the null hypothesis is to be true. The arbitrary probability α determines at what point we cease to accept the null hypothesis, and instead reject it. By doing this we run a small risk α of rejecting the null hypothesis when it is actually true, and this is the Type I error or significance level.

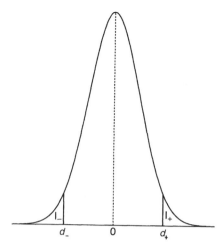

Fig. 3.1 A two-tailed test of the null hypothesis that the variable d is distributed with mean 0. The size of the type I error is set at 5%, shown by the areas marked in the two tails of the distribution.

Figure 3.1 illustrates two cut-offs (d_- and d_+), each of which defines an area in the tail of size $\alpha/2$. This form of significance test is called a two-tailed test, because the null hypothesis can be rejected by values of the test statistic in either tail of the distribution. When comparing two group means, this allows either to be significantly larger (or smaller) than the other.

In certain circumstances it is permissible to use a one-tailed test instead of a two-tailed test. In this case the area α is all in one tail. This means that the null hypothesis can only be rejected for values of the statistic in one direction, and even extreme values in the other direction are ignored. There are situations where this can be justified, e.g. the testing of a new treatment against a conventional treatment where the new treatment has to be an improvement – if it is the same or worse then it is of no value. Nevertheless such situations are relatively unusual, and one-tailed tests should in general be avoided.

A one-tailed test of size α has its cut-off at the same point as a two-tailed test of size 2α, so that if the probability of the observed statistic is between α and 2α, then it is significant by the one-tailed test but not by the two-tailed test. This allows marginal levels of significance to be exaggerated, as the fact that a one-tailed test has been used is often not made sufficiently clear when the results are published.

3.3.2 Alternative hypotheses

A significance test is used to decide whether or not there is a difference between groups. However, when the true difference between groups is small, there is a risk of accepting the null hypothesis when it is false. It is important when planning epidemiological studies to know in advance what difference is being looked for, and how big the risk is of failing to detect it (i.e. accepting the null hypothesis), as this determines how big the study should be.

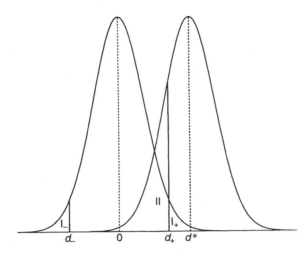

Fig. 3.2 A two-tailed test of the null hypothesis that the variable d is distributed with mean 0, versus the alternative hypothesis that the mean is $d*$. The type I error is set at 5% as in Fig. 3.1, while the type II error is 20%, shown by the area in the left tail of the right distribution.

Figure 3.2 is an extension of Fig. 3.1 and includes information about the magnitude of the difference between groups that is to be sought. This difference is termed $d*$. Like Fig. 3.1, Fig. 3.2 shows the distribution of the observed difference under the null hypothesis, centred on 0, and a second distribution, centred on $d*$, which shows the distribution of the difference if it is actually present. This is known as the *alternative hypothesis*, that the true difference between groups is $d*$.

The cut-offs d_- and d_+ in Fig. 3.2 define two tails for the null hypothesis (marked I_- and I_+ as before) but now d_+ also defines a single tail for the alternative hypothesis (marked II). The area of this latter tail represents the Type II error, also called β, the probability of accepting the null hypothesis when the alternative hypothesis is true. This is the probability of deciding that the group means are the same, when actually they are different.

So areas I_- and I_+ (probability α) on the one hand, and II (probability β) on the other, are the misclassification errors in deciding which hypothesis is appropriate. The quantity $(1-\beta)$, known as the *power* of the experiment, is the probability of accepting the alternative hypothesis when it is true. In a well-designed experiment the power to detect the desired effect will be set to 80% ($\beta=0.2$), 90% ($\beta=0.1$), or even 95% ($\beta=0.05$). This ensures that there is little chance of a non-significant test result when the effect is actually present. Figure 3.2 is drawn with Type I and Type II errors of 0.05 and 0.2 respectively, i.e. a 5% significance level and 80% power.

In planning a study, the choice of $d*$ is of paramount importance. The smaller it is, the larger the sample needs to be to detect it. This can be seen from Fig. 3.2 – as $d*$ gets smaller the two distributions overlap more and the tail area II gets bigger. If $d*$ is large, the tail area II is small but differences smaller than $d*$ may not be detected. Thus a study with an apparent difference between groups may fail to reach significance, and the study is said to be *underpowered.* Pocock[9] points out that this is a weakness of many experimental studies. Equally if $d*$ is too small, implying a very large sample size, the effect may not in practical terms be worth having. To demonstrate that changing a surgical procedure reduces morbidity from say 10% to 9% would require many thousand subjects, yet the improvement would probably not be sufficient to justify the effort.

3.3.3 Power and sample size

Figure 3.2 shows the probability of observing particular values of the difference d between groups under the null hypothesis and the alternative hypothesis. Three values of d are particularly important; the mean under the null hypothesis (0), the mean under the alternative hypothesis ($d*$), and the value at the cut-off point between the two distributions (d_+). If the distribution of d is known, in particular its standard error, the value of d_+ can be defined simply from α the significance level. Assuming a normal distribution, then the value of d_+ is such that it is $Z_{1-\alpha/2}$ standard errors away from 0, where $Z_{1-\alpha/2}$ indicates the point on the normal distribution defining area $\alpha/2$ in the upper tail. So

$$d_+ = Z_{1-\alpha/2}\mathrm{SE}(d) \tag{3.2}$$

where $\mathrm{SE}(d)$ is the standard error of d. However d_+ is also defined from $d*$ and β, i.e.

$$d_+ = d* - Z_{1-\beta}\mathrm{SE}(d) \tag{3.3}$$

where $Z_{1-\beta}$ is the point on the normal distribution defining the cut-off d_+ relative to $d*$. Note that (3.2) and (3.3) assume that the standard error of d is the same under the two distributions, although this is not always the case. Combining (3.2) and (3.3) and eliminating d_+ gives

$$d* = Z_{1-\alpha/2}\mathrm{SE}(d) + Z_{1-\beta}\mathrm{SE}(d)$$

$$= \mathrm{SE}(d)\,(Z_{1-\alpha/2} + Z_{1-\beta}) \tag{3.4}$$

In general the standard error of d is proportional to $1/\sqrt{n}$ where n is the sample size. So eqn (3.4) shows that the power ($1-\beta$) is determined by $d*$, α, and n (as it affects the standard error). Of these, α is the fixed significance level (Fig. 3.1). Thus to alter the power, only $d*$ or n can be changed. If for example $d*$ is made larger, this has the effect of shifting the distribution of $d*$ in Fig. 3.2 to the right, while leaving d_+ where it is. As a result, the left tail of the $d*$ distribution, the type II error, is reduced in size, and the power increases. Reducing $d*$ has the opposite effect – the distribution shifts to the left, the size of the left tail increases, and the power is reduced.

Changing n, the sample size, also alters the power. If n is doubled say, then the standard error of d shrinks by 30%, and this reduces the widths of the distributions. In particular the cut-offs d_- and d_+ move 30% closer to 0. Thus if $d*$ remains unchanged the distance between it and d_+ increases, so that the tail defining the type II error gets smaller and the power is increased. This is illustrated in Fig. 3.3, where doubling n reduces the type II error from 20% (in Fig. 3.2) to half the type I error, i.e. about 2.5%.

Eqn (3.4) is the fundamental equation linking n, $d*$, α and β, and all the formulae that appear in Section 3.4 are derived from it. Kelsey et al.[2] and Campbell et al.[10]

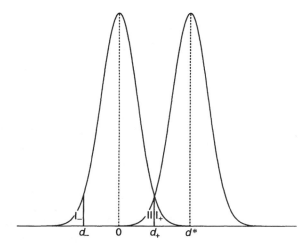

Fig. 3.3 A two-tailed test of the null hypothesis that the variable d is distibuted with mean 0, versus the alternative hypothesis that the mean is d^*. The sample size is twice that shown in Fig. 3.2, so that although the type I error is unchanged at 5%, the type II error is reduced from 20% to 2.5%.

provide a summary of the formulae, with examples, for all except the correlation formulae which are developed here. Table 3.1 gives, for a series of values for α and β, the corresponding values of $Z_{1-\alpha/2}$, $Z_{1-\beta}$ and $(Z_{1-\alpha/2}+Z_{1-\beta})^2$ – the latter term appears in many of the formulae in Section 3.4.

3.3.4   Types of response variable

The derivation of (3.4) uses as its test statistic d, the difference between the means of the response variable in two groups. There are actually three different types of response variable as they affect (3.4), and they need to be distinguished. The first is continuous measurements such as cholesterol intake or systolic blood pressure. Here the standard error of d is obtained from the standard deviation of the measurement, and two different forms of SE(d) apply according to whether or not the measurements in the two groups are paired (matched). A slightly different situation arises when the response variable being compared in the two groups is binary, i.e. a rate or proportion, for example the colon cancer incidence rate or the proportion with brown eyes. As explained earlier, the standard error of a proportion depends on the magnitude of the proportion, so that SE(d) in (3.4) takes a different form. The third case is the testing of a correlation between two variables, and here d is the correlation to be detected. The null hypothesis, that $d=0$, is equivalent to the absence of a correlation between the two variables. The standard error of d in this case is a function of the correlation to be detected. Each of these three forms of alternative hypothesis is considered in turn in Section 3.4.

3.3.5 Transformations

The calculation of power in eqn (3.4) assumes a normal distribution for d. If d is based on a continuous variable, then it is important for the variable to be (at least reasonably) normally distributed. If it is not, then the distribution of d may not be normal either, and in addition and more importantly, the standard error of d may be inflated. This has the effect of increasing the size of sample required.

For this reason, it is worthwhile checking that the variable is reasonably normal, and if not, transforming it to a new scale which is. This is particularly relevant for many of the nutrients commonly investigated in nutritional epidemiology, whose distributions tend to be skew to the right. For example, Nelson et al.[8] found that in up to half of the 30 nutrients they studied (depending on the gender and age of the subjects), a logarithmic transformation improved the efficiency of the comparison.

A logarithmic transformation is very commonly used to remove right skewness, but there are other alternatives which may be more suitable in particular situations. If X is the variable as measured, then four possible convenient transformations of X can be considered, arranged here in order of increasing adjustment; square root, $\sqrt{X}$; logarithmic, $\log_e X$; inverse square root, $1/\sqrt{X}$; and inverse, $1/X$. Each transformation stretches the left tail of the distribution and shortens the right, so that if X has a right skew distribution one of these transformations will be best for removing the skewness.

There is a simple way of seeing which transformation reduces the skewness most, as follows; first calculate the mean and standard deviation (SD) of X and its four transformations. Then antilog the mean of log X to obtain the geometric mean of X; call it $\dot{X}$. Now scale the standard deviations of the five forms of X using $\dot{X}$, as follows: $SD(X)/\dot{X}$; $2\,SD(\sqrt{X})/\sqrt{\dot{X}}$; $SD(\log_e X)$; $2\,\sqrt{\dot{X}}\,SD(1/\sqrt{X})$; $\dot{X}\,SD(1/X)$. These five quantities all represent the coefficient of variation (CV) of X, and can be multiplied by 100 to give percentages. The smallest value among the five CVs indicates the transformation which best removes the skewness in X. It may be that the CVs are all very similar, in which case the choice of transformation is not critical. Nevertheless, it gives an indication of where skewness is present and how best it can be removed.

It should be noted that three of the four transformations cannot be used for data which are zero or negative (as log 0 and 1/0 are infinite). If there are data with zero values they must be made positive. This is best done by adding a small amount, ε, to all the data, perhaps trying more than one value of ε to ensure that the result is not too sensitive to its precise choice.

3.3.6 Non-response and drop-out

Virtually all studies are less than 100% successful in recruiting subjects. Also, longitudinal studies tend to lose further subjects as they progress. All the calculations for sample size given in the next section assume a 100% response rate, so that the numbers given need to be scaled up to cater for non-response. If, for example, a response rate of 80% is expected, then the number obtained should be divided by 80/100, increasing it by 25%. A further adjustment may also be advisable for longitudinal studies, to cover drop-out. Due to uncertainties about the likely response rate, it is wise to treat all sample size calculations as approximate, and to view them only as a minimum requirement for study size.

3.4 Types of study

3.4.1 Ecological studies

Ecological studies are distinct from other forms of epidemiological study in that the unit of measurement is a group rather than an individual (see Chapter 12). For discussions of power and sample size it is the number of groups, not the numbers of individuals in each group, which is important.

The basis of the grouping may be geographical, e.g. by country, state, or county; it may be temporal, e.g. by year of birth, age group, or month of the year; or it may be cultural, e.g. by religion, migrant status, or social class. Ecological studies often represent an early stage in the pursuit of a causal relationship, so that the data are routinely collected statistics obtained for other purposes, which are then linked together. For example, Barker and Osmond[11] demonstrated a strong correlation between infant mortality rates in the 1920s and coronary heart disease rates in the 1970s across 212 local authority areas in the UK, using published data.

Many ecological studies have correlated national or regional cause-specific incidence rates or mortality rates with the corresponding intakes of specified foods or nutrients to look for an association. If a correlation, d^*, is to be detected at significance level α (two-tailed) with power $(1-\beta)$, then the number of groups (i.e. countries or regions) required for this is given by

$$n = \frac{(Z_{1-\alpha/2} + Z_{1-\beta})^2}{d^{*2}/(1-d^{*2})} + 5 \tag{3.5}$$

As an example, set the significance level α to 5%, the power $(1-\beta)$ to 90%, and assume we want to detect a correlation d^* of 0.5. This gives $(Z_{1-\alpha/2} + Z_{1-\beta})^2 = 10.5$ from Table 3.1, from which $n = 36.5$ or 37 rounded up to the nearest whole number. Thus, to detect a correlation of 0.5 with 90% power at 5% significance requires at least 37 distinct groups.

An alternative question might be: what correlation is likely to be detectable for given α and $(1-\beta)$ if n points are available? Eqn (3.5) can be rearranged as

$$d^* = \sqrt{\frac{(Z_{1-\alpha/2} + Z_{1-\beta})^2}{(Z_{1-\alpha/2} + Z_{1-\beta})^2 + n - 5}} \tag{3.6}$$

If just 20 points are available, what correlation can be detected for the same α and $(1-\beta)$? The answer from (3.6) is $d^* = 0.64$. Finally, it may be that with α and n known, the question is: what is the power of the study to detect a correlation of d^*? Rearranging (3.5) again gives

$$Z_{1-\beta} = \sqrt{\frac{d^{*2}(n-5)}{1-d^{*2}}} - Z_{\alpha/2} \qquad (3.7)$$

Suppose n is 22 and α is 5%, what power does the study have to detect $d^* = 0.3$? The answer from (3.7) is $Z_{1-\beta} = -0.66$. This is negative, which means that the power is less than 50%. $Z_{1-\beta}$ can be converted to the power $(1-\beta)$ using normal distribution tables. For this example the power is 25%. Table 3.1 includes some values for $Z_{1-\beta}$ which can be interpolated or extrapolated.

By their very nature, ecological studies often use existing data, so that the power calculation to determine sample size (3.5) may be irrelevant if n is already fixed. Eqn (3.7) is probably of greater value as it shows how likely the study is to detect a specified association. Other forms of ecological study may involve a comparison between one set of groups (or clusters) and another, the aggregated version of the comparison of two groups of individuals. The formulae for this are given in the next section. Note that for ecological studies the sample size should be interpreted as being the number of clusters, not the number of individuals, in each half of the comparison.

3.4.2 Cross-sectional studies

Cross-sectional studies are the simplest form of epidemiological study involving individuals, and they investigate relationships at a single point in time (see Chapter 13). Because they lack a temporal element they are generally unable to provide evidence of causality, so that subsequent retrospective or prospective studies and/or experimental studies are required to test whether the relationships are causal.

There are three general forms of relationship that might be looked for in a cross-sectional study – a difference between groups in the level of some variable, a difference between groups in the *rate* of a condition, and an association (correlation) between two variables in the sample.

Table 3.1   Values of $(Z_{1-\alpha/2}+Z_{1-\beta})^2$ for various $Z_{1-\alpha/2}$ and $Z_{1-\beta}$. The corresponding values of $Z_{1-\alpha/2}$ and $Z_{1-\beta}$ and the power are also shown. The term $(Z_{1-\alpha/2}+Z_{1-\beta})^2$ appears in eqns (3.5), (3.6) and (3.8) of Section 3.4.

		Type II error β	0.5	0.2	0.1	0.05
Type I error α	$Z_{1-\alpha/2}$	Power	50%	80%	90%	95%
		$Z_{1-\beta}$	0.00	0.84	1.28	1.64
0.1	1.64		2.7	6.2	8.6	10.8
0.05	1.96		3.8	7.8	10.5	13.0
0.02	2.33		5.4	10.0	13.0	15.8
0.01	2.58		6.6	11.7	14.9	17.8

In addition to the question of sample size, there is also in nutritional epidemiology the important question of what type of dietary intake assessment to use. The existence of within-subject variance in dietary intake means that assessments based on one day or only a few days may be poor at categorizing individual intakes. However, the number of subjects can be increased to compensate for this. There is a trade-off between the number of subjects, n, and the number of days per subject, k.

To decide on the optimal choice of n and k, three distinct types of study need to be identified – group comparisons, ranking of individuals, and assessing an individual's usual intake.[8] In the simplest case of group comparisons, the best form of assessment is a cheap 1-day method (i.e. $k=1$), allowing the number of subjects, n, to be maximized.[12]

The second type of study involves the ranking of individuals for dietary intake, where the aim is to make the coefficient of attenuation (Equation 3.1) sufficiently near unity to ensure that subjects in the extremes of the distribution are correctly identified. Nelson et al.[8] show that 7 days of weighed intake are adequate for some nutrients, but there are other nutrients which require substantially more days than 7 and others still for which a weighed intake is not appropriate at all.

The third type of study, assessing an individual's usual intake, is irrelevant in an epidemiological context and is not considered further here.

Nutritional epidemiologists are insufficiently aware of the distinction that needs to be drawn between studies comparing group means and studies ranking individuals. There is no benefit in using an expensive method of assessment to compare group means, as a cheap method applied to a large number of subjects is more efficient. Conversely, studies that relate the intakes of individuals to other variables should ideally use a 7-day (or more) weighed intake, or some other validated form of dietary assessment (see Chapters 6 and 8).

Continuous response variables

The sample size required to compare the means of two groups involves four quantities; d^* the difference between the groups to be detected, σ the standard deviation of the variable, the significance level α, and power $1-\beta$. The formula can be simplified by expressing d^* as a fraction f of the standard deviation σ so that $f = d^*/\sigma$. The sample size n required *for each group* is then given by

$$n = 2\, \frac{(Z_{1-\alpha/2} + Z_{1-\beta})^2}{(d^*/\sigma)^2} = 2\, \frac{(Z_{1-\alpha/2} + Z_{1-\beta})^2}{f^2} \tag{3.8}$$

A study is set up to determine whether nutritionists (being fitter) have a higher energy intake than epidemiologists. The standard deviation σ of energy intake is about 2 MJ, so to be sure of detecting a difference d^* of 1 MJ with 80% power at 5% significance requires

$$n = 2\, \frac{7.8}{(1/2)^2}$$

$$= 63$$

subjects in each group, or 126 altogether. The value of 7.8 in the numerator comes from Table 3.1.

Eqn (3.8) is a very widely used power calculation formula, to the extent that a simplified version has a paper named after it.[13] If the first two terms are combined, assuming 5% significance and 80% power, then the sample size for each group is simply

$$n = 16/f^2 \qquad (3.9)$$

In the example $f = 0.5$, so n is 64 compared to the more accurate figure of 63. For 90% power the factor 16 in eqn (3.9) should be replaced by 21, and for 95% by 26.

It may be that subjects in one group are easier or cheaper to recruit than in the other. Assume that for each subject in one group there are r subjects in the other group. In this case the sample size given by eqn (3.8) or (3.9) should be multiplied by $(r + 1)/2r$ to give the smaller group size, while the larger group is r times larger. Note that when the groups are of equal size this scaling factor is 1.

On the assumption that nutritionists are cheaper to recruit than epidemiologists, twice as many nutritionists as epidemiologists are to be recruited (i.e. $r = 2$). The scaling factor for eqn (3.8) is then 3/4, and the required numbers of epidemiologists and nutritionists are 48 and 96 respectively. Thus the total sample is 144 as compared to 126 for equal numbers in the groups, with the increase in numbers offset by the cost saving.

Eqns (3.8) and (3.9) assume that the two groups being compared are unmatched. For *matched* groups the same formulae apply except that the factor 2 should be omitted. Thus the matched version of (3.9) is given by: $n = 8/f^2$.

Eqns (3.8) and (3.9) derive the sample size given the power and the difference to be detected. There are two other useful questions that may be asked: (a) what size of difference would be detected given the sample size and power, and (b) what is the power of the study to detect a given difference knowing the sample size? The difference to be detected, expressed as a fraction f of the standard deviation σ, is given by

$$f = (Z_{1-\alpha/2} + Z_{1-\beta})\sqrt{\frac{2}{n}} \qquad (3.10)$$

while the power can be derived from

$$Z_{1-\beta} = f\sqrt{\frac{n}{2}} - Z_{1-\alpha/2} \qquad (3.11)$$

As mentioned earlier, beware of occasions when $Z_{1-\beta}$ is negative, as this means that the power is less than 50%.

Binary response variables

Eqn (3.8) applies with little modification to the comparison of proportions. The variance of the proportion p is known to be proportional to $p(1-p)$, so this replaces σ^2 in (3.8). Also, since the value of p differs under the null hypothesis and the alternative hypothesis, there are two separate variances to consider. Schlesselman[14] suggests using the average of the two proportions to calculate the variance. Let p_0 be the proportion in one group and p_1 in the other, so that the difference in proportion is given by $d* = p_1 - p_0$. Also let $\bar{p} = (p_0 + p_1)/2$ and $f = \dfrac{d*}{\sqrt{\bar{p}(1-\bar{p})}}$. Then the required sample size n

for each group is as given in eqn (3.8), and unequal group sizes are handled using the multiplier $(r+1)/2r$ as before.

The proportions or rates in the two groups may be related in terms of the *relative risk* (RR). In cross-sectional studies this is simply the ratio of the proportion in one group to that in the other, i.e. $RR = p_1/p_0$. So if the required relative risk to be detected is known, and the proportion in the baseline p_0 is also known, then p_1 and f can be calculated and substituted into (3.8).

A study is set up to determine the relative risk of achilles tendon rupture in squash players as compared to badminton players.* If the lifetime risk of rupture is known to be 1% in badminton players and a relative risk of 5 is to be detected, how many ex-players from each sport need to be questioned? The baseline risk p_0 is 0.01, so that $p_1 = 0.01 \times 5 = 0.05$. This makes $\bar{p} = 0.03$, $d^* = 0.04$, and $f = 0.23$. For significance 5% and power 95%, giving the value 13.0 for $(Z_{1-\alpha/2} + Z_{1-\beta})^2$ from Table 3.1, then

$$n = 2 \; \frac{13.0}{0.23^2}$$

$$= 492$$

To estimate the size of difference that might be detected, or the power of the study, given the other parameters, use eqns (3.10) and (3.11) as before.

Correlation as response variable

To look for correlations in cross-sectional studies, the formulae in Section 3.4.1 are applicable (eqns (3.5), (3.6), and (3.7)), where n represents the number of individuals to be sampled in the whole group, and d^* is the correlation to be detected.

If one of the variables being correlated is a nutrient intake, then the true correlation will be attenuated due to the presence of within-subject error in the nutrient intake estimate (see Section 3.2.2). Thus, if the true correlation to be detected is 0.5, and the coefficient of attenuation (3.1) is 0.8, then the correlation likely to be observed is $0.5 \times 0.8 = 0.4$. In this case the *attenuated* correlation should be used in the formula, to scale up the required sample size appropriately.

3.4.3 Case-control studies

To investigate causality in epidemiological studies it is important to include a temporal element relating the cause and the effect. The case-control study (or retrospective study) is a relatively cheap way to do this, which works backwards in time from the effect to the cause. Cases with the disease are identified (the effect) and controls are obtained to compare them with. The exposures of the cases and controls to the agent under investigation (the putative cause) are then compared, and if the exposures are sufficiently different then this supports the case for a causal link.

In addition the controls may be *matched* to the cases, either on an individual or group basis. For more details of the design and analysis of case-control studies see Chapter 15.

---

* While writing the first edition of this chapter the author had his leg in plaster, recovering from a ruptured achilles tendon, sustained playing badminton.

An important deficiency of case-control studies is that they cannot compare directly the rates of disease in the cases and controls, and so cannot estimate the relative risk. This is because the two groups are sampled from the population using different sampling fractions[15] (and Chapter 2). However, they do allow the *odds ratio* to be calculated, which is the ratio of the odds of cases being exposed to the agent and the equivalent odds for controls. In situations where the disease is rare, the odds ratio is a reasonable estimate of the relative risk.

The simplest form of case-control study is one where the cases and controls are either exposed or unexposed. The proportions of controls and cases so exposed are denoted by p_0 and p_1 respectively, and to calculate sample size p_0 needs to be estimated from previously published data. The value for p_1 can then be obtained from p_0 and the odds ratio (OR) to be detected, using the formula

$$p_1 = p_0 \, OR \, / \, (1 + p_0 [OR-1]) \tag{3.12}$$

For generality assume that r controls are chosen per case, analogously to eqn (3.8). Then given p_0 and p_1 the weighted mean proportion is calculated as

$$\bar{p} = (p_1 + r p_0) / (1 + r) \tag{3.13}$$

and as before $d^* = p_1 - p_0$ and $f = \dfrac{d^*}{\sqrt{\bar{p}(1-\bar{p})}}$. Eqn (3.8) multiplied by the factor $(r+1)/2r$ then gives the required number of cases.

Suppose that in an unmatched case-control study $p_0 = 0.25$, $r = 1$, and an odds ratio of 2 is to be detected with 90% power at 5% significance. The value of p_1 from (3.12) is

$$p_1 = 0.25 \times 2/(1 + 0.25 \times 1)$$

$$= 0.4$$

so that $\bar{p} = 0.325$, $d^* = 0.15$, and $f = 0.32$. Then from (3.8) and Table 3.1,

$$n = 2 \; \frac{10.5}{0.32^2}$$

$$= 205$$

is the number of cases required, together with an equal number of controls.

There will be situations where the number of cases is restricted, perhaps due to the rarity of the disease. In this case it is useful to know the power available to detect a given odds ratio when the sample size n is known. This comes from (3.11) with an adjustment for unequal group sizes:

$$Z_{1-\beta} = f \sqrt{\frac{nr}{r+1}} - Z_{1-\alpha/2} \tag{3.14}$$

and $Z_{1-\beta}$ can be converted to a probability with normal distribution tables.

Another alternative is that both the power and the sample size are known, and the question then is: what size of odds ratio can be detected? This is known as the *smallest detectable risk*, and is discussed in detail by Schlesselman.[15] The relevant formulae are too complicated to include here, but an equivalent effect can be obtained by substituting a series of different values for the odds ratio into eqn (3.8), and seeing which gives a sample size close to the known value.

The discussion so far has assumed that the cases and controls are unmatched. If they are matched on an individual basis, then they need to be analysed in terms of concordant and discordant matched pairs, and the calculation of sample size should take this into account. Assume that P is defined as

$$P = OR/(1+OR)$$

p_0 and p_1 are as before, and $Q = 1-P$, $q_0 = 1-p_0$, and $q_1 = 1-p_1$. Then n, the sample size for each group (and hence the number of matched pairs), is given by

$$n = \frac{(Z_{1-\alpha/2}/2 + Z_{1-\beta}\sqrt{PQ})^2}{(p_0 q_1 + p_1 q_0)(P - 0.5)^2} \tag{3.15}$$

Using the same example as before, find the number of subjects needed to detect an odds ratio of 2 when $p_0 = 0.25$. As before, $p_1 = 0.4$, and $P = 2/(1+2) = 0.67$. Assuming 5% significance and 90% power gives

$$n = \frac{(1.96/2 + 1.28\sqrt{0.67 \times 0.33})^2}{(0.25 \times 0.60 + 0.4 \times 0.75)(0.67 - 0.5)^2}$$

$$= 193$$

This compares with the figure of 205 obtained using eqn (3.8) for unmatched cases and controls, so that the matching reduces the number of subjects required by some 6%.

Schlesselman[15] discusses the issue of matched pairs in more detail, and gives formulae for the situation of multiple controls per case. Breslow and Day[16] cover exposures at more than two levels.

3.4.4   Cohort studies

The main difference between a cohort study (or prospective study) and a case-control study is that a cohort study moves forward in time from the cause to the effect. A sample of a population is drawn, and data about exposure to the agent of interest are collected. Then the sample is followed up for a sufficiently long time for cases of disease to occur. These cases can then be compared either with *all* the non-cases (i.e. controls) or else a sample of them, as regards their exposure. See Chapter 14 for more details.

Unlike a case-control study, a cohort study is able to estimate relative risk, since the sampling fractions of the cases and controls are known. If p_0 is the proportion of unexposed subjects that get the disease and p_1 is the corresponding proportion for exposed subjects, then $p_1 = p_0 RR$, where RR is the relative risk. Also required is r, the ratio of the number of unexposed subjects to exposed subjects in the population. The only other requirement then is to define $\bar{p}$, the mean proportion of subjects getting the disease, from eqn (3.13).

With these changes in definition, eqns (3.8) and (3.14) can be applied to cohort studies. In general, r is rather greater than 1, so that the total sample size required, $n(1+r)$, is larger than for a case-control study. For example consider a ten-year prospective study to measure the protective effect of a high fibre diet on colon cancer. Note that here the relative risk to be detected is less than not greater than 1, because a protective effect is sought. A high fibre diet is defined as being in the top fifth of intake, so that $r = 4:1$, and assume the ten-year colon cancer incidence rate p is 0.01. The relative risk to be detected is 1/3, with a power of 80% at 5% significance. Given RR and eqn (3.13) p_0 can be calculated as

$$p_0 = \bar{p}(1+r)/(RR+r) \tag{3.16}$$

so that $p_0 = 0.0115$, $p_1 = 0.0038$, $d^* = 0.0077$, and $f = 0.0077/\sqrt{0.01 \times 0.99} = 0.0773$. From (3.8), adjusted for unequal groups,

$$n = \frac{4+1}{2 \times 4} \times 2 \; \frac{7.8}{0.0773^2}$$

$$= 1632$$

and the total sample required, $n(1+r)$, is over 8000 subjects.

3.4.5 Experimental studies

Experimental studies, unlike the other types of epidemiological study discussed so far, involve an *intervention*. Subjects at risk of some disease are allocated, usually randomly, to receive either a live treatment or a placebo treatment, and their subsequent progress over a period of time is monitored. Chapter 16 discusses experimental studies in more detail.

Assume for simplicity that subjects are either exposed (treated) or unexposed (placebo), and that they either succumb to the disease (cases) or they do not (controls). In this sense the design is similar to a case-control study, except that the selection is by exposure rather than outcome. The sampling fraction used to obtain the two treatment groups is by definition the same, as they have an equal chance of being assigned to the two groups. Thus the proportion developing the disease can be estimated, and the relative risk as well.

As before, eqn (3.8) can be applied, where p_0 is the proportion of placebo subjects succumbing to the disease, and $p_1 = p_0 RR$ (where RR is the relative risk). A vitamin A supplement is to be tested to see if it will reduce mortality in lung cancer patients by 10% (i.e. $RR = 0.9$) for 5% significance and 95% power. The proportion of deaths p_0 over a year is known to be 50%, so that $p_1 = 0.45$, $d^* = 0.05$, $\bar{p} = 0.475$, $f = 0.05/\sqrt{0.475 \times 0.525} = 0.1$ and

$$n = 2 \times \frac{13.0}{0.1^2}$$

$$= 2600$$

subjects are required in each arm of the study.

These are the simplest designs of experimental study. More complex designs may have more than two treatment arms, or they may be group sequential designs which allow for the study to be stopped before the end point if a clear treatment effect has emerged early. See Pocock[9] for practical details concerning the design and conduct of experimental studies.

References

1. Abramson, J. H. (1984) *Survey methods in community medicine.* Churchill Livingstone, Edinburgh.
2. Kelsey, J. L., Thompson, W. D. and Evans, A. S. (1986) *Methods in observational epidemiology.* Oxford University Press, New York.
3. Prentice, A. M., Black, A. E., Coward, W. A., Davies, H. L., Goldberg, G. R., Murgatroyd, P. R., *et al.* (1986) High levels of energy expenditure in obese women. *Br. Med. J.* **292**: 983–7.
4. Black, A. E., Goldberg, G. R., Jebb, S. A., Livingstone, M. B. E., Cole, T. J. and Prentice, A. M. (1991) Critical evaluation of energy intake data using fundamental principles of energy physiology. 2. Evaluating the results of published surveys. *Eur. J. Clin. Nutr.* **45**: 583–99.
5. Snedecor, G. W. and Cochran, W. (1980) Statistical methods. 7th edn. Iowa State University Press, Iowa.
6. Liu, K., Stamler, J., Dyer, A., McKeever, J. and McKeever, P. (1978) Statistical methods to assess and minimize the role of intra-individual variability in obscuring the relationship between dietary lipids and serum cholesterol. *J. Chron. Dis.* **31**: 399–418.
7. Liu, K., Cooper, R., McKeever, J., *et al.* (1979) Assessment of the association between habitual salt intake and high blood pressure: methodological problems. *Am. J. Epid.* **110**: 219–26.
8. Nelson, M., Black, A. E., Morris, J. A. and Cole, T. J. (1989) Between- and within-subject variation in nutrient intake from infancy to old age: estimating the number of days required to rank dietary intakes with desired precision. *Am. J. Clin. Nutr.* **50**: 155–67.
9. Pocock, S. J. (1983) *Clinical trials: a practical approach.* Wiley, Chichester.
10. Campbell, M. J., Julious, S .A. and Altman, D. G. (1995) Estimating sample sizes for binary, ordered categorical, and continuous outcomes in two group comparisons. *Br. Med. J.* **311**: 1145–8.
11. Barker, D. J. P. and Osmond, C. (1986) Infant mortality, childhood nutrition, and ischaemic heart disease in England and Wales. *Lancet* **i**: 1077–81.
12. Cole, T. J. and Black, A. E. (1983) Statistical aspects in the design of dietary surveys. In: *The dietary assessment of populations.* MRC Environmental Epidemiology Unit Scientific Report. **4**: 5–7.
13. Lehr, R. (1992) Sixteen s squared over d squared: a relation for crude sample size estimates. *Stat. Med.* **11**: 1099–102.
14. Schlesselman, J. J. (1974) Sample size requirements in cohort and case-control studies of disease. *Am. J. Epid.* **99**: 381–4.
15. Schlesselman, J. J. (1982) *Case-control studies: design, conduct, analysis.* Oxford University Press, New York.
16. Breslow, N. E. and Day, N. E. (1980) *Statistical methods in cancer research.* Vol. 1. *The analysis of case-control studies.* International Agency for Research on Cancer, Lyon.

4. Covariate measurement errors in nutritional epidemiology: effects and remedies

David Clayton and Caroline Gill

4.1 The problem and some terminology

This chapter reviews the implications for dietary epidemiology of the inaccuracy of measurements in this field. It discusses the effects of measurement error and the extent to which these can be offset by appropriate statistical methods. Finally, the implications for the design of studies are discussed.

Figure 4.1 illustrates the problem we face in chronic disease epidemiology. A series of variables which are possibly related to a disease process are denoted by $z(t)$, this notation indicating that these will usually vary over time, t. In statistics these variables are simply called *covariates*, while in epidemiology they are called exposures or confounders, depending on their status in the analysis. The distinction between exposure and confounder may be understood most clearly by analogy with experimental science: an exposure is a factor which one would wish to vary in a systematic experiment, while a confounder is a factor which one would prefer to have held constant in the experiment. The fact that epidemiology relies, for the most part, on observational studies in which confounders cannot be held constant, necessitates statistical analyses which seek to re-create the ideal experiment. Since, in the natural experiment observed, several (even many) influences may vary simultaneously, the 'experiment of nature' is a factorial experiment – one in which several factors of interest are studied at the same time.

In nutritional epidemiology, the difficulties of estimating the separate effects of different foods and nutrients is particularly challenging. There are many possibly relevant variables and these are often strongly interrelated. A topical example is the separation of the effect of fat intake from the total caloric intake, since people with more 'fatty' diets also tend to have higher total energy intakes.

The classification of a covariate as either an exposure or confounder is not a stable one. When two factors, z_1 and z_2, are related to disease and to each other and z_1 is of primary interest, z_1 is the exposure and z_2 the confounder. In another analysis, their roles may be reversed.

It may also not be clear when a variable should be considered as a confounder and corrected for in the analysis, and when it should be ignored. Here the decision is dictated by the ideal experiment which the statistical analysis seeks to mimic. In the example of fat consumption and total energy intake, it may be appropriate to carry out

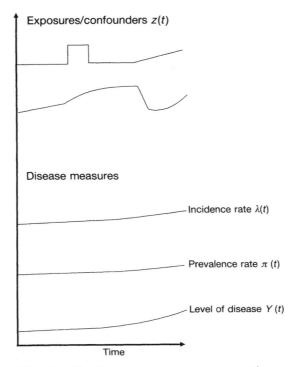

Fig. 4.1   The disease–exposure process over time.

an analysis in which energy intake is treated as a confounder and fat intake is regarded as the exposure of interest. This analysis simulates an experiment in which total energy intake is held constant and fat intake is varied. Such an experiment would be difficult to carry out in practice – the calories lost from reducing fat intake would have to be replaced by increasing intake of some other nutrient. When interpreting statistical analyses of multifactorial problems it is important to bear such considerations in mind. The problems are rendered particularly acute in nutritional epidemiology by the difficulty of making accurate measurements of diet.

All analytical approaches to the problem of confounding require, either implicitly or explicitly, a model for the joint effect of two or more exposures or confounders upon disease. The nature of this model, and the methods for drawing inferences about it, depend upon the outcome measure of the disease process. Outcome measures are usually of three types:

(1) the observation of an event, usually the first clinical sign of a disease (incidence);
(2) the recording of presence or absence of disease at a point in time (prevalence);
(3) the measurement of level of disease on a metric scale.

The arguments for preferring incidence to prevalence data are well known. The most serious limitation of prevalence data is that they may be influenced by a relationship between the presence of disease and subsequent mortality and migration. Studies which record a metric measure of the disease level (for example, blood pressure) suffer the same difficulties of interpretation, unless the disease level is measured repeatedly in a longitudinal study.

Modern epidemiology is largely concerned with processes for which it is impossible to build deterministic models or theories. Instead we must rely on models which relate covariate levels to the probability of outcome. For event data the most useful probability measure of the disease process is the probability per unit time, or 'hazard rate', of event occurrence. This is a function of time and is often denoted in the statistical literature by $\lambda(t)$ (see Fig. 4.1). For first occurrence of disease this is an incidence rate, while with mortality endpoints it is a mortality rate. In prevalence studies, the corresponding measure is the probability of disease presence, $\pi(t)$. For metric measures, statistical models allow for random errors of measurement of the level of disease, usually by assuming that the observed measurement has a probability distribution with mean equal to the true level but with variability (error) around this value. In Fig. 4.1 the mean level is denoted by $Y(t)$.

4.2 Modelling disease–covariate relationships

Most elementary treatments of epidemiological theory concentrate upon simple binary comparisons of exposed versus non-exposed groups. Dietary intakes, however, represent a continuum of exposure and in this chapter we shall concentrate upon models for a smooth dose–response relationship between intake and disease.

At some time of observation, t_{OBS}, the disease measure – $\lambda(t_{OBS})$, $\pi(t_{OBS})$, or $Y(t_{OBS})$ – depends upon the entire history of exposure up to t_{OBS}. This is referred to as the *covariate history*. Only certain aspects of the covariate history will be relevant to later disease, although we often do not know which aspect is directly relevant. For example, a disease may be affected by nutrition in childhood with later diet being largely irrelevant. In the case of cancer, considerations of latency would suggest that exposure in the period immediately before the incidence of disease must be irrelevant and that analysis should concentrate upon earlier exposure.

If sufficient knowledge (or, at least, a working hypothesis) is available, it is possible to define a summary measure of the relevant exposure history at t_{OBS}. This shall be denoted by $z^*(t_{OBS})$. In nutritional epidemiology, this is that summary measure of the dietary history which is relevant to the incidence of disease at t_{OBS}. The asterisk serves to remind us that this may differ substantially from the measured intake. For this reason, observed relationships between measured intakes and disease will reflect the underlying causal relationships rather imperfectly.

In statistical analysis, we adopt a mathematical model for the relationship between $z^*(t_{OBS})$ and the measure of disease. Such models involve unknown constants, or parameters which control the strength and form of the relationship. Usually available data do not justify other than rather simple models, such as:

(1) linear dose-response relationships between level of exposure and outcome;
(2) additive or multiplicative models for joint effect of two factors.

These are the relationships implied by multiple regression models and this chapter will consider only models of this general form. If biological knowledge were to suggest other dose-response relationships, the same principles would apply, if not some of the detailed results. Correct analysis requires careful examination as to whether the data support the model assumed for the dose-response relationship.

The statistical theory surrounding regression models has become highly developed in recent years. Although developed originally for the case of metric outcome measures, the modern theory includes variants for binary outcomes (logistic regression), ordered categorical measures of outcome (ordinal regression), and event occurrence over time (proportional hazards, or 'Cox' regression).

A widespread misconception is that these methods represent a philosophically different approach to the analysis of epidemiological data from that of older methods based upon the idea of stratification. In fact these older methods are special cases of the modern modelling approach. The greater generality of the regression modelling approach lends itself particularly to computer implementation, and software is widely available. In the epidemiological literature progressively more complex analyses are being performed and reported.

A limitation with this methodology, only widely appreciated quite recently, is that regression models only allow for random influences or errors on the disease side of the equation. The fact that exposures and confounders are subject to measurement error is ignored. In these circumstances the regression model is a mathematical model for the relationship between the measurements of the covariate history and the disease outcome. While this is quite appropriate for actuarial prediction of future disease from measured characteristics of individuals, the fitted model may be a serious distortion of the causal relationship between true covariate history and disease. One aim of this chapter is to urge some caution in the interpretation of statistical analyses in these circumstances. We shall also discuss the possibilities for inferring the true causal relationship from epidemiological studies, and explore the implications of these considerations for their design.

4.3   Measurement errors and bias in epidemiological studies

Figure 4.2 illustrates the possible influence upon the relationship between observed exposure and observed disease status in epidemiological studies.

Path 1 represents the true relationship between relevant exposure and disease. In the absence of confounding, this will reflect the causal relationship.

Path 2 represents the relationship between true relevant exposure and the observed surrogate.

Path 3 allows for measurement error of disease status or onset time.

The remaining paths allow for the major sources of bias which have been widely recognized to distort epidemiological findings:

Path 4 represents influences of disease status upon the measurement of exposure. This leads to information bias, the most widespread example of which is recall bias in case-control studies. Such influences present serious problems in nutritional epidemiology; for example early disease may influence diet or, at least, the reporting of diet.

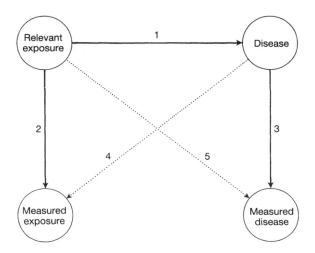

Fig. 4.2 Path diagram showing the possible influences on the observed disease–exposure relationship.

Path 5 allows the exposure to influence the recording of disease status. Examples include referral or investigation bias arising because certain groups may be more likely to be diagnosed than others, and bias arising from direct effects of early disease on physiology or behaviour. In nutritional epidemiology, such paths are most likely to arise out of indirect relationships with socio–economic status – more affluent groups may be better investigated and diagnosed and their diet differs from that of the less wealthy. This could induce a spurious relationship between diet and disease which would disappear if it were possible to correct for the confounding effect of socio–economic status.

Paths 4 and 5 represent *differential misclassification*. They have been widely recognized as having the potential to lead to seriously erroneous findings. In particular, they may create an apparent relationship when no true relationship exists (i.e. when path 1 is truly absent). For this reason, in the design of any study, the epidemiologist must take every possible step to exclude such influences. If attempts are unsuccessful, it is unlikely that any degree of sophistication of analysis will salvage useful results.

The realization that epidemiological studies may yield biased results even in the absence of differential misclassification has come more recently. In particular, *symmetric misclassification* (errors of measurement of exposure unrelated to disease state indicated by path 2), although incapable of introducing spurious relationships where no true relationships exist, may distort the true causal relationship. The most frequently occurring distortion arising from exposure measurement error is attenuation of effect – the observed relationship is weaker than the underlying true relationship. This has implications for the design, analysis, and interpretation of studies.

More serious distortion may be caused by an inability to accurately measure strong confounders. A statistical analysis which attempts to control for confounding by stratification according to the observed level of the confounding variable will be misleading, since the stratification will fail to achieve its goal of holding the true confounder constant within strata. Two forms of distortion may occur:

(1) *residual confounding*, in which the inability to measure accurately the confounder means that the correction for confounding is incomplete;
(2) *spurious or exaggerated confounding*, in which the relationship between exposure and confounder is exaggerated by the measuring instrument.

An example of exaggerated confounding could be the relationship between fat intake and total energy intake. If this relationship is exaggerated by errors of measurement, a naïve correction of the relationship between fat intake and disease for the confounding effect of energy intake may be misleading.

Since there is no likelihood that such measurement errors can be excluded from epidemiological studies, the question is raised of whether one should only report relationships between observed quantities and discuss their implications for underlying causal models informally, or follow statisticians in social science in attempting to model underlying causal pathways. The remainder of this chapter discusses some possibilities and associated problems of the latter approach.

4.3 Covariate measurement error in linear regression

We have discussed above how regression methods allow for random influences or recording errors on outcome measures. In epidemiology, an equally serious problem is the discrepancy between the true value of the relevant history, $z^*(t_{oBS})$, and an imperfect measure, $x(t_{oBS})$, say. The difficulty is particularly acute since we are often unsure what aspect of the covariate history is relevant – if fat intake is implicated in breast cancer, should we be interested in lifetime intake, recent intake, childhood intake . . . ?

This section briefly reviews the problem of exposure measurement error in the simple case of a linear regression relationship between covariate z^* and metrically measured disease outcome y. The observed relationship is between y and x, but the causal relationship between y and z^* is of more interest to the epidemiologist. These are not usually the same! The results outlined below are well known in the statistical literature, but their implications for epidemiology have only recently been widely discussed.

Consider first the case where we assume a linear relationship between level of disease and true relevant exposure. Since all quantities now refer to the time of observation, t_{oBS}, this may be omitted from the notation. The (causal) model for the relationship between relevant exposure and measured disease outcome must allow for random error of measurement of disease level. We assume the recorded level to have some probability distribution (perhaps a normal distribution) with expected (E) (mean) value determined by relevant exposure according to the linear dose–response relationship:

$$E(y) = Y = \alpha + \beta z^* \tag{4.1}$$

and with variance $(y) = \sigma^2$. The parameter β determines the slope of the line and, therefore, the strength of the dose–response relationship.

Unfortunately this model cannot be fitted directly since the true exposure, z^*, is unknown except for the flawed measure, x. To progress further we need to model the

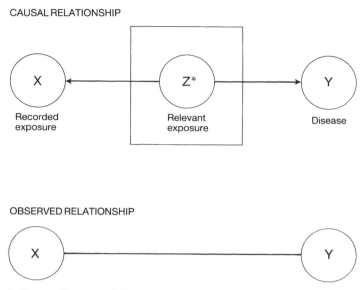

Fig. 4.3 Influence diagram of the causal and observed disease–exposure relationship.

process of exposure measurement. This measurement error model specifies the conditional probabilities of observations x given true exposures x^*, $\text{Prob}(x|z^*)$. This model specifies the distribution of measured exposures amongst individuals who share the same true relevant exposure.

Figure 4.3 represents the problem as an influence diagram. The disease outcome, y, and the measured exposure, x, are both causally related to the true relevant exposure, z^*. We only directly observe the relationship between x and y. To understand why this is not the same as the relationship between z^* and y gives insight into the potential for more accurate inference.

A simple analysis of the data is to plot disease level, y, against measured exposure, x. How would we expect this plot to appear given the model outlined above? Since y is not causally related to x, but only to z^*, it follows that the mean value of y for persons with the same measured exposure, x, depends on the mean true exposure in that group. Naïvely we might think that this is simply x, but more usually it is not! The measurement error model gives the probability distribution of measured exposure given true exposure, $\text{Prob}(x|z^*)$, but we need the distribution of true exposure amongst people with the given measured exposure, $\text{Prob}(z^*|x)$. The shape of this distribution is given by a fundamental theorem of probability theory – Bayes theorem:

$$\text{Prob}(z^*|x) \propto \text{Prob}(x|z^*)\,\text{Prob}(z^*) \tag{4.2}$$

$\text{Prob}(x|z^*)$ is the measurement error model and $\text{Prob}(z^*)$ is the overall distribution of true exposure in the study group. If both these distributions are known (or can be estimated), Bayes theorem allows estimation of the distribution of true exposure for people with given measured exposure. The mean or expected value of this distribution is written as $E(z^*|x)$, and is referred to as the *Bayes estimate* of z^* (the true exposure) given x (the measured exposure).

The Bayes estimate is usually 'shrunk' towards the population mean exposure; i.e. the mean true exposure is less extreme than the measured exposure. When the measured exposure is high the mean true exposure is rather lower and when the measured value is low the mean true exposure is rather higher. The reason for this is the same as for the well-known phenomenon of *regression to the mean*. We will discuss this and the important special cases in which it does *not* occur below. For the present, we will examine its effect upon the observed relationship. Figure 4.4 illustrates this in a plot of outcome versus exposure for four points. The circles represent measured exposure while the crosses represent mean true exposures. A line fitted to the crosses estimates the correct disease–exposure relationship, and this is stronger than the relationship between disease and measured exposure, corresponding to the line through the circles.

The regression to the mean which leads to the discrepancy between the observed relationship and the true relationship arises as follows. The group of people who share the same measured exposure, x, are a mixture of persons whose true exposure was more extreme than x and persons whose true exposure was closer to the population mean than x. However, if the distribution of true exposure is bell-shaped, so that there are progressively fewer individuals in each band of exposure as we depart from the mean, it follows that individuals with true exposures less extreme than x will predominate. Thus, the mean true exposure will be intermediate between the measured exposure and the population mean exposure. Note that the effect is crucially dependent on the shape of the distributions of exposure and of measurement error. Sometimes errors of measure-

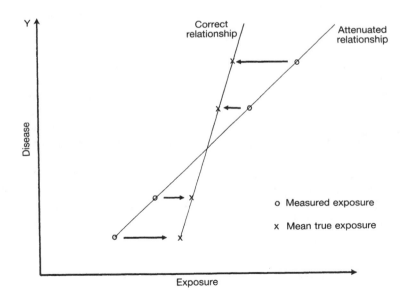

Fig. 4.4   Graph showing the attenuated disease–exposure relationship resulting from 'regression to the mean'.

ment do not lead to this effect. In such cases, the measurement errors are referred to as *Berksonian* after a paper by Berkson[1] which pointed out these results. One case is when the measurement error and the measured value are uncorrelated, and the distribution of measurement errors is symmetric. This case is sometimes referred to as *control knob error* since it would arise if the experimenter sets the control knob of some apparatus to deliver some level of stimulus (the measured value), but the true stimulus delivered differs from the nominal value by a random error, symmetrically distributed above and below zero. In these circumstances, the mean stimulus delivered, $E(z^*|x)$, is identical to the nominal stimulus, x. In epidemiology, two examples of this situation are as follows:

1. Prentice[2] suggested that the estimates of radiation dose received by atom bomb survivors are subject to Berksonian errors. The dose is calculated from information concerning the location of the individual at the time of the explosion. While these estimates are subject to considerable error, it remains likely that the mean dose for individuals with the same measured dose will not be too far wrong.
2. Of more relevance to nutritional epidemiology is the case of 'ecological' studies of diet and disease. Plotting community disease rates against estimated mean intake yields the same regression relationship as would be obtained from individual data, if each individual's intake were estimated by the community mean. Although this strategy clearly leads to very considerable exposure measurement error, the errors are Berksonian and do not lead to distortion of the relationship. (Ecological studies, however, have other difficulties!)

Berksonian errors occur when the measurement error is uncorrelated with the measured exposure. More commonly in analytical epidemiological studies exposure measurement errors are not Berksonian. It would more often be reasonable to assume that measurement error is uncorrelated with true exposure. The next section explores the possibility of correcting for the resultant distortion of the relationship in the statistical analysis.

4.5 Correcting for measurement error

When measurement errors are uncorrelated with true exposure, we have shown that the correct relationship may still be estimated providing we can calculate the Bayes estimate of the true exposure, $E(z^*|x)$. This can be calculated if we know (or reliably estimate) both the distribution of true exposure and the distribution of measurement error.

This is particularly easy when both these distributions can be assumed to be normal. Let the true exposures, z^*, be normally distributed with mean μ and variance σ^2, and let the measurement errors be normally distributed (independently of z^*) with mean 0 and variance τ^2. In these circumstances there is a simple linear shrinkage of the Bayes estimates of exposure towards the mean – the distance between the expected true exposure and μ is a constant proportion, ρ, of the distance between the measured exposure and μ. Algebraically,

$$E(z^*|x) - \mu = \rho(x - \mu) \tag{4.3}$$

The 'shrinkage factor', ρ, is determined by the relative magnitudes of true variability of exposure, σ^2, and of measurement error, τ^2:

$$\rho = \frac{\sigma^2}{\sigma^2 + \tau^2} \qquad (4.4)$$

The square root of ρ is the coefficient of correlation between the measured exposure and the true exposure and ρ is the correlation between two independent measurements of the same underlying exposure.

It follows that the induced relationship between y and x remains a straight line relationship, but the slope is reduced by the factor ρ. If ρ is known, the regression coefficient in the underlying causal model may be estimated, either by calculation of the regression coefficient of y on x and subsequently scaling it up by division by ρ, or by regression of y on Bayes estimates of the true exposure, z^*. These two approaches will yield identical results.

In practice ρ is rarely known, although in some circumstances it may be estimable from test–retest reliability data. If repeated measures are taken on the same individual, and it may be assumed that the measurement errors on the different occasions are uncorrelated with each other, then ρ is simply the coefficient of intra-class correlation between different measurements on the same individual. In nutritional epidemiology, however, the independent errors assumption is unlikely to hold and the intra-class correlation coefficient will overestimate ρ.

When validation studies are available which use several methods on several spaced occasions, it is possible to obtain estimates of measurement variances and covariance by, for example, assuming that different methods on different occasions do not have correlated errors. A full review of the selected methods for the analysis of such studies is given by Dunn.[3]

When it is believed that the relevant exposure is the average of the dietary intake of some nutrient over many years, then test–retest studies carried out over a relatively short period may underestimate measurement error, and it may only be possible to informally estimate ρ. As an aid to this, Table 4.1 relates ρ to the percentage of individuals who could be classified in the correct third of the distribution of true exposure using the measured exposure.

When we cannot assume normal distributions, the problem is more difficult although, if the relevant distributions are known, the correct relationship is always estimable. In practice the difficulty will be lack of good data concerning these distributions.

4.6   Scale bias

The discussion above has assumed that there is no systematic bias in measures of the true exposure. Formally this model for measurement error can be written

$$x = z^* + e$$

where e, the measurement errors, are normally distributed with zero mean and variance τ^2. We have further assumed that the errors, e, are uncorrelated with true exposure, z^*, and with this assumption the total variance of the measured exposure x, is the sum of variances of true exposure and measurement error, $\sigma^2 + \tau^2$. This model underlies the

Table 4.1 Correct classification by thirds of the exposure distribution.

ρ	% Correctly classified
0.1	42.8
0.2	46.5
0.3	51.4
0.4	54.8
0.5	59.2
0.6	63.2
0.7	67.9
0.8	73.4
0.9	81.0

usual analyses of validity and reliability studies, and the two variance components may be estimated using the analysis of variance. However, in nutritional epidemiology these simple assumptions are all too often violated, leading to systematic biases.

One form of systematic bias is *location bias*, in which the mean of the measured exposures is not equal to the mean of the true exposures. This requires a minor elaboration of our model,

$$x = \delta + z^* + e$$

where δ is the location bias. Under this model the variance of the observed measurement is still $\sigma^2 + \tau^2$ and the analysis of validity and reliability studies is little changed, save for the need to quantify the location bias. While this form of bias could have serious consequences in studies involving population comparisons, it can be ignored for comparisons within populations, since all subjects will share it.

A more serious form of bias is caused by a relationship between the measurement error and the true exposure. For example, it might be that subjects with a high total energy intake under-report their food intakes and/or subjects with low total energy intake over-report consumption. Such behaviours would lead to a compression of the apparent range of intakes – that is to a *scale bias*. If the relationship between measurement error and true exposure is a linear regression, then our measurement error model becomes

$$x = \delta + \gamma z^* + e$$

where deviation of γ from 1 indicates *scale bias*. As before, we may continue to assume that e is independent of z^* since the dependence of measurement error on true exposure is accounted for in the parameter γ.

Such scale biases would seem to be quite prevalent in nutritional epidemiology. Clearly, the consequence of a scale bias in the measurement of exposure is a further distortion of relationship between exposure and disease outcome. The correction for the effects of measurement error now requires estimation of a further parameter of the measurement error model: the scale bias, δ, in addition to the variance components σ^2 and τ^2. This is a more difficult task than estimating the variance components in the simpler models. The variance of the measured exposure is

$$\gamma^2 \sigma^2 + \tau^2$$

and the parameters could be estimated from a validity study, if a totally accurate 'gold standard' measurement of exposure were available. In practice, such measurements are not available and estimation of the parameters requires more elaborate reliability studies involving several types of measurement, at least one of which must be assumed to have no scale bias. It will also be necessary to assume independence of the errors in some or all of the repeated measurements. Analysis of such studies can be carried out using covariance structure analysis, a statistical method more usually applied in the context of *path analysis* in the behavioural sciences and implemented in computer programs such as LISREL and EQS.[4,5,6]

4.7 Calibration

The difficulties implicit in specification and estimation of the measurement error model have led some researchers to explore more empirical methods. In recent years these have come to be described as *calibration*, but a similar procedure has been known for many years in the statistical literature[7] as the *method of instrumental variables*. In the most accessible version of the method, the study group is classified into say, deciles on an initial measure of exposure, and mean true exposure in subgroups may be estimated by the mean of a second measure. An 'ecological' analysis relating this estimate of group exposure to the mean disease level in the subgroups will yield the correct relationship, providing that the errors in the second measurement are unrelated to the errors in the first. If the errors are correlated, then the regression to the mean is not complete and some distortion of the relationship will remain. This approach was used by McMahon *et al.*[8] in studying the relationship between blood-pressure and cardiovascular disease. Table 4.2 shows blood-pressure for groups classified according to an initial, or baseline, measurement. Regression of disease rates for these groups against the mean baseline blood-pressure would yield an incorrect slope since the range of variation of long-term average blood-pressure is overestimated. Use of a further measure 2–4 years later will lead to a much improved estimate. In nutritional epidemiology, however, the assumption of uncorrelated measurement errors may not be justified and regression-to-the mean estimated from repeated measurements in this way may not correctly estimate long-term intakes. The term 'calibration' arises because, in this method, the main study method provides an initial estimate of the relationship, and the statistical test of its significance. Later analysis using a second measurement in a subsample, can be thought of as calibrating the relationship. In the example discussed above, calibration was achieved by grouping on the main study measurement and using the second measurement to assess true mean exposure within groups. An alternative approach is *regression calibration*, in which the regression line of calibration measurement upon main study measurement is used to the same effect.[9,10] Under the assumptions outlined above, the fitted values from this regression estimate the expected

Table 4.2 Diastolic blood pressure (DBP) in five categories.[8]

Baseline DBP	Number of subjects	Mean DBP in category: at baseline	at 2 years	at 4 years
–79	1719	70.8	75.7	76.2
80–89	1213	83.6	83.0	83.9
90–99	566	93.5	90.2	90.3
100–109	186	103.4	99.2	98.5
110–	92	116.4	107.3	104.7
Range:		47.7	31.6	28.5

true exposure for given measured exposure. Using these values in place of the measured exposures in the main study achieves the required calibration.

Some simple algebra shows that this procedure is equivalent to estimation of the regression coefficient of disease outcome on true exposure by dividing the 'naïve' regression coefficient for outcome on measured exposure in the main study by the regression coefficient for calibration measurement versus main study measurement in calibration study.

For calibration methods to successfully correct the disease–exposure relationship, several assumptions must be made.

1. As indicated above, errors of measurement of the calibration measurement and the main study measurement must be uncorrelated with one another in the calibration study.
2. There must be no scale bias in the calibration method. Note that it is not necessary to assume no scale bias in the main study method, since calibration simultaneously takes account of any such bias if the calibration method itself is free of it.
3. The distributions of measurement errors and of true exposures must be the same in the calibration study as in the main study. In practice the best way to ensure this is to perform an *internal* calibration study – a sub-study in a representative sample of the main study population.

Although calibration methods seem to avoid further strong modelling assumptions, this is only apparent – there are other hidden assumptions. For example, regression calibration requires linear regression between disease and true exposure, between calibration measures and main study measurement, and between disease and main study measurement. These three assumptions are only consistent with one another in rather special circumstances – when the distributions of true exposure and measurement errors are both normal. While it seems likely that the method is tolerant to a modest degree of non-normality, it could not be expected to perform well with grossly non-normal distributions such as arise, for example, for intakes of some micronutrients (see also Chapter 3, Section 3.3.5, on transformation).

4.8   Regression models for incidence and prevalence data

The results set out in the last section have been known for many years. More recently, similar results have been shown to hold for relative risk regression models for the occurrence of events in time[2,11] and for logistic regression models for prevalence studies and case-control studies.[12] This section briefly reviews the results for regression analyses of incidence data. Similar results hold for logistic regression analyses of prevalence data.

In recent years, the analysis of event data has been dominated by the relative risk regression model introduced by Cox.[13] In the present notation this may be written:

$$\text{Incidence rate } (t_{OBS}) = \lambda_0(t_{OBS})\theta(z^*(t_{OBS});\beta) \qquad (4.5)$$

The incidence rate at t_{OBS} is expressed as the product of a 'baseline' incidence rate, $\lambda_0(t_{OBS})$, and a relative risk term, $\theta()$ which is a function of the relevant exposure history. Again, regression coefficients, β, express the strength of the relationship between exposure(s) and risk of disease occurrence. The most convenient relative risk function, and that most frequently available in current computer software, is the log-linear function:

$$\theta(z^*;\beta) = \exp \beta z^* \qquad (4.6)$$

or

$$\log \theta(z^*;\beta) = \beta z^* \qquad (4.7)$$

This model implies that a one-unit change in exposure confers a relative risk of $\exp \beta$ at every point on the scale. As in the case of a metric disease measure, if the measure of the relevant exposure history is flawed, there will be an induced relationship between the measured exposure, x, and subsequent incidence of events. In the same way as a linear regression relationship between true exposure, z^*, and disease level, y, induces a (rather weaker) relationship between measured exposure, x, and y, the relative risk model for the effect of exposure upon incidence induces an attenuated risk relationship between measured exposure and incidence. The derivation of the degree of attenuation follows very similar lines as before. A group of persons with the same measured exposure, x, will in fact have had varying true exposures, z^*, and so will experience varying relative risks, $\theta(z^*;\beta)$. The average relative risk for such persons is *not* $\theta(x;\beta)$ but a rather less extreme value. The size and pattern of discrepancy between the observed relationship and the underlying causal relationship depends on the magnitude of measurement error in relation to the true variability of exposure. Again one special case leads to simple equations; if true exposure and measurement error are both normally distributed with variances σ^2 and τ^2 respectively, and incidence is related to true exposure in the log-linear manner discussed above, the relationship between incidence and measured exposure follows exactly the same log-linear relationship, but with a regression coefficient which is reduced by the factor ρ. The same is true for logistic regression of case-control studies when the distributions of true exposure *within case and control populations* are normal.

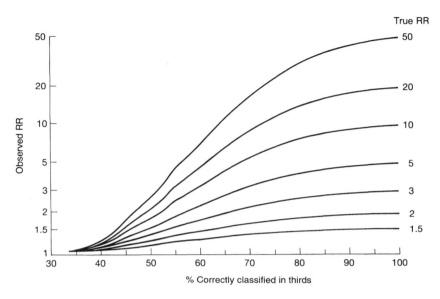

Fig. 4.5 Graph showing the effect of exposure misclassification upon observed relative risk.

Since many epidemiologists do not find regression coefficients and correlation coefficients very intuitive, these relationships are explored in terms of comparisons between thirds of the exposure distribution in Fig. 4.5. Each curve shows, for a causal relationship of given strength, the rate ratio for the top versus the bottom third of the distribution of measured exposure plotted against the accuracy of the measurement, expressed in terms of our ability to correctly classify subjects into thirds of the exposure distribution. The seven curves shown represent underlying true rate ratios of 1.5, 2, 3, 5, 10, 20, and 50. It would appear that the attenuation is not too serious when we can correctly classify at least 75% of subjects into thirds of the distribution.

When the measure of disease outcome is metric, and we are prepared to assume normality for all distributions, then a full model for the relationship between disease and exposure, incorporating measurement errors for exposure, can be fitted using software for path analysis. However, for disease outcome measures which are binary or which are records of the occurrence of events, the theoretical difficulties are more serious[14,15], and no general software is available at present. In such applications, calibration methods are popular, although they are only completely accurate in rather special circumstances.[9,10]

4.9   Confounder measurement errors

The relationships set out in sections 4.4, 4.5 and 4.6 between regression models in z^* and regression models in x may be extended to the case where there are confounders or multiple exposures. Indeed, it can be argued that this is the only case in which formal correction for the effects of covariate measurement error is required. With a single covariate, the effect of non-differential measurement error is to attenuate the exposure–disease relationships, and calibration has no relevance to the problem of statistical significance testing. However, with two or more variables, the situation becomes more complex. Even in the case of a single exposure and a single confounder, the discrepancy between the exposure effect as estimated by conventional methods and the true 'causal' effect depends upon:

(1) the size of the effect of the confounder;
(2) strength of association between exposure and confounder;
(3) measurement of error for the exposure;
(4) range of variation of exposure in the study group;
(5) measurement error for the confounder;
(6) range of variation of the confounder;
(7) correlation between measurement errors of exposure and confounder.

If a confounder is measured with error, any control for confounding in the analysis is flawed. If confounder measurement error is independent of exposure measurement error, then we have the phenomenon of *residual confounding*. The coefficient of the exposure variable is adjusted in the correct direction but by an insufficient amount.

If confounder measurement error is correlated with exposure measurement error, then the bias may go in either direction. In particular we may overestimate the correlation between exposure and confounder and, as a result, overcorrect for the effect of the confounder. The potential for this type of error has not been widely recognized, yet it remains a strong possibility in nutritional epidemiology – the methods of measuring diet are very likely to lead to strongly correlated measurement errors, as is the use of current diet as a surrogate for diet during the period relevant to the development of disease.

Further difficulties arise if the error variance is related to the level of true exposure. It has been shown that this may lead to spurious curvature of dose–response relationships and spurious interaction (effect modification).

In principle, and given sufficient data, these distortions may be corrected in the analysis, using multivariate extensions to methods described in earlier sections. In particular, path analysis is a statistical method explicitly designed for such situations, and has been widely used in the behavioural sciences. Such analyses depend upon many assumptions, some of them not easily testable, and have not found favour in epidemiology. Calibration methods, which seem more intuitive and less mathematical, have been preferred.

Calibration by grouping does not extend naturally to the case of several covariates, since it would be necessary to define many groups to adequately span all dimensions. However, regression calibration extends easily and naturally.[10] The calibration equations to be used in the main study are estimated in the calibration study, by regressing the calibration measurements of each covariate in turn against the main study measurements of *all* covariates. Note that extraneous covariates such as season, which may be related to the covariate measurement process but which one would not wish to include in the analysis for disease outcome, can be included in these calibration equations.

4.10 Concluding remarks

For the sake of clarity this chapter has oversimplified some of the statistical problems, and there is need for more research in this area. We have shown that correct estimation of exposure/disease relationships requires us to have knowledge of:

(1) the probability distribution of measurement errors
(2) the distribution of true exposures and confounders in the population studied.

We have also shown that both distributions may be multivariate. Then it will be necessary to consider not only the variability of each component but also their interrelationship. While simple results are available if the distributions are multivariate normal, the development of statistical methods based on weaker assumptions is a considerable challenge. For the present, the multivariate normal results serve as a yardstick for gauging the seriousness of the measurement error problem.

The discussion has concentrated on the problem of bias arising as a result of covariate measurement error, and upon techniques for its removal. The problem of the effect of such corrections on the precision of estimation has been left to one side. Clearly, extra measurements collected in quite small substudies whose primary purpose is to correct, or calibrate, relationships demonstrated in a larger study cannot be expected to lead to increased precision. Indeed, in general there will be some loss of precision as a result of errors introduced by the calibration process. If calibration is intended, some thought needs to go into the planning of calibration substudies to ensure that this is not too serious.[16]

Even the simplest model requires knowledge of its parameters and the estimation of the magnitude of measurement errors presents serious problems to the nutritional epidemiologist. Ideally this requires validation studies to be carried out on subsamples of the study population, but this is not possible in a field in which no error-free 'gold standard' measurement is available. To some extent this lack can be redressed by reliability studies in which several different measuring instruments are used on several occasions. Inference from such studies depends upon the validity of assumptions made in modelling measurement errors. While these may be checked to some extent, there is considerable danger in extrapolation. For example, results of a reliability study with repeated measures over a 1-year period could not be applied with any confidence to inference concerning the relationship between disease and dietary intakes over 20 years or more. This problem is particularly acute when it is not possible *a priori* to identify the relevant exposure.

Conventional concerns over information bias ensure that case-control studies are not the method of choice in nutritional epidemiology. The need to study measurement error whilst simultaneously studying diet/disease relationships provides additional rationale for advocating long-term prospective studies with repeated measures of diet. To minimize the intercorrelation between measurement errors on different occasions, the repeated measurements should be well separated in time. The use of more than one measuring instrument, at least in subsamples, is essential.

The main requirement of calibration studies in subsamples is that such studies should use, as far as is possible, unbiased measurements in a representative subsample.

Additionally, the errors in calibration measurements should not tend to repeat errors in the main study measurements they aim to calibrate. High test–retest reliability is not essential, although it does allow calibration studies to be smaller in size. It is the quality of measurements made in 100% of subjects which ultimately dictate the power of the study and for this purpose measurement methods should be chosen with the aim of accurately ranking subjects with respect to intake. For these main study measurements, it is lack of bias which is essential. There is no single 'best' method of measuring diet in free-living populations, and if progress is to be made in this difficult area, it will come from study designs which exploit the best characteristics of all available methods appropriately.

References

1. Berkson, J. (1950) Are there two regressions? *J. American Statistical Assoc.* **45**: 164.
2. Prentice, R. L. (1982) Covariate measurement errors and parameter estimation in a failure time regression model. *Biometrika.* **69**: 331–42.
3. Dunn, G. (1989) *Design and analysis of reliability studies.* Edward Arnold, London.
4. Plummer, M. and Clayton, D. (1993) Measurement error in diet: an investigation using covariance structure models, part i. *Stat. Med.* **12**: 925–36.
5. Plummer, M. and Clayton, D. (1993) Measurement error in diet: an investigation using covariance structure models, part ii. *Stat. Med.* **12**: 937–48.
6. Kaaks, R., Riboli, E., Esteve, J., van Kappel, A. L. and van Staveren, W. A. (1994) Estimating the accuracy of dietary questionnaire assessments: validation in terms of structural equation models. *Stat. Med.* **13**: 127–42.
7. Kendall, M. G. and Stuart, A. (1979) *The advanced theory of statistics.* Vol. II. 4th edn. MacMillan, New York.
8. McMahon, S., Peto, R., Cutler, J., Collins, R,. Sorlie, P., Neaton, J., *et al.* (1990) Blood pressure, stroke, and coronary heart disease. *Lancet.* **335**: 765–74.
9. Rosner, B., Willett, W. C. and Spiegelman, D. (1989) Correction of logistic regression relative risk estimates and confidence intervals for systematic within-person measurement error. *Stat. Med.* **8**: 1051–69.
10. Rosner, B., Spiegelman, D. and Willett, W. C. (1990) Correction of logistic regression relative risk estimates and confidence intervals for measurement error: the case of multiple covariates measured with error. *Am. J. Epid.* **132**: 734–45.
11. Armstrong, B. G. and Oakes, D. (1982) The effects of approximation in exposure assessment on estimates of exposure response relationships. *Scand. J. of Work, Envir., and Hlth.* **8**(Suppl 1): 20–30.
12. Armstrong, B. G., Whittemore, A. S. and Howe, G. R. (1989) Analysis of case-control data with covariate measurement error: application to diet and colon cancer. *Stat. Med.* **8**: 1151–63.
13. Cox, D. R. (1972) Regression models and life tables. *J. Royal Statistical. Soc. Series B.* **33**: 187–202.
14. Clayton, D. (1992) Models for analysis of cohort and case-control studies with inaccurately measured exposures. In: Dwyer, J. H., Feinleib, M., Lipert, P. and Hoffmeister, H. (ed.), *Statistical models for longitudinal studies of health.* Oxford University Press, Oxford.
15. Carroll, R. J., Ruppert, D. and Stefanski, L. A. (1995) *Measurement error in non-linear models.* Chapman and Hall, London.
16. Plummer, M., Clayton, D. and Kaaks, R. (1994) Calibration in multi-centre cohort studies. *Int. J. Epid.* **23**: 419–26.

Part B   The measurement of exposure and outcome

Introduction

At the core of any nutritional epidemiological study, no matter how well designed or cleverly analysed, is the matter of measurement of exposure and outcome. Inappropriate or inaccurate measurements will lead to spurious conclusions (either false positive results or a failure to detect relationships which exist) and will waste precious resources. The focus of this section is therefore to consider how best such measurements can be made, and how the errors associated with the measurements can themselves be measured and taken into account during analysis. Measurement error in relation to specific epidemiological study designs is discussed further in Part C.

The breadth of the presentations in this section is intended to help readers think about how errors relating to many different types of variables may interact to undermine the ability to detect diet–disease relationships. Corroboration of findings based on different types of measurements taken at different stages in the causal pathway (dietary measurements, biochemical measurements, genetic susceptibility) will only be likely if all the measurements are as accurate as possible and the errors associated with those measures are clearly described. The validity of measurements is a key issue running through this section, and the likely consequences of mis-measurement with undescribed errors is discussed extensively.

Techniques for measuring diet, and their associated problems, are described in Chapter 6. The particular role that food composition tables play in relation to errors of estimates of nutrient intakes is discussed in Chapter 5. In Chapter 7 readers will find an appreciation of the ways in which biochemical markers can be used both to enhance the objectivity of some measures of diet (e.g. use of urinary nitrogen measurements to detect dietary under-reporters) and to elucidate steps along the causal pathway (e.g. measures of glutathione peroxidase in relation to the role of dietary selenium as part of an anti-oxidant defence network); special attention is paid to the pitfalls and limitations of biochemical measurements. Chapter 8 is devoted to the validation of dietary measurements and a consideration of how to assess and cope in analysis with the errors which are likely to arise.

The section is considerably expanded from the first edition and includes new material on the measurement of socio-demographic and psycho-social variables (Chapter 9), anthropometry (Chapter 10), and genetic influences (Chapter 11). These measurements may include direct measures of nutritional status (e.g. height and weight), or susceptibility to a dietary factor (e.g. cellular vitamin receptor activity).

In any nutritional epidemiological study, confounding may be as important as misclassification in misinterpreting findings. For example, if income level is a potentially important confounder of the relationship between educational background and response to nutrition education in a secondary prevention trial of CHD (because the dietary changes needed to reduce CHD risk are too expensive for subjects on low income to support), it is vitally important that income as well as education be measured without error (Chapter 9). Similarly, the failure of some subjects to respond to intervention may have to do with genetically determined variations in response to dietary factors (Chapter 11). An awareness of the range of factors which may interact with one another will spell the success or failure of a study. In planning studies, it is up to individual researchers to make themselves aware of the scope of interactions which may take place, and to ensure that all of the appropriate variables are measured in the best possible way.

5. Food consumption, nutrient intake, and the use of food composition tables

Clive E. West and Wija A. van Staveren

5.1 Introduction

Food consumption data are collected for a variety of purposes. The most relevant to nutritional epidemiology are:

(1) estimation of adequacy of the dietary intake of population groups;
(2) investigation of relationships between diet and health and nutritional status;
(3) evaluation of nutrition education, nutrition intervention, and food fortification programmes.

In general, data obtained on food consumption by individuals or groups of individuals is converted to intake of nutrients. This conversion process can be achieved either by analysing the foods consumed directly or by using food composition tables. Table 5.1 classifies the most commonly used dietary survey methods on the basis of whether chemical analysis of food samples or food tables are used to estimate nutrient intake.

The methods using direct analysis are considered to be the most accurate and most appropriate for examining the effect of changes in nutrient intake on parameters of

Table 5.1 Classification of the most commonly used methods for measuring nutrient intake.[42]

Use of chemical analysis	Characteristics of method		
	Use of food composition tables		
	Record methods	Interview methods	Short-cut methods
Duplicate portion technique	Precise weighing	Recall	Record
Aliquot sampling technique	Weighed inventory	Dietary history	Recall
Equivalent composite	Present intake recorded in household measures		

nutritional status over a period of time. However, for observational studies of large populations, these methods are too cumbersome, costly, and time consuming. Methods based on the use of food composition tables are more often used.

Food composition tables, or nutrient databases, which are their electronic/magnetic equivalent, are available in many countries. However, there may still be a need to carry out food analyses under a number of circumstances, including:

(1) when the content of a nutrient or other food component is not available in an existing food table;
(2) when there is no information available on which foods are important sources of a nutrient/other food component of interest;
(3) when there is no information on the loss or gain of nutrients in foods during preparation by the methods being used by the population under investigation;
(4) when it is necessary to check the comparability of the various food composition tables being used in a multicentre study.

5.2   The use of food analysis in determining nutrient intake

Of all the dietary survey methods available, the duplicate portion technique is regarded as the most accurate, although its accuracy depends on being able to obtain a sample that is identical to the food consumed by the subject under study. This is probably more difficult when composite foods such as a stew or a food with a lot of free fat is being consumed.[1] In addition, it may not be possible to include small items in the duplicate portion[2] either because the observer is unaware that they have been eaten, such as snacks between meals, or because they are not available. Often the cook may not have prepared sufficient for a complete duplicate portion and the food prepared for the subject under study would be consumed in its entirety by the subject or shared with the duplicate portion thus resulting in reduced food intake by the subject.

In the aliquot sampling technique, the weights of all foods eaten and all beverages drunk, usually with the exception of water, are recorded and aliquot samples, e.g. one-tenth of all foods and beverages consumed, are collected daily. Subsequently, the combined aliquot samples collected over the survey period are chemically analysed. Errors can arise in this method, in addition to those inherent in the duplicate portion method, from the recording of weights and volumes. However, the method is often preferred to the duplicate portion technique because less food is required and only one analysis is required for the entire survey period.

In the equivalent composite technique, which is hardly ever used, the weights of all foods eaten and all beverages drunk are recorded, as for the aliquot sampling technique. At the end of the survey period, a sample of raw foods equivalent to the mean daily amounts of food eaten by an individual during the survey period is taken for analysis. Errors over and above those experienced with the aliquot sampling technique arise from the analysis of raw foods as opposed to foods as consumed (see Section 5.3.7) and from qualitative differences between foods in the composite and those eaten. The method is cheaper than the duplicate portion and aliquot sampling techniques and it is relatively easy to collect the food samples, although this process cannot commence until the average consumption of foods over the whole period of study has been calculated.

There are two additional problems with all three of these techniques. The first is that the techniques are very difficult to validate in an absolute way, and differential mis-classification may occur in the collection of samples in free-living populations. Nevertheless the duplicate portion technique is the method to which all other methods should be compared. Secondly, the accuracy of the results will depend on the accuracy of the analyses, as does the accuracy of results based on the use of food composition tables. Thus, good laboratory practice is essential in order to obtain satisfactory results (see Section 5.3.5).

5.3 Food consumption tables and nutrient databases

Nutritional epidemiological studies may want to look at nutrient intake as well as food consumption data. It is necessary, therefore, to be able to convert information on food consumption into intake of nutrients. Thus, the needs of the nutritional epidemiologist are not always identical with other users of the tables, such as medical practitioners and dietitians involved in giving dietary advice, or those involved in food production and preparation at various levels. Therefore, it is essential that the needs of the epidemiologist are taken into account when food composition tables/nutrient databases are being constructed. Guidelines for the preparation of food composition tables have been prepared by Southgate[3] and by Greenfield and Southgate.[4] The requirements of food composition tables, particularly relevant to the nutritional epidemiologist, are outlined below.

5.3.1 Foods included in the table

To be able to calculate nutrient intake, the foods delivering the nutrients of interest should be included in the table. If the foods are not included, information on their nutrient content could be obtained from other sources, including other tables or by analysing foods especially for the study. However, if the number of foods on which information is not available is very large, methods based on direct analysis could be considered (see Section 5.2). The number and nature of foods required will depend not only on the population or individuals under study, but also on the information being sought. A study of the energy intake of a group of farm workers in a traditional rural area would require fewer foods than an international case-control study of cancer at a particular site aimed at estimating the intake of 13 vitamins. First, because the range of foods consumed by the farm workers would be much narrower than that consumed by those in the international study. Secondly, because information on fewer foods would be required for measuring energy intake only, than for measuring energy and vitamin intake. In addition, more detailed descriptions of the foods would be required for the study on vitamin intake because foods differ more markedly in their content of individual vitamins than in their energy value. The vitamin content of plants, for example, is more dependent than the energy value on variety, degree of maturity, part of the plant, method of food preparation, and the method and duration of storage.

Indeed, the naming and general description of foods is a very important aspect of constructing a food composition table, not only for epidemiological purposes.

It is important that a food is labelled unequivocally and that all those involved in a study understand what is meant by the food described. For international studies, a thesaurus can be used to relate the locally used name to that by which the food is known in other countries. For unprocessed plants and animals, the scientific name will assist in identification while for plants, the variety should also be given. Prepared foods are more difficult to name because some proprietary names have restricted use while some describe products with different formulations. The problem is even more complicated for cooked dishes because the composition of a named dish varies between countries, regions, and even households. Thus, the name on its own is quite often not sufficient to characterize and identify a cooked dish. Another approach to studying foods from different countries has been developed by Eurofoods and its successors FLAIR EUROFOODS-ENFANT and COST 99 (EUROFOODS). It involves grouping foods together on the basis of their similarities. A food coding system based on 14 major food groups has been agreed upon by representatives from 17 countries. The 14 groups were subdivided into 2500 subcategories and the system developed has been revised. The result is called EUROCODE 2 and is part of a food coding and descriptor system.[5] The latest information on EUROCODE 2 can be obtained from the homepage of COST 99 EUROFOODS on the World Wide Web (http://food.ethz.ch:2000/cost99.html).

5.3.2 Nutrients included in the table

The nutrients to be included in the food composition table will depend on the purpose of the study. It should also be remembered that it is sometimes better to estimate the intake of nutrients not from food intake, but indirectly using biological markers. Thus, sodium and chloride intake are often measured more readily by measuring excretion in the urine, but such estimates can be subject to large errors. More sodium chloride is lost through perspiration in a hot climate or during physical exertion than during sedentary work in a temperate climate and there is increased loss of water and electrolytes during fever, vomiting, and diarrhoea. Even though intake can be estimated from excretion, it is still necessary to estimate intake of electrolytes using food tables to be able to determine which foods in the diet are sources of such electrolytes. The use of biological markers for estimating nutrient intake is discussed further in Chapter 7.

5.3.3 Methods of expression of nutrients

Increasing attention has been paid in recent years to how data are presented in food composition tables. Although it may not matter how nutrients are expressed for many epidemiological studies, it is becoming important for an increasing proportion of studies. For example, a study on the role of vitamin A and carotenoids in lung cancer requires more information than the vitamin A activity expressed in retinol equivalents. At the very least, vitamin A and provitamin A activity is required separately. Perhaps information on provitamin A should be divided into the various provitamin A carotenoids, and it may also be desirable to have information on other carotenoids present. Unfortunately, much of the information desired may not be available. Thus, the original study design may have to be re-examined or more analytical work carried out before the study can proceed. Other problems related to the method of expression of nutrients may arise from the long-standing convention of using protein values derived by applying a factor to measured total nitrogen values and from the calculation of energy values using energy conversion factors.[6] In order to overcome ambiguities in the naming of nutrients and also to allow the transfer of data among food composition tables, INFOODS has developed a system for identifying food components referred to as tags.[7] The latest information on this system is available on the World Wide Web via the INFOODS home page (http://www.crop.cri.nz/crop/infoods/infoods.html).

5.3.4 Methods used for the estimation of nutrients

The basic principle is that the method used should provide information that is nutritionally appropriate. Traditionally, carbohydrate was estimated by difference: that is, by directly measuring the percentage of protein (from the nitrogen content), fat, ash, and water, and deducting these from 100 to give the percentage of carbohydrate. This method is clearly inadequate for all nutritional purposes because it combines in one value all the different carbohydrate species: sugars, starch, and components of dietary fibre, together with all the errors in the other determinations. Nutritionists require much more detailed information, because the metabolic effects of all the components are quite different.[8] The biological action of related nutrients was referred to above with respect to vitamin A and carotenoids (Section 5.3.3) because the method of expression of a nutrient is often related to the analytical method used to obtain the data. This is also so for the vitamers of other vitamins including vitamin B6 (pyridoxal, pyridoxal phosphate, and pyridoxamine), folic acids (with a side chain with one, three, or seven glutamic acid residues), vitamin D (D2 or D3), vitamin E (various tocopherols and tocotrienols), and vitamin K (with various numbers of saturated and unsaturated isoprene units in the side chain). The problem of biological availability is addressed in Section 5.3.8.

5.3.5 Data quality

If you ask someone whether they want to use high quality food composition data for their epidemiological study, the answer will invariably be 'yes'. Thus, the question is really whether the data are of sufficient quality to answer the question being asked; and a number of specific aspects need to be addressed.

Naming and description of foods

The question that has to be addressed is whether the food being consumed is similar to that described in the food composition table (see Section 5.3.1). Describing foods precisely is a difficult task and much effort is required to ensure that foods are described adequately. For this purpose, INFOODS has developed guidelines for describing foods[9] and the Food and Drug Administration has developed a faceted food vocabulary which enables many aspects of a food to be described. Information on this can be obtained from the Langual homepage on the World Wide Web (http://food.ethz.ch:2000/Langual/langhome.html).

Origins of foods

A plant food being consumed and the same plant food in the table should be 'sufficiently similar' with respect to soil type, method of husbandry, fertilizer treatment, harvesting, and post-harvesting treatment. Animal products should take into account locality, methods of husbandry, and methods of slaughter. The definition of 'sufficiently similar' will depend on the nature of the study being carried out.

Sampling framework of food on which data are included in the food table

If information is available on data in the food composition table with respect to a description of the sampling process, place and time of sampling, number of samples, origin of samples, and state of sample when purchased, it should be possible to judge whether the sample is representative of the food as a whole, of a subset of the foods, or whether the data apply merely to the food analysed. With cooked foods, the cooking procedures and recipe should be known (see Section 5.3.7). Some data in food composition tables are based on analyses on pooled samples and this may influence the value of the data obtained. In addition, information on treatment of samples before analysis may be important. Before analysis, inedible material is usually removed and details of the portion taken for analysis should be known. For example, a Frenchman would never think of eating brie with the hard outside coat, but many people from other countries would have no qualms in doing so. This type of difference may mean that the food analysed is not the same as that being consumed in a particular epidemiological study.

Quality of food analysis

Differences in sampling techniques and the quality of the analytical work *per se* are usually the most important reasons for differences in analytical data in food composition tables. Differences in the methods used can be important (see Section 5.3.4), but this is usually over-emphasized. When compared with the traditional methods of titrimetry and gravimetry, modern methods of instrumental analysis, such as high performance liquid chromatography and atomic absorption spectrometry, are more convenient and allow more samples to be analysed but are not necessarily intrinsically more accurate. The problem of the quality of food analysis as a source of variation between data in different food composition tables was recognized by EUROFOODS, who organized an interlaboratory trial in 1985 in which 20 leading laboratories in Europe and the USA participated.[10] Each laboratory received a well homogenized dried sample of six foods and was requested to perform analyses of dried weight by a prescribed vacuum method, and of protein, fat, available carbohydrates, total dietary fibre, and ash by its own routine method. The results obtained were far from satisfactory. There were large between-laboratory coefficients of variation (CV) for dietary fibre (ranging from 23% for French beans to 84% for biscuits), which could be explained by the use of different methods. The CV for protein ranged from 2.8% for egg to 6.4% for wheat and rye, but recalculation of these values using uniform Kjeldahl factors reduced these CVs to 2.7, 4.7, and 5.2%, respectively. It could be concluded that leading laboratories in different countries may produce widely different values for proximate constituents in common foods. Thus, there is a need for better standardization of methods and for the essential elements of good laboratory practice to be followed. These include:

(1) replicate analyses carried out as a matter of course;
(2) analysis of reference materials such as those provided by the Association of Official Analytical Chemists in the United States and by the Community Bureau of Reference of the European Commission;
(3) regular use of standards;
(4) recovery of added standards;
(5) analysis of concealed replicates;
(6) exchange of samples between laboratories;
(7) collaborative tests of methodological protocols;
(8) comparison of values obtained with literature values.[8]

Information on sources of data

It is important to have information on the source of the data in a food composition table to be able to check its appropriateness for the study and to confirm its authenticity. Data in food composition tables can be original analytical values, imputed, calculated, or borrowed.[4,11] Original analytical values are those taken from published literature or unpublished laboratory reports. This latter category includes original calculated values, such as protein values derived by multiplying the nitrogen content by the required factor, and 'logical' values, such as the content of cholesterol in vegetable products, which can be assumed to be zero. Imputed values are estimates derived from analytical values for a similar food or another form of the same food. This category includes those data derived by difference, such as moisture and, in some cases, carbohydrate, and values for chloride calculated from the sodium content. Calculated values are those derived from recipes by calculation from the nutrient content of the ingredients corrected by the application of preparation factors. Such factors take into account losses or gain in weight of the food or of specific nutrients during preparation of the food (see Section 5.3.7). Borrowed values are those derived from other tables or databases without referring to the original source. When a value for the content of a specific nutrient in a food is not included, there is an 'absent' value and, when a table has no values for a particular nutrient, the value is regarded as being 'not included'. The proportion of the various types of data differs between tables and for different nutrients.[12] In some tables, such as the McCance and Widdowson tables in the United Kingdom[13] and the tables in the United States[14], most data are based on analyses that have been carried out especially for inclusion in the tables. Details of the tables can be obtained on the World Wide Web (http://www.inform.umd.edu). In other tables, such as those in the Netherlands, where sources of the data are given in the references[15], information on how the data have been acquired can also be obtained. However, this is not the case for all tables of food composition.

5.3.6 Missing values in food composition tables

In general, original analytical data provides information of the highest quality for inclusion in a food composition table with only such data. Thus, tables often have missing values, which are usually represented by zeros. It is important to realize that missing values in a food table can lead to an underestimate of the intake of a nutrient, especially when there are no values for a nutrient in those foods that make a significant contribution to the supply of that nutrient in the diet. If it is not possible to arrange for foods to be analysed, data can be sought in the literature, imputed, sought from other tables, or estimated as outlined in Section 5.3.5. Alternatively, the intake of a particular nutrient could be estimated by direct analysis (Section 5.3.2), excretion (Section 5.3.2), or by the use of biological markers (Chapter 7).

5.3.7 Nutrient losses and gains during the preparation of foods

The content of nutrients per unit weight of food changes when foods are prepared; such losses and gains can be classified in two ways. The first is related to yield, when the primary ingredients at the pre-cooking stage are compared with the prepared food at the cooking stage and also with the food as consumed at the post-cooking stage. The second is related to changes in the amount of specific nutrients when foods are prepared. In a perfect world, original analytical data would be available for foods at all stages of preparation. However, it is often necessary to make estimates based on the use of factors for calculating the nutrient content of prepared foods from raw ingredients.[16]

5.3.8 Bioavailability

The concept of bioavailability has developed from observations that have shown that measurements of the amount of a nutrient consumed do not necessarily provide a good index of the amount of a nutrient that can be utilized by the body. The bioavailability of a nutrient can be defined as the proportion of that nutrient that is available for utilization by the body.[17] This is not simply the proportion of a nutrient absorbed, and cannot be equated with solubility or diffusibility in in vitro-simulated physiological systems. Bioavailability is not a property of a food nor of a diet per se, but is the result of the interaction between the nutrient in question with other components of the diet and with the individual consuming the diet. Because of the many factors influencing bioavailability, tables of food composition cannot give a single value for a nutrient's bioavailability. Most research up until now has centred upon inorganic constituents, particularly iron, but the concept is applicable to virtually all nutrients. Iron incorporated into haem is more readily absorbed than non-haem iron, and these two forms of iron are sometimes listed separately in food composition tables. But such information does not take into account, for example, the effect of ascorbic acid on non-haem iron absorption. In the coming years, it can be expected that much more work will be carried out on bioavailability than in the past, because of its key role in relating functional nutritional status to nutrient intake.

5.3.9 Ease of use of food composition tables

As well as possessing the attributes outlined above, a food composition table is easier to use if the format allows ready access to the information available. This is not only true for tables in the written form but also for those in a magnetic/electronic form. For the latter, the format in which data are made available to the user depends more on the database access software available (see Section 5.4) than on the way data are stored. Although there is no one correct way of constructing a food table or nutrient database, those contemplating constructing such a table or database are urged to consult the guidelines prepared by Greenfield and Southgate.[4]

5.3.10 Food composition and nutrient databases available

When planning a nutritional epidemiological study, a decision needs to be made as to which table or database will be used. In the first instance, consideration will be given to using national tables/databases because these are more likely to include data on the foods available in the country. However, for international studies, or for those in which it is planned to compare the data with that obtained in another study, consideration may be given to using international tables/databases.

National food composition tables and nutrient data banks

Most people are aware of the tables/databases available in their own countries but are less aware of those available in other countries. A bibliography of food composition tables was published by FAO.[18] To allow people in Europe to know what information is available, a series of inventories of food composition tables and nutrient databases was prepared by EUROFOODS.[19,20] This task is being continued by COST 99 (EUROFOODS), and details can be found via their World Wide Web home page (see bottom of Section 5.3.1). Details of the major food composition tables in Europe with English translations of the introductions, where appropriate, were also prepared under the auspices of EUROFOODS.[5] The INFOODS Secretariat has prepared an international directory of food composition tables which lists tables published throughout the world,[21] and the latest version can be seen on their World Wide Web home page (see bottom of Section 5.3.3).

International food composition tables

At the present time, the main sources of international data on food composition are the tables published by FAO for various regions including Africa,[22] East Asia,[23] and the Near East,[24] and for amino acids.[25] A table for use in tropical countries was prepared by Platt.[26] In addition, there are regional tables such as that prepared by the Caribbean Food and Nutrition Institute[27] for use in the English-speaking Caribbean, by INCAP and ICNND for use in Central America,[28] and by West, Pepping, and Temalilwa[29] for East Africa. However, a number of initiatives are under way to make data on food composition more internationally available. In 1985, EUROFOODS carried out a study to investigate the feasibility and methodology of developing an easily accessible database of food composition data derived from tables and databases currently existing in various European countries. The construction of such a merged database was found to be technically feasible. The problems encountered were tedious but not difficult and were related mostly to language and terminology. There are also questions related to copyright, but these are not technically insurmountable.[30,31] The major problems are financial because national governments are not prepared to finance such a database. Efforts in this area have been made by INFOODS, the International Food Data Systems Organization, which was established in 1983 under the aegis of the

United Nations University to promote international cooperation in the acquisition, quality improvement, and exchange of data on the nutrient composition of foods.[32] (See their World Wide Web home page referred to earlier.) It has convened a number of working groups, which have prepared a series of guidelines on the preparation of food composition tables and nutrient databases[4], on compiling data for food composition databases[33], on identifying food components for data interchange[7], for describing foods[9], and for exchanging data between nutrient databases[34], and on the needs of those who use food composition tables.[35] More recently, The Food and Agricultural Organization of the United Nations (FAO) is also developing new activities in the area. Further information can be obtained from the FAO Director of the Food Policy and Nutrition Division in Rome. EUROFOODS has also produced a number of documents including several which have been referred to earlier.[5,10,12,19,20,36,37,38]

Databases for non-nutrients

Databases for non-nutrients have not been developed to the high degree of sophistication found with those for nutrients. Non-nutrients are a diverse group of substances including 'pseudo-nutrients', such as cholesterol, taurine, and choline; innate natural toxins, such as cyanogenic glycosides; toxins of microbial origin, such as aflatoxin; contaminants, such as polychlorinated biphenyls; and food additives, including emulsifiers, colouring agents, and flavours. As yet, few epidemiological studies have used non-nutrient databases but it can be expected that, as the number and diversity of such databases increase in the coming years, so will the number of studies based on them. There is no readily available inventory of non-nutrient databases.

5.4   Calculation of nutrient intake from data on food intake and on the composition of foods

Up until about 30 years ago, the conversion of food consumption data into estimates of nutrient intake had to be done manually – a laborious and time consuming task. With the advent of mainframe computers, much of the work, especially for larger surveys, could be and in fact has been done on such machines. As with many applications previously confined to mainframe computers, much of the work has now passed on to microcomputers, because of their ready accessibility and ease of use. Data on food and nutrient intakes often subsequently are transferred to a mainframe computer where it can be combined with other survey data for further analysis.

5.4.1   Entry and checking of data

Before proceeding to calculate nutrient intake from data on food consumption, it is necessary to ensure that mistakes that have crept into the data set during collection, coding, aggregation, transcription, and storage, are reduced to an acceptable level. Errors associated with the collection of data on food consumption are discussed in other chapters in this book, and those associated with food composition data are discussed earlier in this chapter. Such problems will therefore not be discussed further here. Regardless of the method used for the collection of data on food consumption, consideration should be given to how the data will be entered into the computer. Suitable forms should be designed for the collection of data. These can be on paper or in a personal computer-based program that can save time and eliminate errors associated with transcription of data from paper to the computer. The use of carefully prepared forms, with information to guide those collecting the data, can reduce the chance of error during the collection of data and, if a separate process, during entry into the computer. Common errors associated with the collection of data include:

(1) recording of data on the wrong subject's form, or incorrect assignment of subject's identification number;
(2) incorrect identification of food;
(3) recording of wrong (sometimes improbable) amounts of food;
(4) omission of data on parts of meals, entire meals, or entire days.

Common errors associated with the entry of data include:

(1) reading errors, which are sometimes associated with illegible handwriting or data that have been altered at the time of collection;
(2) wrong identification numbers being assigned to subjects and entered;
(3) transcription errors often arising from inversion of digits, transposition of amount and food code, or addition/omission of zero values, which give rise to incorrect amounts or food codes;
(4) omission or double entry of data on parts of meals, entire meals, or entire days;
(5) lines or segments of data are shifted, resulting in misreading of data in the data file;
(6) data are erased or lost once entered into the computer.

Because the collection and entry of data are subject to both human and machine error, procedures need to be developed to ensure that the quality of data is as high as possible. Editing and error-checking routines should be incorporated in the data entry process and subsets of data entered into the computer should be compared with the original written records. Where mistakes are found, the extent of the error should be determined, because it could involve data of the previous (or next) subject or day, or that previously (or subsequently) entered by the operator involved. In addition to such checks, frequency distributions of all amounts of food and food codes should be carried out.

5.4.2 Calculation of nutrient intake

The conversion of food consumption to nutrient intake requires computer software and a nutrient database. Great care should be taken to ensure that the software chosen meets the needs of the study adequately. There has been an explosion in the number of software packages available in recent years and there are many to choose from[39] but it is often difficult to make a choice. Apart from the usual criteria that are used to select a computer program, such as compatibility with the computer(s) available, user-friendliness, speed of operation, etc. it is necessary that the program can accept the type of data that are being collected and can produce the type of output required. In recent years, many programs have been developed for use not only with mainframe computers but also for personal computers. For example, the Komeet program has been developed in the authors' laboratory for use with personal computers (for information contact Ben Scholte by fax on + 31 317 315884 or + 31 317 483354). As is necessary, there was close cooperation between the users and the developers of the software. As time goes on, the collection of dietary information will become more automated, as outlined by Arab.[40] With such automation the need for coding foods is unnecessary. It is hoped that further automation will lead to reduced costs and increased quality of the data.

5.4 Food groups and food scores

Foods may be categorized into groups, based on biological characteristics, function in meals or the daily food pattern, or based on their nutrient value. In food composition tables, categorization is based mainly on biological characteristics and/or function within a meal in order to facilitate food identification and the retrieval of comparative foods. For this reason, each food group is allocated a specific code, thus allowing the amount of food in these food groups and the contribution of each food group to the intake of a specific nutrient to be assessed. In the EUROCODE (see Section 5.3.1), there are 14 main food groups and there are subgroups based on species for animal foods and variety for plant foods, plus data on methods of food preparation. In some tables, particularly those for educational purposes, there are subgroups based on the content of specific nutrients such as high fat and low fat dairy products.

Some methods for assessing food consumption, in particular the dietary history and food frequency methods, enquire about the consumption of groups of foods, and not about individual foods. For example, questions on vegetable consumption are directed towards the consumption of dark green leafy vegetables, carrots and pumpkins, and other vegetables. Division of vegetables into these groups is, to some extent, based on their carotene content. Generally, foods are not classified in such a way in food composition tables or nutrient databases. Therefore, specific entries have to be created in the nutrient database to provide appropriate food composition data on such food groups. Values of food composition can be calculated from the weighted mean of the most commonly eaten foods in the food groups. This method has the disadvantage that it is less accurate and, if at a later date there is interest in other nutrients such as trace elements, or in bioavailability, the grouping of foods used may not be appropriate. For this reason and in order to be able to repeat a study, it is important that the method of compiling the food groups is clearly documented.

When assessing nutrient intake, two types of nutrient can often be distinguished: those nutrients that are found in small quantities in a large number of foods, such as iron and many B vitamins, and those that are found in large quantities in a small number of foods, such as cholesterol and vitamin A. It is very difficult to estimate the intake of the latter type of nutrient by many of the conventional methods because of the large day-to-day variation. Thus, specific food frequency methods need to be developed (Chapter 6). Although such estimates are not generally very precise, food and nutrient scores may indicate whether average daily intake is adequate.[41] These scores are calculated as follows:

Food score   = Frequency × Portion size

Nutrient score = Food score × Nutrient composition

Generally, the time interval chosen is 1 day, 1 week, or 1 month.

5.6   Concluding remarks

The disadvantage of using food composition tables and nutrient databases is that each value in the table/database is the average of a value for a limited number of samples of each food. As explained in Section 5.3.4, sampling errors are large, especially for mixed dishes and meals. These errors contribute to the total error and variation in results from dietary intake studies, but as long as no measure of spread is given for values in food composition tables, it will not be possible to calculate what proportion of random error is attributable to variation in food composition. This variation differs from food to food and from nutrient to nutrient. It is well-known that differences in water content are the main cause of variation in the content of other nutrients. Thus, data on the nutrient composition of foods containing large amounts of water are always subject to large variation. The least variable nutrient is probably protein and the other proximate constituents. Table 5.2 presents data in which analysed and calculated values for energy and proximate constituents of an experimental diet are compared. The data indicate that the differences are all within 10 per cent, which is not sufficient for a metabolic ward study but suggest that data derived from using food composition tables are probably adequate for epidemiological studies aimed at classifying individuals or groups of individuals on the basis of their nutrient intake.

Variation in the vitamin content of foods is generally much greater than that for macronutrients. Therefore, an assessment of the vitamin content of a diet based on data in food composition tables/nutrient databases is, for most vitamins, not very reliable. At best, classification of intake into high and low is all that can be done. This

Table 5.23 Differences between the composition of a one-day experimental diet determined by analysis of a duplicate portion and by the use of food composition tables.*

	Analysed a	Calculated c	Difference c-a	Difference c-a in %	Difference c-a in energy %
Energy (kJ)	8895	9050	155	1.7	
Protein (g)	60	64.9	4.9	8.1	0.5
Fat (g)	103	110.7	7.7	7.5	2.6
Carbohydrate (g)	233	220.0	−13.0	−5.6	−3.2
Mono and disaccharides (g)	108	103.1	−4.9	−4.5	−1.2

* Unpublished data cited in van Staveren and Burema[43]

Table 5.3 Provitamin A content of frequently eaten Indonesian vegetables and fruits in different food composition tables. (Modified from De Pee et al.[44])

Foods			Provitamin A content		
Indonesian name	English name	Scientific name	Indonesian tables[45]	Recent data in literature[46] RE* / 100 g food as eaten	Analysed[47]
Bayam	Spinach	*Amaranthus viridis*	914	207	640
Daun katuk	Leaf sweet shoot	*Sauropus androgynus*	1556	608	1889
Daun melinjo	Jointfir spinach leaf	*Gnetum gemon*	1500	608	289
Daun singkong	Cassava leaves	*Manihot utulissima*	1650	1055	1776
Kangkung	Water spinach	*Ipomoea aquatica*	945	214	492

* RE – Retinol Equivalents

is illustrated by recent work on the provitamin A content of foods in Indonesia as shown in Table 5.3.

For minerals, tables/databases are also of limited value, although calcium may be an exception because the main source of calcium in many cultures is milk and milk products, and the calcium content of milk products is relatively constant.

The situation for minerals is complicated by the large variation in the mineral content of foods and also by the wide variation in the biological availability of minerals in different diets and in different people. The whole subject of bioavailability is one that, as yet, has hardly been addressed.

Thus it can be concluded that food composition tables/nutrient databases can be of great value in epidemiological research, but knowledge of how they are constructed and their limitations is necessary to make intelligent use of them. In general, it is better to use food composition tables compiled for local use. However, for international studies, data on food composition should be comparable and the efforts of organizations such as INFOODS and EUROFOODS are directed towards this goal.

References

1. Thomas, R. U., Rutlege, M. M., Beach, E. F., Moyer, E. Z., Drummond, M. C., Miller, S., et al. (1950) Nutritional status of children. XII. Accuracy of calculated intakes of food components with respect to analytical values. *J. Am. Diet. Assoc.* **26**: 889–96.
2. Leitch, I. and Aitken, F. C. (1950) Technique and interpretation of dietary surveys. *Nutr. Abstr. Rev.* **19**: 507–25.
3. Southgate, D. A. T. (1974) *Guidelines for the preparation of tables of food composition.* p. 57ff. Karger, Basel.
4. Greenfield, H. and Southgate, D. A. T. (1992) *Food composition data: production, management and use.* Chapman and Hall, Hampshire, UK.
5. Arab, L., Wittier, M. and Schettler, G. (1987) *European food composition tables in translation.* pp. viii and 155. Springer-Verlag, Heidelberg.

6. Southgate, D. A. T. and Durnin, J. V. G. A. (1970) Caloric conversion factors: an experimental evaluation of the factors used in the calculation of the energy value of human diets. *Br. J. Nutr.* **24**: 517–35.

7. Klensin, J. C., Feskanich, D., Lin, V., Truswell, A. S. and Southgate, D. A. T. (1989) *Identification of food components for INFOODS data interchange.* United Nations University Press, Tokyo.

8. Southgate, D. A. T. (1985) Criteria to be used for acceptance of data in nutrient databases. *Ann. Nut. Metab.* **29**(Suppl. 1): 47–53.

9. Truswell, A. S., Bateson, D., Madafiglio, K., Pennington, J. A. T., Rand, W. M. and Klensin, J. C. (1991) INFOODS guidelines for describing foods: a systematic approach to describing foods to facilitate international exchange of food composition data. *J. Food Comp. Anal.* **4**: 18–38.

10. Hollman, P. C. H. and Katan, M. B. (1988) Bias and error in the determination of common macronutrients in foods: an interlaboratory trial. *J. Am. Diet. Assoc.* **88**: 556–63.

11. Greenfield, H. and Southgate, D. A. T. (1985) A pragmatic approach to production of good quality food composition data. *ASEAN Food J.* **1**: 47–54.

12. Meyer, B., Van Oosten-Van der Goes, H. J. C., van Staveren, W. A. and West, C. E. (1988) Missing values in European food composition tables and nutrient databases: preliminary results of a survey. *Food Sci. Nutr.* **42F**: 29–34.

13. Paul, A. A. and Southgate, D. A. T. (1978) *McCance and Widdowson's the composition of foods.* 4th edn. Her Majesty's Stationery Office, London.

14. USDA (1976) *Composition of foods, Agricultural Handbook No. 8.* United States Department of Agriculture, Washington (the latest version is available on the World Wide Web).

15. NEVO (1989) *NEVO tabel: Nederlands voedingsstoffenbestand.* NEVO (Stichting Nederlands Voedingsstoffenbestand), CIVO-instituten, Zeist and Voorlichtingsbureau voor de Voedings, Gravenhage.

16. Bergström, L. (1985) *Nutrient losses and gains in the preparation of foods.* Report 32/94. National Food Administration, Uppsala, Sweden.

17. Southgate, D. A. T. (1989) Bioavailability: conceptual issues and significance for the nutritional sciences. In: Kim Wha Young (ed.) *Proceedings of the 14th International Congress of Nutrition,* pp. 777–80. The 14th ICN Organizing Committee, Seoul.

18. FAO (1975) *Food composition tables: updated annotated bibliography.* FAO, Rome.

19. EUROFOODS (1985) Review of food composition tables and nutrient data banks in Europe. *Ann. Nut. Metab.* **29**(Suppl. 1): 11–45.

20. West, C. E. (1990) *Inventory of European food composition tables and nutrient database systems.* National Food Administraiton, Uppsala, Sweden.

21. Heinize, D., Klensin, J. C. and Rand, W. M. (1988) *International directory of food composition tables.* 2nd edn. INFOODS Secretariat, Massachusetts Institute of Technology, Cambridge, MA.

22. Wu Leung, W. T., Busson, F. and Jardin, C. (1968) *Food composition table for use in Africa.* US Dept. of Health, Education, and Welfare, Bethesda, Md, and FAO, Rome.

23. Wu, Leung, W. T., Butrum, R. and Chang, F. H. (1972) *Food composition table for use in East Africa.* US Dept. of Health, Education, and Welfare, Bethesda, MD, and FAO, Rome.

24. Pollachi, W., McHargue, J. S. and Perloff, B. P. (1982) *Food composition tables for the Near East.* FAO Food and Nutrition Paper No. 26. FAO, Rome and USDA, Washington.

25. Pollachi, W., McHargue, J. S. and Perloff, B. P. (1972) *Amino acid content of foods and biological data of proteins.* 2nd edn. FAO, Rome.

26. Platt, B. S. (1962) *Tables of representative values of foods commonly eaten in tropical countries.* Medical Research Council Special Report Series No. 302. Her Majesty's Stationery Office, London.

27. Caribbean Food and Nutrition Institute (1974) *Food composition tables for use in the English-speaking Caribbean.* Caribbean Food and Nutrition Institute, Kingston, Jamaica.

28. Wu Leung, W. T. and Flores, M. (1961) *INCAP-ICNND food composition table for use in Latin America*. INCAP, Guatemala and Bethesda, Md: National Institutes of Health.

29. West, C. E., Pepping, F. and Temalilwa, C. R. (1988) *The composition of foods commonly eaten in East Africa*. Wageningen Agricultural University, Wageningen.

30. Castenmiller, J. J. M., Southgate, D. A. T. and West, C. E. (1996) *Constructing a nutritional database for use in Europe*. Discussion paper for COST Action 99 meeting, 8–9 March 1996, Stuttgart. Wageningen Agricultural University, Wageningen.

31. Buss, D. H. and West, C. E. (1996) *Sharing European food composition table values: future needs for cooperation between users and compilers in different countries*. Discussion paper for COST Action 99 meeting, 8–9 March 1996, Stuttgart. Wageningen Agricultural University, Wageningen.

32. Rand, W. M. and Young, V. R. (1984) Report of a planning conference concerning an international network of food data systems (INFOODS). *Am. J. Clin. Nutr.* **30**: 144–51.

33. Rand, W. M., Pennington, J. A. T., Murphy, S. P. and Klensin, J. C. (1991) *Compiling data for food composition databases*. United Nations University Press, Tokyo.

34. Klensin, J. C. (1992) *Food composition data interchange handbook*. The United Nations University Press, Tokyo.

35. Rand, W. M., Windham, C. T., Wyse, B. W. and Young, V. R. (1988) *Food composition data: a user's perspective*. United Nations University Press, Tokyo.

36. West, C. E. (ed.) (1985) Eurofoods: towards compatibility of nutrient data banks in Europe. *Ann. Nut. Met.* **29**(Suppl. 1): 1–72.

37. Fox, K. and Stockley, L. (1988) EUROFOODS: Proceedings of the Second Workshop. *Food Sciences and Nutrition*. **42F**: 1–82.

38. Becker, W. and Danfors, S. (1990) *4th Eurofoods Meeting May 31–June 3, 1989. Uppsala, Sweden: Proceedings*. Swedish National Food Administration, Uppsala.

39. University of Washington Computer Services (1989) *Computer programs and databases in the field of Nutrition*. University of Washington Computer Services, Seattle, WA.

40. Arab, L. (1988) Analyses, presentation, and interpretation of results. In: Cameron, M. E. and van Staveren, W. A. (ed.) *Manual on methodology for food consumption studies*. Oxford University Press, Oxford.

41. Bazzarre, T. and Myers, M. (1979) The collection of food intake data in cancer epidemiology studies. *Nutr. Cancer*. **5**: 201–14.

42. Van der Haar, F. and Kromhout, D. (1985) Food intake, nutritional anthropometry and blood chemical parameters in three selected Dutch school children populations. *Meded. Landbouwhogeshool Wageningen*. **5**: 78–9.

43. Van Staveren, W. A. and Burema, J. (1985) Food consumption surveys: frustrations and expectations. *Näringsforskning*. **29**: 38–42.

44. De Pee, S., West, C. E., van Staveren, W. A. and Muhilal. Vitamin A intake of breastfeeding women in Indonesia: critical evaluation of a semi-quantitative food frequency questionnaire. Submitted for publication.

45. Hardinsyah, and Briawan, D. (1990) *Penilaian dan perencanaan konsumsi pangan (Food composition: calculation and planning)*. 140 pp. Institut Pertanian Bogor, Fakultas Pertanian, Bogor, Indonesia.

46. West, C. E. and Poortvliet, E. J. (1993) *The carotenoid content of foods with special reference to developing countries*. USAID-VITAL, Washington, DC.

47. Xu Chao, Hulshof, P. J. M., van de Bovenkamp, P., Muhilal, and West, C. E. Validation of a method for the determination of carotenoids and its application to Indonesian foods. Submitted for publication.

6. Assessment of food consumption and nutrient intake

Michael Nelson and Sheila A. Bingham

6.1 Introduction

A major challenge facing the nutritional epidemiologist is the correct measurement of dietary exposure.[1] An apparently straightforward task is fraught with difficulties, and plagued by a seemingly endless list of factors which will introduce error into the simplest measurement. If the aim is to measure current diet, the Heisenberg uncertainty principle rears its head: as you stop something to measure it, you change its behaviour. If the aim is to measure past dietary exposure, then one is reliant on the memory, conceptual abilities, and ruthless honesty on the part of respondents. There are particular problems associated with the measurement of diet within single populations where there is little dietary variation between individuals but large measurement error associated with each individual assessment. It would seem that no direct measure of what people eat will provide a true picture of their dietary habits. And this is before one considers the error introduced by the use of food composition tables (see Chapter 5).

Nevertheless, in the absence of truly objective measures of diet, it is the task of the nutritional epidemiologist to obtain the best measure of diet possible. This chapter is devoted to an exploration of how such measurements can be obtained with the minimum of error. Equally important, it addresses the question of how best to measure the error itself, as a knowledge of the size of the error in dietary assessments will provide valuable information about the likely attenuation of risk estimates based on imprecise measurements. Two bibliographies of almost 300 dietary validation and calibration studies have recently been published.[2,3]

Section A looks at measures of diet available at the household level. It outlines methods for assessing household diets, and explores ways in which household data can be manipulated for epidemiological purposes. Section B looks at measures of diet in individuals. It questions in a positive way the notion that 'current' is equivalent to 'valid' by examining the relationship between current records and external standards which offer scope for assessing the validity of dietary records. (The design and implementation of validation studies is described in Chapter 8.) Section B concludes with a discussion on the assessment of past diet, using a variety of techniques, and addresses the problems of deciding which measures are appropriate in which circumstances.

SECTION A   HOUSEHOLD BASED SURVEYS

6.2   Introduction

Measures of exposure relevant to nutritional epidemiology are often collected at the household level in the course of monitoring food consumption, health, or expenditure for non-epidemiological purposes. In consequence, there already exist large bodies of data which are sufficient in their own right for epidemiological analysis. For example, the British National Food Survey provides detailed information on food acquisition at the household level. This has been used in conjunction with existing health statistics to examine the aetiology of appendicitis.[4] To have collected this data *de novo* would have been a long and costly exercise.

Data available at national level are discussed in Chapter 12. This section focuses on data collected at the household level, as this can be more economical than individual surveys (see Section B) for obtaining information for ecological studies. It also opens possibilities for assessing diet–disease relationships in a number of different subgroups within the population if the distribution of food and nutrients within households can be properly assessed. Use of existing health data is discussed elsewhere.[5]

6.3   Characteristics of household data

Aggregate data based on surveys of groups of people rather than individuals can be used in ecological, geographical, and community trial studies to assess diet–disease relationships. The unit in which these data are collected is usually the household, although information can be usefully collected at the institution level.[6] These studies often shed light on the diversity of food consumption patterns between communities at far less cost than individual surveys. They can also provide opportunities to aggregate data along regional or socio–economic lines. Such studies are often carried out by government or other bodies for non-epidemiological purposes, but can provide a ready-made database with epidemiological applications. Their principal drawback is that the relationships between diet and disease cannot be assessed at the level of the individual, although techniques exist for estimating the distribution of food[7] and nutrients.[8] They are therefore more appropriate for hypothesis generating studies rather than for testing specific hypotheses concerning the causation of disease in particular individuals (see Chapter 12 for more detailed discussion of ecological studies). Special problems occur when estimating individual intakes in households where members eat from communal vessels.[9,10]

Many household food consumption studies focus on economic rather than nutritional aspects of diet.[11,12,13] This is not adequate for most nutritional epidemiological studies: to be of use, they must have as their basis:

(1) the quantitative measurement of food acquired for consumption over a given time period;
(2) a reasonable level of disaggregation of food items or groups;
(3) information on the number, age, and gender of people sharing the food. This is

needed to standardize estimates of food availability for purposes of comparison between groups.

Questions about the distribution of food within the group, and the importance of the age structure in comparing groups are discussed later in Section 6.4.1.

6.4   Techniques, uses, and limitations

There are four principle methods of assessment at the household level which have been used: food accounts, inventories, household recall, and list-recall.[14] They vary in respondent and interviewer burden, and each has its advantages according to the degree of accuracy required at the household level, the degree of literacy and numeracy within the population, and the extent to which food is consumed from outside the household or institution food supply.

6.4.1   Food account method

This method is based upon the household. The main respondent (housewife, or person responsible for food purchasing and/or preparation), or the interviewer, keeps a detailed record of the quantities of food entering the household, including purchases, food from allotments or gardens, gifts, payments in kind, and other sources. In its most widely used form, no attempt is made to assess changes in stocks (see Inventory method, Section 6.4.2). The method assumes that within a given category of household composition, over a sufficient number of households, there is no change in the *average* levels of food stocks, although it is recognized that some households will acquire more food than they consume over the survey period, while others will acquire less and use existing stocks to make up for any shortfalls in acquisition. Efforts are made to estimate the proportion of the diet consumed from outside the household food supply (usually in the form of a menu diary kept for or by each household member), some surveys attempting to measure directly the food consumed outside the home. The nutrient content of the diet can be estimated using appropriate nutrient conversion tables. Preparation losses and waste are estimated, and the diet obtained outside the home is assumed to have a composition similar to the home food supply.

The longest running of these surveys is the British Household Food Consumption and Expenditure Survey (The National Food Survey (NFS)), conducted annually for half a century.[15] The Survey was begun in 1940 to monitor the nutritional quality of the diets of urban working class households[16,17] in order to assess the value of the wartime food policy, but by 1950 it had been extended to cover virtually all sectors of the population. In its original form it included a larder inventory (see 6.4.2)[18], but this was dropped in 1952, and the survey continued essentially unchanged[19] until 1992, when assessments of sweets, soft drinks, alcohol, and foods eaten away from home were included.[20] Reports are published annually, and these provide an excellent unbroken record of British food habits since 1950. The published results afford opportunities to conduct time trend[21,22], social class[23,24], and regional[25] analyses in relation to epidemiological questions, and some methodological issues in its use have been discussed by Derry and Buss[26] and Nelson and co-workers.[27]

Across Europe, a large number of household budget surveys (HBS) have been conducted. Although the frequency and level of detail of the information on food varies widely[28] they provide an extremely useful database for within- and between-country epidemiological analysis. Considerable efforts are being made to find a common grouping of foods which would allow direct comparisons between countries.[29,30]

Surveys are carried out typically every five years, although in some countries they are conducted annually. Sampling is usually based on census or geographical (postcode) data, using a stratified or cluster approach. Some countries replace non-compliant households in the sample, whereas others do not. In every country, certain households are excluded, but the exclusion criteria vary between countries (e.g. in Sweden house-holders over 74 are excluded, in Poland the self-employed are excluded). Cooperation rates range from 11% (in Belgium) to 97% (in Cyprus), although in most countries well over half of those invited participate. The cooperation rate has important implications for the generalizability of the results, and the extent to which the findings may be compared with health data for similar regions or population subgroups, or between countries. Kemsley[31] examined the effect of non-response in the British NFS, showing that when the results were re-weighted to the characteristics of the entire sample (based on census data describing the non-responding households), the national averages for food and nutrient consumption remained essentially unchanged. The effect of differ-ential non-response by income group was not assessed.

The length of time for which information is recorded will affect the level of precision for the estimates of food consumption and nutrient intake. Most surveys record data for between one and four weeks, although some last for two to three months, or even longer. Longer recording periods will in theory improve the representativeness of the findings in each household and improve estimates of consumption for small subgroups within the community. There may, however, be fatigue effects.

The level of disaggregation of food data varies widely, from as few as 46 groups in Italy to as many as 500 in the Netherlands. Fewer food groups will result in less precise estimates of nutrient contents of the diet, and fewer opportunities to test epidemiological hypotheses.

Studies vary in the ways in which waste and pet foods are handled, and in making allowance for purchases of bulk items. Particularly difficult issues arise around the recording of foods eaten away from home, the consumption of food by visitors, and the recording of alcoholic beverages (more often just by price than by quantity) and vitamin and mineral supplements (usually omitted). These may affect the completeness of the estimates of food consumption and energy and nutrient intake differentially between population subgroups, making comparisons within countries (let alone be-tween countries) less viable.

Results can be calculated in terms of average consumption per person, or can take into account differences in requirements by expressing consumption as a percentage of dietary reference values. The latter method has the advantage of taking into account differences between age and gender structure in different segments of the community, but the reference values differ to some extent between countries.[32] The way in which consumption of food by visitors or outside the home is handled will also influence the final estimates of intake or adequacy. Uniform factors applied to account for waste (e.g. in the British NFS it is assumed that 10% of food is wasted) do not distinguish between items like cooking oil (for which wastage may be high) and meat (for which it is likely to be low).

All surveys collect data on the socio–economic background of each household. It is possible therefore to aggregate the data in a wide variety of ways (e.g. according to region, household income group, population density, age of housewife). Increasingly, the basic data on food acquisitions, nutrient intakes, and socio–economic and demographic information is being stored on magnetic media and being made available for research purposes.

Strengths and limitations

The principal strengths of the HBS data are their availability and (in some countries) continuity. They are accessible and cheap for analysing food and nutrient consumption trends in epidemiological studies. With the availability of the data on magnetic media, detailed geographical[4] or income group[33] comparisons can be undertaken. Because the surveys are undertaken routinely on behalf of the government, it may be possible to include special studies on a subsample (e.g. milk consumption in children).

The limitations of the HBS deserve close attention in order to avoid misinterpretation of results based on its analysis.

1. *Validity of the method*: HBS estimates of consumption are typically between 5% and 25% below national accounts based on food disappearance data (food balance sheets), taking into account imports, exports, and food moving in and out of stocks.[27,28] The source of the discrepancy may lie in the extent to which food balance sheets tend to overestimate availability. However, two surveys have compared the average level of purchases in the British National Food Survey with average consumption estimated independently, one in elderly single women[34] and one in families with two adults and two or three children.[27] These studies suggest that the NFS tends to stimulate overpurchasing, i.e. foods are purchased in excess of requirements during the survey week. For many groups of households, it is likely that the degree of overpurchasing is roughly equal to the amount consumed outside the home, so that when average food or nutrient availability is calculated, it approximates the actual level of consumption (less any waste). The overpurchasing, however, appears to be greater in households on low incomes[35] and amongst the elderly[34], so comparisons between income or age groups are likely to be less reliable than those between regions (assuming no major demographic differences in population structure), or over time within given groups of households of a consistent socio–economic mix.

2. *The data provide information on households, not individuals*: In the calculation of dietary adequacy, HBS tacitly assume that nutrient is distributed to individuals within households according to the dietary reference values, but this is likely to overstate the dietary adequacy of some groups (such as women and young girls) and understate it in others (men and boys).[36] Alternatives to the dietary reference values can be used for estimating nutrient distribution within families in epidemiological studies[9,10,36,37,38], but the reliability of these approaches needs further assessment.

Recently, statistical techniques have been used for modelling within household food and nutrient distribution.[7,8] The results from the modelling exercise have been compared with existing data on food consumption and nutrient intake in nationally

Table 6.1 Differences between household budget survey (HBS) data and dietary reference measures used for validation purposes.

	HBS	Dietary reference measure
Data source	Household	Individual
Data type	Food acquisition data	Food consumption (repeat 24 hr recall; weighed inventory; household measures)
Sources of error:		
Food stuffs	Mainly unprocessed Listed separately and used in cooking (e.g. oil)	Mainly ready to eat Incorporated in foods, do not appear separately (e.g. flour)
Food composition data	Relates to foods as purchased – preparation losses – vitamin and mineral losses	Relates to foods as eaten – preparation losses – recipe variations
Waste	Estimated by survey of preparation losses and household food waste	Measured as individual plate waste but not at preparation stage
Distribution within households	Estimated by modelling	Estimated by factors (man values, family values)
Reporting bias	Over-reporting likely overall, but individual households who over-report are difficult to identify. May be regional or socio–economic biases in over-reporting	Under-reporting likely, under-reporting not always in the same households. Extreme under-reporting can be identified.

representative samples of individuals[39,40,41], and there has been good agreement. There are problems in the validation of such models, and these are summarized in Table 6.1. An important issue concerns the validity of the reference measures themselves. For example, if energy intake based on a seven-day weighed record of individual diet (the reference measure) is less than 1.2 times Basal Metabolic Rate (BMR), the subject may be regarded as having under-reported their usual intake[42] and might be legitimately excluded from the analyses. If a particular subset of the reference group is thereby excluded[43] (e.g. overweight subjects tend to under-report intake more often than normal weight or lean subjects), then the reference group may no longer be directly comparable to the HBS sample for purposes of validation. A large number of data sets on individuals are available for comparison with British HBS data.[44]

3. *The data must be aggregated over groups of households*: Because no measure is made of changes in larder stocks, the results for a single household over one or two weeks are unlikely to represent the usual consumption levels in that household. (The exception to this may be in some developing countries or low income groups where the range of foodstuffs is narrow, food acquisition is frequent, and storage facilities are minimal.) The reliability of results for small groups of households may be poor if the between-household variability is large, and any analysis of small groups should ensure that the grouping of the households does not depend in any way on the apparent level of purchase (or expenditure).[33] Aggregated household data cannot be used to estimate disease risk to individuals within households having high or low consumption of a particular food or nutrient.

4. *The data are confined to food brought into the home*: Although the analyses of nutrient adequacy may take into account the amount of food consumed outside the home, this amount is probably an underestimate, as foods eaten between meals are not taken into account.[35] Comparisons between large regions are likely to be less subject to differential misclassification. Time trend analysis may be viable provided the proportion of meals eaten outside the home does not change appreciably over time. When comparing smaller groups of households or assessing differences between household types, it is necessary to ensure that any differences observed are not due to differences in the proportion of the diet consumed away from home.

5. *Exclusion of sweets, chocolates, alcoholic beverages, soft drinks, and vitamin and mineral supplements*: Apart from vitamin and mineral supplements, these foods can be regarded primarily as sources of energy. If comparisons between groups include an analysis of energy, fat, or carbohydrate, attempts must be made to ensure that these missing items are unlikely to provide a significantly different proportion of energy or nutrient in the different groups. HBS are therefore arguably better for monitoring trends in protein, dietary fibre, and mineral and vitamin consumption (where supplements do not make substantial contributions to intake), taking into account the limitations of the food composition tables (see Chapter 5).

6.4.2   Inventory method

The inventory method is similar in nature to the food account method, in that respondents are asked to keep records of all foods coming into the house. In addition, a larder inventory is carried out at the beginning and end of the survey period. This was the method used by the NFS prior to 1952, including the first study on urban working class households.[16] The ability of respondents to provide accurate inventory data is good.[45]

6.4.3   Comparison of food account and food inventory methods

Both the food inventory and the food account method are appropriate to communities in which a high proportion of food is purchased rather than home produced, and where the level of literacy is high. Where the interviewer has regular access to the respondent, it may be possible to obtain information by recall concerning the amounts of foods removed from stores.

The principal advantage of the food inventory over the food account method is that it provides a direct measure of the amount of food and nutrient available for consumption within a single household. In contrast to the food account method, this allows single households to be identified on the basis of the nutrient available to the household members, and so to correlate food or nutrient availability (making appropriate assumptions concerning distribution within the household) with disease occurrence within the household.

Most household surveys cover a period of one or two weeks. This may be associated in the food account method with an initial reaction to 'stock up' on items.[27,34,46] This can be taken into account in the food inventory method by subtracting from the total available those foods which have been acquired but not consumed. However, the food inventory may draw to respondents' attention items in the larder which would otherwise have remained unused, and may therefore distort the usual purchasing pattern.[6,47]

6.4.4 Household record

In the household record method, the foods available for consumption (whether raw or processed) are weighed, or estimated in household measures, allowing for preparation waste (e.g. discarded outer leaves, peel, trimmed fat). Any food consumed by visitors is estimated and subtracted from the total, and an allowance should also be made for food waste (food prepared but not consumed), either by collecting the waste directly (which is likely to underestimate the true waste[48]), or by estimating the proportion of the total prepared food believed to be wasted. The technique is often a combination of recall and record, and a recommended approach has been outlined.[6] Briefly, the interviewer calls in the morning, establishes the household composition, and asks the respondent to recall the quantities of food used to prepare breakfast. The foods to be used in the preparation of lunch can then be weighed or recorded in household measures. An afternoon interview allows the waste at lunch to be estimated, and the foods for the evening meal to be measured and recorded.

Uses and limitations

The technique is well suited to populations in which a substantial proportion of the diet is home-produced rather than pre-processed. It lends itself for use in populations where the level of literacy is variable or low, as the number of visits to each household can easily be tailored to obtain the necessary degree of detail. Because the technique provides a direct measure of food available for consumption and makes no assumptions about changes in food stocks, it can be used, like the inventory method, to identify households with particular consumption characteristics (subject, of course, to a knowledge of the day-to-day or week-to-week variability in consumption within households).

As with other household food assessment methods, no information is obtained concerning the distribution of foods to individuals within the household, nor about consumption of foods outside the home. (An elaboration of the household record method, the semi-weighed technique, has been described by Nelson and Nettleton[49], in which household consumption is measured at the preparation stage, and distribution to individual household members is described in household measures). As it is more likely to be used in less developed countries where literacy is low, there may be seasonal variations in consumption which need to be taken into account. This is especially important in epidemiological studies where regional comparisons are undertaken and recording takes place in different regions at different times of the year, or where it is proposed to examine diet–disease relationships within households.

6.4.5 List-recall method

This is a structured survey in which the respondent is asked to recall the amount and cost of food obtained for household use over a given period, usually one week. In addition to food purchases and acquisitions, it takes into account the use of food. It can therefore be used to provide an estimate of food costs, and for nutritional epidemiological purposes, net household consumption of both foods and nutrients. The technique has been used in the United States food consumption surveys.[50]

Uses and limitations

The technique is well suited to populations in which most food is purchased rather than home-produced. It is relatively quick and cheap as it requires only a single interview. It is helpful to notify the respondent of the study in advance, in order that he or she may keep records of purchases (such as supermarket receipts) to aid the recall, but this may have the effect of distorting food consumption patterns. The information on food use helps to overcome problems about movement of foods into and out of stock, but distortions in recall which are characteristic of any memory based survey will inevitably influence the outcome, although perhaps less so than in individual surveys. Problems persist concerning foods eaten away from home, consumption of food by visitors, and distribution of nutrients within families.

Studies on the validity and reliability of list-recall surveys have been reviewed by Burk and Paso[51] and Öhlin *et al.*[2] These suggest that list-recall methods give values some 20% lower than inventory methods. Conversely, comparison of the 1955–65 United States household food consumption survey results with food disappearance data showed that the list-recall gave values some 5–10% higher. This lack of consistency in comparative validity suggests that substantially more work needs to be done to characterize the nature of the error in list-recall surveys.

6.5   Using household surveys in epidemiological studies

Household food consumption surveys provide a powerful yet economical tool for obtaining information about the food consumption characteristics of a wide cross-section of the population. In most instances the data have already been collected at the expense of government, so the costs to the epidemiologist are enormously reduced and relate solely to the collection of non-nutritional information and analysis of the data.

Household food surveys fail in two major areas: completeness of data, and knowledge of distribution of food and nutrient within households. In addition, little is known about the within-household repeatability of measurements, and the extent to which differential biases in recording between population subgroups, regions, and between countries may influence epidemiological comparisons. It is worth considering ways in which these problems can be addressed.

Lack of completeness: This relates to foods not recorded, foods obtained and eaten away from home, food consumed by visitors, and waste. Where data have already been collected, as in HBS, the investigator is restricted in interpretation of data by the assumptions inherent in the survey design. If the opportunity is available to undertake a household survey *de novo*, however, then it may be possible to collect data on *all* food consumed, not just those items under the purview of the respondent. This requires a record from every individual within the household, in household measures, of foods obtained and eaten away from home, and of foods such as chocolate, sweets, soft drinks, and alcoholic beverages which may not be included in the record of household food acquisitions or consumption. For children, the responsibility for the record would have to lie with an adult. Information concerning the consumption of food by visitors should also be obtained, again if possible in household measures. Collection of this information will substantially improve the quality of the data for relatively little effort on the part of the respondents. It also enables a more accurate calculation of the proportion of food in the diet obtained from outside the household food supply. The data resulting from the introduction of such measurements would need to be compared with the outcomes from assessment of individuals' complete diets. The matter of waste remains a thorny one, and until less invasive techniques are established, we will have to rely on existing estimates.[27,48]

Lack of knowledge about the distribution of consumption within households: It is clear that nutrient distribution is not in accordance with dietary reference values[36,38], and the DRVs provide no clues as to the distribution of foods within the households. The semi-weighed technique mentioned above[49] has addressed this problem by recording the diet of every household member individually. While the technique may be too labour intensive to consider using in a large epidemiological study, it could be used to determine within-household food and nutrient distribution in a subset of households from a larger survey in which household food acquisition data were being obtained. This would then allow a more accurate estimate of distribution of food consumption and nutrient intakes within a given sample. This could considerably enhance the value of a geographical study, for instance, by allowing diet–disease comparisons to be made in a number of age–gender subgroups. The modelling techniques described in Section 6.4.1 offer some further opportunities for analysis, but they require further examination and development.

Comparisons between countries using HBS data are fraught with problems related to food grouping and conversion from estimates of food acquisition to nutrient intakes. This problem now forms the core of the DAFNE (Data Food Networking) project coordinated by Prof. A. Trichopoulou at the National Centre for Nutrition, National School of Public Health, Athens, Greece. Involving 11 European countries (Belgium, Germany, Great Britain, Greece, Hungary, Ireland, Italy, Luxembourg, Norway, Poland, Spain), the project aims to report by the end of 1996 on the first phase of the work.

One final point worth mentioning is that virtually no studies have been carried out to assess the ideal period for recording household food data, nor to assess the within-household variability in purchases of food and nutrient distribution. Most studies in industrialized countries obtain data from each household for a period of one or two weeks. The variability of nutrient intake, and more so, the variability of food consumption, means that for a given period of recording, the error in the estimate of intake or consumption will differ substantially between nutrients or foods. For a given difference in intake or consumption between groups of households, the ability to demonstrate a significant risk of disease in relation to diet is inversely related to the size of the within-household variability. New nutritional epidemiological studies based on households should attempt to assess within- as well as between-household variance in consumption or intake. Any analysis which includes estimates of the distribution of foods or nutrients within households should also consider the errors associated with such estimates.

SECTION B   INDIVIDUAL SURVEYS

6.6   Introduction

Nutritional epidemiology provides the only direct approach to the assessment of risks from diet in most chronic disease. The majority of nutritional epidemiological studies require detailed information on diet and nutrient intake from large numbers of subjects. The aim is to characterize present diet (e.g. in cohort studies) or the diet at a time in the past which coincides with the induction of disease (e.g. case-control studies), although recent dietary factors which influence the progress of disease may also be of interest. The choice of prospective or retrospective methods (Table 6.2) will be dictated in part by the study design, and in part by available resources, respondent skills, etc. Where doubts exist concerning subjects' abilities to recall past diet accurately, the investigator may need to make assumptions regarding associations between current and past diet. Very few studies have addressed the question of methodology and validity of recall of diet in the distant past.

Virtually all methods depend on the ability of the subject to provide accurate information, none of which is easily corroborated. It is therefore necessary to establish the validity of the responses obtained. Ideally, a valid external measure (such as a

Table 6.2   Advantages and disadvantages of prospective and retrospective methods of dietary assessment

Method	Advantages	Disadvantages
Prospective	Current diet Direct observation Daily variation described Length of recording can be varied to suit study needs	Labour intensive for respondent and data entry Requires respondent skills (numeracy and literacy) Under-reporting likely in some population subgroups Expensive
Retrospective	Quick Cheap Low subject motivation Lower literacy and numeracy skills than prospective methods Good cooperation Can be posted	Reliant on memory Conceptualization skills needed to describe accurately frequency of consumption and food portion sizes Observer bias possible Reported diet may be a distortion of usual diet May lack measure of day-to-day variation in diet Requires regular eating habits Dependent on food composition tables

validated estimate of consumption or biochemical marker of intake) can be used to assess the validity of the measurements. Alternatively, internal markers of validity (in which the subject is asked for the same information in different ways) may be used, but the weakness of this approach is that a bias in one aspect of measurement may be carried over to another. The purpose of the validation process is to assess the extent to which subjects may be misclassified using the chosen measuring instrument. Some studies which assess measurement error are limited to measures of repeatability, an important part of the validation process, but not in itself sufficient to show whether differential misclassification is likely to affect the interpretation of results in an epidemiological study. A full discussion of the validation process is given in Chapter 8.

6.7   Methods for assessment of present or recent diet

There are many methods in use for the measurement of diet in cohort, cross-sectional, and intervention studies, where the aim is to assess contemporaneous diet. Details, together with practical advice on equipment, timing, protocols, etc. are given elsewhere[14,52,53] but methods generally consist either of the collation of observations from a number of separate days' investigations, as in records, checklists, and 24-hour recalls, or attempts to obtain average intake by asking about the usual frequency of food consumption, as in the diet history and food frequency questionnaires (FFQ). In all methods of dietary assessment, some estimate of the weight of food consumed is required and, for the determination of nutrient or other food component intake, either an appropriate description for use with food tables or an aliquot for chemical analysis is necessary (see Chapter 5).

6.7.1   Food frequency questionnaires (FFQ)

Of all methods, FFQ are the most frequently used in cohort studies in epidemiology. They are designed to assess usual eating habits, over recent months or years, and comprise a list of foods most informative about the nutrients or foods of interest. Instruments vary from very short questionnaires with only nine food items to assess a single nutrient (calcium)[54] in a study of osteoporosis[55]; a 13-item telephone interview to assess fat intake[56]; to comprehensive food lists numbering 190 items or more for assessing a wide variety of nutrients[57–61] in studies on vascular disease and cancer. The choice of a questionnaire approach to dietary assessment may relate to the limitation of resources for dietary recording in relation to the number of subjects. It is important to recognize, however, that a weighed record or full diet history is not always necessary for measuring a limited range of nutrients, and that the ability to rank subjects reliably, according to usual intake, demands more than a single 24-hour recall.

Questionnaires have generally been of the frequency and amount type (FAQ), in which subjects are asked to say how often they usually consume an item of food or drink, and how much they typically have on the days they consume it. Some attempts have been made at classifying subjects according to nutrient intake on the basis of frequency of consumption alone[62–66].

Various methods to assess portion sizes may be used, for example fitting average portion weights derived from other data to the respondents' chosen food and frequency selections[67,68] or asking subjects to describe amounts in terms of household measures or standard portions. To assess the frequency of food consumption, accompanying the food list is a multiple response grid in which respondents attempt to estimate how often selected foods are eaten. Up to 10 categories ranging from never or once a month or less, to six times per day is a usual format. Because responses are standardized, FFQ can be analysed in comparatively short periods of time so that large numbers of individuals can be investigated relatively inexpensively, for example in cohort studies. Generally, only one response to a FFQ has been obtained from each individual during study follow-up of several years in published results from existing cohorts. Their primary aim is often to characterize subjects according to their position in the distribution of intake for purposes of grouping or ranking, although absolute levels of consumption may also be of interest. These methods commonly have a highly structured format and if appropriately designed may be completed by the respondent without the need for an interviewer.

The basic principles of questionnaire design have been outlined in Chapter 2, Appendix 1, and it is worth restating the major points in relation to FFQs.

1. The purpose of the questionnaire should be clearly defined: to assess food consumption or nutrient intake, frequency or amounts, group means or individual intakes, one nutrient or a range of nutrients, etc.
2. The foods included in the questionnaire should be the minimum number which includes the major sources of nutrient for the majority of subjects. Extraneous questions take up valuable time and provide little information.
3. Questions on frequency and portion size should be closed rather than open. This reduces coding time and transcription errors, and reduces the number of question-naires which have to be rejected because the responses are incomplete or cannot be adequately interpreted.
4. Frequency categories should always be continuous, e.g. 'Never', 'Less than once per month', 'One to two times per month', 'Three to four times per month', followed by categories indicating the number of days per week on which the item was consumed. Other groupings of frequency may be appropriate according to the items being measured, but there should never be gaps, e.g. 'Once or twice per month', 'Once or twice per week', 'Every day', as the sensitivity of the questionnaire will be reduced, and respondents will be frustrated if they cannot find a response which they believe corresponds to their own habits.
5. Portion sizes should reflect known consumption patterns in the population, and the questionnaire should allow for a sufficient range of expression of portion size to enable subjects with the same frequency of consumption but different portion sizes to be adequately distinguished. Use of 'standard' portions applied equally to all subjects will reduce sensitivity.[69]
6. Aids to the assessment of portion size are desirable in the form of photographs, line drawings, or models of portions (neutral shapes) of foods.
7. Questionnaires may be either interviewer- or self-administered according to the needs of the study. Self-administered questionnaires require more careful preparation and

pre-testing. A useful way of overcoming limited interviewer resources is to design a questionnaire which is self-administered, but to include in the study protocol an opportunity for the responses to be reviewed and any queries clarified in a face-to-face or telephone interview.

Every questionnaire should be rigorously pre-tested to ensure that the meanings of the food names and the portion size descriptors are clear to the subjects, and that the method for recording responses is unambiguous. Questionnaires must also be validated against a reference measure of known accuracy. The matter of questionnaire validation, a vital stage in the design of many nutritional epidemiological studies, is covered in depth in Chapter 8.

The main advantages of questionnaires are their ease and uniformity of administration (which can overcome problems of interviewer bias), their low cost (especially if self-administered), and their use with samples which are geographically widespread (through the use of postal questionnaires). The primary disadvantages are the amount of work required for their development and validation, and the level of imprecision in the estimates of usual food consumption or nutrient intake.

6.7.2   Diet histories

The diet history is usually conducted by trained interviewers who obtain detailed information on usual foods consumed, portion sizes, recipes, and frequency of food consumption over the recent past. This method is less commonly used in epidemiology due to the necessity for face-to-face interviews and consequent costs, but it is the most frequently used method for the assessment of diet in clinical dietetics.[53]

The research diet history, attributed to Burke[70], consists of a three part assessment: a detailed face-to-face interview to assess usual consumption of a wide variety of foods; a cross-check food frequency list; and a 3-day record. Most allusions to the 'diet history' in the literature refer to the interview alone, and the food frequency list and 3-day record, used by Burke as markers of internal validity, tend to be forgotten. The diet history is typically a detailed interview to establish 'usual' food consumption patterns. Often starting with a 24-hour recall, the interviewer probes carefully for food consumption meal by meal, seeking day-to-day and seasonal variations to build up the 'usual' pattern. As with the 24-hour recall, aids to memory and conceptualization, in the form of food lists and photographs or models, contribute significantly to the accuracy of the assessment. Interviews often last for one to two hours, and are best recorded on prepared forms that allow for the meals, foods, and variations to be noted clearly and systematically. Interviewer training is vital, both to ensure that diet histories are complete and that differences between interviewers are minimized. (It is not acceptable for untrained interviewers to undertake diet histories, however straightforward they may at first appear.)

The diet history has numerous theoretical and practical advantages over prospective methods and over 24-hour recalls and questionnaires. A single, extended interview can provide detailed information about meal patterns, food consumption, and nutrient intake for an individual. Depending upon the quality of the food composition tables used to calculate nutrient intake, diet histories can provide data on the usual intakes of

a wide variety of nutrients. Subject involvement is kept to a minimum
or numeracy skills are needed. The information is representative of diet o.
periods, regarding both the interval and point in time, which can be varied to sui
needs of the study. Particular attention can be paid to foods or nutrients that may be of
special interest (for example, sources of dietary selenium), or which are notoriously
under-reported (such as sweets and alcohol). An individual's consumption of foods
which may be important sources of nutrient but which are eaten relatively infrequently
(liver and offal, for example), or which are highly seasonal in nature, is better assessed
by diet history than by other methods.

The disadvantages of the diet history are common to those relating to other recall
methods as regards memory, conceptualization, regular habits, etc. Moreover, the
complexity of the procedure makes it particularly prone to interviewer bias, and
subjects are likely to recall diet which relates to the immediate past and which may not
necessarily correspond to the period of interest. Diet histories may also exaggerate the
regularity of dietary habits[14], and do not provide information about day-to-day
variations in diet. Assessment of the likely error of misclassification is more difficult
than in prospective methods, requiring both repeat measures within individuals using
the diet history, and comparison with a more 'objective' external standard. However,
the diet history may be a poorly standardized technique, subject to observer bias, and
therefore not robust to changes in interviewer.[71]

The repeatability of diet histories is generally good for assessing group means of
energy and macronutrients for periods up to two years before the interview[72-74],
although the repeatability of ranking is less consistent, correlations for repeat
interviews ranging from 0.57 to 0.9 in the study by Reshef and Epstein[73], and up to
0.92 in the study by Morgan[74], to as low as 0.13 for protein in a study of elderly
subjects.[75] The results for micronutrients are generally poorer than those for
macronutrients.[75,76] Beyond two years, it becomes difficult to separate sources of
error relating strictly to repeatability from factors which relate to real changes in diet
over time.[77]

Relative validity has been measured in relation to weighed records. Mean intakes
by diet history are usually higher than by weighed intake[76,78,79], although not
always.[14,75,80] Diet history data are suitable for evaluation using the approach of
Goldberg et al.[42] to identify under-reporters, as it represents usual intake[81], although if
the diet history is consistently underestimating energy intake in relation to a robust
standard such as energy expenditure measured in a respiration chamber[82] then a high
proportion of subjects may be excluded from the analysis as 'under-reporters'. Whether
diet histories overestimate or underestimate true intakes, comparisons between group
means will be as reliable as for any other method providing the groups are balanced in
relation to potential confounders such as age, gender, or BMI.

Correlations between individuals' estimates of intake based on histories and weighed
records sometimes show poor agreement, in part because of the variation between
individuals in the factors which determine the success with which they are likely to
complete the two types of assessment, and in part because diet histories are designed to
assess 'usual' diet while weighed records assess diet for a limited period only. Morgan
et al.[74] showed only modest correlations for energy, fat, and fat fractions between diet
histories and 4-day records (0.27 to 0.42). In a study comparing 30-day records kept by

spouses with the diet histories of 16 men[76], correlations ranged from 0.24 for fibre to 0.63 for Vitamin C.

The awareness that weighed records cannot be regarded as an unquestioned reference measure suggests that part of the lack of agreement between diet histories and weighed records is due to imprecision in the determination of the reference measure. This raises the possibility that diet histories may actually perform better as a tool for ranking subjects than has been believed previously. More thorough validation studies are needed to discover the truth of this possibility. However, those that have been conducted with biomarkers suggest that subjects are as prone to make errors with this method as with others.[71,83]

The repeatability and relative validity of diet histories suggest that the method is robust enough to be of value in epidemiological studies, either to compare group means or to rank subjects according to levels of current or recent food consumption or nutrient intake. The probable error in ranking is more difficult to judge than when using methods which provide information on within-subject day-to-day variations in diet, because the sources of error are less readily amenable to measurement. A particular advantage of the diet history method in epidemiological studies is that the comprehensive assessment of diet allows for a measure of seasonal variation in diet, and for assessment of nutrient interactions or confounding to be taken into account at the level of the individual, which may not be feasible with single 24-hour recall data, and may be overlooked with questionnaire techniques.

6.7.3 24-hour recalls

Interviewed or written information about the previous day's intake, the 24-hour recall, is commonly used in cross-sectional investigations. In this the actual foods consumed are described, and information on portion weights obtained. This method may be more costly because the wide variety of foods consumed (at least 10 000 different food items are available in most westernized food supplies) requires estimation of portion sizes and individual computer coding. For individual dietary assessments, multiple 24-hour recalls may be needed, depending on the level of precision required and nutrient to be studied (see Section 6.9.2).

Originally attributed to Wiehl[84], the technique for administering a 24-hour recall is deceptively simple. Each subject is asked, through a systematic repetition of open-ended questions, to recall and describe all food and drink consumed in the 24 hours prior to the interview. The respondent may be asked either to recall diet from the first thing upon waking up to the time of the interview, and then to recall diet from exactly 24 hours previously until going to bed; or to recall consumption of the previous day (midnight to midnight). The detail of description must be consistent with the food tables upon which nutrient calculations are to be based, and the interviewer must be thoroughly familiar with the food habits of the population from which the sample has been drawn. Photographs or food portion models portraying portion sizes (preferably based on surveys of weighed food consumption within the population) are likely to improve estimation of portion size, and respondents should be given as wide a latitude as possible to describe portions in their own terms, rather than the interviewer suggesting measures with which the respondent may be unfamiliar. Interviews should be conducted in the subject's native language where this will facilitate more complete and accurate responses. It is essential that interviewers receive adequate training in the technique, as it is easy to bias subjects' responses through ill-judged or leading questions, or by failing to probe adequately for items not mentioned initially.

The Nordic Cooperation Group of Dietary Researchers suggests a recommended procedure which is intended to minimize differential misclassification and facilitate the collection of representative results[14]:

1. subjects should be given no prior warning that they will be interviewed, as they may choose to alter their habits;
2. the recall should be conducted as an interview (either in person or by telephone);
3. the interview should take place in a quiet, relaxed atmosphere, and in so far as possible should follow the same format for every subject;
4. in the sample as a whole (and within any strata on which data will be analysed), interviews should be evenly distributed over the days of the week;
5. the order of recall should commence with the first food or drink taken in the day (or, for night workers, from midnight to midnight);
6. the interviewer should ask neutral questions, and be aware of combinations of foods likely to be eaten together in order to be able to probe effectively for items not mentioned;
7. aids to description of portion sizes should be provided;
8. an open-ended form with pre-coded foods listed may aid speed of recording and subsequent coding.

The principal advantages of the 24-hour recall are its speed and ease of administration. This allows large numbers of subjects to be interviewed with the minimum of resources, and compliance is usually excellent because of the small amount of information required from each respondent. This has made its use particularly attractive in very large-scale studies such as NHANES III.[85]

The principal limitation of the 24-hour recall is that it does not provide a reliable estimate of an individual's intake due to day-to-day variation. A single 24-hour recall from each subject cannot be used to rank subjects reliably.[86] If used for this purpose in epidemiological studies, the ability to describe significant relationships between diet and disease risk will be severely reduced (although not entirely lost). This holds true even if subjects are grouped according to their intake (high, medium, and low) based on their 24-hour recalls, as the degree of misclassification will persist. The problem is confounded by the fact that 24-hour recall results exhibit the 'flat-slope' syndrome[87]: subjects with true low intakes tend to report higher than usual intakes, and those with true high intakes tend to report lower than usual intakes. While this may not significantly influence the mean, the variation in intakes between subjects is further underestimated. The problem can in part be overcome by obtaining repeat 24-hour recalls[88] (see Section 6.9.2), but the advantages in terms of cost and inconvenience quickly begin to evaporate and make other techniques more attractive.

The validity of group mean nutrient intakes based on 24-hour recalls has been assessed by comparing results with weighed records[61,89,90,91], diet histories[61,86,92,93,94] and biological markers.[95] The results are not consistent, sometimes overestimating[91] and sometimes underestimating[90] intake in relation to dietary energy and nutrients. The differences in outcome may be due in part to the use of different reference measures, varying from 16-day weighed records[61] to 7-day recalls.[96] The repeatability of 24-hour results on a group basis is generally good[86,93,97], but this does not imply validity.

24-hour recalls are most appropriate for measuring current diet in groups of subjects, and are therefore particularly well suited to studies where differences between group means are to be assessed, either cross-sectionally or longitudinally. The number of subjects needed in a study is a function of the likely size of the difference between means, and the within- and between-subject variance (which will vary with the nutrient in question) (see Chapter 3 and Nelson et al.[98]).

If information on variation in diet within or between individual subjects is needed, as few as two repeat measures may help to elucidate the likely extent of misclassification of individuals[99,100], although the more repeats, the better the classification is likely to be. Non-consecutive days are more likely to provide a better estimate of variance than consecutive days.[101] Techniques for estimating within subject variance have been described[101-103] to allow for regression to the mean effects and to adjust for the 'flat-slope' syndrome (see Chapter 4), thereby enhancing the use of single 24-hour recall data. It is not appropriate to use the technique of Goldberg et al.[42] to identify 24-hour recall data in which energy intakes are $< 1.2 \times BMR$[104], as a one-day record is not necessarily representative of usual intake, and low intakes are more likely to be described as untypical.[105]

6.7.4 Records

In these methods, subjects are taught to describe and give an estimate of the weight of food immediately before eating, and to record any leftovers. Records are generally written by the participants, although verbal records, with descriptions recorded on tape cassettes have been obtained.[71,106] Information about the weight of food consumed may be obtained either by asking subjects to weigh out food onto the plate as it is being served, or portions of food are described in terms of household measures, volume models, photographs, average portions, units, or pack sizes. As with the 24-hour recall, generally these descriptions are incorporated into computer systems for coding food records to obtain information on nutrient intake. When sufficient days' observations are collected on each individual, this method is commonly used for the purposes of validation of individual results obtained by other methods such as FFQ used in cohort studies (see Sections 6.7.1–3 and Chapter 8). However, at least 7 days data are necessary and the time taken for analysis is considerable. Few large scale cohorts have included this method for collection of data. Nevertheless, in newer cohort studies, where a high proportion of participants in large scale cohorts agree to complete diaries, they are suitable for use in nested case-control studies.[61] Food diaries are also commonly used for surveillance[40], multicentre cross-sectional investigations[107], small cohorts[108,109], and intervention studies.[110]

6.7.5 Checklists

This method potentially avoids problems in the estimation of the frequency of food consumption in FFQ (see Section 6.9.3), and yet is a record completed daily which can be pre-coded for rapid data entry. In one published version[106], the checklist took the form of a booklet which comprised one page of instructions, one of an example, and seven pages (one for each day over one week) of the checklist. The checklist was a printed list of foods on which subjects were asked to check off which foods they had eaten, counting half for a small portion, and two for a large portion at the end of each day. A space was left for subjects to record foods not present on the printed list, but otherwise the list was pre-coded for nutrient analysis. The list of 160 foods was largely that used for a FFQ, and where possible, 'units' (slices, cups, etc.) were specified.

6.8 Food composition tables

Many hypotheses concerning diet and health relate to the content of foods, such as nutrients, contaminants such as aflatoxins, heterocyclic amines, or to non-nutritive food constituents. An estimate of the content of these items in each food eaten is also required in order to obtain intake, unless biomarkers are available (see Section 5.3.2) Tables of food composition include information about the average nutrient content of the most commonly consumed foods for most nutrients. They are less comprehensive with regard to food contaminants and non-nutritive constituents. If there is inadequate food table information, 'precise weighing' may be necessary, for example if food composition tables with values for cooked foods are not available. In 'precise weighing', raw ingredients, the cooked food, meal, or snack, plus the individual portions must all be weighed, and aliquots collected for chemical analysis. This method is very different from records outlined above and it is usual for skilled field-workers to carry out this survey, rather than the subjects themselves.

6.9 Measurement error in dietary assessments

Methods of measuring diet are associated with both random and systematic error. Bias in the overall average may well be due to errors in reports from some individuals in the distribution (differential misclassification), rather than a systematic rendering of biased information from all individuals (non-differential misclassification). Errors arise from the use of food tables, assessment of the frequency of food consumption, portion size, daily variation, and failure to report usual diet, either due to changes in habits whilst taking part in an investigation, or misreporting of food choice or amount. (See Chapter 5 for errors associated with the use of food tables.)

6.9.1 Assessment of portion size

On balance, there appears to be little or no systematic bias in group averages of nutrients obtained by records with estimates of food, compared with group averages obtained by weighed dietary records. Nevertheless, despite the absence of overall bias in a population, the estimation of portion size rather than direct weighing is associated with imprecision at the individual level and for different foods. In general, this is in the order of 50% (coefficient of variation) for foods, but less, about 20%, for nutrients, probably due to cancellation of error from the use of food tables. Table 6.3 shows a summary of comparisons between estimated and direct weights of food. Models and

Table 6.3 Coefficients of variation of differences in estimated versus measured weights of food eaten.

Foods		Nutrients
Household measures	Photographs	
1–96[a]	9–44[f]	7–11[h]
13–32[b]	30–50[g]	11–16[i]
16–53[c]	10–26[c]	19–28[j]
21–70[d]	0–45[k]	0–30[m]
21–91[e]	3–49[l]	

(a) Minimum value cookies, maximum casseroles;[166] (b) Minimum value heaped tablespoons, maximum level teaspoons;[167] (c)[168] (d) Minimum value corn bread, maximum sugar;[169] (e) Minimum value drinks, maximum cake;[170] (f)[171] (g)[172] (h) Minimum value energy, maximum iron;[173] (i) Energy 11%, protein 16%;[174] (j) Minimum value protein, maximum vitamin C;[175] (k) Minimum value boiled potato, maximum cornflakes;[111] (l) Minimum value quiche, maximum broccoli; (m) Minimum value iron, maximum value saturated fatty acids.[69]

photographs may incur less error in the estimation of portion weights, at least when compared with estimations from household measures and dimensions. The use of information from prepacked foods is associated with smaller errors, 2–5%.

When using photographs, there is a tendency for some foods to bias towards average weight, while for others weight may be consistently over or underestimated.[69,111] Where choices are given, these should encompass the full range of food quantities consumed.[111,112]

Table 6.4 shows that the percentage of subjects within ±10% of the value based on weighed records of consumption is greatly increased compared with the studies where household measures of food portion were used. Furthermore, the remaining error associated with the reliance on household measures data is small compared with that from daily variation (see Section 6.9.2). This indicates that the variance and therefore ranking of individuals within a distribution of nutrient intake seems little affected whether or not weighed data or household measures are used.

6.9.2 Daily variation

Individuals do not consume the same food from day to day and substantial error is introduced when diet is assessed from a single day's dietary investigation. Daily variation is one of the main factors in reducing precision of individual estimates in record and 24-hour recall methods of assessing diet. The variability from day to day is closely related to the nutrient under study. The early descriptions of record techniques specified that subjects should be observed for seven days and this practice has been followed for nearly 50 years. Nevertheless, when only the average intake of a group of individuals is required for cross-sectional studies, it is difficult to justify gathering this amount of data, even for the more variable nutrients such as cholesterol, or polyunsaturated fatty acids. A 3- to 4-day record or 24-hour recall, randomized to cover seasonal and weekday variations, seems to be the optimum, there being little decrease in

Table 6.4 Percentage of subjects whose nutrient intakes estimated from household measures is within ± 10 of the value based on weighed records of consumption.

Nutrient	Study		
	Bransby et al.[173]	Eppright et al.[175]	Nettleton et al.[176]
Energy	71	33	92
Protein	49	41	87
Fat	41	37	71
Carbohydrate	82	37	89
Calcium	69	35	100
Iron	35	–	84
Thiamin	–	32	87
Ascorbic Acid	–	29	79
No.	49	25	38

– indicates value not published

the difference between averages that can be detected from a given sample size if the number of observations on each subject is increased to 7 days (Table 6.5). In some circumstances, a 1-day record or 24-hour recall collected from a large number of subjects may suffice for the assessment of group means, although it is generally more useful to obtain at least two days of repeat measures to be able to estimate the within-subject component of error.

Longer periods of observation on each individual are necessary for cohort and dietary validation studies. Table 6.5 shows the number of recording days necessary to classify 80% of subjects correctly into the extreme thirds of the distribution, based on data from three population groups. The actual number of records in any specific population will depend on the ratio of average within-person daily variation and the between-person variation. Nevertheless, it is clear from Table 6.5 that, whereas a 7-day record is probably sufficient to classify into thirds of the distribution for energy and energy-yielding nutrients, longer periods are necessary for items such as alcohol, some vitamins and minerals, and cholesterol. Only if a less precise estimate of individual mean intakes is acceptable, and correct classification into extreme fifths of the distribution is adequate, would a 7-day record be sufficient for these more variable food constituents. If habitual diet is to be assessed, consecutive observations are less satisfactory than those spread over, for example, the course of several months in one year, or over several years in a cohort study. In the UK EPIC cohort for example, follow-up repeat 7-day diaries are obtained 18 and 48 months after the first 7-day diary is completed.[106]

6.9.3 Frequency of food consumption

Compared with records of food consumption, FFQ typically overestimate consumption, particularly of vegetables, but also of energy and energy yielding nutrients.[61,113,114]

Table 6.5 Number of daily food records necessary to correctly classify 80% of men into the extreme thirds of the distribution P < 0.05.

	British Civil Servants (Marr[177])	Random selection of British men (Bingham et al.[178])	Random selection of Swedish men*
Energy	7	5	7
Protein	6	5	7
Fat	9	9	7
Carbohydrate	4	3	3
Sugar	2	2	–
Dietary fibre	6	10	–
P:S ratio	11	–	–
Cholesterol	18	–	–
Alcohol	4	–	14
Vitamin C	–	6	14
Thiamin	–	6	14
Riboflavin	–	10	–
Calcium	–	4	5
Iron	–	12	9

* Callmer, Personal communication. 58 × 7-day weighed records from middle-aged men randomly selected in Stockholm, Sweden.

The cause of this is uncertain, but may result from the use of lists. Restriction of the choice of food into a comparatively short list of around 150 foods or less, means that error associated with estimation of amounts of single items is more likely to be biased than when the full variety of foods is analysed, for example in a 24-hour recall or record of food consumption. Participants using the FFQ may also have difficulty in choosing the correct category of how often food is consumed, so that over-estimation of the numbers of time foods are eaten over a defined period of time occurs. For example, too many main dish items compared with days in the week may be selected in error.

6.9.4   Under-reporting

Many FFQ are not designed to assess total dietary intake, and information relating only to the food or nutrient of interest at the time of study is obtained. In one prospective study for example, the FFQ covered only 80 food items and covered 83% of mean total energy intake.[115] The term under-reporting particularly applies to methods which attempt to assess total energy intake. This problem has primarily been demonstrated by biomarkers and has relied on three techniques to establish completeness of dietary data: doubly-labelled water to assess usual energy expenditure; urinary nitrogen excretion to assess protein intake; and an estimate of energy expenditure (Basal Metabolic Rate or BMR) based on body weight, age, and gender.[42] These are described in more detail in Chapter 7.

In early reports, energy expenditure assessed from doubly-labelled water was unexpectedly low, 1.4 times basal metabolic rate (BMR) on average in a small group of sedentary women.[116] In women of normal weight, energy intake from weighed dietary records agreed with energy expenditure data, but in obese women, energy intake assessed from 7-day weighed records was about 2 MJ (465 kcal) per day lower than expenditure, suggesting that overweight women do not report their habitual food intake.[117] In a later study, energy expenditure also exceeded energy intake measured from 7-day records in 31 normal individuals, on average by 20%.[118] As a ratio to BMR, energy intake was 1.46 ± 0.31, and energy expenditure was 1.82 ± 0.24, greater than previously found in sedentary women.[116] Reported energy intakes agreed with energy expenditure in about one-third of these subjects, predominantly those who were at the higher end of the distribution of energy intake.[118]

The doubly-labelled water method is too expensive for routine use for validation of dietary intake measurements. Twenty-four hour urine nitrogen excretion provides a more economical alternative. Isaksson first proposed that 24-hour urine nitrogen (N) should be used as an independent validity check on dietary survey methods.[119] This has been used to validate dietary survey methods used to estimate average dietary intakes of groups in a number of population studies in Gothenberg.[119] Further studies from this group have confirmed the difficulties of dietary assessments of patients in clinical work. For example, reported protein intake in obese subjects (from a diet history) was only 46 g, but on the basis of 24-hour urine collections it was 87 g.[120] In another study, subjects who were overweight or diabetic seemed to report their prescribed diet rather than what they were actually eating as judged by their urine N excretion.

Twenty-four-hour nitrogen excretion can also be used to validate individual estimates of usual diet, provided that sufficient collections are obtained (Chapter 7). In a study of the validity of different methods of dietary assessment, 160 women were studied at home on four occasions (seasons) over the course of one year, and at each session the participants were asked to complete four days of weighed food records. The volunteers were also asked to provide two 24-hour urine collections on each occasion so that over the year each individual provided 16 days of weighed dietary records, and eight 24-hour urine collections. The completeness of the urine collections was assessed using the PABAcheck method (Chapter 7) and only those that were complete were used to validate the dietary assessments. Average N intake from the 16-day weighed records (mean $\pm$ SD) was 11.2 ± 2.3 g per day, and that from N excretion in the complete 24-hour urine 9.84 ± 1.78 g per day, so that the average ratio of urine N to dietary N (UN/DN) was 0.91 ± 0.09. This was rather greater than the ratio of 0.81 ± 0.05 expected if the average results from all individuals were valid.[106] To determine which, if any, of the individual results were valid, the ratio of urine to dietary N was ranked and data was examined in fifths of the distribution of the urine to dietary nitrogen ratio. Means of this ratio ranged from 0.76 in the lower fifth of the distribution to 1.13 in the upper fifth. Examination of correlations between urine and dietary N, ratios of energy intake to BMR (EI/BMR), correlations of the ratio of energy intake to BMR with the urinary to dietary N ratio, body mass index (BMI), and body weight, indicated that mean values from the 20% of individuals assigned to the top fifth were different from data from the 80% of individuals assigned to the other four fifths.[106] All data were therefore considered separately for individuals in the top fifth and for individuals in the other

Table 6.6 Means (se) of daily intake of nutrients and foods from individuals grouped into top versus other four fifths of the distribution according to their urine to dietary nitrogen ratio from 16-day weighed records, and anthropometric and biological data on the same individuals.

Numbers	Lower four fifths 125		Top fifth 31		P value, Top versus lower four fifths
	Mean	se	Mean	se	
Nutrients and foods					
Energy MJ	8.14	0.04	6.65	0.23	<0.001
Protein g	71	0.2	60	1.7	<0.001
Fat g	80	0.3	62	2.5	<0.001
Starch g	113	0.9	100	4.8	<0.05
Sugars g	115	0.1	88	5.2	<0.001
Calcium mg	997	21	781	35	<0.001
Vitamin C mg	100	3.5	94	7.7	ns
NSP g	16.1	0.03	14.6	0.85	ns
Alcohol g	9	1	8	2	ns
Total cereals g	258	3	212	12	<0.05
Breakfast cereals g	23	0.1	14	3	<0.01
Cakes g	34	0.4	25	3	<0.01
Milk g	256	5	150	20	<0.001
Eggs g	24	0.3	18	2	<0.01
Fats (including butter) g	16	0.2	11	1	<0.001
Sugars and confectionery g	29	0.8	20	3	<0.01
Meat g	95	0.5	96	7	ns
Fish g	32	0.4	30	4	ns
Vegetables g	271	3	269	19	ns
Fruit g	202	4	212	27	ns
Anthropometry					
Weight kg	64.25	0.80	71.99	2.67	<0.05
Height m	1.63	0.01	1.64	0.01	ns
BMI kg/M^2	24.00	0.29	26.59	0.97	<0.05
Biological variables					
UN/DN ratio	0.86	0.007	1.13	0.022	<0.001
Urine N g	9.76	0.16	10.89	0.30	<0.01
Dietary N g	11.38	0.17	9.69	0.28	<0.001
EI/BMR ratio	1.46	0.02	1.15	0.04	<0.001
Urine K mmol	71.7	1.54	75.37	4.09	ns
Diet K mmol	83.23	1.56	73.82	2.97	<0.01
UK/DK ratio	0.867	0.011	1.025	0.037	<0.001

four fifths of the distribution in urine to dietary N ratio. Table 6.6 shows mean body weight and intakes of foods and nutrients for the 80% of individuals classified as having valid records compared with those in the top fifth who were classified as under-reporters. Not only were individuals in the top fifth heavier with a lower energy intake to BMR ratio than the others, but their intakes of energy and all energy yielding nutrients calculated from weighed records were significantly lower than those from individuals in the other fifths. On average there was an 18 g difference in reported fat consumption between the average values reported in the top and the other four fifths according to the urine to dietary N ratio. Mean consumption of cakes, breakfast cereals, milk, eggs, fats, and sugars was also significantly lower in those individuals classified in the top fifth of the distribution. However, there was no difference in reported consumption of meat, fruits, vegetables, and potatoes between these under-reporters and the other 80% of the population who gave valid records, nor in intake of vitamin C or carotene.

Figure 6.1 shows box plots (with medians, mid ranges and extreme values) for total grams of fat for the records which were valid and those which were not. There are clear differences between the two. However, differences in mean intake of macronutrients between under-reporters and those who give valid records are reduced by techniques of energy adjustment (see 6.10). Figure 6.1 shows that the medians and mid ranges for the two groups are similar; average values were 37 (sd 5) % for valid records, and 35 (sd 3) % for the under-reporters. Hence, bias in reports of food intake obtained from methods of dietary assessment can be assessed from 24-hour urine nitrogen. Only some, not all, nutrients and foods may be under-reported, and differences in means are reduced by energy adjustment. Overweight individuals in particular are likely to under-report the amount they eat. This problem is not confined to weighed dietary records, since it has been documented with all methods of dietary assessment, including 24-hour recalls[119–121], weighed records[117,118], diet histories[122,123], and FFQ designed to assess total diet[61], although in general it is more likely to occur with 24-hour recalls than with diet histories and records.[53]

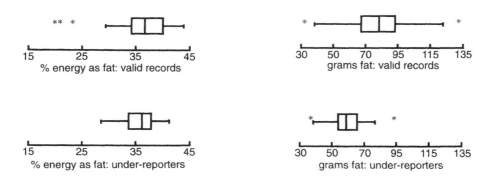

Fig. 6.1 Box plot showing median, interquartile range, and extreme values for % energy from fat and total grams of fat based on 125 valid records and 31 under-reporters.

6.9.5   Problems associated with retrospective methods

A number of aspects of the disadvantages with retrospective methods listed in Table 6.2 warrant further discussion. First, responses are dependent upon subjects' ability to remember food consumption accurately, which varies in an unsystematic way from person to person. It can be said generally that children under the age of about 12 and elderly people are less likely to recall diet well, although age need not always be a barrier.[124] Children under 12 should not be asked to recall their diets without the help of an adult. Subjects over the age of 60 should be given a simple mental ability test (such as the Hodkinson Abbreviated Mental Test Score)[125] in order to ensure that basic memory skills are intact, although some tests may not separate groups sufficiently to elicit differences in response to FFQs.[126] The problem of memory relates primarily to the omission of foods, particularly sauces and condiments, which may contribute significantly to micronutrient intakes in some diets. The number of foods recalled is often correlated with the total intake of energy and nutrients[127], and important differential misclassification will occur between those with good memories and those with poor memories. It could nevertheless be argued that in a case-control study, for example, the distribution of people with good and bad memories is likely to be similar amongst both cases and controls, and that the only effect will be attenuation of relative risk estimates. This may not be true if the disease itself or drug treatment affects memory differentially in cases and controls. Validation of retrospective measures of diet in hospitalized patients is particularly problematic.[128]

Like memory, conceptualization skills, or the ability to relate actual consumption to descriptions of portion sizes and estimates of frequency, will vary substantially between individuals. Children under 12 are again likely to be poor at conceptualization, even when visual aids in the form of photographs, portion models, or actual food models are used. Some aid to describe portion sizes is usually beneficial.[69,111] Particularly when regional differences in diet are being assessed, what may be regarded as a small portion in one area may be medium in another; an 'average' portion for a woman is typically smaller than an 'average' portion for a man.

Observer bias can take two forms. First, one observer may ask a different set of questions from another. This problem is more likely in regional or multinational studies in which different interviewers are used in different areas to save on time and travel costs. It may be overcome in part by adequate training[129] or calibration of multi-centre measuring devices.[130] Second, in case-control studies, the interviewer may change the emphasis of questions if he or she is aware of the hypothesis being tested. This problem can be addressed by blinding the observer to the status of the patient (if that is a possibility, i.e. the cases are not all being interviewed in hospital and the controls at home). Where this is not possible, a more structured interview can reduce the problem, or it may even be an advantage to substitute a self-completing questionnaire with a follow-up interview if observer bias is likely to be a severe problem. (Ideally, of course, cases and controls should always be measured in the same environment – see Chapters 2 and 15).

Subjects may distort their reported diet for several reasons. First, they may not wish to confess to the consumption of certain types of foods, particularly sweets and alcohol which are notoriously under-reported, often by 50% or more. Second, subjects may more generally wish to report a diet which they believe will be acceptable in the eyes of the interviewer (for example, reporting less consumption of fried foods and more of fruit and vegetables). These distortions may be greater in a face-to-face interview than when filling in a self-completing questionnaire or using a computer terminal interactively. Third, people often idealize their consumption by reporting a diet that they *believe* reflects what they usually do or would like to achieve, but which in fact represents their activity only a small proportion of the time. This is of particular concern in subjects who are overweight, where the level of consumption reported has been shown to be inversely proportional to their weight.[131] Distortions of this type can only be brought to light by careful validation using methods which are free from error due either to reporting or recording.

Most retrospective methods do not provide a measure of day-to-day variation in diet. The exception is repeat 24-hour recalls[88,129], but these are in essence the application of a retrospective method to the assessment of current diet. Given that a diet history or questionnaire will to some extent misclassify individuals according to their true intake, it is important to have a measurement of error associated with each individual's estimate of mean intake. Repeat interview or application of questionnaire will provide an estimate of error associated with the measuring tool but not with the variability of each individual's intake. Thus, retrospective techniques are generally less effective than prospective techniques in identifying within-subject sources of measurement error, and it is therefore more difficult to adjust for attenuation of risk in epidemiological analyses. Approaches to this problem are discussed in Chapter 8.

All of the retrospective methods, apart from the 24-hour recall, require that subjects have sufficiently regular habits for the concept of 'usual' intake to have meaning, to allow successful completion of an interview or questionnaire in which regular frequency of consumption is the key to accuracy. Subjects whose diets consist primarily of a small number of foods eaten very regularly are more likely to have their dietary intakes assessed accurately than subjects who eat a wide variety of foods relatively infrequently.[132] Interview or questionnaire responses give no immediate clues as to the true characteristics of the subject's diet, and differential misclassification may occur in regional or international comparisons of diet if meal patterns and the availability of foods differ substantially between areas.

Finally, it is important to remember that all estimates of nutrient intakes based on retrospective methods are dependent upon food composition tables. The problems inherent in their use are discussed in detail in Chapter 5.

6.10   Energy adjustment

One reason for attempting to correct for energy intake in dietary assessments is to reduce extraneous variation from the general correlation of nutrients with total energy intake, brought about by differences in body size and hence (in sedentary populations) energy expenditure.[67] In addition, in validation studies, the relation between results from one method and another is sometimes improved by energy adjustment.[67,133] Furthermore, there are significant differences in absolute macronutrient intake between individuals who give valid records and those who do not; these differences are

Table 6.7 Mean (se) differences in absolute and energy adjusted nutrients between individuals who under-reported dietary intake, and those who did not.

Nutrient	Valid records n = 125		Under-reporters n = 31		P
	Mean	se	Mean	se	
Absolute intakes					
Energy MJ	8.14	0.04	6.65	0.23	<0.001
Protein g	71	0.2	60	1.7	<0.001
Fat g	80	0.3	62	2.5	<0.001
Carbohydrate	231	4.3	191	8.2	<0.001
Energy adjusted intakes					
Protein	69	0.8	67	1.4	>0.05
Fat	77	0.9	65	0.9	>0.05
Carbohydrate	223	2.7	225	4.0	>0.05

substantially reduced after energy adjustment, although the overall mean within a population is not altered. Table 6.7 shows absolute and energy adjusted[67] intakes of fat, carbohydrate, and protein in a group of women shown to give either valid records or underestimates.[106] Differences between under-reporters and those who gave valid records were no longer significant after energy adjustment. The effect of energy adjustment depends on the correlation between the nutrient concerned and energy intake, and also on the correlation between the errors of measurement for these two quantities. The latter is heavily dependent on the dietary method used. Hence, the relation between FFQ and weighed records can be much improved by energy adjustment, but to a lesser extent between weighed records and 24-hour recalls. Energy adjustment is inappropriate (and without effect) if there are zero correlations between energy intake and the nutrient concerned, for example in the case of carotene.[134] To what extent energy adjustment reduces measurement error of fat and carbohydrate from under-reporting in prospective studies is uninvestigated, due to lack of a biomarker of intake of these nutrients. However, 24-hour urine N is a biomarker for protein intake, which is also under-reported, and correlations between intake of protein and 24-hour urine N were not improved by energy adjustment (see Section 6.11).

6.11 Effects of measurement error on validity

Methods of dietary assessment have different types of error structure, so that the magnitude of the error varies according to the method and may not always be predictable. For this reason, 'relative validation' studies are conducted prior to use of a particular method, particularly in large prospective studies in order that the extent of measurement error can be determined and reduced if possible (see Chapter 8).

Table 6.8 Correlations between dietary nitrogen, potassium, carotene, and vitamin C intake from different methods of dietary assessment and biomarkers of these nutrients, in 156 individuals classified as having given valid reports of habitual food intake or as under-reporters.

All values	Valid n = 125	Under-reporters n = 31	All n = 156	Energy adjusted n = 156
Correlations between 24 h urine nitrogen (N) versus				
N from 16 day weighed record	0.87	0.78	0.69	0.69
N from FFQ	0.27	0.50	0.24	0.49
N from 24 h recall	0.26	−0.31	0.10	0.09
N from 7 day diary	0.70	0.60	0.65	0.67
Correlations between 24 h urine potassium (K) versus				
K from 16 day weighed record	0.82	0.74	0.76	0.76
K from FFQ	0.28	0.28	0.25	0.41
K from 24 h recall	0.52	0.53	0.51	0.54
K from 7 day diary (7DD)	0.70	0.57	0.66	0.64

Correlations between dietary carotene and vitamin C from different dietary methods and plasma carotenoids and vitamin C

	Weighed record	FFQ	24 h recall	7 day checklist
Lutein	0.36	0.03	0.05	0.21
β-cryptoxanthin	0.20	−0.02	−0.03	0.07
Lycopene	0.33	0.17	0.08	0.21
α-carotene	0.62	0.42	0.19	0.34
cis-carotene	0.35	0.14	0.00	0.13
β-carotene	0.48	0.15	0.08	0.28

	Weighed records	FFQ	24 h recall	7 day diary
Vitamin C:				
Including supplements (n = 156)	0.51	0.35	0.34	0.22
Non-supplement users (n = 127)	0.49	0.26	0.26	0.22

Generally, methods are compared with results from records of food consumption, but some biomarkers have been shown in metabolic studies to closely agree with habitual intake and can be used as an independent reference to assess the extent of measurement error associated with different methods (see Chapter 7). When used to assess the relative validity of different dietary methods, biomarkers generally confirm that records of food consumption are more likely to rank subjects correctly when estimating habitual diet than other methods such as FFQ.[106,135–138] Table 6.8 shows correlations between dietary nitrogen and potassium intake from different methods of dietary assessment and the biomarkers of habitual diet of 24-hour urine nitrogen and potassium in individuals classified as having given valid reports of habitual food intake or under-reporters according to 24-hour urine N (see Chapter 7). Records and check-lists consistently gave better correlations with the biomarkers than FFQ when all subjects were considered together, and when valid reports were separated from results from individuals who had under-reported, as judged by comparisons with 24-hour urine N.[106,134] Energy adjustment improved the correlation between results from different methods, especially the FFQ, and biomarkers for N and K, but the overall ranking of methods was maintained.

Substantial effort has gone into assessing the reproducibility and validity of ques-tionnaires. Reproducibility measures help to assess the contribution of within-subject error to misclassification of subjects based on questionnaire responses in studies where rank order is important (e.g. case-control and cohort studies). In the absence of these measures, the degree of attenuation of risk estimates will be understated, and therefore the true relative risk underestimated. Most reproducibility studies show correlations between repeat nutrient intake assessments consistently above 0.5[57–59,73], although this is not always so.[139] These errors in repeatability are substantial, and in the process of validation, when questionnaire results are compared with those from a reference measurement, the estimate of within-subject variance should be distinguished from the errors associated with the imprecision or bias in the questionnaire (see Chapters 4 and 8). Flegal and Larkin[140] recommend additional analysis to identify which com-ponents of measurement (e.g. frequency or amount) are contributing to the errors.

Öhlin et al.[2] have summarized the findings from many studies comparing FFQ performance with a variety of reference measures. A sample of validation studies is summarized in Table 6.9. It can be seen from the ranges of values for the correlation coefficients shown in Table 6.9 that a large number of items in a questionnaire is no guarantee of better agreement with the reference measure, and that macronutrients are not consistently better correlated with the reference measures than micronutrients. Most of the values shown are Pearson correlations, which may not be the best measure of agreement between methods, and which is certainly not appropriate for some of the higher values shown for non-normally distributed variables such as alcohol intake or P/S ratio (even after log transformation). Further discussion of techniques for evaluating agreement between questionnaire responses and standards is presented in Chapter 8.

Alternative reference measures for validation have been used recently to overcome problems of reference mismeasurement. Bingham et al.[61] have used urinary nitrogen excretion to identify subjects whose reference measure (16-day weighed food record) are likely to be below their true intake, and considered them separately from the comparisons with results from other methods. There is no marked improvement in level of agreement between the FFQs and the 16-day weighed food record in this study compared to others in Table 6.9. Rothenberg[137] used urinary nitrogen as a reference measure and showed that the correlation between dietary protein and urinary nitrogen excretion was better with the 4-day food record than with the FFQ, especially if the subjects reporting incomplete urine collections were excluded from the analysis. Horwath and Worsley[141] used an inventory of foods in the cupboards and refrigerators of elderly subjects to show good agreement between frequency of eating as reported in a FFQ and the presence of food in the house (kappa range: 0.33 (cauliflower) to 1.00

Table 6.9 Summary of selected validation studies.

Authors	Sample	Test measure	Reference measure	Nutrients (r_{min} r_{max})
Balogh et al., 1968[179]	Israeli men, aged 40–59	'short' DH interview (n = 14)	DH (n = 48) 7-day WI	Energy, animal protein, fat, SFA, PUFA (0.69 PUFA, 0.94 fat)
Morgan et al., 1978[74]	Canadian women, n = 400	DHQ	4-day HM	Energy, fat, SFA, 18:1, 18:2, cholesterol (0.34 energy, 0.42 cholesterol)
Jain et al., 1980[76]	US men, n = 16	DHQ	30-day record kept by spouse	Energy, protein (total, animal, vegetable), fat (total, animal, vegetable), 18:1, 18:2, cholesterol, fibre, vitamin C (0.24 fibre, 0.61 cholesterol)
Jain et al., 1982[180]	US women, aged 40–59, n = 50	69 item SA	DH	Energy, protein (total, animal, vegetable), fat (total, animal, vegetable), 18:1, 18:2, cholesterol, fibre, vitamin C (0.50 cholesterol, 0.64 energy)
Barasi et al., 1983[181]	Welsh women aged 18–75 n = 103	27 item SA	4-day WI	Dietary fibre (total, cereal, fruit/vegetable) (0.34 fruit/veg, 0.69 cereal)
Stuff et al., 1983[182]	US pregnant women, n = 40	105 item	7-day HM	Energy, protein, fat, carbohydrate, calcium, phosphorus, iron (r_I: 0.42 protein, 0.66 phosphorus)
Yarnell et al., 1983[183]	Welsh men, n = 119	54 item SA	7-day WI	Energy, protein, fat, SFA, carbohydrate, sucrose, dietary fibre, cereal fibre, vitamin C, alcohol (0.27 carbohydrate, 0.75 alcohol)
Gray et al., 1984[184]	California, aged 58–95 men n = 19, women n = 31	56 item SA	DH	Vitamins A and C (0.43 A, 0.38 C)
Shepherd et al., 1985[185]	UK men and women, n = 33	15 item SA	7-day urine sodium	Salt (0.66)
Willett et al., 1985[57]	US female nurses, aged 34–59, n = 173	61 item SA	28-day WI (4 × 7-day) over 1 year	Energy, protein, fat, SFA, PUFA, cholesterol, carbohydrate, sucrose, crude fibre, vitamins A, B_6, C (0.18 protein, 0.53 vitamin C)
Cummings et al., 1987[186]	California women, aged 65+, n = 37	34 item	7-day HM	Calcium (0.76)

Table 6.9 (*cont.*)

Authors	Sample	Test measure	Reference measure	Nutrients (r_{min} r_{max})
Nelson et al., 1987[187]	UK women, aged 25–64, n = 56	22 item SA	24-hour urine iodine	Iodine(0.24, 0.50)
Willett et al., 1987[188]	US, men n = 12, women n = 15	61 item SA	1 year HM record	as per 1985 plus 18:1, vitamins B_1, B_2, niacin, Ca, P, K, Fe (0.38 vitamin C, 0.76 fat)
Nelson et al., 1988[54]	UK women, aged 65–74, n = 30	9 item	7-day WI	Calcium (0.69)
	aged 72–90 men n = 13 women n = 15		5-day DD	Calcium (0.76)
Pietinen et al., 1988a[59]	Finnish men, aged 55–69, n = 190	276 item SA	24-day WI (12 × 2-day)	Energy, protein, fat, SFA, MUFA, PUFA, cholesterol, carbohydrate, starch, sucrose, dietary fibre, alcohol, vitamins A, C, D, E, Na, K, Ca, Mg, Cu, Zn, Se, Pb, % energy from protein, fat, carbohydrate, alcohol, P/S ratio (0.38 fat % energy, 0.80 alcohol)
Pietinen et al., 1988b[58]	Finnish men, aged 55–69 n = 190	44 item SA	24-day WI (12 × 2-day)	Energy, fat, SFA, PUFA, vitamins A, C, E, Se, dietary fibre, % energy from fat, carbohydrate, P/S ratio (0.33 Se, 0.81 P/S ratio)
Boutron et al., 1989[60]	French men and women, aged 30–79, n = 40	190 item by meal (n = 20) by food (n = 20)	14-day HM	Energy, protein (total, animal, vegetable) fat, SFA, MUFA, PUFA, carbohydrate, saccharose, sugar, starch, dietary fibre, alcohol (0.08 fat, 0.90 alcohol)
Stigglebout et al., 1989[189]	Dutch women, aged 30–49, n = 82	30 item	DH	Retinol, beta-carotene (0.54 retinol, 0.59 beta-carotene)
O'Donnell et al., 1991[138]	UK, aged 25–64, men n = 24, women n = 28	196 item SA	16-day WI (4 × 4-day)	Energy, protein, fat, SFA, PUFA, carbohydrate, sucrose, dietary fibre, vitamins A, B_1, B_2, C, D, E, niacin, folate, carotene, % energy from fat P/S ratio (0.26 Vitamin D, 0.73 alcohol)
O'Brien et al., 1991[190]	UK, aged 60–75, men n = 14, women n = 15	133 item SA	7-day WI	Energy, fat, SFA, retinol, carotene, vitamins A, C, E (0.45 vitamin E, 0.59 fat)
Tjønneland et al., 1993[143]	Denmark, aged 40–64, men n = 23, women n = 63	92 item SA	Adipose tissue biopsy	Individual fatty acids as a percent of total fatty acid. (r_s: 0.07 mono-unsaturated, 0.55 C20:5n-3 (EPA))

Table 6.9 (*cont.*)

Authors	Sample	Test measure	Reference measure	Nutrients (r_{min} r_{max})
Bingham et al., 1994[61]	England, aged 50–64, women n = 156	FAQ1 FAQ2 24 h recall 1 24 h recall 2 7d checklist 7d checklist + portion sizes 7d estimated record	16-day WI (4 × 4) with urinary N validation	Energy + 14 nuts: (0.39 K, 0.90 alc) (0.13 protein, 0.89 alcohol) (0.21 protein, 0.63 sugars) (0.21 carotene, 0.65 sugars) (0.48 carotene, 0.90 alcohol) (0.29 retinol, 0.87 alcohol) (0.35 retinol, 0.88 alcohol)
Rothenberg, 1994[137]	Sweden, aged 70, men n = 34, women n = 42	257 item FAQ	4d HM 4 × 24h urine N	Energy + 11 nuts: (0.35 sugars, 0.60 energy, fat) Nitrogen: vs. FAQ: 0.19 vs. 4d HM: 0.47
Andersen et al., 1995[191]	Norway, aged 18, boys n = 13, girls n = 36	190 item FAQ	7d WI	Energy + 17 nuts: (0.14 vit D, 0.66 MUFA)

DD – Duplicate diet
DH – Diet history (after Burke)
DHQ – Diet history questionnaire
HM – Household measures food record
WI – Weighed food record
SA – self-administered (otherwise interview administered)
SFA – saturated fatty acids
MUFA – monounsaturated fatty acids
PUFA – polyunsaturated fatty acids
18:1 – Oleic acid
18:2 – Linoleic acid

(cold meats and plain biscuits)). Hammond et al.[142] used a 14-day food checklist in children to validate a FFQ completed by parents. Tjønneland et al.[143] used adipose tissue biopsies to assess the validity of measures of per cent fatty acids in the diet based on FFQ responses, ranging from 0.1 for monounsaturated fatty acids as per cent of total in men to 0.53 for C20:5n-3 (EPA) in both men and women.

It is clear from these data and those in Table 6.9 that the validity of questionnaire estimates of nutrient intake (or food consumption) varies between items and between communities. There are as yet no clear-cut reasons why questionnaires perform as differently as they do with the groups to be assessed (apart from the more obvious technical limitations concerning inadequate assessment of frequency of consumption or portion size), although newer analyses of the sources of error may help to clarify these issues. The variability in the findings emphasize the need to assess the performance of a questionnaire in *every* new study population, not to assume that its performance will mimic that in a previous investigation, and to consider the use of novel reference measures. It is also imperative that any reference measure is itself evaluated (e.g. completeness of dietary records, completeness of 24-hour urine collections), although this in itself raises questions about the generalizability of the results of a validation study (see Chapter 8).

6.12   Assessment of intake in the distant past

The aim in many case-control studies is to assess dietary exposure at the time relevant to the initiation of disease. While it is in practice possible to simply ask questions concerning the time in question (and Moore et al.[144] have devised a scheme to assist subjects in remembering the characteristics of a particular period in the past), it is difficult to know (a) how well the responses correspond with the true intake in the past, and (b) the extent to which recent diet may have biased responses. A number of studies have addressed these questions, and the results are summarized in Table 6.10. The ages shown for the samples in the Table are those when the original dietary assessment was made.

The results show that the level of agreement between recall and original diet varies considerably between studies. The values given in the table are correlation coefficients, unadjusted for energy intake[57], with the exception of Thompson et al.[3] who report kappa statistics. Correlations are of the order of 0.5–0.8 in the studies by Van Leeuwen et al.[82], Byers et al.[145], Bakkum et al.[146], and Goldbohm et al.[147], and generally lower in the studies by Rohan and Potter[148], Jensen et al.[37], Wu et al.[149], Willet et al.[150], and Sobell et al.[151] The low values in the latter studies suggest that some attempts to assess past diet may lead to such extensive misclassification of subjects as to substantially understate risks associated with diet in case-control studies. Assessment of variance in both the recalled and original estimates of intake[147,149–151] can be used to adjust both the correlations (see Chapters 4 and 8) and risk estimates[152] upwards.

It is also striking from the studies[137,146,148,149] in which current as well as past diet was assessed that the recalled diet agrees more closely with the current diet than with the past diet. This suggests that the current diet is having a strong influence on the recalled diet. Moreover, the original diet correlates as well with the current diet as it does with the recalled diet, suggesting that the extent of misclassification (and attenuation of risk estimates) would be as great using the recalled diet as it would be using the current diet, although the sets of individuals who were misclassified would be slightly different in the two analyses, and there are no reports of the differences in risk calculated using the three measures of diet (original, recalled, and current). Indeed, in the first Bakkum study[146], for three out of four nutrients, any estimate of risk associated with past diet would have been more likely to be detected using an assessment of current diet rather than recall of the distant past. The only potential advantage of using recall from the distant past in a case-control study, therefore, would be the probable identification of individuals whose diets had changed radically over the intervening period, but Lindsted and Kuzma[153] (in an analysis of foods rather than nutrients) found that the extent of misclassification was likely to remain the same in cases and controls, and that change in diet was *negatively* associated with an ability to recall accurately. This has been confirmed by Thompson et al.[154], who have shown in both men and women that the influence of current diet on recall is greatest for those whose diets have changed the most.

Thus, while the recall of diets in the distant past is theoretically an attractive measurement to make, it has yet to be demonstrated that it has advantages over risk analyses based on current diet. Substantially more work needs to be carried out to identify the most useful way in which a meaningful recall of diet in the distant past can be achieved.

6.13 Problems of retrospective assessment in population subgroups

Dietary assessment in epidemiological studies of population subgroups such as children and the elderly may present special problems. In children, the problem relates primarily to the ability to recall both the types and amounts of foods consumed and their ability to conceptualize portion sizes. Livingstone *et al.*[155] compared energy intakes based on diet histories and weighed intakes to energy expenditure estimated using doubly-labelled water in 3–18 year-olds. Diet histories were conducted with parents present. Whereas the weighed records showed an increasing tendency to underestimate intake with increasing age, the diet histories tended to overestimate intake (except in 18-year-olds), the size of the error for the group means being generally smaller than for the weighed records. Individual agreement was more variable for the weighed records than for the diet histories. Studies in Ghanaian 4–6 year-olds[100] suggest that with parental help, estimates of intake based on 24-hour recall validated against weighed records or precise weighing are no worse than in adults (correlations ranging from 0.60–0.80). In Senegalese weanlings[99], however, agreement with weighed records of consumption were less good (intraclass correlation coefficient ranging from 0.06 for energy to 0.78 for vitamin A), but the poorer level of agreement may relate to the alteration in food consumption practices necessitated by the weighing procedure (separate servings rather than the traditional consumption from the communal pot). There is some recent evidence of a capability in children of 8–10 years to recall diet over 24 hours such that the group means agree well with those based on parental diet histories, but correlations are low for energy (0.22) and protein (0.25).[156] Use of taped records may improve agreement.[124]

In the elderly, several studies have been carried out to assess the validity of intakes reported retrospectively. Dietary histories with 3-day diaries and checklists were compared with 3-day weighed records to assess validity in the SENECA study.[157] The reported level of intake was typically 10–15% higher based on the diet history. Correlation coefficients ranged from 0.18 (Vitamin A) to 0.79 (water), the values being of a similar order to those reported for other age groups. The findings were confirmed in a study of elderly Norwegian women.[158] Rothenberg[137] compared FAQs with food records (FR) in 76 elderly Swedes and concluded that the FAQ gave a better estimate of energy intake than the FR, based on validation which used urinary nitrogen as an external marker. Van Staveren and colleagues[159], however, were concerned about the effects of memory on 24-hour recall in some elderly subjects, and recommend the use of a combination of techniques including FAQ and FR. The recent British study of diet in the elderly has opted for 4-day weighed records, notwithstanding concerns about under-reporting.[160]

Table 6.10 Summary of questionnaire validation studies of diet in the distant past.

Reference	Sample	Assessment methods and date		Nutrients and correlations			
		Original	Recall	Nutrient	Recall vs original	Recall vs current	Current vs original
Van Leeuwen et al., 1983[82]	Dutch, aged 25–65, men n=44, women n=56	7-day WI 1977	DH 1981	Energy	0.68	—	—
				Protein	0.47	—	—
				Fat	0.68	—	—
				Cholesterol	0.51	—	—
				Carbohydrate	0.64	—	—
				Dietary fibre	0.54	—	—
				Alcohol	0.82	—	—
Rohan and Potter, 1984[148]	Australian, aged 30–74, men n=37, women n=33	141 item FAQ	141 item FAQ	Energy	0.62	0.87	0.58
				Protein	0.25	0.82	0.48
				Fat	0.52	0.84	0.53
				Cholesterol	0.32	0.78	0.35
				PUFA	0.34	0.61	0.48
				Starch	0.66	0.77	0.45
				Sugar	0.61	0.91	0.53
				Dietary fibre	0.52	0.74	0.52
				Alcohol	0.87	0.89	0.91
				Retinol	0.48	0.67	0.48
				Iron	0.38	0.74	0.41
Jensen et al., 1984[37]	Danish, aged 18–50, n=79	28-day FPR 1954–57 1964–66	DH 1982	Energy	0.42	0.63	0.41
				Protein	0.31	0.55	0.38
				Fat	0.40	0.66	0.45
				Carbohydrate	0.33	0.64	0.35
Byers et al., 1987[145]	US, men n=232, women n=91	129 item FAQ 1975–79	47 item FAQ 1984–85	Fat	0.50	—	0.50
				Vitamin A	0.61	—	0.49
				Dietary fibre	0.61	—	0.53
Wu et al., 1988[150]	US, men n=378, women n=495	47 item FAQ 1972	47 item FAQ 1983	Energy*	0.33	0.54	0.32
				Fat*	0.33	0.53	0.30
				PUFA*	0.25	0.58	0.19
				Cholesterol*	0.37	0.55	0.32

Study	Subjects	Method 1	Method 2	Nutrient				
Bakkum et al., 1988[146]	Dutch, aged 58–65, men n=37	DH 1971–72	DH 1984–85	Energy	0.54		0.70	0.75
				Protein	0.65		0.66	0.77
				Fat	0.59		0.74	0.50
				Carbohydrate	0.52		0.75	0.78
	aged 67–82, men n=22, women n=24			Energy	0.69		0.69	0.63
				Protein	0.50		0.47	0.31
				Fat	0.64		0.67	0.55
				Carbohydrate	0.63		0.79	0.52
Willett et al., 1988[149]	US, aged 34–59, women n=150	61-item FAQ1 1980–81 +4×7d WI	116-item revised FAQ2 1984	FAQ2 vs:	WI	FAQ1		
				Energy	0.37	0.54	–	–
				Protein	0.29	0.47	–	–
				Fat	0.37	0.48	–	–
				Carbohydrate	0.47	0.60	–	–
				MUFA	0.37	0.49	–	–
				PUFA	0.43	0.56	–	–
				Sucrose	0.50	0.61	–	–
Sobell et al., 1989[151]	US, interview, men n=90	7d FR 1971–1975	98-item FAQ 1985	Energy	0.50		–	–
				Protein	0.54		–	–
				Fat	0.61		–	–
				Carbohydrate	0.45		–	–
				Calcium	0.40		–	–
				Thiamin	0.41		–	–
	Mail, men n=126			Energy	0.14		–	–
				Protein	0.16		–	–
				Fat	0.27		–	–
				Carbohydrate	0.20		–	–
				Calcium	0.28		–	–
				Thiamin	0.18		–	–
Goldbohm et al., 1994[147]	Dutch, men n=59, women n=48	3×3d FR 1987	150-item FAQ	Energy	0.74		–	–
				Protein	0.61		–	–
				Fat	0.72		–	–
				Carbohydrate	0.77		–	–
				Calcium	0.60		–	–
				Thiamin	0.40		–	–

* results for men only; women's results very similar
FAQ – Food frequency and amount questionnaire
FR – Food consumption record in household measures

DH – Diet history
FPR – Food purchasing record
WI – Weighed inventory

Other studies have analysed problems of assessment specifically in relation to constraints that may be associated with low income, education, or occupation[161-165], all potential sources of differential misclassification.

6.14 Concluding remarks

There are three main components to the error generated in measurements of diet: that associated with the method of assessment itself (its repeatability); that associated with variation in diet over time; and that associated with the ability of the respondent to provide the information required (the main source of differential misclassification). These three components should be identified in every analysis of disease risk, in order to appreciate the extent of attenuation that may be occurring. Failure to assess the components of error, and to undertake proper validation of methods, significantly reduces the ability to interpret the results from nutritional epidemiological studies.

References

1. (1994) First International Symposium on Dietary Assessment Methods. *Am. J. Clin. Nutr.* (Suppl. 1).
2. Öhlin, A., Ahlander, E-M., Ekberg, A. and Bruce, Å. (1994) *Bibliography on validations of dietary assessment methods*. National Food Administration, Uppsala, Sweden.
3. Thompson, F. E., Moler, J. E., Freedman, L., Clifford, C. and Willett, W. C. (1994) *Dietary assessment calibration/validation studies register*. National Cancer Institute, Bethesda, Maryland.
4. Barker, D. J. P., Morris, J. A. and Nelson, M. (1986) Vegetable consumption and acute appendicitis in 59 areas in England and Wales. *Br. Med. J.* **292**: 927–30.
5. Lilienfeld, D. E. and Stolley, P. D. (1994) *Foundations of epidemiology*. 3rd edn. Oxford University Press, Oxford.
6. Flores, M. and Nelson, M. (1988) Methods for data collection at household or institutional level. In: Cameron, M. E. and van Staveren, W. A. (ed.) *Manual on methodology for food consumption studies*. Oxford University Press, Oxford.
7. Zintzaris, E., Kanellou, A., Trichopoulou, A. and Nelson, M. (1996) The validity of household budget survey (HBS) data: estimation of individual food availability in an epidemiological context. *J. Hum. Nutr. Diet.* (In press.)
8. Chesher, A. (1995) Person type specific nutrient intakes from National Food Survey Data. Unpublished report prepared for the Ministry of Agriculture, Fisheries, and Food. London.
9. Hudson, G. J. (1995) Food intake in a west African village. Estimation of food intake from a shared bowl. *Br. J. Nutr.* **73**: 551–69.
10. Dop, M. C. (1995) *African children's intake from the family common pot: how can we measure it?* [abstract]. Second International Conference on Dietary Assessment Methods. Harvard School of Public Health.
11. Department of Employment. (1995) *Family expenditure survey 1993*. HMSO, London.
12. Community Council of Greater New York. (1982) *A family budget standard*. Budget Standard Service of New York Community Council, New York.
13. Montreal Diet Dispensary. (1982) *Budgeting for basic need*. Montreal Diet Dispensary, Montreal.

14. Cameron, M. E. and van Staveren, W. A. (ed.) (1988) *Manual on methodology for food consumption studies.* Oxford University Press, Oxford.

15. Ministry of Agriculture, Fisheries, and Food. (1991) *Household food consumption and expenditure 1990, with a study of trends over the period 1940–1990.* HMSO, London.

16. Ministry of Food. (1951) *The urban working-class household diet 1940–1949.* HMSO, London.

17. Ministry of Food. (1956) *Studies in urban household diets 1944–1949.* HMSO, London.

18. Ministry of Food. (1952–1954) *Domestic food consumption and expenditure: 1950–1952.* HMSO, London.

19. Ministry of Agriculture, Fisheries, and Food. (1955–1990) *Household food consumption and expenditure: 1953–1988.* HMSO, London.

20. Ministry of Agriculture, Fisheries, and Food. (1994) *Household food consumption and expenditure 1992.* HMSO, London.

21. Ingram, D. M. (1981) Trends in diet and breast cancer mortality in England and Wales 1928–1977. *Nutr. Cancer.* **3**: 75–80.

22. Key, T. J. A., Darby, S. C. and Pike, M. C. (1987) Trends in breast cancer mortality and diet in England and Wales from 1911 to 1980. *Nutr. Cancer.* **10**: 1–9.

23. Marmot, M. G., Adelstein, A. M., Robinson, N. and Rose, G. A. (1978) Changing social class distribution of heart disease. *Br. Med. J.* **2**: 1109–12.

24. Low Income Project Team. (1996) Low income, food, nutrition, and health: strategies for improvement. A report by the Low Income Project Team for the Nutrition Task Force. Department of Health, London.

25. Bingham, S., Williams, D. R. R., Cole, T. J. and James W. P. T. (1979) Dietary fibre and regional large bowel cancer mortality in Britain. *Br. J. Cancer.* **40**: 456–63.

26. Derry, B. J. and Buss, D. H. (1984) The British national food survey as a major epidemiological resource. *Br. Med. J.* **288**: 765–7.

27. Nelson, M., Dyson, P. A. and Paul, A. A. (1985) Family food purchase and home food consumption: comparison of nutrient contents. *Br. J. Nutr.* **54**: 373–87.

28. Vassilakou, T. and Trichopoulou, A. (1992) Overview of household budget surveys in 18 European countries. *Eur. J. Clin. Nutr.* **46** (Suppl 5): S137–S153.

29. Lagiou, A., Valaora, A., Vassilakou, T. and Trichopoulou, A. (1992) Comparability of food availability data in household budget surveys in European Community countries. *Eur. J. Clin. Nutr.* **46** (Suppl 5): S35–S136.

30. Poortvliet, E. J., Klensin, J. C. and Kohlmeier, L. (1992) Rationale document for the Eurocode food coding system. *Eur. J. Clin. Nutr.* **46** (Suppl 5): S9–S24.

31. Kemsley, W. F. F. (1976) *Statistical news no. 35.* HMSO, London.

32. Ralph, A. (1993) Dietary reference values. In: Garrow, J. S. and James, W. P. T. (ed.) *Human nutrition and dietetics.* 9th edn. Churchill Livingstone, Edinburgh.

33. Nelson, M. and Peploe, K. A. (1990) Construction of a modest-but-adequate food budget for households with two adults and one preschool child: a preliminary investigation. *J. Hum. Nutr. Diet.* **3**: 121–40.

34. Platt, B. S., Gray, P. G., Parr, E., Baines, A. H. J., Clayton, S., Hobson, E. A., *et al.* (1964) The food purchases of elderly women living alone: a statistical inconsistency and its investigation. *Br. J. Nutr.* **18**: 413–29.

35. Nelson, M. (1983) PhD Thesis. University of London.

36. Nelson, M. (1986) The distribution of nutrient intake within families. *Br. J. Nutr.* **55**: 267–77.

37. Jensen, O. M., Wahrendorf, J., Rosenquist, A. and Geser, A. (1984) The reliability of questionnaire-derived historic information and temporal stability of food habits in individuals. *Am. J. Epid.* **120**: 281–90.

38. Wheeler, E. F. (1992) Intrahousehold food and nutrient allocation. *Nutr. Res. Rev.* **4**: 69–82.

39. Department of Health. (1989) *The diets of British schoolchildren.* Report on Health and Social Subjects No. 36. HMSO, London.
40. Gregory, J., Foster, K., Tyler, M. and Wiseman, M. (1990) *The dietary and nutritional survey of British adults.* HMSO, London.
41. Gregory, J., Collins, D. L., Davies, P. S. W., Hughes, J. and Clarke, P. C. (1995) *National diet and nutrition survey: children aged 1½ to 4½ years.* HMSO, London.
42. Goldberg, G. R., Black, A. E., Jebb, S. A., Cole, T. J., Murgatroyd, P. R., Coward, W. A., et al. (1991) Critical evaluation of energy intake data using fundamental principles of energy physiology. 1. Derivation of cut-off limits to identify under-recording. *Eur. J. Clin. Nutr.* **45**: 569–81.
43. Pryer, J. A. Vrijheid, M., Nichols, R. and Elliott, P. (1994) Who are the 'low energy reporters' in the Dietary and Nutritional Survey of British Adults? *Proc. Nutr. Soc.* **53**: 235A.
44. Wenlock, R. W. (1991) The generation and use of nutritional data by the Department of Health. in: Margetts, B. M. and Nelson, M. (ed.). *Design concepts in nutritional epidemiology.* 1st edn. Oxford University Press, Oxford. pp. 130–152.
45. Crockett, S. J., Potter, J. D., Wright, M. S. and Bacheller, A. (1992) Validation of a self-reported shelf inventory to measure food purchase behavior. *J. Am. Diet. Assoc.* **92**: 694–97.
46. Sudman, S. and Ferber, R. (1971) Experiments on obtaining consumer expenditures by diary methods. *Am. Stat. Assoc.* **66**: 725–35.
47. Hollingsworth, D. F. and Baines, A. H. J. (1961) *A survey of food consumption in Great Britain.* Family Living Studies, A Symposium. Studies and Reports No. 63. Geneva: International Labour Office, Geneva.
48. Wenlock, R. W., Buss, D. H., Derry, B. J. and Dixon, E. J. (1980) Household food wastage in Britain. *Br. J. Nutr.* **43**: 53–70.
49. Nelson, M. and Nettleton, P. A. (1980) Dietary survey methods. I. A semi-weighed technique for measuring dietary intake within families. *J. Hum. Nutr.* **34**: 325–48.
50. United States Department of Agriculture. (1983) *Food consumption: households in the United States, seasons and years 1977–78.* Nationwide food consumption survey 1977–78. Report No. 4–6. US Government Printing Office, Washington D.C.
51. Burk, M. C. and Pao, M. (1976) *Methodology for large-scale surveys of household and individual diets.* Home Economics Research Report No. 40, Agricultural Research Service, US Department of Agriculture, US Government Printing Office, Washington D.C.
52. Bingham, S. A. (1987) The dietary assessment of individuals: methods, accuracy, new techniques and recommendations. *Nutr. Abs. Rev.* **57**: 705–42.
53. Black, A. E. (1982) The logistics of dietary surveys. *Hum. Nutr: Appl. Nutr.* **36A**: 85–94.
54. Nelson, M., Hague, G. F., Cooper, C. and Bunker, V. W. (1988) Calcium intake in the elderly: validation of a dietary questionnaire. *J. Hum. Nutr. Diet.* **1**: 115–27.
55. Cooper, C., Barker, D. J. P. and Wickham, C. (1988) Physical activity, muscle strength and calcium intake in fracture of the proximal femur in Britain. *Br. Med. J.* **297**: 1443–6.
56. Coates, R. J., Serdula, M. K., Byers, T., Mokdad, A., Jewell, S., Leonard, S. B., et al. (1995) A brief, telephone-administered food frequency questionnaire can be useful for surveillance of dietary fat intakes. *J. Nutr.* **125**: 1473–83.
57. Willett, W. C., Sampson, L., Stampfer, M. J., Rosner, B., Bain, C., Witschi, J., et al. (1985) Reproducibility and validity of a semi-quantitative food frequency questionnaire. *Am. J. Epid.* **122**: 51–65.
58. Pietinen, P., Hartman, A. M., Haapa, E., Rasanen, L., Haapakoski, J., Palmgren, J., et al. (1988b) Reproducibility and validity of dietary assessment instruments. II. A quantitative food frequency questionnaire. *Am. J. Epid.* **128**: 667–76.
59. Pietinen, P., Hartman, A. M., Haapa, E., Rasanen, L., Haapakoski, J., Palmgren, J., et al. (1988a) Reproducibility and validity of dietary assessment instruments. I. A self-administered food use questionnaire with a portion size picture booklet. *Am. J. Epid.* **128**: 655–66.

60. Boutron, M. C., Faivre, J., Milan, C., Gorcerie, B. and Esteve, J. (1989) A comparison of two diet history questionnaires that measure usual food intake. *Nutr. Cancer.* **12**: 83-91.

61. Bingham, S. A., Gill, C., Welch, A., Day, K., Cassidy, A., Khaw, K. T., *et al.* (1994) Comparison of dietary assessment methods in nutritional epidemiology: weighed records *v.* 24 h recalls, food-frequency questionnaires and estimated diet records. *Br. J. Nutr.* **72**: 619-43.

62. Wiehl, D G. and Reed, R. (1960) Development of new or improved dietary methods for epidemiological investigations. *Am. J. Publ. Hlth.* **50**: 824-8.

63. Marr, J. W., Heady, J. A. and Morris. J. N. (1961) Towards a method for large-scale individual diet surveys. Proceedings of the 3rd International Congress of Dietetics, London, 10-14 July, 1961. Newman Books. 85-91.

64. Abramson, J. H., Slome, C. and Kosovsky, C. (1963) Food frequency interview as an epidemiological tool. *Am. J. Publ. Hlth.* **53**: 1093-101.

65. Hankin, J. H., Rhoads, G. G. and Glober, G. A. (1975) A dietary method for an epidemiologic study of gastrointestinal cancer. *Am. J. Clin. Nutr.* **28**: 1055-61.

66. Chu, S. Y., Kolonel, L. N., Hankin, J. H. and Lee, J. (1984) A comparison of frequency and quantitative dietary methods for epidemiologic studies of diet and disease. *Am. J. Epid.* **119**: 323-34.

67. Willett, W. C. (1990) *Nutritional epidemiology.* Oxford University Press, New York.

68. Thomas, B. (ed.) (1994) *Manual of dietetic practice.* Blackwell Scientific, Oxford.

69. Nelson, M., Atkinson, M. and Darbyshire, S. (1996) Food photography 2. Use of food photographs for estimating portion size and the nutrient content of meals. *Br. J. Nutr.* **76**: 31-49.

70. Burke, B. S. (1947) The diet history as a tool in research. *J. Am. Diet. Assoc.* **23**: 1041-6.

71. Black, A. E., Jebb, S. A., Bingham, S. A., Runswick, S. and Poppitt, S. (1995) The validation of energy and protein intakes in post-obese subjects. *J. Hum. Nutr. Diet.* **8**: 51-64.

72. Trulson, M. F. and McCann, M. B. (1959) Comparison of dietary survey methods. *J. Am. Diet. Assoc.* **35**: 672-81.

73. Reshef, A. and Epstein, L. M. (1972) Reliability of a dietary questionnaire. *Am. J. Clin. Nutr.* **25**: 91-5.

74. Morgan, R. W., Jain, M., Miller, A. B., Choi, N. W., Matthews, V., Munan, L., *et al.* (1978) A comparison of dietary methods in epidemiologic studies. *Am. J. Epid.* **107**: 488-98.

75. Bazzarre, T. L. and Yuhas, J. A. (1983) Comparative evaluation of methods of collecting food intake data for cancer epidemiology studies. *Nutr. Cancer.* **5**: 201-14.

76. Jain, M., Howe, G. R., Johnson, K. C. and Miller, A. B. (1980) Evaluation of a diet history questionnaire for epidemiologic studies. *Am. J. Epid.* **111**: 212-19.

77. Dawber, T. R., Pearson, G., Anderson, P., Mann, G. V., Kannel, W. B., Shurtleff, D., *et al.* (1962) Dietary assessment in the epidemiologic study of coronary heart disease: the Framingham study. 2. Reliability of measurement. *Am. J. Clin. Nutr.* **11**: 226-34.

78. Young, C. M., Chalmers, F. W., Church, H. N., Clayton, M. M., Tucker, R. E., Werts, A. W., *et al.* (1952) A comparison of dietary study methods. I. Dietary history vs seven-day record. *J. Am. Diet. Assoc.* **28**: 124-8.

79. Huenemann, R. L. and Turner, D. (1942) Methods of dietary investigation. *J. Am. Diet. Assoc.* **18**: 562-8.

80. Black, A. E. (1981) Pitfalls in dietary assessments. In: Howard, A. N. and McLean-Baird, I. (ed.) *Recent advances in clinical nutrition.* John Libbey, London.

81. Jarvinen, R. (1995) *Validity of dietary history interview data.* [abstract]. Second International Conference on Dietary Assessment Methods. Harvard School of Public Health.

82. Van Leeuwen, F. E., de Vet, H. C. W., Hayes, R. B., van Staveren, W. A., West, C. A. and Hautvast, J. G. A. J. (1983) An assessment of the relative validity of retrospective interviewing for measuring dietary intake. *Am. J. Epid.* **118**: 752-8.

83. Heitman, B. L. and Lissner, L. (1995) Dietary under-reporting by obese individuals. Is it specific or non-specific? *Br. Med. J.* **311**: 986–9

84. Wiehl, D. G. (1942) Diets of a group of aircraft workers in Southern California. *Millbank Memorial Fund Quarterly.* **20**: 329–66.

85. Kohlmeier, L. (1992) Dietary methodology considerations for NHANES III. *Vital Health Stat.* 4. Mar: 81–4.

86. Rasanen, L. (1979) Nutrition survey of Finnish rural children. VI. Methodological study comparing the 24-hour recall and the dietary history interview. *Am. J. Clin. Nutr.* **32**: 2560–7.

87. Rasanen, L. (1982) Validity and reliability of recall methods. In: Report to the EEC workshop on methods of evaluating nutritional status with empasis on food consumption studies. Wageningen.

88. Balogh, M., Kahn, H. A. and Medalie, J. H. (1971) Random repeat 24-hour dietary recalls. *Am. J. Clin. Nutr.* **24**: 304–10.

89. Linusson, E. E. I., Sanjur, D. and Erickson, E. C. (1974) Validating the 24-hour recall method as a dietary survey tool. *Arch. Latinamer. Nutr.* **24**: 277–94.

90. Acheson, K. J., Campbell, I. T., Edholm, O. G., Miller, D. S. and Stock, M. J. (1980) The measurement of food and energy intake in man – an evaluation of some techniques. *Am. J. Clin. Nutr.* **33**: 1147–54.

91. Potischman, N., Carroll, R. J. and Swanson, C. A. (1995) *24-hour recalls and diet records: differences in dietary intakes and other methodological considerations.* [abstract]. Second International Conference on Dietary Assessment Methods. Harvard School of Public Health.

92. Emmons, L. and Hayes, M. (1973) Accuracy of 24-hour recall of young children. *J. Am. Diet. Assoc.* **62**: 402–15.

93. Karvetti, R. L. and Knuts, l. R. (1981) Agreement between dietary interviews. *J. Am. Diet. Assoc.* **79**: 654–60.

94. Borrelli, R., Cole, T. J., Di Biase, G. and Contaldo, F. (1989) Some statistical considerations on dietary assessment methods. *Eur. J. Clin. Nutr.* **43**: 453–63.

95. Johansson, G., Callmer, E. and Gustafsson, J. A. (1992) Validity of repeated dietary measurements in a dietary intervention study. *Eur. J. Clin. Nutr.* **46**: 717–28.

96. Hebert, J. R., Ockene, I. S., Merriam, P., Botelho, L. and Ellis, S. (1995) *Development and testing of a seven day dietary recall.* [abstract]. Second International Conference on Dietary Assessment Methods. Harvard School of Public Health.

97. Posner, B. M., Borman, C. L., Morgan, J. L., Borden, W. A. and Ohls, J. C. (1982) The validity of a telephone administered 24-hour dietary recall methodology. *Am. J. Clin. Nutr.* **36**: 546–53.

98. Nelson, M., Black, A. E., Morris, J. A. and Cole, T. J. (1989) Between- and within-subject variation in nutrient intake from infancy to old age: estimating the number of days required to rank dietary intakes with desired precision. *Am. J. Clin. Nutr.* **50**: 155–67.

99. Dop, M. C., Milan, C. and N'Diaye, A. M. (1994) The 24-hour recall for Senegalese weanlings: a validation exercise. *Eur. J. Clin. Nutr.* **48**: 643–53.

100. Ferguson, E. L., Gibson, R. S. Opare-Obisaw, C. (1994) The relative validity of the repeated 24h recall for estimating energy and selected nutrient intakes of rural Ghanaian children. *Eur. J. Clin. Nutr.* **48**: 241–52.

101. Rutishauser, I. H. E. (1995) *Is one replicate enough to reliably estimate the population variance ratio?* [abstract]. Second International Conference on Dietary Assessment Methods. Harvard School of Public Health.

102. Junkins, E. A. and Karpinski, K. F. (1995) *Comparison of multivariate classification procedures with current methodology of adjustment for intraindividual variability in the evaluation of dietary intakes.* [abstract]. Second International Conference on Dietary Assessment Methods. Harvard School of Public Health.

103. Kott, P. S. (1995) *Using multi-day CSFII data and the ISU method to remove within-person variability from a 1-day dietary data set.* [abstract]. Second International Conference on Dietary Assessment Methods. Harvard School of Public Health.

104. Webb, K. L. (1995) *Apparent under-reporting in two Australian dietary surveys – the implications.* [abstract]. Second International Conference on Dietary Assessment Methods. Harvard School of Public Health.

105. Wilcox, A. J. and Gartside, P. S. (1995) *Validity of 24-hour dietary recall data from NHANES II examinees.* [abstract]. Second International Conference on Dietary Assessment Methods. Harvard School of Public Health.

106. Bingham, S. A., Cassidy, A., Cole, T., Welch, A., Runswick, S., Black, A. E., *et al.* (1995) Validation of weighed records and other methods of dietary assessment using the 24 h urine technique and other biological markers. *Br. J. Nutr.* **73**: 531–50.

107. Keys, A. (1970) Coronary heart disease in seven countries. *Circulation.* Supplement 1 to vols 41 and 42.

108. Braddon, F. E. M., Wadsworth, M .E. J., Davies, J. M. C. and Cripps, H. A. (1988) Social and regional differences in food and alcohol consumption in Britain. *J. Epid. Comm. Hlth.* **42**: 341–9.

109. Thorogood, M., Mann, J., Appley, P. and McPherson, K. (1994) Risk of death from cancer and ischaemic heart disease in meat and non-meat-eaters. *Br. Med. J.* **308**: 1667–70.

110. MacLennan, R., Macrae, F., Bain, C., Battistutta, D., Chapuis, P., Gratten, H., *et al.* (1995) Randomized trial of intake of fat, fiber, and beta carotene to prevent colorectal adenomas. *J. Nat. Cancer Inst.* **87**: 1760–6.

111. Nelson, M., Atkinson, M. and Darbyshire, S. (1994) Food photography 1. The perception of food portion size from photographs. *Br. J. Nutr.* **72**: 649–63.

112. Lucas, F., Nivarong, M., Villeminot, S., Kaaks, R. and Clavel-Chapelon, F. (1995) Estimation of food portion sizes using photographs. *J. Hum. Nutr. Diet.* **81**: 65–74.

113. Krebs-Smith, S. M., Heimendinger, J., Subar, A. F., Patterson, B. H. and Pivonka, E. (1993) Estimation of fruit and vegetable intake using FFQ: a comparison of instruments. (abstract) *Am. J. Clin. Nutr.* **59** (Suppl 1): 283S.

114. Black, A. E., Prentice, A. M., Goldberg, G. R., Jebb, S. A., Bingham, S. A., Livingstone, M. B. E., *et al.* (1993) Measurements of total energy expenditure provide insights into the validity of dietary measurements of energy intake. *J. Am. Diet. Assoc.* **93**: 572–9.

115. Gaard, M., Tretli, S. and Loken, E. (1995) Dietary fat and the risk of breast cancer: a prospective study of 25 892 Norwegian women. *Int. J. Cancer.* **63**: 13–17.

116 Prentice, A. M., Coward, W. A., Davies, H. L., Murgatroyd, P. R., Black, A. E., Goldberg, G. R., *et al.* (1985) Unexpectedly low levels of energy expenditure in healthy women. *Lancet.* **ii**: 1419–22.

117. Prentice, A. M., Black, A. E., Coward, W. A., Davies, H. L., Goldberg, G. R., Murgatroyd, P. R., *et al.* (1986) High levels of energy expenditure in obese women. *Br. Med. J.* **292**: 983–7.

118. Livingstone, M. B. E., Prentice, A. M., Strain, J. J., Coward, W. A., Black, A. E., Barker, M. E., *et al.* (1990) Accuracy of weighed dietary records in studies of diet and health. *Br. Med. J.* **300**: 708–12.

119. Isaksson, B. (1980) Urinary nitrogen output as a validity test in dietary surveys. *Am. J. Clin. Nutr.* **33**: 4–6.

120. Steen, B., Isaksson, B. and Svanborg, A. (1977) Intake of energy and nutrients and meal habits in 70-year-old males and females in Gothenburg, Sweden: a population study. *Acta. Med. Scand.* **611**(Suppl): 39–86.

121. Warnold, I., Carlgren, G. and Krotkiewski, M. (1978) Energy expenditure and body composition during weight reduction in hyperplastic obese women. *Am. J. Clin. Nutr.* **31**: 750–63.

122. Heitman, B. L. and Lissner, L. (1995) Dietary under-reporting by obese individuals – is it specific or non-specific. *Br. Med. J.* **311**: 986–9.
123. Vissner, M., de Groot, L. C. P. G., Deurenburg, P. and van Staveren, W. J. A. (1995) Validation of dietary history method in a group of elderly women using measurements of total energy expenditure. *Br. J. Nutr.* **74**: 775–85.
124. Van Horn, L. V., Gernhofer, N., Moag-Stahlberg, A., Farris, R., Hartmuller, G., Lasser, V. I., *et al.* (1990) Dietary assessment in children using electronic methods: telephones and tape recorders. *J. Am. Diet. Assoc.* **90**: 412–16.
125. Hodkinson, H. M. (1975) *An outline of geriatrics.* Oxford University Press, Oxford.
126. Centonze, S., Misciagna, G., Cisternino, A. M. and Guerra, V. (1995) *Short-term recall of usual diet and current cognitive difficulties in a cohort of free-living elderly population in southern Italy.* [abstract]. Second International Conference on Dietary Assessment Methods. Harvard School of Public Health.
127. Epstein, L. M., Reshef, A., Abrahamson, J. H. and Bialik, O. (1970) Validity of a short dietary questionnaire. *Israel. J. Med. Sci.* **6**: 589–97.
128. Levine, J. A., Madden, A. M. and Morgan, M. Y. (1987) Validation of a computer-based system for assessing dietary intake. *Br. Med. J.* **295**: 369–72.
129. Beaton, G. H., Milner, J., Corey, P., McGuire, S., Cousins, M., Stewart, E., *et al.* (1979) Sources of variance in 24-hour dietary recall data: implications for nutrition study design and interpretation. *Am. J. Clin. Nutr.* **32**: 2546–59.
130. Kaaks, R., Plummer, M., Riboli, E., Estève, J. and van Staveren, W. (1994) Adjustment for bias due to errors in exposure assessments in multicenter cohort studies on diet and cancer: a calibration approach. *Am. J. Clin. Nutr.* **59**(Suppl): 245S–250S.
131. Keen, H., Thomas, B. J., Jarrett, R. J., and Fuller, J. H. (1979) Nutrient intake, adiposity and diabetes. *Br. Med. J.* **1**: 655–8.
132. Nomura, A., Hankin, J. H. and Rhoads, G. G. (1976) The reproducibility of dietary intake data in a prospective study of gastrointestinal cancer. *Am. J. Clin. Nutr.* **29**: 1432–6.
133. Bingham, S., Plummer, M. and Day, N. E. (1995) Energy adjustment in dietary surveys. Letter. *Br. J. Nutr.* **74**: 141–3.
134. Bingham, S. and Day, N. E. (1996) Use of biomarkers to validate dietary assessments and the effect of energy adjustment. *Am. J. Clin. Nutr.* (In press.)
135. Porrini, M., Gentile, M. G. and Fidanza, F. (1995) Biochemical validation of self-administered FFQ. *Br. J. Nutr.* **74**: 323–33.
136. Yong, L. C., Forman, M., Beecher, G. R., Graubard, B. I., Campbell, W. S., Reichman, M. E., *et al.* (1994) Relationship between dietary intake and plasma concentration of carotenoids in premenopausal women. *Am. J. Clin. Nutr.* **60**: 223–30.
137. Rothenberg, E. (1994) Validation of the food frequency questionnaire with the 4-day record method and analysis of 24-h urinary nitrogen. *Eur. J. Clin. Nutr.* **48**: 725–35.
138. O'Donnell, M. G., Nelson, M., Wise, P. H. and Walker, D. M. (1991) A computerised diet questionnaire for use in health education. *Br. J. Nutr.* **66**: 3–15.
139. Hankin, J. H., Kolonel, L. N. and Hinds, M. W. (1984) Dietary history methods for epidemiologic studies: application in a case-control study of vitamin A and lung cancer. *J. Nat. Cancer Inst.* **73**: 1417–21.
140. Flegal, K. M. and Larkin, F. A. (1990) Partitioning macronutrient intake estimates from a food frequency questionnaire. *Am. J. Epid.* **131**: 1046–58.
141. Howarth, C. C. and Worsley, A. (1990) Assessment of the validity of a food frequency questionnaire as a measure of food use by comparison with direct observation of domestic food stores. *Am. J. Epid.* **131**: 1059–67.
142. Hammond, J., Nelson, M., Chinn, S. and Rona, R. J. (1995) Validation of a food frequency questionnaire for assessing dietary intake in a study of coronary heart disease risk factors in children. *Eur. J. Clin. Nutr.* **47**: 242–50.
143. Tjønneland, A., Overvad, K., Thorling, E. and Ewertz, M. (1993) Adipose tissue fatty

acids as biomarkers of dietary exposure in Danish men and women. *Am. J. Clin. Nutr.* **57**: 629–33.

144. Moore, J. V., Prestridge, L. L. and Newell, G. R. (1982) Research technique for epidemiologic investigation of nutrition and cancer. *Nutr. Cancer.* **3**: 249–56.

145. Byers, T., Marshall, J., Anthony, E., Fiedler, R. and Zielezny, M. (1987) The reliability of dietary history from the distant past. *Am. J. Epid.* **125**: 999–1011.

146. Bakkum, A., Bloemberg, B., van Staveren, W. A., Verschuren, M. and West, C. E. (1988) The relative validity of a retrospective estimate of food consumption based on a current dietary history and a food frequency list. *Nutr. Cancer.* **11**: 41–53.

147. Goldbohm, R. A., van 't Veer, P., van den Brandt, P. A., van 't Hof, M. A., Brants, H. A., Sturmans, F., *et al.* (1995) Reproducibility of a food frequency questionnaire and stability of dietary habits determined from five annually repeated measurements. *Eur. J. Clin. Nutr.* **49**: 420–9.

148. Rohan, T. E. and Potter, J. D. (1984) Retrospective assessment of dietary intake. *Am. J. Epid.* **120**: 876–87.

149. Willett, W. C., Sampson, L., Browne, M. L., Stampfer, M. J., Rosner, B., Hennekens, C. H., *et al.* (1988) The use of a self-administered questionnaire to assess diet four years in the past. *Am. J. Epid.* **127**: 188–99.

150. Wu, M. L., Whittemore, A. S. and Jung, D. L. (1988) Errors in reported dietary intakes. II. Long-term recall. *Am. J. Epid.* **128**: 1137–45.

151. Sobell, J., Block, G., Koslowe, P., Tobin, J. and Andres, R. (1989) Validation of a retrospective questionnaire assessing diet 10–15 years ago. *Am. J. Epid.* **130**: 173–87.

152. Freudenheim, J. L. and Marshall, J. R. (1988) The problem of profound mismeasurement and the power of epidemiological studies of diet and cancer. *Nutr. Cancer.* **11**: 243–50.

153. Lindsted, K. D. and Kuzma, J. W. (1989) Long-term (24 years) recall reliability in cancer cases and controls using a 21-item food frequency questionnaire. *Nutr. Cancer.* **12**: 135–49.

154. Thompson, F. E., Metzner, H. L., Lamphiear, D. E. and Hawthorne, V. M. (1990) Characteristics of individuals and long-term reproducibility of dietary reports: the Tecumseh Diet Methodology Study. *J. Clin. Epid.* **43**: 1169–78.

155. Livingstone, M. B. E., Prentice, A. M., Coward, W. A., Strain, J. J., Black, A. E., Davies, P. S., *et al.* (1992) Validation of estimates of energy intake by weighed dietary record and diet history in children and adolescents. *Am. J. Clin. Nutr.* **56**: 29–35.

156. Haraldsdóttir, J. and Hermansen, B. (1995) Repeated 24-h recalls with young school-children. A feasible alternative to dietary history from parents? *Eur. J. Clin. Nutr.* **49**: 729–39.

157. Nes, M., van Staveren, W. A., Zajkas, G., Inelmen, E. M. and Moreiras-Varela, O. (1991) Validity of the dietary history method in elderly subjects. Euronut SENECA investigators. *Eur. J. Clin. Nutr.* **45**(Suppl 3): 97–104.

158. Nes, M., Frost-Andersen, L., Solvoll, K., Sandstad, B., Hustvedt, B. E., Løvø, A., *et al.* (1992) Accuracy of a quantitative food frequency questionnaire applied in elderly Norwegian women. *Eur. J. Clin. Nutr.* **46**: 809–2.

159. van Staveren, W. A., de Groot, L. C., Blauw, Y. H. and van der Wielen, R. P. (1994) Assessing diets of elderly people: problems and approaches. *Am. J. Clin. Nutr.* **59**(Suppl 1): 221S–223S.

160. Hughes, J. M., Smithers, G., Gay, C., Clarke, P. C., Smith, P., Lowe, C., *et al.* (1995) The British national diet and nutrition survey of people aged 65 years or over: protocol and feasibility study. *Proc. Nutr. Soc.* **54**: 631–43.

161. Ammerman, A. S., Haines, P. S., DeVellis, R. F., Strogatz, D. S., Keyserling, T. C., Simpson, R. J. Jr, *et al.* (1991) A brief dietary assessment to guide cholesterol reduction in low-income individuals: design and validation. *J. Am. Diet. Assoc.* **91**: 1385–90.

162. Birkett, N. J. and Boulet, J. (1995) Validation of a food habits questionnaire: poor performance in male manual laborers. *J. Am. Diet. Assoc.* **95**: 558–63.

163. Suitor, C. J. W., Gardner, J. and Willett, W. C. (1989) A comparison of food frequency and diet recall methods in studies of nutrient intake of low-income pregnant women. *J. Am. Diet. Assoc.* **89**: 1786–94.

164. Suitor, C. W. and Gardner, J. D. (1992) Development of an interactive, self-administered, computerized food frequency questionnaire for use with low-income women. *J. Nutr. Educ.* **24**: 82–6.

165. Webb, C. A. and Yuhas, J. A. (1988) Ability of WIC clientele to estimate food quantities. *J. Am. Diet. Assoc.* **88**: 601–2.

166. Young, C. M., Hagan, G. C., Tucker, R. E. and Foster, W. D. (1952) A comparison of dietary study methods. II. Dietary history vs. seven-day record vs. 24 h recall. *J. Am. Diet. Assoc.* **28**: 218–21.

167. Lockwood, M. J., Riding, K. H. and Keen, H. (1968) The spoonful as a dietary measure. *Nutrition.* **22**: 7–14.

168. Rutishauser, I. H. E. (1982) Food models, photographs or household measures? *Proc. Nutr. Soc. Aust.* **7**: 144.

169. Bollard, J. E., Yuhas, J. A. and Bollard, T. W. (1988) Estimation of food portion sizes: effectiveness of training. *J. Am. Diet. Assoc.* **88**: 817–20.

170. Blake, A. J., Guthrie, H. and Smicklas-Wright, H. (1989) Accuracy of food portion estimates by overweight and normal weight subjects. *J. Am. Diet. Assoc.* **89**: 962–4.

171. Morgan, S., Flint, D. M., Prinsely, D. M., Wahlqvist, M. L. and Ponsh, A. E. (1982) Measurement of food intake in the elderly by food photography. *Proc. Nutr. Soc. Aust.* **7**: 172.

172. Brock, K. and Ellery, C. (1982) Quantitative dietary assessment in human populations: the development and assessment of food photographs to aid in the use of a food frequency questionnaire. *Proc. Nutr. Soc. Aust.* **7**: 169.

173. Bransby, E. R., Daubney, C. G. and King, J. (1948) Comparisons of results obtained by different methods of individual dietary survey. *Br. J. Nutr.* **2**: 89–110.

174. Todd, K. S., Hudes, M. and Calloway, D. H. (1983) Food intake measurement problems and approaches. *Am. J. Clin. Nutr.* **37**: 139–46.

175. Eppright, E. S., Patton, M. B., Marlatt, A. L. and Hathaway, M. L. (1952) Dietary study methods. V. Some problems in collecting dietary information about groups of children. *J. Am. Diet. Assoc.* **28**: 43–8.

176. Nettleton, P. A., Day, K. C. and Nelson, M. (1980) Dietary survey methods. 2. A comparison of nutrient intakes within families assessed by household measures and the semi-weighed method. *J. Hum. Nutr.* **34**: 349–54.

177. Marr, J. W. (1981) Individual variation in dietary intake. In: Turner, M. (ed.) *Preventive nutrition and society*. Academic Press, London.

178. Bingham, S., McNeil, N. I. and Cummings, J. H. (1981) The diet of individuals: a study of a randomly chosen cross-section of British adults in a Cambridgeshire village. *Br. J. Nutr.* **45**: 23–35.

179. Balogh, M., Medalie, J. N., Smith, H. and Groen, J. J. (1968) The development of a dietary questionnaire for an ischaemic heaeart disease survey. *Israel. J. Med. Sci..* **4**: 195–203.

180. Jain, M. G., Harrison, L., Howe, G. R. and Miller, A. B. (1982) Evaluation of a self-administered dietary questionnaire for use in a cohort study. *Am. J. Clin. Nutr.* **36**: 931–5.

181. Barasi, M. E., Burr, M. L. and Sweetnam, P. M. (1983) A comparison of dietary fibre intake in South Wales estimated from a questionnaire and weighed dietary records. *Nutr. Res.* **3**: 249–55.

182. Stuff, J. E., Garza, C., O'Brian-Smith, E., Nichols, B. L. and Montandon, C. M. (1983) A comparison of dietary methods in nutritional studies. *Am. J. Clin. Nutr.* **37**: 300–6.

183. Yarnell, J. W. G., Fehily, A. M., Millbank, J. E., Sweetnam, P. M. and Walker, C. L. (1983) A short questionnaire for use in epidemiological surveys: comparison with weighed dietary records. *Hum. Nutr.: Appl. Nutr.* **37A**: 103–12.

184. Gray, G. E., Paganini-Hill, A., Ross, R. K. and Henderson, B. E. (1984) Assessment of three brief methods of estimation of vitamin A and C intakes for a prospective study of cancer: comparison with dietary history. *Am. J. Epid.* **119**: 581–90.

185. Shepherd, R., Farleigh, C. A. and Land, D. G. (1985) Estimation of salt intake by questionnaire. *Appetite.* **6**: 219–33.

186. Cummings, S. R., Block. G., McHenry, K. and Baron, R. B. (1985) Evaluation of two food frequency methods of measuring dietary calcium intake. *Am. J. Epid.* **126**: 796–802.

187. Nelson, M., Quayle, A. and Phillips, D. I. W. (1987) Iodine intake and excretion in two British towns: aspects of questionnaire validation. *Hum. Nutr.: Appl. Nutr.* **41A**: 187–92.

188. Willett, W. C., Reynolds, R. D., Cottrell-Hoehner, S., Sampson, L. and Browne, M. L. (1987) Validation of a semi-quantitative food frequency questionnaire: comparison with a 1-year diet record. *J. Am. Diet. Assoc.* **87**: 43–7.

189. Stiggelbout, A. M., van der Giezen, A. M., Blauw, Y. H., Blok, E., van Staveren, W. A. and West, C. E. (1989) Development and relative validity of a food frequency questionnaire for the estimation of retinol and beta-carotene. *Nutr. Cancer.* **12**: 289–99.

190. O'Brien, C. and Nelson, M. Validity of a dietary questionnaire for assessing anti-oxidant vitamin intake. (Unpublished.)

191. Andersen, L. F., Nes, M., Lillegaard, I. T., Sandstad, B., Bjørneboe, G. E. and Drevon, C. A. (1995) Evaluation of a quantitative food frequency questionnaire used in a group of Norwegian adolescents. *Eur. J. Clin. Nutr.* **49**: 543–54.

7. Biochemical markers of nutrient intake

Chris J. Bates and David I. Thurnham, with Sheila A. Bingham, Barrie M. Margetts, and Michael Nelson

7.1 Prediction of nutrient intakes from the values of biochemical markers of nutrient status

It is a reasonable assumption that any valid biochemical, functional, or clinical index of status of an essential nutrient (i.e. any essential component of the diet) or non-nutrient is likely to be related over at least part of the entire range of observed values, to the amount that is present in the diet. Such an index is, therefore, at least potentially a marker of nutrient or other food constituent intake. The usefulness of biomarkers is illustrated in a follow-up study of markers of aflatoxin exposure in relation to liver cancer. The range of aflatoxin contamination of foods is very great, so that use of food tables of average levels of contamination is unlikely to pick up individual exposure. Relative risks of cancer from aflatoxin consumption were only 0.9 and insignificant (confidence intervals 0.4–1.9) for individuals classified as having had high dietary exposure, as assessed by an interview of the frequency of consumption of 45 foods. However, aflatoxin exposure biomarkers in urine samples obtained from individuals in the cohort were able to detect substantial significant relative risks for liver cancer in the order of 6–19. Relative risks were to 59.4 (16.6–212.0) in individuals positive for urine biomarkers of both aflatoxin and hepatitis B.[1]

However, it cannot be assumed that there will be a close or simple relationship between the amount in the diet and the values that can be obtained by laboratory or other quantitative measurements of status indices. Indeed, the primary intention in developing these indices has been not to predict or estimate the amount in the diet, but rather to estimate the amount present in, or available to, the essential and vulnerable tissues of the body, in order to define different states, namely deficiency, adequacy, or possibly overload, at the tissue level. Thus, independent measurements of intake, of biochemical status, and of functional or clinical status indices when added together, give three different windows on the level of 'nutrient adequacy' of the individual (or group of individuals) being studied. Epidemiological studies might independently investigate the three questions: (i) whether diet affects risk; (ii) whether biochemical status affects risk; and (iii) whether functional status affects risk. The answers could be different in each case, but agreement between two independent measures, say diet and risk, and biomarkers of diet and risk, allows greater confidence in the validity of both sets of results. Biomarkers may also be used to validate the accuracy of dietary assessment methods but prior detailed studies under controlled conditions, for example a metabolic suite, are necessary to ascertain that the predictability of the biomarker in humans consuming varying diets is at least as good as the dietary intake method which is being validated. Few biomarkers of dietary intake have been studied in this way.

Although there are links between them, in the sense that each window can be partly observed from the other two, the view from each is different and the overlap of views is only partial. In addition, the degree of overlap differs for different nutrients, and for different types of indices (e.g. urinary nutrients versus plasma levels, versus blood cell levels, versus tests to probe metabolic pathways), so that it is difficult to generalize about the extent to which intakes can be predicted from status values. In the following section, a brief discussion of some of the factors and, in particular, the potential errors and confounders that blur the relationship between status values and nutrient intakes, is attempted. It should be recognized at the outset that the quantitative and statistical aspects of these relationships have hitherto received very little attention in published studies, so that although we can, in some instances, give an approximate value for the mean intake of a nutrient by a defined human group, as predicted from the mean biochemical index value, we have virtually no data describing the precision of such estimates, especially for micronutrients. In many instances, the best that can be attempted at present is a very approximate subdivision into 'deficient' and 'acceptable' intakes, or perhaps into 'low', 'medium', and 'high' intakes, in terms of their relationships to the (also poorly-defined) limits of long-term nutrient requirements. In the following discussion it should also be recognized that comparisons between mean values for groups or populations of subjects should, by the law of averages, yield closer correlations (e.g. of intakes versus status values) than can be obtained by similar comparisons between individuals.

7.1.1 Validity and reproducibility*

The factors that determine the quality of laboratory data are central to any discussion of quality control in clinical chemistry. The assay procedures used must be sufficiently sensitive, sufficiently robust, sufficiently free from short-term fluctuations and long-term drift, and sufficiently free from interference by other sample components (especially the variable ones) to yield a reliable data set. Many vitamins are unstable to heat, light, oxygen, etc. and therefore decay during storage (to different extents in different solutions and matrices, and it is difficult to predict the extent of decay from any known values of storage time and temperature). It is therefore especially important to define an optimum storage schedule, e.g. acidification with a metal-chelating acid for vitamin C, addition of vitamin C as preservative for folate, elimination of light-exposure for riboflavin, elimination of haemolysis for vitamin A.

Validity implies that the data are true, unbiased measures of the variable. As nutrition is an international discipline, it is important that results in one laboratory are comparable with another, and attention to this aspect of concurrent validity should not be neglected.

---

* For consistent use of language throughout the book, we have used the term 'validity' when a clinical chemist would use the word 'accuracy', and 'reproducibility' when the clinical chemist would use 'precision'.

Reproducibility (or precision) implies reliability and expresses the variability of results obtained when a single sample is measured many times. In practice, a mean and standard deviation are calculated from several measurements on a sample (commonly 20) and used to obtain the coefficient of variation ($CV = SD/\bar{x} \times 100$). It is ideally calculated for samples at the bottom, middle, and top of the reference range. The CV represents the sum of all the laboratory factors that can influence a result, and ideally should not be greater than 5%. The simplest methods will have the lowest CVs, while those with many steps and requiring a high level of technical skill will be higher. Automation should be used wherever possible because this will lower the CV and, generally speaking, results obtained where the CV is greater than 10% should be examined very carefully. Low CVs may not be obtained when a new method is first used because factors influencing the variance in the technique may not be known, but measuring a CV makes one aware of potential problems and with time and experience, sources of error will be identified and removed and the CV will improve. The more experienced a laboratory or worker with a particular method, the lower the CV is likely to be. Reproducibility, therefore, is a measure of good laboratory practice.

Validity and reproducibility are both important in any biochemical measurement. Validity may appear to be more difficult to achieve because most biochemical measurements involve many stages when bias may enter the procedure and consistently raise or lower the end result. When national quality control schemes were introduced, measurements of the same material by different methods produced different results, indicating differences in the accuracy of different methods. However, as time passed reproducibility in the participating laboratories improved and, as it did so, differences between the means obtained by different methods fell; that is, as the quality of work in laboratories improved (as measured by CV), so relative validity between methods also improved. This discussion does not include the variability or bias that may be attributable to within-subject variance, or differential misclassification between subjects. For a fuller discussion on laboratory quality control the reader is referred to Whitehead.[2]

Provided that exactly the same method is used to calibrate the relationship between dietary intake and the status index values (as subsequently used to predict the intake of new individuals or groups from the original calibration), then the absolute accuracy of the index values may be of minor importance, provided the calibration is stable and precise. However, it is very important to realize that apparently minor differences in laboratory protocol, which may not be at all apparent from the published descriptions or worksheets, may have a profound effect on the quantitative relationships between nutrient intakes (or tissue levels) and the index values that are obtained by a particular laboratory. A very clear example of this problem is manifested in the differences in values obtained between the Glatzle et al.[3] and Beutler[4] techniques for the assay of riboflavin status by the activation coefficient of glutathione reductase (both of these are widely used variants). At least part of the explanation for this particular difference became apparent from the subsequent studies of Garry and Owen[5] and of Thurnham and Rathakette.[6] However, the problem in more general terms is one of the major pitfalls that can be encountered if a 'calibration' curve obtained in one laboratory is then used uncritically in another, even if the assay protocols appear to be identical on paper.

Reference materials

For most of the substances measured by the clinical chemist there are reference materials available. These are commercially available serum/plasma samples in which the concentrations of the component materials are known having been analysed by one or more reference laboratories. Unfortunately, the nutritional biochemist may not have these available because the methods are used by too few people to be commercially justifiable. This situation is changing for some analytes such as folate, vitamin B_{12}, retinol, carotenoids, vitamin E, and some trace elements, but there is nothing to suggest that reference materials for the other vitamins will appear in the near future.

In the absence of standard reference material, attempts should be made to prepare the laboratory's own reference material. This should be as close as possible in its physical form to the substance that is routinely analysed. Compromises have to be made for unstable substances, hence, for vitamin C the authors' reference materials are plasma and standard extracts in metaphosphoric acid, although lyophilized plasma was found to be satisfactory over 12 months at 4°C (unpublished data). For retinol and carotene, portions of normal plasma stored at −20°C proved satisfactory over 6 months[7] but −70°C or lower, or the use of lyophilized plasma,[8,9] is necessary for storage over longer periods. For the riboflavin assay, haemolysates (1 part erythrocytes: 19 parts water) containing the glutathione reductase enzyme are stable when stored at −50°C or lyophilized at 4°C (unpublished). By routinely including such materials in every batch of samples analysed, the routine performance of assays can be monitored and early indications of more subtle drifts in the data can be picked up.[6] Such procedures help to maintain precision and prevent or reduce drift to a minimum, but of course the longer the study, the more difficult this becomes, particularly if the quality control standards are themselves unstable. Ideally, the reference material should be calibrated by an unambiguous procedure such as mass spectrometry/isotope dilution.

7.1.2 Temporal variations in the biochemical, functional and clinical status indices and factors affecting choices

It is clearly important to know whether a particular index will respond rapidly to fluctuations in nutrient intake (or indeed to other factors that may change in the short term, e.g. diurnal cycles or metabolic adjustments by hormonal mechanisms), or whether it will respond more slowly, over weeks or months, so that a single measurement will portray an integrated response of dietary intake (or tissue status) over a period of time, but be less affected by particular meals, or ingestion of supplements at a particular time (Table 7.1).

Limitations both of space and of accurate data preclude any details or comprehensive discussion of this complex subject, but the following generalizations may be useful:

Faecal analysis Clearly this would not be considered as an option for vitamin status assays, because most vitamins are extensively metabolized, or otherwise destroyed, especially in the large bowel. Some, namely the B vitamins and vitamin K, can be produced there in considerable amounts, but the proportion that is then available for absorption by the host may be small.

Table 7.1 Choice of biochemical markers or indices for nutrients subdivided by their temporal relationships with dietary intake.

Compartment	Nutrients[b]	Comments
Short term indices*		
Faeces	Inorganic ions Lipids	Balance studies only; for lipids one needs to consider endogenous production and contributions of colonic bacteria
Urine[a]	B-vitamins [not folate or B_{12}], Vitamin C	Greatest variation and therefore predictive power at moderate-to-high intakes
	Na^+, K^+, $(Ca^{2+}$, $Mg^{2+})$	
	Halides, sulphate, selenium	
	Nitrogen, urea, creatinine, 3-methyl histidine, sulphur amino acids	All require complete collections, adequate days for desired precision
Bile salts	Cholesterol	Metabolic ward study only
Breath	Fibre (hydrogen, methane)	Validity uncertain
Serum/plasma[c]	All vitamins, but mainly used for vitamin B_6 (pyridoxal phosphate), vitamin C and the fat-soluble vitamins	Intake range for predictive power varies between nutrients, e.g. wide for water-soluble vitamins, narrow for vitamin A
	Some inorganic nutrients	Variable predictive power between nutrients
	Cholesterol, cholesteryl esters, phospholipids, triglycerides, free fatty acids	May be affected by recent diet (TG, FFA). Total FA can be measured, better analysed in subfractions separately
Medium/long-term indices†		
Red cells[d]	Vitamins B_1, B_2, B_6 B_1, B_6, niacin, folate Se Cu^{2+} Fatty Acids	Enzyme activation indices Total co-factor concentration Glutathione peroxidase Superoxide dismutase
White cells[d]	Vitamin C Zn, Se Fatty Acids	Entire 'buffy coat' generally used; separated cell types probably better Monocytes; may be only short term indicator
Hair, toe-nails finger-nails	(Zn, Cu and other 'trace' elements)	Controversial interpretation
Cheek cells	Phospholipid fatty acids	Validity uncertain
Adipose tissue	Fatty acids	Useful in metabolic and experimental studies

For balance studies involving organic anions or cations, faecal analysis may be essential, and in such cases the measurement of transit time (for example by faecal markers) will be needed to relate the amount recovered in the faeces to that in the ingested food. Present understanding of the origins of faecal lipid and nitrogen and their relationship with dietary intake is limited. Faecal lipid levels are derived from maldigested and malabsorbed dietary intake, endogenous secretions, and from colonic bacteria, and levels of output may be quite different in different subjects despite similar intakes (Murphy, unpublished data). Faecal analyses are difficult, laborious, and demanding in terms of subject cooperation; their usefulness in most types of epidemiological studies is limited.

Urine analysis For water-soluble substances that are readily transported into the renal glomerular filtrates, e.g. the water-soluble vitamins and a range of inorganic ions, the analysis of a well defined urine collection may be informative, particularly about recent dietary intake. Clearly, at equilibrium the difference between the net amount of a nutrient that is absorbed and the amount retained in the tissues must equal the amount excreted in the urine plus other, usually minor, excretory routes. For those nutrients (like iron) which cannot be removed by this route, there has to be a strict control of net absorption, but for those that can be removed (like the water-soluble vitamins and alkali metals), the renal excretion route is continually adjusting the balance, and ensures an appropriate level of retention, provided that the kidneys are functioning correctly. A new bolus of intake in an already saturated subject will produce a bolus of urinary excretion, generally beginning in less than an hour, so that a 6-hour urine collection may then reflect quite accurately the dietary intake over the same period. However, this generalization presupposes that only a small proportion of the nutrient intake is either stored in the tissues or is metabolized.

For instance, in the case of water-soluble vitamins the amount recovered in the urine exhibits a much closer relationship with intake and a more sensitive response to changes in intake when the previous long-term intakes (and body stores) are above the 'saturation threshold' for the nutrient in that individual or group. Therefore, the urinary excretion of vitamins like thiamin, riboflavin, and vitamin C tend to reflect intake fairly well when the intakes are moderate to high when compared with requirements, but the variation in excretion is much less informative when the intake is

---

* Responding within hours or days to changes in intake, especially in the upward direction. Note that serum/plasma indices may have both short and medium-term components.

† Responding within weeks or perhaps months to changes in intakes; unresponsive to short term fluctuations. Red cell indices may respond more slowly than white cell indices, but this depends whether individual nutrients can enter or leave during the lifetime of the cell. Hair and finger- or toe-nail indices are medium or long term, depending whether or not specific zones are anlaysed separately. All of these medium/long-term indices are most responsive at the lower end of the intake-range. Adipose tissue levels will reflect intake over the last 2–3 years.

ª Urine usually requires acidification and refrigeration to prevent bacterial growth and preserve labile nutrients, such as vitamin C.

ᵇ Indices in parentheses are not strongly recommended, because of difficulties of adequate sample collection or interpretation.

ᶜ The choice between serum and plasma often depends on arbitrary historical factors, for instance, many clinical chemistry measurements have been validated with serum, but not yet with plasma. Some anticoagulants interfere with certain assays, but the clotting process may also interfere with the natural distribution of nutrients between cells and extracellular fluid.

ᵈ Certain haematological indices, polymorphonuclear cell lobe counts, etc. are sensitive to certain nutrient deficiencies, e.g. folate, B_{12}.

habitually low. Indeed, one approach to the definition of requirements is the measurement of a break-point between the small slope of increase of urinary excretion with increasing intake when the tissues are unsaturated, and the much larger slope when saturation is surpassed.[10,11]

Use of urine analyses in an epidemiological study presupposes that the subjects are able and willing to provide a satisfactory sample, and that the nutrients of interest are stable, or can be satisfactorily preserved. A complete 24-hour urine sample is usually more informative than, say, a random or 'overnight' sample, but is much more difficult to collect. Young infants or demented elderly and certain other human groups are obviously unable to cooperate. Bacterial growth will destroy organic nutrients and unstable substances like vitamin C may require a combination of acidification and cold storage after collection. These constraints frequently tip the balance of choice in favour of blood-sampling. Severe tissue-depletion can be detected by the percentage recovery of an oral test dose of the nutrient in the urine for some nutrients, but this older method has now been largely superseded by blood analysis.

Blood analysis   Blood has the advantages of rapid sampling, with a minimum amount of active participation by the subject. It can provide several fractions representing different compartments and hence presents a wide choice both of analytical possibilities and timescale viewpoints. Although some nutrient assays can, with advantage, be performed on whole blood (e.g. 'red cell' folate), the vast majority employ an initial separation procedure to look at a single compartment within the blood sample.

The most common choice of sampling compartment is plasma or serum, and this is also the most responsive to recent dietary intake, or at least to intestinal lumen contents assuming that absorption is normal. Serum can have certain advantages over plasma, namely of avoiding anticoagulant additives (which may interfere with certain assays) and of 'clean' storage in the frozen state (without the formation of insoluble protein precipitate). However, it has the disadvantages of contamination with platelet contents, of a possibly greater risk of haemolysis, which can seriously affect certain assays, and it entails losing both the red and white cells in the clotted fraction. With respect to temporal variations, serum or plasma often exhibit major fluctuations following meals because nutrients are usually transported from the site of absorption to the tissues via the acellular compartment of the bloodstream, but there will also be an equilibrium set up with tissue nutrient levels, and this will exhibit longer term fluctuations, if tissue status fluctuates. Thus, plasma or serum nutrients usually exhibit rather complex kinetics, with two or more input compartments, representing (i) the gut lumen; and (ii) the tissue pool, in even the simplest case. For those nutrients which are absorbed rapidly into the plasma pool and are then distributed more slowly to intracellular compartments, it may be advantageous to collect fasting blood samples, to avoid short-term fluctuation caused by recent dietary intake.

It is an oversimplification to say that plasma levels only reflect recent intake, whereas other compartments only represent long term status, although it would be true to say that plasma levels can often respond rapidly (and transiently) to the intake of nutrient-rich foods or supplements, just as urinary excretion does. Of course, for certain nutrients (e.g. calcium) the homeostatic control mechanisms are so tight that variations in intake over a huge range have a negligible effect on plasma levels, and in the case of vitamin A, for instance, plasma levels depend primarily on the steady-state level of retinol-binding protein. Thus, plasma retinol levels reflect tissue vitamin A status only when tissue stores are very low (i.e. moderate-to-severe deficiency in functional terms), whereas plasma retinyl ester levels normally reflect only very recent intake, while the chylomicrons are transporting them from the site of intestinal absorption to the liver, for storage, or for release as the retinol–RBP complex.

The second possible choice of compartments within an anticoagulated blood sample is the red cell compartment, whose advantages, especially in the water-soluble vitamin field, have become increasingly evident during the past couple of decades. Erythrocytes contain a variety of enzyme systems that depend on B vitamin-derived cofactors, and these have proved very sensitive to variations in tissue and body status of individual vitamins, in a manner that has made them eminently suitable for status-index development. Thus, the total red cell concentrations of vitamin-derived cofactors, or the extent of stimulation of specific enzymes by their vitamin-containing coenzymes (e.g. glutathione reductase by flavin adenine dinucleotide) have yielded status assays that are robust, very sensitive at the borderline of deficiency, and an accurate reflection of body stores. Another approach is the use of red cell enzyme stimulation tests. Here, activity of a red cell enzyme is measured in the presence and absence of its appropriate vitamin coenzyme. In nutritional adequacy, the added coenzyme has little effect on the overall enzyme activity, so the ratio of the two measurements is very close to unity. However, in vitamin deficiency, added coenzyme increases enzyme activity to a variable extent, depending on the degree of deficiency. The test thus measures the extent to which the red cell enzyme has been depleted of coenzyme, and the result is expressed either as the Activation Coefficient (AC, or 'α'), where

$$\text{Activation Coefficient (AC)} = \frac{\text{Activity of the coenzyme-stimulated enzyme}}{\text{Activity of unstimulated enzyme}}$$

or as Percentage stimulation, where

$$\text{Percentage stimulation} = \frac{\text{Stimulated activity} - \text{Basic activity}}{\text{Basic activity}} \times 100$$

(e.g. TPP effect for thiamin). Table 7.2 gives values for activation coefficients for four vitamins. If the question of risk concerns intakes that can usefully be classified as normal, marginal, or deficient, then functional tests of this type may have value in nutritional epidemiological studies.

For certain vitamins, individual red cells can exhibit gains or losses during their lifetime, although these losses are measured in weeks rather than in hours or days (as would be the case with plasma or urine responses). (It is worth noting that dietary supplements of riboflavin, thiamin and pyridoxine may alter the results of red cell enzyme tests within days, as vitamin-deficient red cells may take up vitamins within

Table 7.2 Erythrocyte enzyme stimulation tests of nutritional status.

Vitamin	Enzyme/coenzyme	Status measured by activation coefficient	Interpretation	General comments
Thiamin*	Transketolase/ thiamin pyrophosphase	1.00–1.25	Normal or marginal status except when basic transketolase activity is low, then probably chronic deficiency.	Unstable enzyme. Must be stored at −70°C or measured fresh
		>1.25	Biochemical deficiency; high values likely to be acute deficiency	Values of 1.15–1.25 may be considered as intermediate risk
Riboflavin	Glutathione reductase/Flavin adenine dinucleotide	1.00–1.30 1.30–1.80 >1.80	Normal status Marginal/deficient status Deficient status associated with intake below 0.5 mg riboflavin/day	Very stable enzyme. Good indicator of tissue status, but unreliable in situations of negative nitrogen balance or glucose 6-phosphate dehydrogenase deficiency[12]
Pyridoxine	Aspartate aminotransferase/ pyridoxal phosphate	1.00–1.50 1.50–2.00 >2.00	Normal status Marginal status Deficient status	Many modifications of method exist. There is disagreement on thresholds. Uncertain stability at −20°C for more than a few days
Biotin	Pyruvate carboxylase	No human data available.†		Deficiency rare in man

* Unlike the other red cell enzymes used for B vitamin status, the basal (unstimulated) activity of transketolase is an important index, which should be recorded together with the activation coefficient, for joint interpretation.
† Limited data available from studies in pigs.[13] Recent studies have explored the alternative use of lymphocyte propionyl CoA carboxylase.[14]

24 hours.) For other vitamins (e.g. red cell folate), the level is determined even before the cell is released from the bone marrow, and it then remains constant until the cell is eventually destroyed. Thus, red cell folate can provide a reasonably good long-term reflection of dietary intake and of tissue levels, but it is insensitive to short term fluctuations.

The third possible choice within the bloodstream is the white cell complex. 'Complex' is the operative word, because different white cell types (granulocytes, lymphocytes, platelets, etc.) may not only concentrate many nutrients to different degrees according to the cell type, but they may also exhibit quite different temporal changes in varying situations. For instance, the measurement of 'buffy coat', i.e. total white cell content, of vitamin C can, in certain circumstances, be a good reflection of tissue vitamin C levels, but it may also be severely confounded by a big influx of new granulocytes, e.g. during surgery or acute infection. The exploration of white cells as a biopsy tissue for nutrient status monitoring is at an early stage of development. Provided that new methods of cell-type purification and sensitive assay procedures can overcome the existing problems of contaminated populations and large blood volume requirements, white cell based status assays may become increasingly useful. Like the red cell compartment, white cells tend to reflect integrated intakes, although their turnover is somewhat more rapid than that of red cells and they may therefore be able to detect medium to long-term fluctuations of intake.

Other compartments   Breast milk can also provide a useful set of nutrient indices that tend to reflect circulating (plasma) levels and recent nutrient intakes for many nutrients. However, there may also be major effects of the stage of the infant's feeding cycle and stages of lactation that will complicate interpretation and this creates a need for carefully controlled sampling protocols. In some cases (e.g. vitamin A), milk levels can show a wider range of sensitivity than plasma levels, because of the near absence of the retinol binding protein (buffering capacity).

Saliva, semen, or term-placental nutrient levels   These can give information about some nutrients, but have not been widely used.

Fat biopsies   These have been shown to be reasonable markers of long-term fatty acid intake, and may be useful for some fat-soluble vitamins, although the latter have not yet been sufficiently well validated.

Hair, finger-nails, and toe-nails   Levels of trace elements in hair or in finger-nails or toe-nails have been explored, but there is wide disagreement about their usefulness as indices either of status or of intake. More refined technical procedures and a better control of sampling protocols are required in this field.

Table 7.3 has attempted to indicate which biochemical indices are most usefully predictive of intakes for each micronutrient and over what broad range of intakes the relationship is best. To some extent, the choice is necessarily idiosyncratic and personal because the ability to assess the available tests depends on the expertise and equipment available. In addition to considering the 'deficient' and 'normal intake' ranges, Table 7.3 includes some indications of those indices that can recognize the use

Table 7.3 Feasibility of predicting intakes from the biochemical index values of specific nutrients.

Nutrient	Range of intakes*	Feasibility[†]	Choice of index
Vitamins:			
Vitamin A	Low	+(L)	Plasma retinol, RDR, MRDR[a]
	Intermediate	0	
	High (T)	+(S/L)	Plasma vitamin A (mainly esters)
Vitamin D	Low	+[b](L)	Plasma 25-hydroxycholecalciferol
	Intermediate	+[b](L)	
	High (T)	+(S/L)	Plasma vitamin D
Vitamin E	Low	?[c]	
	Intermediate	+(L)	Plasma vitamin E:cholesterol ratio
	High	+(L)	
Vitamin K	Low	? +(L)	Blood clotting (prothrombin) time[d]
	Intermediate	+(S/L)	
	High	? +(S/L)	Plasma vitamin K
B-vitamins (general)	Low	+(L)	Red cell enzyme activation tests; plasma or red cell levels
	Intermediate	+(S/L)	Plasma or red cell levels; urinary levels
	High	+ +(S/L)	Plasma or urinary levels
B-vitamins (specific):			
Thiamin	Low	+(L)	Red cell transketolase or thiamin level
Riboflavin	Low	+ +(L)	Activation of erythrocyte glutathione reductase
Vitamin B_6	Low	+(S/L)	Plasma pyridoxal phosphate or urine pyridoxic acid, or red cell transaminases
Folate	Entire range	+(S/L)	Serum (S/L) or red cell (L) folate
Vitamin B_{12}	Entire range	+(S/L)	Serum vitamin B_{12}
Vitamin C	Low	+(L)	Buffy coat vitamin C
	Intermediate	+ +(S/L)	Plasma or buffy coat vitamin C
	High	+(S/L)	Plasma or urinary vitamin C
Cations:			
Na^+ and K^+	Entire range	+ + +(S)	Urinary levels
Ca^{2+} and Mg^{2+}	Low/intermediate	+[e](S)	Urinary levels
Fe^{2+}	Entire range	+/−[f](L)	Serum ferritin, red cell protoporphyrin; transferrin saturation
Zn^{2+}	Entire range	+/−[f](S/L)	Plasma Zn^{2+}
Cu^{2+}	Low	+/−[f](S/L)	Red cell superoxide dismutase
Ultra trace: (Mn^{2+}, Cr^{2+} etc.)	Entire range	+/−[f](S/L)	Plasma levels

Nutrient	Range of intakes[*]	Feasibility[†]	Choice of index
Anions:			
F^-, Cl^-, I^-	Entire range	$+++$(S)	Urinary level
I^-	Low	$+$(L)	Plasma thyroid hormone levels
$Se^{2-}(SO_3^{2-})$	Entire range	$++$(S)	Urinary level
	Entire range	$+$(S/L)	Plasma, platelet, hair and toe-nail Se
	Low	$+$(L)	Red cell glutathione peroxidase
$S^{2-}(SO_4^{2-})$	Entire range	$++$(S)	Urinary levels
PO_4^{3-}	Low/intermediate	$+$(S)	Urinary levels
Lipids:			
Fatty acids[g]	Entire range	$++$(S/L)	Cholesteryl esters, phospholipid of cell membranes, such as erythrocytes and monocytes For long term marker: adipose tissue
Cholesterol[h]	Low	$+$(S/L)	Plasma level, LDL
Protein:			
Nitrogen	Entire range[i]	$++$(S/L)	Urinary level

[*] Uses approximate and arbitrary subdivisions: a) 'low' i.e. intakes that are below the RDA and include the biochemical, functional, and clinical deficiency ranges; b) 'intermediate', i.e. intakes that yield adequate status including the RDA, up to the maximum that could be obtained from a sensible balanced diet; c) 'high' i.e. intakes that can only be obtained by taking supplements, including amounts that are in the pharmacological and in some cases potentially toxic (T) ranges.

[†] Arbitrary subdivisions: 0, not feasible, usually because there is no index that is sensitive over this range; $+/-$, poor predictive power; $+$, fair predictive power; $++$ or $+++$, good predictive power; ?, insufficient information; S, short term reflection of intake (hours or days); L, long term reflection of intake (weeks or months); S/L, may reflect either short or long-term intakes.

[a] RDR, Relative dose response, the increase in plasma retinol after a test oral dose. MRDR, Modified relative dose response: see Section 7.3.1.

[b] Assumes that the contribution from sunlight is very small.

[c] Deficiency only encountered in conjunction with a metabolic abnormality; natural human diets do not normally cause overt deficiency.

[d] Or recent variants with improved sensitivity.

[e] Complicated by interference, especially with protein.

[f] Complicated by many other factors, e.g. availability from food matrix, acute phase response for serum ferritin and plasma Zn. Faecal analysis would give better estimates of intake, but this is generally impractical. Hair and finger- or toe-nail analyses may give some long-term information .

[g] The best markers of intake are those fatty acids that can not be synthesized endogenously (n6;n3 families). Recent studies have shown good associations between fish oil intake and levels in monocytes.[15] Dietary fatty acids influence levels of serum cholesterol and of cholesterol in lipoprotein fractions.

[h] The relationship between dietary cholesterol and serum cholesterol is complex. Keys *et al.*[16] and Hegsted *et al.*[17] have formulae that predict this relationship. Plasma cholesterol rises less steeply as dietary cholesterol intake increases. A recent study [18] has shown that change in cholesterol is strongly influenced by initial levels and that the effect of dietary modification on serum cholesterol was greater in the upper third and lower in the lower third of intake. Other studies have suggested the opposite. Predicting dietary cholesterol intake from serum cholesterol may well result in substantial misclassification. As about 65 per cent of cholesterol is carried in LDL, the relationship between dietary cholesterol and LDL cholesterol is similar to that for total cholesterol.

[i] Tissue catabolism when subjects are in negative energy balance will lead to overestimate of intake based on urinary excretion. Extrarenal losses may influence predictive power of urinary measure.

of dietary supplements, i.e. intakes above the range provided from food alone. Because such supplements might be overlooked during the completion of a diet history or other diet record, it is sometimes important to choose a status index or marker that can recognize 'pharmacological' intakes, and flag the subjects involved. Naturally, the intermittent use of supplements may have only a transient effect on many of the available indices, and could therefore go unrecognized.

Other status indices include 'functional tests' of metabolic pathways, in which a loading dose of a pathway precursor is given, usually by mouth, after which the appearance of metabolic intermediates, usually in the urine, is monitored. This approach can distinguish between long-term dietary inadequacy and adequacy, but it is generally insensitive to short-term dietary variations. As these tests usually require collection of timed urine samples, they add significantly to the time taken to see subjects, and their use in epidemiological studies needs careful evaluation in terms of both compliance and cost:benefit.

Clinical deficiency signs (or physiological abnormalities, e.g. dark adaptation decline) usually represent the extreme lower end of status and intake ranges. Although clinical investigations are very important in defining the status of an individual or population, they frequently have the disadvantage of poor specificity. They are therefore useful only in recognizing prolonged periods of dietary deficiency, and they require biochemical evidence, together with evidence of an improvement during supplementation, to confirm the diagnosis. In some cases, the reversal of clinical deficiency signs (e.g. oedema in beri-beri) may be very rapid, but in others (e.g. mouth signs in riboflavin deficiency) it may be slow and uncertain, because of secondary local infections that require separate treatment.

Finally, no discussion of the temporal aspects of the relationship between dietary nutrients and the status indices that represent the levels in various body compartments would be complete without some discussion of repeat measures. The necessity for time-averaged estimates in dietary measurements is obvious because no nutrient (except in laboratory animal chow perhaps!) is present at exactly the same concentration in all foods, in all meals, on all days of the week, and at all seasons of the year. The extent of variability itself varies enormously between nutrients[19] so that the number of days of diet estimation that are needed for a predetermined constant degree of precision for estimation of usual long-term intakes also varies greatly between different nutrients. The advantage of repeated dietary measurements on the same individual at intervals during an epidemiological study is that the risk of percentile group misclassification is greatly reduced. It is thus possible to verify the initial classification of individuals in extreme groups of intake by means of a second or subsequent repeat estimate. Likewise, the repetition of biochemical index measurements at intervals during a longitudinal study not only ensures a greater certainty in the classification of individuals by their long-term mean status values, but it also permits the estimation of within-subject variations in status, which can then be compared with the between-subject variation. Clearly, if between-subject variation is large in comparison with the within-subject variation, the between-subject status classification achieved will be more precise and should have a better predictive power then if the within-subject variability is large compared with between-subject variation. Thus, studies that attempted to separate between-subject from within-subject variation for intakes and biochemical indices for riboflavin and vitamin C in elderly people[20,21] demonstrated quite different patterns for these two nutrients, which may have implications for their predictive power in such a population.

7.1.3   Complicating factors in the relationships between dietary nutrient intakes and status indices

A wide variety of complicating factors remains even when the fundamental physiological factors, such as limits on intestinal mucosal transport rates, tissue and renal threshold saturation levels, feedback control of absorption, etc. have all been recognized and defined. A theoretical relationship could then be drawn between the amount of a nutrient in the diet and the amount expected in various tissue or body fluid compartments, with appropriate mathematical treatments of the flux rates through the different body compartments to describe the complex temporal relationships between them. These factors will blur the relationship between intakes and status indices in free-living people (Table 7.4).

The first complication is that of between-subject variations in nutritional physiology and metabolism. This can, of course, occur either at the level of absorption, tissue distribution of uptake, turnover, excretion, or indeed subsidiary elements of these processes. Clearly, it is the combination of individual variations in intake, nutrient deposition, and susceptibility to specific (nutrient-linked) disease, that forms the first and uppermost layer of the science of nutritional epidemiology. Beneath this layer there are important interactions that complicate these relationships:

1. Nutrients may interact with each other, either in the food or in the intestinal lumen, or they may interact with enzymes or with binding proteins or with other secreted substances. One example of a 'beneficial' interaction is that of food folate polyglutamates with polyglutamylhydrolase (conjugase) enzyme in the intestinal lumen, which liberates the monoglutamate and short chain polyglutamates in the form that can then be absorbed. Another is the interaction of vitamin B_{12} with intrinsic factor, which is essential for its absorption. An example of a 'non-beneficial' interaction is that of divalent cations with phytate and other polyvalent anionic substances in food, which thereby diminish nutrient availability. Table 7.5 lists some chemical changes and interactions that may affect the availability of nutrients in food.

The relationships between certain nutrients in the diet and their biochemical index values may also be affected by other nutrients in the diet or in the body. Thus, for instance, vitamin B_6 status indices are greatly affected by dietary protein levels independently of vitamin B_6 intake; other nutrients may compete with each other for absorption, e.g. zinc versus iron. Some nutrients may arise from two or more very different routes, e.g. vitamin D from either the dietary vitamin or ultra-violet light acting on vitamin D precursors in the skin; niacin arising from dietary niacin co-enzymes or tryptophan; vitamin A arising from dietary vitamin A or carotenoids. In such cases it is often difficult to define the relative contributions of the two (or more) sources, whose efficacy may vary independently under different conditions.

2. A wide variety of substances, particularly drugs and xenobiotics, can alter the absorption, disposition, or metabolism of individual nutrients in various different ways.

Some drugs may have wide ranging general effects (such as purgatives, diuretics, anti-diuretics, inducers of microsomal drug oxidation enzymes); others may have more specific effects on certain nutrients (e.g. folate antagonists). Many of these interactions are only partly mapped at the present time. For instance the interactions of antiepileptic drugs, antimalarials, antibiotics, etc. with specific nutrients are only partially under-stood. The effect of smoking on nutrient status (major effects on vitamin C and carotene levels) could be considered a special case of xenobiotic interactions, and alcohol, likewise, has a variety of effects on nutrient status indices. Clearly, with the increasing use of drugs in human medicine, drug–nutrient interactions are becoming of increasing significance in modulating the relationship between nutrient intakes and status.

3. Gender, physiological stage (pregnancy, lactation), and age can affect not only the true requirements for nutrients, but also their distribution between body compart-ments, and hence the performance of certain (e.g. enzyme and metabolic pathway) indices, in ways that may complicate the intake–status index relationships. Long-term

Table 7.4 Points of measurement at which discrepancies between dietary estimates and biochemical index values may arise.

Point of measurement	Reasons for discrepancy
Diet estimate	Inaccurate recording/recall techniques. Inappropriate time-period for records. Inaccurate or inappropriate food table nutrient values; variations in nutrient content between apparently similar food items; variations in manufacturing techniques, etc. Variations in storage losses, cooking losses, plate wastage, etc.
Absorption	Variation in fundamental bioavailability of the different chemical forms of nutrients. Interactions between nutrients and food components (positive or negative) within the GI tract. Interactions between nutrients and secreted substances in GI tract (digestive enzymes, binding proteins, etc.) Effects of gut flora: contributing to or destroying certain nutrients. Physiological variations in absorptive capacity; feedback control of absorption by size of tissue load for some minerals; effects of transit time, intraluminal concentration and bolus effects, etc.
Disposition, metabolism, and turnover	Variations in distribution between the different tissues (usually via the bloodstream); temporal effects, involving various body pools and rates of transfer between them. Variations in degradative pathways. Variations in excretory pathways: renal, biliary, enterohepatic circulation, etc. Effects of xenobiotics. Effects of medical conditions.

adaptations to very low or very high intakes may disturb the 'natural' relationships between intake and status indices. These are encountered more frequently for mineral nutrients than for vitamins.

4. Disease processes may upset these relationships, and again produce potentially misleading changes. For instance, any substance that is affected by changes in acute-phase protein status in the bloodstream will show alterations during infection and inflammation that do not reflect either changes in intake or changes in general tissue nutrient status. The increase in plasma ferritin level during the acute phase reaction, for example, does not reflect iron status in the way that the ferritin levels do in a healthy subject. Retinol-binding protein is a negative acute-phase reactant, which therefore decreases in concentration in plasma during inflammation and infection. Such changes have often been recognized, and low retinol concentrations have been incorrectly interpreted as 'poor' vitamin A status, i.e. diminished body stores.[22] Buffy coat vitamin C levels become reduced during the leukocytotic response to infection because the normal balance between white cell populations in the bloodstream is temporarily altered. Table 7.6 lists some of these changes, which can clearly have a major effect on the relationships between normal intake and status indices and thus confuse inter-pretation. Disease processes that affect the intestine or kidneys will clearly affect nutrient absorption and renal excretion respectively; diseases affecting the liver may likewise affect the metabolism of nutrients and of their plasma binding proteins; diseases of the immune system may also have profound effects on nutrient balance. Some nutrients (e.g. vitamin C and vitamin E) appear to be destroyed at a rate that is at least partially determined by their involvement in tissue-protective reactions and these, in turn, may be affected by diseases, especially those in which oxidative processes play an important part. however, the quantitation of such effects remains poorly defined.

Diseases that affect nutrient status may, of course, be either inherited or acquired, and of these a proportion may be ameliorated by high intakes of the nutrients affected, e.g. where there is impaired absorption, impaired transport or impaired conversion to the active metabolite (cofactor, etc.). Such 'nutrient-responsive errors of metabolism', which occur both for vitamins (e.g. pernicious anaemia, due to impaired absorption of vitamin B_{12}) and minerals (e.g. acrodermatitis enteropathica, due to impaired absorption of zinc) naturally represent gross departures from the 'normal range' of relationships between intake and status indices. The correct and early diagnosis of disease can be critical, both for the attainment of adequate nutritional status and also for the prevention of irreversible degenerative damage in certain tissues.

Another type of interaction that can affect the relationship between nutrient intake and status indices is exemplified by glucose-6-phosphate dehydrogenase deficiency, which virtually abolishes the increase in activation coefficient of glutathione reductase during riboflavin deficiency in subjects with this enzyme deficiency. It appears that, when a genetic abnormality increases the demand by the red cell, the organism can override the normal redistribution of cofactor. Table 7.6 lists some examples both of inborn errors and of other disease states that affect nutrient status independently of intake. Such a list obviously cannot be comprehensive because of the wide range of potential interactions between functional derangement and nutrient status index values.

Table 7.5 Chemical changes, interactions, and *de novo* synthesis, which may affect the availability of nutrients in food.

Nutrient	Process	Effect	Possible sources of variation
Carotenoids	Cleavage to retinol in the mucosa	Conversion to Vitamin A	Amount of carotenoids, vitamins A and E, fat and possibly protein, in the diet
Vitamin A esters	De-esterification by lipases	Conversion to free retinol	May affect availability of vitamin A in infants
Vitamin K	Synthesis of menaquinones by intestinal flora	Possible contribution to vitamin K status	Variations in gut flora
Thiamin	Destruction by thiaminases	Losses	Food preparation methods; raw fish
Thiamin and niacin	Interactions with mycotoxins	?Reduced availability	Mycotoxin contamination of foods, especially rice
Folate	Removal of polyglutamyl side chain	Increased availability	Varies with food preparation methods, and probably also between individuals
Vitamin B$_{12}$	Release from protein-bound forms in food. Adsorption to salivary haptocorrins and gastric intrinsic factor	Greatly enhanced availability	Essential for adequate absorption; failure of intrinsic factor typically results in pernicious anaemia. Affected by several abnormal medical conditions, which tend to increase with age

All multivalent metal ions	Interaction with phytate and other organic polyanions in food	Usually diminished availability	Balance between animal and plant foods; levels of dietary protein and other enhancers of absorption
Calcium	Induction of calcium-binding protein by vitamin D	Enhanced absorption	Determinants of vitamin D status (sunlight; diet sources); determinants of hormone balance; specific disease states
Iron	Interactions with chelating or reducing agents, e.g. ascorbate, protein, etc.	Enhanced absorption	Meal composition. Absorption also controlled by body stores, limiting excessive absorption
Zinc, copper	Interactions with protein, etc.	Enhanced absorption	Competition between metal ions and interaction of each metal with food chelators
Lipids	Cis to trans isomers	Reduced availability	Heating and hydrogenation of oils in formation of margarines
Protein	Maillard reaction; protease inhibitors in legumes	Reduced availability; reduced absorption	Food preparation methods

Table 7.6 Some examples of disease states that may affect nutrient status indices independently of intake.

Disease	Nutrient indices that may be altered (usually lowered)
Pernicious anaemia	Vitamin B_{12} (secondary effect on folate)
Vitamin-responsive metabolic errors	Usually B-vitamins (e.g. vitamins B_{12}, B_6, riboflavin, biotin, folate)
Tropical sprue	Vitamins B_{12} and folate (local deficiencies); protein
Steatorrhoea	Fat-soluble vitamins, lipid levels, energy
Abetalipoproteinemia	Vitamin E
Thyroid abnormality	Riboflavin, iodine, lipid levels, energy
Diabetes	Possibly vitamin C, zinc, and several other nutrients, lipid levels
Infections, inflammation, acute phase reaction	Vitamin C, vitamin A, and several other nutrients, lipids, protein, energy
Measles, upper respiratory tract infections, diarrhoeal disease	Especially vitamin A, lipid levels, protein
Renal disease	Increased retention or increased loss of many circulating nutrients, lipid levels, protein
Cystic fibrosis	Especially vitamin A, lipid levels, protein
Various cancers	Lowering of vitamin indices
Acute myocardial infarction	Lipid levels affected for about 3 months
Malaria, haemolytic disease, hookworm, etc.	Iron, vitamin A, lipid
Huntington's chorea	Energy
Acrodermatitis enteropathica; various bowel, pancreatic or liver diseases	Zinc, lipid levels, protein
Hormone imbalances	Mineralocorticoid, parathyroid hormone, thyrocalcitonin (effects on the alkali metals and calcium), lipid levels affected by oral contraception and oestrogen therapy

7.2 Markers of dietary intake: inorganic nutrients

7.2.1 Sodium and potassium

There is tight homeostatic control of the blood levels of sodium and potassium, and blood levels do not therefore reflect dietary intake except at the extremes of deficiency or excess that are associated with acute clinical signs. In health, urine is the major route of excretion of sodium and potassium.

The urinary excretion of sodium is generally a good indicator of dietary intake[19,23] because faecal excretion of sodium is minimal, in the order of 2–4 mmol per day.[24,25] In temperate climates it is assumed that skin losses of sodium are minor, so that on an average basis, 24-hour urine excretion of sodium can be shown to account for 95–98% of dietary intake when this is directly analysed rather than calculated from food tables. However, the within-person variability in sodium excretion is in the order of 30% and substantial numbers of observations are needed to gain precision in the overall mean for individuals.[26,27] This low level of precision, together with the difficulty of ensuring complete 24-hour urine collections, accounts for some of the poor agreement between individual estimates of diet and individual estimates of urine sodium excretion. Table 7.7 shows that some workers have shown low correlation coefficients, in the order of 0.4 for short periods of observation.[23] At least 7 days of observation of both urine and diet are needed before reported correlation coefficients of 0.8 emerge, for example in the data of Holbrook.[24] This is as predicted by Liu and Stamler[27] who suggested that at least eight 24-hour urine collections were needed to achieve a diminution of the true correlation coefficient by less than 10%. Due to difficulties in calculating intake of sodium from food tables, not unexpectedly, comparisons between calculated intakes of sodium and urine excretion show poorer agreement than comparisons with direct analysis (Table 7.7).

Faecal excretion of potassium is somewhat larger and more variable than sodium and, compared with sodium, faecal losses constitute a greater proportion of dietary intake, from 5–13 mmol per day in Western populations, or 11–15% of the dietary

Table 7.7 Correlations between estimates of intake of sodium and potassium from weighed records or analysis of duplicate portions, and output as 24-hour urine excretion.

Days of diet records	Days of urine collections	Na	K	Number and gender of subjects (reference)
Analysed diet				
28	28	0.76	0.82	28, M, F[24]
28	7	0.81	0.49	8, M, F[31]
3	3	0.31	0.56	9, M, F[23]
Calculated diet				
28	28*	0.96	0.95	8, M, F[29]
16	8*	0.30	0.73	160, F[30]
16	4	0.40	0.50	52, M, F[32]
7	3	–	0.42	44, M, F[33]
7	7	0.42	0.23	8, F[31]
3	3	0.04	0.40	9, M, F[23]
6	1	0.61	0.62	55, M, F[34]
7	1	0.25	0.26	794, M[35]
7	1	0.36	0.26	834, F[35]

* Protocol included PABA as a marker of completeness of collection of 24h urine samples.

intake.[24,26,28] The faecal loss may vary between different populations depending on faecal weight, so that up to 30% of the dietary intake may be lost by this route in South African populations.[25] However, the correlation between intake and excretion of potassium can be high even when dietary intakes are calculated from food tables rather than analysed, when sufficient 24-hour urines are obtained. Studies which have obtained at least eight 24-hour urine collections, validated for their completeness, have shown correlations of at least 0.7 between calculated intake and excretion,[29,30] The within-person variation in potassium excretion is in the order of 24%, and Table 7.7 shows that the agreement between diet and urine is less good and more variable with fewer days of collection. When only single 24-hour urine collections are available and dietary intake is calculated rather than analysed, the agreement between the two values may be weak, with correlation coefficients in the order of 0.3–0.4.

Other factors also contribute to the poor agreement between 24-hour urine excretion and dietary intake. The difficulties of obtaining complete collections have been mentioned, and the PABA marker has been developed for the purposes of validating dietary assessments with 24-hour urine estimations of nitrogen (see Section 7.4.2). When used to validate 24-hour urine specimens for estimation of sodium excretion in blood pressure studies, regression coefficients were larger in the subgroup of individuals whose 24-hour collections were classified as complete by the PABA technique than in the analysis of the group as a whole.[36] Heavy perspiration in non-adapted individuals could detract further from the closeness of the relation between intake and excretion, and secretion into breast milk of approximately 7.8mEq (180 mg) sodium and approximately 12.8 mEq (500 mg) potassium per litre, is also a significant diversion. Severe and prolonged diarrhoea causes major losses.

Replacement of 24-hour urine collections with overnight or casual urine specimens in epidemiological studies has been extensively discussed. Values for 24-hour excretion extrapolated from 8-hour collections have been used to assess group compliance with study protocols in low salt intervention studies in hypertension.[37] Liu and Stamler[27] suggest that full 24-hour specimens are necessary for estimation of individual sodium and potassium output, and estimated the correlation between mean 24-hour urine sodium excretion and true mean overnight sodium excretion to be 0.72. They suggest that multiple measurements of the sodium/potassium to creatinine ratios might be feasible for assessing the relation between blood pressure and electrolyte excretion.[27]

Table 7.8 shows correlations between output as assessed from 8 24-hour urines and output from a single 24-hour urine, and from eight repeat overnight urines in UK men. Unfortunately, repeat overnight collections were much less satisfactory than even one single 24-hour urine collection when compared with eight 24-hour urines; in the case of sodium, for example, correlations between excretion from all 24-hour collections and a single 24-hour collection was 0.60 but only −0.093 for the first overnight, which did not improve (0.035) when eight overnight collections were obtained.[38]

In other studies, correlations between overnight, random, and true electrolyte excretion vary between populations; Ogawa found correlations in the order of 0.8 between overnight and 24-hour collections[39], as did He et al.[40] in Chinese men, whereas Yamori found the greatest agreement (correlation coefficients in the order of 0.8) for evening collections, with less good agreement between overnight and 24-hour

Table 7.8 Correlation coefficients (r) between repeat overnight and 24-hour urine collections for sodium and potassium.[38]

	8 24-hour collections versus:		
	Single 24-hour collection	First overnight collection	8 overnight collections
Sodium	0.600	−0.093	0.035
Potassium	0.614	0.028	0.355

collections (correlation coefficient 0.6).[41] In a German population, Khalaf *et al.*[42] found that correlations with 24-hour urine collections were higher for day rather than night collections. Attempts to substitute partial for 24-hour urine collections therefore require independent validation studies in the population to be surveyed.

7.2.2 Calcium, phosphorus, and magnesium

These alkaline earth metals are less completely absorbed than the alkali metals and, although the net amount of them that is absorbed virtually equals the amount excreted in the urine for a subject in balance, the prediction of intakes from the amount in the blood or excreted in the urine can only be approximate and in broad categories. This is because the percentage of calcium that is absorbed varies between from about 70% at very low intakes, to about 30% at daily intakes of 2 g in adults.[43] At intakes below 200 mg/day the subject is generally in negative balance, i.e. urinary excretion exceeds absorption, and above this breakpoint there is a linear increase, albeit with considerable scatter.[43] Much of this scatter is due to a major dependence of calcium excretion on salt and protein intake. There is a strong homeostatic control of plasma calcium levels and the amount in plasma is not generally a useful predictor of intake, although there are, of course, transient increases following meals or supplements.

The extent of absorption of dietary magnesium is similar in magnitude to that of dietary calcium, i.e. around 50% of intake and, like calcium, the plasma level is held remarkably constant[27,28], although the mechanism of this homeostasis is not well understood. Thus, urinary magnesium is the best available, although approximate and poorly-validated index of dietary intake.

The absorption of phosphorus from the diet is normally around 50–70%, rising to around 90% when the intake is low, or is from a good source, such as human milk.[46] The absorbed phosphorus must be renally excreted at balance, so the amount in the urine should generally be a fairly good reflection of recent intake. However, there are several unavailable forms of phosphorus (e.g. phytates) that can complicate this relationship.

7.2.3 Iron

Iron is not excreted to any significant extent in the urine and therefore there have to be alternative ways of ensuring that tissue overload cannot occur, especially as iron is potentially a very toxic element. The main way that this is achieved is by strictly limiting the extent of absorption to the amount that is required either for replacement (mainly the net requirement for haemoglobin synthesis), or for storage.

In addition to the control that is exerted upon intestinal absorption according to the subject's existing iron load, there is also a wide variation in the availability of different types of dietary iron, which is further complicated by potential interactions with other food components.[47] Thus, a fairly constant amount (approximately 25%) of haem iron in food is absorbed, but absorption of non-haem iron may vary between 1 and 40%, even in individuals with similar iron status, depending on the dietary amounts of protein, ascorbate, and other acids that enhance absorption, and of phytates and certain types of fibre or protein that may inhibit it. The overall result is that none of the conventional indices of iron status (serum iron, per cent saturation of transferrin, serum ferritin, or free erythrocyte protoporphyrin) can yield an entirely satisfactory estimate of iron intakes, at least on an individual basis. The best of the available indices, at reflecting a wide range of long-term intakes on a population basis, is serum ferritin, because this can reflect iron overload as well as iron deficiency. However, raised serum ferritin levels can also result from situations (i) where haemoglobin synthesis is inhibited (e.g. by lead poisoning); (ii) by the acute phase reaction; and (iii) in liver damage associated with iron overload; so that it needs to be interpreted with care. Very low serum ferritin levels, coupled with raised erythrocyte protoporphyrin levels, raised levels of circulating transferrin receptor, and a low per cent saturation of transferrin, are diagnostic of a long-term insufficiency of intake. However, as noted above, this only implies insufficiency of available iron, not necessarily of total dietary iron. Similarly, low haemoglobin levels may reflect low dietary iron, but many other factors, including low intakes of vitamin B_{12}, folic acid, helminthic infestation, haemoglobinopathies, and a variety of diseases will reduce circulating haemoglobin, and higher iron intakes above the levels required for adequate haemoglobin formation will not be reflected in raised haemoglobin levels.

7.2.4   Zinc, copper, and other trace metals

Although a small part of the dietary intake of zinc is excreted in the urine, the amount in this compartment has not proved very useful, either for measuring status or for predicting intakes. At intakes typical of Western diets (7–15 mg/day) the percentage absorption of dietary zinc measured by tracer studies is around 50–70%, but most of this is re-excreted via the intestine, and only 5–10% appears in the urine.[48] Serum zinc is a poor indicator of status, and an equally poor indicator of intake, although it can probably distinguish between the extremes of intake for population groups. The zinc content of specific white cell types may prove better indicators of long-term status, but these seem unlikely to prove to be much better markers for intake. As with iron, the total amount of zinc in a diet is poorly correlated with the amount that is utilizable by the body. Apart from the faecal index, status indices for transition elements tend to reflect the biological availability, rather than the total amounts in the diet.[49] Food table values rarely distinguish between total and available amounts of nutrients such as zinc and iron in foods, and this represents a further bar to accurate prediction.

Measurements of zinc status based on hair or nail clipping analysis do not correlate well with zinc intake or other measures of zinc status.

What has been written above about zinc and iron is also true, in general terms, about the other trace metal nutrients: copper, manganese, chromium, molybdenum, vanadium, etc. There are no biochemical markers for these metals to reflect their intakes accurately. Even the measurements of status and of human requirements remains very difficult, and the search for markers here is in its earliest stages. A study by Gallagher *et al.*[50] compared between-subject variation between biochemical status indices for calcium, copper, iron, magnesium, and zinc, and also compared mean values of these indices between two groups of women with different long-term intakes. Little, if any, discernible effect of dietary intake on the biochemical index values was observed.

In studies of the relationship between copper intake and tissue markers, both the copper-dependent enzyme superoxide dismutase in erythrocytes[51] and the copper–protein complex caeruloplasmin in serum[52], have been shown to be associated with copper intake. Unfortunately, both of these markers may be influenced by non-dietary factors[53], although superoxide dismutase seems the more useful, being less affected by acute phase status. Measurements of copper in hair and urine (a minor excretory route) are of little value in assessing either copper intake or status.

7.2.5 Iodine, selenium, and other anionic elements

Of the electronegative elements, the halide ions (chloride, fluoride, and iodide) may exhibit the best reflection of intakes, because a very high proportion of the intake appears rapidly in the urine. Provided that renal clearance is normal and that other routes of removal, mainly perspiration and breast milk, are allowed for, the urinary content virtually equals intakes for these substances, so they do accurately reflect intakes over the short term.

The relationship between selenium intake and biochemical markers is reasonably good[54], although somewhat less close than is the case for halides. Urine is the major route of excretion and provides a reasonable marker of intake.[55] Plasma levels reflect intake to a degree provided the range of variation is large; red cell selenium or glutathione peroxidase activity are markers of medium-term status and therefore of longer-term intakes. Hair and toe-nail levels have been employed as long-term status indicators and are thus alternative possibilities, although contamination of hair samples by shampoos must be controlled for.

Non-dietary factors such as age, smoking, and alcohol use are associated with reduced levels of markers, but the extent to which this may reflect reduced intakes is not clear. Important interactions between selenium-dependent enzyme systems and other components of the body's antioxidant defences (for example vitamins E, C, and β-carotene) may necessitate a broader examination of these factors in studies assessing the effects of selenium on disease risk.

Free sulphate in the diet is freely absorbed and freely excreted in the urine. Sulphur in other forms, such as amino acids, sulphated polysaccharides, etc., is generally converted to sulphate during turnover and is excreted via the urinary pathway, so that urinary sulphate should provide information about intake. However, little direct confirmation exists.

7.3 Markers of dietary intake: vitamins

7.3.1 Retinol and carotenoids (vitamin A)

Retinol   Vitamin A is a fat-soluble vitamin and the name is used to include retinol and some of its metabolites and the provitamin A carotenoids, the most important of which is β-carotene. The vitamin is essential for numerous metabolic processes, particularly vision, growth, cellular differentiation, reproduction, and immunity. The latter function in particular has attracted much attention recently because studies have suggested that even mild deficiency may be clinically important and responsible for much of the morbidity in Third World countries.[22] Carotenoids are present in vegetables and fruits and provide more than 90% of Third World vitamin A requirements; retinol and its derivatives are only present in foods of animal origin.

It was estimated from available evidence about two decades ago that, of the dietary carotenoids in a Western diet, an average of one-sixth of the β-carotene and one-twelfth of the other dietary carotenoids are converted to vitamin A in the intestinal mucosa.[56] This is, of course, an approximation, which undoubtedly varies considerably between individuals and different food types. Thus, carotenoids in oily solution or in fruit juices such as mango are more efficiently utilized than carotene in carrots – the 'typical' carotenoid source in Western diets. With the recent increase in interest in carotenoids for their intrinsic properties, independent of conversion to vitamin A, there is bound to be a resurgence in interest in their dietary availability. As the amount ingested increases, from typical dietary levels toward pharmacological intakes, the percentage absorbed falls sharply, but the total amount absorbed continues to increase.

The two main biochemical markers of vitamin A that need to be considered are plasma retinol and the 'relative-dose-response' (RDR) test[57] which reflect only the lowest segment of the intake scale on a long term basis. In Western countries, where vitamin A deficiency is now very rare, dietary intake of this vitamin is only a very minor determinant of its plasma levels. This was demonstrated in the recent survey of UK adults[35], in which the cross-sectional correlation between vitamin A intakes and plasma vitamin A was non-significant for women, and explained only 1% of the variance in plasma vitamin A for men (Table 7.9(a)). Similar findings were observed in toddlers (Table 7.9(b)).[60] The RDR or MRDR tests are believed to be more informative at intermediate status and intake levels[57] but are more difficult to perform and have not been used for normal Western populations.

Ninety per cent of the body's vitamin A is stored in the liver, 9% in other tissues, and 1% is present in the plasma. Furthermore, retinol present in the plasma is homeostatically controlled and only represents that in the liver at the two extremes. Plasma retinol is very low when the liver is virtually exhausted but when there is 10–30 μg retinol/g liver, plasma retinol rises to a plateau that remains relatively constant until the liver becomes saturated at 300 μg/g.[61] Therefore, plasma retinol concentrations below 0.70 μmol/l are regarded as borderline vitamin A status and those below 0.35 μmol/l as deficient[62] (see Table 7.10).

It is widely accepted that plasma retinol below 0.35 μmol/l is associated with low liver reserves and clinical signs of deficiency, although malaria infection and acute-phase reaction may also result in low plasma values without associated clinical signs

Table 7.9(a) Cross-sectional correlations between dietary intake of nutrients and biochemical indices (markers) in the UK adult survey (Gregory *et al.*).[35]

Nutrient (in food)[a]	Biochemical index[b]	No. of subjects (M/F)	Correlation coefficients	
			Male	Female
			r (P)	*r* (P)
Iron	Haemoglobin	788/821	−0.04 (NS)	−0.02 (NS)
Iron	Serum ferritin	793/689	0.02 (NS)	0.04 (NS)
Folate	Red cell folate	745/673	0.22 (<0.01)	0.18 (<0.01)
Vitamin B_{12}	Serum vitamin B_{12}	825/755	0.11 (<0.01)	0.10 (<0.01)
Carotenes	Plasma β-carotene	880/902	0.20 (<0.01)	0.38 (<0.01)
Carotenes	Plasma α-carotene	880/902	0.41 (<0.01)	0.43 (<0.01)
Retinol	Plasma vitamin A	881/906	0.10 (<0.01)	0.01 (NS)
Vitamin E	Plasma vitamin E	881/906	0.20 (<0.01)	0.14 (<0.01)
Vitamin E	Plasma tocopherol/cholesterol	856/773	0.29 (<0.01)	0.27 (<0.01)
Riboflavin	Erythrocyte glutathione reductase activation coefficient	874/888	−0.23 (<0.01)	−0.31 (<0.01)

[a] Data given refer to nutrients from food sources only, calculated from 1 week of weighed intake data per subject. The publication includes some additional information relating to all sources, including supplements.
[b] One blood sample from each subject collected after, but not necessarily immediately after, the completion of the diet record (not necessarily a fasting sample). NS, not significant. P>0.05

of deficiency.[22,70-72] In contrast, it is advised that the so-called borderline category, 0.35–0.70 μmol/l, should be interpreted with caution because such values may be associated with inadequate protein intake, parasitic infestation, liver disease, and other conditions.[61-63]

Measurements of retinol are done on a lipid solvent extract of plasma using HPLC,[73-75] and both retinol and carotenes are stable in stored plasma/serum provided samples are not haemolysed and are handled with appropriate care. The temperature of storage should be −50°C or below if stored beyond 6 months but −20°C is satisfactory for 3–6 months.[9,76]

Retinol is transported in plasma in a 1:1 molar combination with retinol binding protein (RBP). Immunoassay and other techniques can be used to measure RBP but the only advantage may be slightly greater stability of the protein over retinol in plasma after long periods of storage.[61] The existence of RBP depleted of retinol is also evidence of vitamin A deficiency.

Relative dose response (RDR)

The control of retinol transport by RBP has provided the basis of a functional test for retinol stores. In vitamin A deficiency, there is continued synthesis of RBP, which remains in the liver as apoRBP. The RDR is like a loading test, in that a blood sample is taken and a loading dose of retinol is given followed by a second sample of blood after 5 hours. The effects differ from the conventional loading test in that the plasma

Table 7.9(b) Cross-sectional correlations between dietary intake of nutrients and biochemical indices (markers) in the UK pre-school child survey (Gregory *et al.*).[60]

Nutrient (in food)[a]	Biochemical index[b]	No. of Subjects (M/F)	Correlation Coefficients			
			Male		Female	
			r	(P)	r	(P)
Total iron	Haemoglobin	463/460	0.10	(NS)	0.04	(NS)
Total iron	Serum ferritin	452/452	0.06	(NS)	0.05	(NS)
Haem. iron	Haemoglobin	453/457	0.04	(NS)	0.14	(<0.01)
Haem. iron	Serum ferritin	445/446	0.02	(NS)	0.08	(NS)
Folate	Red cell folate	371/351	0.06	(NS)	0.19	(<0.01)
Total carotenes	Plasma retinol	398/395	0.06	(NS)	0.03	(NS)
Retinol	Plasma vitamin A	398/395	0.06	(NS)	0.10	(NS)
Vitamin E	Plasma α-tocopherol	398/395	0.06	(NS)	0.13	(<0.05)
Riboflavin	Erythrocyte glutathione reductase act. coefficient	408/396	−0.29	(<0.01)	−0.31	(<0.01)
Vitamin C	Plasma vitamin C	369/354	0.43	(<0.01)	0.39	(<0.01)
Vitamin D	Plasma 25(OH) vit. D	365/350	0.06	(NS)	0.18	(<0.01)

[a] Where specified, the data refer to nutrients from food sources only calculated from 4 days of weighed intake data per subject. The publication includes some additional information relating to all sources, including supplements.
[b] One non-fasting blood sample from each subject was collected some time after the diet record.
NS = Not significant, (P > 0.05)

response is greatest in deficient subjects. The presence of apoRBP in the deficient liver readily combines with the incoming retinol and emerges into the plasma. If the preloading concentration of retinol is increased by more than 20%, this indicates a deficient liver retinol below 20 µg/g. There is very little increase in plasma retinol in the person with normal vitamin A status.

This method has the disadvantage of needing two blood samples and a 5 hour wait in between. A modification to this has been proposed (MRDR test) in which the load of retinol would be replaced by dehydroretinol and a single blood sample drawn after a set interval. Dehydroretinol is not normally present in the diet and therefore, using HPLC techniques to separate the two isomers, its concentration could be expressed as the percentage of the total of the two isomers. Initial experiments in both rats and humans have appeared promising[77], but a recent study[59] claimed that the MRDR test may be less sensitive than the original RDR test, for moderate deficiency. More work is needed to determine whether these techniques are useful for assessing subclinical retinol deficiency in epidemiological studies. Another vitamin A status test which is undergoing evaluation, is the conjunctival impression cytology (CIC) test for reduced numbers of goblet cells in the conjunctival epithelium. Two recent studies[78,79] have questioned its earlier promise for human populations, and its role as a marker of dietary intake remains uncertain.

Table 7.10 Criteria for assessment of fat-soluble vitamin status in adults for the recommended methods.

Vitamin	Measurements	Level of risk			References
		High Risk	Medium Risk	Acceptable	
Retinol (vitamin A)	Plasma retinol (μmol/l)	<0.35	0.35–0.70	>0.7	61, 63, 64
	Relative dose response, (percent change)	>20		<20	61
Cholecalciferol (vitamin D)	Plasma 25-hydroxychole-calciferol (nmol/l)	<12.5 (<25.0*)	12.5–25.00	>25	64, 65
Tocopherol (vitamin E)	α-tocopherol: cholesterol (μmol/mmol)	<2.22		>2.22	66, 67
Phylloquinone (vitamin K)	Clotting time (seconds)	>26	13–26	11–13†	63, 68
	PIVKA - II	>4AU/ml		<0.13AU/ml	69

* Higher risk threshold suggested for subjects who are housebound or similarly restricted during late summer months.
† Recommended clotting time to standardize the wide variety of conditions that exist.[63]

Thus, the prediction of vitamin A intakes from biochemical indices is possible only in the very broad terms of distinguishing long-term deficient intakes from those that are 'adequate'. Another category where blood vitamin A levels become informative is that of excessive intakes and potential toxicity.[80] In lactating women, breast milk vitamin A levels reflect status rather more clearly than blood levels,[81] but the relationship is still not sufficiently precise to be able to predict intakes, except in very broad categories.

Carotenes The only biochemical marker that is currently used for carotenoids is the plasma concentration, which reflects short to medium-term intakes over a wide range. Between-individual variation in the plasma response was found to be 'substantial' in one recent supplementation study.[82] However, Romieu *et al.*[83] observed a significant cross-sectional correlation between dietary carotene intake and plasma β-carotene levels (r = 0.38–0.43) in a group of non-smoking North Americans, and a similar correlation between intake and plasma carotenoids was seen in the UK study of adults[35] (Table 7.9(a)). Evidence from a study by Tangney *et al.*[84] indicated that plasma β-carotene was sensitive to intake but remained relatively constant within individuals, so that it probably reflected fairly long-term habitual intakes.

There is currently considerable interest in carotenes as antioxidants, but until a physiological requirement for substances with this property can be identified, the adequacy or otherwise of these substances in the blood cannot be assessed. All the carotenoids in blood have similar structures and may have similar antioxidant properties. If antioxidant function does prove to be of biological relevance, then the non-provitamin A carotenoids in blood, e.g. lutein[85], may be the more useful markers of dietary intake or status because the rate of conversion of the provitamin A carotenoids can influence their levels in blood. Lutein is as common as β-carotene in most fruits and vegetables.[86] Furthermore, the sex differences noticed with the provitamin A carotenoids do not seem to be as obvious in the non-provitamin A carotenoids.[87,88] There is some recent evidence for interaction between carotenoids during intestinal absorption[89] which may complicate the relationships between intake and blood or tissue levels.

7.3.2   Vitamin D

Following the conversion of 7-dehydrocholecalciferol to vitamin D_3 in the skin, or absorption of dietary vitamin D_3 in the gut, the vitamin is stored in the body fat or metabolized in the liver to 25-hydroxy-cholecalciferol ($25(OH)D_3$). $25(OH)D_3$ circulates in the blood as the main active reservoir, or is metabolized to one or other of the dihydroxy metabolites by the kidney or excreted in the bile. The 1,25-dihydroxy-cholecalciferol ($1,25(OH)_2D_3$) is the active metabolite of vitamin D and maintains calcium levels in the blood, but its levels are influenced by serum calcium, parathyroid hormone, and other D metabolites. Both the 1,25- and 25 vitamin D_3 metabolites can be used to measure vitamin D status, but the higher plasma concentrations and lesser metabolic control of the latter make it by far the better option. Plasma $25(OH)D_3$ concentrations reflect the availability of vitamin D in the body[90] whereas $1,25(OH)_2D_3$ reflects the immediate physiological need. In deficiency, $1,25(OH)_2D_3$ concentrations are low but on supplementation with vitamin D will rise rapidly into the normal range, whereas $25(OH)D_3$ concentrations will remain low until a reserve accumulates. $25(OH)D_3$ is thus a marker of medium to long-term vitamin D availability from both dietary and endogenous sources, and it can be measured directly by HPLC, or by RIA, or competitive binding assay.

   Those factors that might influence exposure to sunlight (time of the year, habit of dress, mobility, season, age, gender, etc.) should be considered when interpreting $25(OH)D_3$ results. There is far less endogenous synthesis of vitamin D during the winter than the summer months at higher latitudes, so there are pronounced seasonal fluctuations in plasma $25(OH)D_3$ in all age groups, and particularly the elderly. Thus, Lawson et al.[65] showed that in elderly people in the UK, a strong cross-sectional relationship existed between winter dietary intakes of the vitamin and winter $25(OH)D_3$ levels because the sunlight contribution was small ($r = 0.55$; $P < 0.02$; $n = 23$), whereas in the summer there was no significant relation between intake and plasma $25(OH)D_3$, but the latter was then strongly related to an 'outdoor score', i.e. to sunlight exposure ($r = 0.62$; $P < 0.01$). Thus, there should be a reasonable prediction of broad categories of intake from measurements of plasma $25(OH)D_3$ in those who are only minimally exposed to sunlight or to other UV light sources, for a period of several months. Persons who restrict their exposure to sunlight need to achieve minimum stores of vitamin D during the summer months to maintain them through the winter. The threshold of 'risk' in such people should be the level associated with osteomalacia (below 12.5 nmol/l) plus a 'safety margin'. Thus, for persons whose potential sunlight exposure is adequate, marginal concentrations of 25(OH)D$_3$ will be 12.5–25 nmol/l, but in the elderly, particularly in the latter part of the summer months, such levels would be considered a high risk.[64,65] (Table 7.10).

Other factors that may affect vitamin D status at the lower end of the intake scale include the increased turnover of the vitamin that may occur in people eating typical Asian diets, which are very low in calcium and high in cereals.[91] Vitamin D levels in breast milk from unsupplemented mothers are very low but they do respond markedly to high level supplementation.[92] Thus, both plasma and breast milk levels of vitamin D and its metabolites will detect excessive intakes, and thus potential toxicity, in human subjects. Very low vitamin D intakes by some breast-fed infants have been associated with rickets or biochemical deficiency; a broad correlation between intake and marker level also exists in this vulnerable age group.

7.3.3 Vitamin E (α-tocopherol)

Vitamin E consists of eight naturally-occurring chromanols made up of four tocols and four tocotrienols. α-Tocopherol has the highest biological activity and is the least resistant to oxidation. Furthermore it is the predominant form of the tocopherols in animal and human tissues, but is not always the one which is most abundant in foods.[93] α-tocopherol is present in a wide variety of different foods but the largest proportion in human diets comes with dietary fat. A large number of biological and chemical methods are available to measure vitamin E[94] but liquid chromatography is the most relevant to the nutritionist measuring vitamin E status. Unfortunately, however, none of the methods currently available will reliably assess the intake of vitamin E in unsupplemented diet for the reasons described below.

Although dietary vitamin E exhibits some relation to blood tocopherol levels over a wide range of intakes, so that vitamin E supplements have a reasonably predictable effect on individuals' plasma, red cell, or white cell vitamin E levels,[95] the predictive power of all the biochemical indices for individual intakes in supplemented diets is only moderate, as can be seen in the weak relationship between intakes and plasma levels in the recent UK adult study[35] (Table 7.9(a)). Here, variations in intake explained only 4% of the variance in total plasma vitamin E, or about 7% of the variance in the tocopherol:cholesterol ratio (which is considered to be a better reflection of status (see below).[66] The correlation observed in the preschool children's survey was even weaker (Table 7.9(b)). This weak correlation is partly because the absorption of the vitamin is incomplete and variable (between 20 and 80% in published studies), and partly because the extent of absorption declines with increasing amounts per meal. A further complication is the variable biological activity of different members of the tocopherol family.[96]

α-Tocopherol in the blood   The measurement of vitamin E status is commonly made by measuring the concentration of tocopherol circulating in the plasma, where values less than 11.6 µmol/l are generally accepted as indicating vitamin E deficiency.[63]

However, tocopherol circulates in the blood predominantly with the low density lipoprotein fraction, and it was pointed out several years ago that vitamin E was closely correlated with total lipid in the blood.[67] Blood lipids comprise mainly cholesterol, triglycerides, and the phospholipids, and vitamin E correlates best with the cholesterol fraction.[66] The molar cholesterol:vitamin E ratio is approximately 200:1 and is found in plasma samples from healthy persons in Third World and developed countries.[97] In addition, a molar ratio of 200:1 for polyunsaturated fatty acid to tocopherol is found in membranes and microsomes of highly oxygenated tissues of heart and lung and the *in vitro* antioxidant efficiency of vitamin E is of a similar order.[98]

We have therefore suggested that the vitamin E:cholesterol ratio is more biologically relevant than vitamin E alone as a marker of vitamin E status.[66,97] Its use prevents the over-estimation of vitamin E deficiency in Third World countries, it enables comparisons between Western countries with different plasma lipid levels[99] and enables comparisons between different age groups within a community.[35,100] Very few persons fall below the high risk threshold of 2.2 µmol α-tocopherol/mmol cholesterol.[66] Furthermore, the assay only requires the additional measure of cholesterol to standardize the results.

Functional tests of vitamin E status The antioxidant properties of vitamin E are believed to protect biological membranes against oxidant damage. This feature was used by Horwitt *et al.*[101] to develop the hydrogen peroxide haemolysis test (erythrocyte stress test) to assess the vitamin E status by the ability of red cells to resist oxidant damage. The hydrogen peroxide haemolysis procedure must be performed in a standardized manner with caution exercised with regard to sample handling, time lapse between sample collection and test, preparation of reagents, incubation temperatures, etc.[63,101,102] Unfortunately, the method lacks specificity[103] and many workers have reported difficulties. Where simultaneous estimations of blood tocopherol and the red cell peroxide haemolysis test have been done, the results suggest that appreciable haemolysis is rarely observed if plasma tocopherol is greater than 11.6 µmol/l. Unfortunately, this agreement between the results of the two tests is only a reflection of the tocopherol concentration in the blood and does not necessarily reflect the vitamin E status of other tissues in the body.[63]

A modification of the peroxide test has recently been suggested in which malonaldehyde (MDA) generated by exposure of red cells to peroxide is measured instead of haemolysis.[102] The authors claim that MDA production more accurately reflects vitamin E deficiency as documented by plasma vitamin E or E:lipid ratios. However, as many features of the MDA and haemolysis tests are common, the MDA procedure suffers from most of the limitations of the hydrogen peroxide haemolysis test.

Platelet vitamin E has also been examined as an index of vitamin E status.[103,104] α-Tocopherol inhibits platelet aggregation and both deficiencies and excess of α-tocopherol have been shown to alter platelet function. Vatassery *et al.*[103] found that platelet α-tocopherol concentrations did not correlate with plasma lipids and reported a linear relationship between platelet α-tocopherol and supplements of DL-α-tocopherol up to 1800 IU/day. They suggested these results indicated that platelet α-tocopherol was a better indicator of vitamin E status than plasma measurements. The first point is worth further investigation but supplementary vitamin E also produces a linear response in plasma concentrations in short term experiments.

Currently, the most useful measurement of vitamin E status is the plasma α-tocopherol:cholesterol ratio (Table 7.10).

7.3.4 Vitamin K

The major dietary form of vitamin K is phylloquinone, derived mainly from plant sources. Its absorption is variable and incomplete because it depends on solubilization within intestinal micelles containing bile salts and the products of pancreatic lipolysis.[105] The development of adequate assay procedures for the very small amounts of vitamin K that are found in human plasma has been achieved only recently, and the limited evidence available suggests a partial, but not very strong relationship with dietary phylloquinone.[106-109] The picture is further complicated by synthesis of vitamin K (menaquinones) in the gut, which may contribute as much as 50 per cent of the total vitamin K in the body. Certainly little evidence exists to suggest that plasma vitamin K can do better than define a very broad classification of group intakes.

The major criterion for assessing the adequacy of vitamin K status in adults is the maintenance of plasma prothrombin concentrations in normal range (1.2–1.8 µmol/l). Prothrombin levels are mostly estimated using tests that determine clotting (prothrombin) time[68] but prothrombin levels can now be measured directly by radioimmunoassay.[110] It has been suggested that the ratio of non-carboxylated:carboxylated prothrombin in plasma may be a useful indicator of marginal vitamin K deficiency in individuals who have not yet developed defects in blood clotting.[69,111] The measurement of abnormal prothrombin by radio immunoassay and its disappearance following injection of vitamin K is also used as a measure of vitamin K status and is claimed to be 1000-fold more sensitive than prothrombin time.[112] Its use in patients with chronic gastro-intestinal disease and/or resection revealed one-third with evidence of deficiency. Abnormalities of vitamin K-dependent decarboxylation are also present in patients with cirrhosis, acute hepatitis, and hepatocellular carcinoma but these do not respond to vitamin K.

Most people have a diet nutritionally adequate in vitamin K_1 plus an unknown amount of K_2 from micro-organisms in the gut.[111] A population group with most evidence of prolonged clotting times is the elderly.[113] Seventy-five per cent of more than 1000 hospitalized elderly had abnormal prothrombin times, but most of these were associated with anticoagulant therapy or hepatic damage.

Low plasma prothrombin levels are also found in newborn infants and, because breast milk contains little vitamin K, intramuscular injections of phylloquinone have been recommended to prevent haemorrhagic disease of the newborn, although there is some controversy about this.[69, 114] The very small amounts of vitamin K that are present in breast milk are sensitive to major changes in maternal intake of the vitamin[92,115] but these variations have not yet been refined to permit them to predict intakes from dietary sources. Since it is the young breast fed infant who is most clearly at risk of developing vitamin K deficiency, it will probably be within the area of lactational and breast milk vitamin K nutrition that future efforts will be concentrated.

7.3.5 Thiamin (Vitamin B₁)

Thiamin deficiency is closely associated with the consumption of milled rice, which is why the deficiency disease beri-beri has been commonly associated with South-East

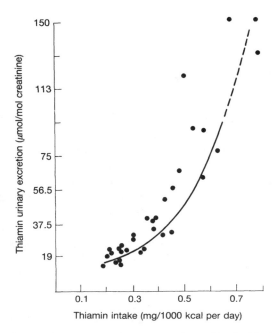

Fig. 7.1 Thiamin intake and urinary excretion. Data collected in the National Nutrition Surveys by the Interdepartmental Committee on Nutrition for National Defence.[120]

Asian countries. However, thiamin is present in a wide variety of foods and it is restriction in food choice that commonly precipitates the disease.

As with most of the water-soluble vitamins, there is no recognizable store of thiamin in the body and the only reserve is that part of the thiamin pool that is functionally bound to enzymes within the tissues. A characteristic urinary excretion pattern has been demonstrated for thiamin (and also riboflavin and vitamin B$_6$)[116] in which an initially slow rise with increasing intakes is followed by a rapid rise at relatively high intakes, after saturating the main tissue compartments and reaching the urinary excretion threshold. Although none of these vitamins exhibits a complete recovery of intake in the urine, even at relatively high intakes, because intestinal absorption becomes the limiting factor, it is nevertheless possible to predict intake fairly precisely at high intakes, at least on a population basis. On an individual level, variations in absorption efficiency tend to blur this relationship. It depends, of course, on the chemical form of the vitamin present in the diet, on the transit time through the gut region of maximum absorptive capacity, etc. Moreover, excretion is increased by infection and exercise[117] and in situations of negative nitrogen balance, although not to the same extent as riboflavin.[118]

Twenty-four-hour urine collections, and dietary intakes, are both tedious and difficult to achieve, and methods to use both shorter timed (4–6 hour) and random urine samples were developed. The thiamin:creatinine ratio is useful for the interpretation of random samples (Table 7.11 and Fig. 7.1) while loading doses of 1–5 mg thiamin administered orally or intramuscularly, and coupled with the

Table 7.11 Criteria for assessment of water-soluble vitamin status in adults: some recommended methods based on concentration measurements.*

Vitamin	Measurement Blood	Measurement Urine	High risk	Medium risk	Acceptable	References
Thiamin	RBC thiamin nmol/l		<90	90–132	132–284	121, 122
		thiamin: creatinine µmol/mol	<10.1	10.1–24.5	>24.5	63
Niacin		NMN: creatinine mmol/mol	<0.4	0.4–1.3	1.3–3.9	123
Pyridoxine	Pyridoxal 5′-phosphate nmol/l		<10.0	10.0–20.0	20.0–165	64, 124, 125
Folate	RBC folate mmol/l		<0.23	0.23–0.34	>0.34	63, 64, 126
	Plasma folate nmol/l		<6.8	6.8–13.4	>13.4	63, 64, 126
Vitamin B_{12}	Serum Vitamin B_{12} pmol/l		<74	74–147	>147	63, 64, 126
Ascorbate	Plasma ascorbate mmol/l		<6.0	6.0–17.0	>17.0	63. 64, 127
	Buffy layer ascorbate pmol/10^6 WBC		<40	40–86	>86	64, 128
	Ascorbate load 15 mg/kg body wt		<14 µmol/l plasma ascorbate at 3 h		>14 µmol/l plasma ascorbate at 3 h	129

* For alternative, red cell enzyme-based analysis, see Table 7.2.

measurement of urinary thiamin over 4 or 24 hours, have been used to make the urinary measurement of thiamin more indicative of tissue saturation. Different workers have suggested that if the proportion of urinary thiamin is below 20% of the administered dose in the subsequent 24 hours, then thiamin deficiency is indicated.[119] However, these two techniques fail to provide continuous quantitative markers of thiamin intake for epidemiological purposes. Measurement of urinary excretion below 0.5 mg/1000 kcal (4200 kJ) deviates from linearity in relation to intake and loses sensitivity; and percentage excretion of an administered dose above 20% says little about the degree of deficiency. A combination of the two techniques may help to develop a scheme for classifying individual intakes into broad categories, but problems remain in epidemiological studies regarding the collection of urine samples.

The newer method for assessment depends on the reactivation of the cofactor-depleted red cell enzyme transketolase *in vitro* (see Table 7.2). This is sensitive over a lower range of intakes, from the 'deficient' to the 'moderate intake' range. While it is possible to 'titrate' deficient individuals with varying amounts of the vitamin *in vivo*, and to observe a fairly close correlation between intakes and status indices, it is also clear that the magnitude of the biochemical response to a given intake varies considerably between individuals. This will limit the accuracy of prediction of individual (long term) intakes from the status index values. Thus values of the transketolase activation coefficient (TKL-AC) above 1.25 are indicative of thiamin deficiency (see Table 7.2), and those near 1.0 suggest that intakes are sufficient to saturate tissues, the values in between suggest a low to moderate intake, but the correlation of TKL-AC and intake within this range may be poor.[130–132] Furthermore, a combination of a TKL-AC below 1.25 and low TKL activity may indicate chronic thiamin depletion. There is some doubt about the stability of haemolysate TKL activity unless storage at −70°C is possible.[64,133,134]

Direct analysis by HPLC of thiamin diphosphate (TPP), the form in which thiamin coenzyme is mainly found in red blood cells, offers an alternative assay to the TKL-AC. While the range of sensitivity is not greater than with TKL-AC, the reliability of the assay is better.[121]

7.3.6   Riboflavin (Vitamin B₂)

Riboflavin is present in meats, cereals, and vegetables, but the richest dietary source is dairy products. Consequently, riboflavin intakes are generally lower in milk-free diets, and hence riboflavin deficiency occurs in many parts of the tropics.[6,135,136]

Urinary riboflavin was the first index to be used extensively for the assessment of riboflavin status.[137,138] As with thiamin, there is a linear relationship between intake and excretion at levels of riboflavin intake in excess of dietary requirements.[56] However, when riboflavin intake falls below tissue requirements there are adaptive improvements in the utilization of riboflavin coenzymes that reduce riboflavin excretion.

The intersection of the excretion curves produced by dietary intakes of riboflavin, below and above the amounts required to saturate the tissues can define requirements[56] provided that the subject is in positive nitrogen balance. Infections or drugs that induce a breakdown of tissue protein will increase urinary excretion.[10] Thus, the measurement of urinary riboflavin is of limited usefulness in situations where low protein intake or chronic infection are common.

As with thiamin, there is a red cell enzyme (glutathione reductase) that is dependent on a cofactor derived from riboflavin. This gives rise to the erythrocyte glutathione reductase stimulation test (activation coefficient) or EGRAC. The measurement is like that of total red cell riboflavin, in being a measure of tissue saturation and long-term riboflavin status. However, it has the advantage of being stable and extremely sensitive and can be easily made on finger-prick samples.[135] The test appears to be independent of age and gender.

The test is sensitive only at low levels of riboflavin intake, and does not correlate particularly well with higher ranges of intake. Thus, there was little correlation between long term riboflavin intakes and several repeated measures of EGRAC in elderly UK subjects.[20] In the recent UK adult survey[35] (Table 7.9(a)) correlation coefficients between −0.13 and −0.31 were observed between riboflavin intakes and the glutathione reductase index.

Bates *et al.*[139] reported a fall in EGRAC values in pregnant Gambian women associated with a fall in body weight during the rainy season (i.e. an apparent improvement in riboflavin status, although other factors suggested that malnutrition increased). Others have shown similar changes in EGRAC (in sick children) that reversed on treatment.[136]

Measurements of EGRAC between 1.00 and 1.30 represent more or less complete saturation of the tissues with riboflavin[140,141] and are obtained in young men on daily intakes of 1.5 mg riboflavin.[142] However, in young women, Belko *et al.*[143] found that amounts of riboflavin between 1.2 and 2.4 mg were required to maintain EGRAC values in this range. EGRAC values of 1.2–1.4 indicate borderline status and were obtained in pregnant women on 1.5 mg in the Gambia and Cambridge.[139] Elderly Guatemalan subjects exhibited borderline values at intakes around 1.3–1.4 mg/d. [144] Activation coefficients around 1.5–2.5 are found in populations consuming minimal intakes of riboflavin, together with evidence of clinical deficiencies.[139,145,146] The EGRAC is thus a useful measure to classify subjects into broad categories of intake and to make comparisons between populations, but its sensitivity becomes poorer as dietary intakes of riboflavin approach the levels that correspond to tissue saturation.

7.3.7 Niacin (Vitamin PP)

Niacin is present in large amounts in most cereals and can also be synthesized from the essential amino acid tryptophan and so deficiencies are uncommon. However, maize is an exception, because the niacin is present in a bound form and is unavailable if the food preparation does not include some form of hydrolysis. The niacin deficiency disease pellagra became common in southern Europe and north Africa following the introduction of maize from the New World and was responsible for a tremendous death toll in the southern states of the USA follow the social and economic upheaval of the American Civil War.[123]

An Indian variety of sorghum known as jowar has also been linked with pellagra[147] and it was pointed out that jowar contains a high content of leucine, which may interfere with tryptophan metabolism by creating an amino acid imbalance. Other workers have also found evidence that leucine interferes with the metabolism of tryptophan, particularly when niacin intake is low.[148]

The most sensitive method for the determination of niacin, niacinamide and closely related compounds in serum, urine, food, tissues, etc. is by microbiological methods.[149] Chemical methods are far less sensitive and require extensive purification.

The most sensitive indicator of niacin status in experimental animals is the tissue concentrations of the NAD(P) coenzymes. In man, it has been suggested that whole blood NAD(P) may serve the same purpose.[150]

The principal urinary metabolite of nicotinamide, and hence the coenzyme NAD(P), is N'-methylnicotinamide (NMN) and this substance forms the basis of the most widely used method of assessing niacin nutritional status.[151] The method has high sensitivity and reproducibility.[149] NMN is measured on a timed urine sample or expressed in terms of the creatinine concentration in random samples.

There are also some other urinary metabolites: N'-methyl-2-pyridone-5-carboxamide and N'-methyl-2-pyridone-3-carboxamide which are more severely reduced in marginal deficiency than NMN and virtually cease to be excreted several weeks before the appearance of clinical signs of deficiency. It has been suggested that a more precise measure of niacin status can be obtained by measuring the pyridones or the ratio of 2-pyridone to NMN.[152,153]

The excretion of NMN expressed as mmol/mol creatinine in random samples of urine is technically simple and a useful guide to niacin status (Table 7.11). The sensitivity of the index in relation to total intake of niacin equivalents (niacin + tryptophan/60) is better at the margins of adequacy and below than it is at higher intake.

7.3.8 Pyridoxine (Vitamin B$_6$)

Pyridoxine is widely available in foods of vegetable and animal origin, the range of intake is wide, and severe deficiencies are rare. The requirement for vitamin B$_6$ is linked to protein intake, and its role in amino acid metabolism.

Several biochemical markers are currently used for vitamin B$_6$ (plasma pyridoxal phosphate levels (PLP), red cell transaminase activation, and urinary excretion of B$_6$ degradation products). Although plasma pyridoxal phosphate levels have gained some popularity, recent studies[154,155] suggest that there is unlikely to be a strong correlation between B$_6$ intakes and index levels and that many confounding factors exist, including recent dietary intake, prolonged fasting concomitant with the release of PLP from glycogen phosphorylase,[156] and conditions associated with a raised plasma alkaline phosphatase that can hydrolyse PLP to pyridoxal (PL) in blood.[124] Incomplete availability of some dietary (e.g. glycosylated) forms of vitamin B$_6$ imposes a further complication.

In vitamin B$_6$ deficiency, the erythrocyte transaminase activation coefficient allows the increase in the catalytically inactive apoenzyme of various PLP-dependant enzymes to be evaluated. It has been shown that two enzymes in erythrocyte lysates, alanine (ALT) and aspartate (AST) aminotransferase (Table 7.2) can be used to assess the degree of PLP unsaturation. ALT is considered the more sensitive but AST is more active and more frequently used.[157] Like other activation coefficients, the test is most sensitive at and below marginal intakes (Table 7.2), and is less valuable for ranking individuals with higher (more normal) intakes.

Two metabolic loading tests have been developed to assess vitamin B_6 status. In the tryptophan load test, the potentially rate-limiting enzyme kynureninase is especially sensitive to vitamin B_6 depletion. The excretion of kynurenic and xanthurenic acids is measured before and after the loading dose of trpytophan. However, there are many factors that interfere with this test[158] and its usefulness is restricted.

In contrast, the methionine load test is less frequently used but there are no reports of artifacts. Three enzymes are involved and, in vitamin B_6 deficiency, a test dose of methionine results in an abnormal accumulation and excretion of homocysteine, cystathionine, cysteine, and cysteine-sulphinic acid and a reduced excretion of taurine.[159] Both of these tests require the collection of timed urine samples, a disadvantage from the epidemiological standpoint.

The concentration of urinary metabolites also reflects recent dietary intake of the vitamin rather than the underlying state of tissue reserves.[160] 4-pyridoxic acid is the main metabolite of PLP and there is some evidence that catabolism increases with age.[63] Loss of sensitivity of the marker at low intakes is problematic.

A recent study[161] compared several of the available biochemical indices of vitamin B_6 status during controlled depletion and repletion with the vitamin. 0.015 mg vitamin B_6/g protein normalised most of the biochemical indices. As with the other B vitamins, there is no single marker for intake with equal sensitivity at all levels of dietary intake, and the use of two or more markers for the same nutrient, if feasible, should help to increase confidence.

7.3.9 *Folate*

Folate deficiency is one of the more frequently occurring vitamin deficiencies found in Western populations. Folate is necessary for purine and pyrimidine synthesis and actively growing tissue raises folate requirements, e.g. in pregnancy and infancy. Vegetables are the most important dietary source of folate but, since folate is easily oxidized, the freshness and vitamin C content influence the folate content. Folate metabolism is also intimately linked with vitamin B_{12} status, which must therefore be considered in interpreting folate measurements (see below).

The most useful tests of folate status are measurements of folate concentrations in serum and red cells. Because folic acid is susceptible to oxidation, suitable antioxidants (e.g. 1.0% sodium ascorbate) must be added to stabilize folate in samples during collection and storage. Red cell folate is a better measure of long term status because it reflects body stores at the time of red cell synthesis, while serum concentrations reflect recent dietary intake (see Table 7.11).[126] However, because of the chemical and biological complexity of the dietary folates, and the wide variety of factors that determine their bioavailability,[35] only broad categories of intake can be predicted, e.g. for population groups. Experience with the elderly UK subjects[162] shows that their red cell folate levels were more closely related to their dietary folate intake than was plasma folate. This appears to confirm the suggestion that red cell folate measures long term integrated status. In UK surveys[35,60] (Tables 7.9(a),(b)) the correlation (*r*) between dietary folate and red cell folate ranged from 0.06–0.22, due in part to the relatively short-term measure of intake, and in part due to the lack of specificity in the food assay for available forms of folate.

For a complete picture of folate status, both serum and red cell folate should be measured, together with serum vitamin B_{12}, to exclude any involvement of that vitamin in folate metabolism.

In vitamin B_{12} deficiency the metabolism of folate intermediates is blocked, serum folate is normal or high, but red cell folate is low because the deficiency also blocks the tissue uptake of folate.[163,164]

In recent years, radioassay kits have superseded microbiological assays in the measurement of folate and vitamin B_{12}. The former are simpler to perform and are not affected by antibiotics. However, the performance of the different commercially available kits can vary enormously.[165] It is important for laboratories which use the kits to participate in external quality assurance schemes to verify their performance.[166]

An alternative measure of folate status utilizes formiminoglutamate (FIGLU), a product of histidine metabolism that is normally metabolized by formiminotransferase to 5-formiminotetrahydrofolate. Excretion of FIGLU in folate deficiency is elevated in urine and is particularly elevated following a histidine load.[167] The assay is specific for folate deficiency but offers no advantage over serum or red cell folate assays. Similarly, macrocytic anaemia may indicate folate deficiency but again, these measurements provide no information on the continuum of intake above the levels needed to prevent signs of anaemia from appearing.

7.3.10 Cyanocobalamin (Vitamin B₁₂)

Vitamin B_{12} is only present in foods of animal origin, therefore people who are most likely to be at risk of this deficiency are those living wholly on vegetable foods. However, absorption of this vitamin depends upon an intrinsic factor, a binding protein secreted in the stomach. Hence, old age, hypochlorhydria, gastrectomy, and pernicious anaemia, which all influence the production of this protein can give rise to failure of vitamin B_{12} absorption. Thus, biochemical markers lose their sensitivity to dietary intake in these circumstances.

Vitamin B_{12} influences the metabolism of folate – apparently by starving the tissues of formyl tetrahydrofolate. When vitamin B_{12} status is poor, serum folate may be normal or high, but erythrocyte folate may be low, because vitamin B_{12} is also necessary for uptake of folates by tissue.[164]

Vitamin B_{12} status can only be estimated from serum levels, not from red cell levels (Table 7.11). Although in normal subjects dietary vitamin B_{12} is considered to possess good bioavailability, the correlation between dietary intake and serum levels is generally not very strong ($r = 0.09–0.12$ in the UK adult study,[135] Table 7.9(a)). One possible reason for this is that body stores of B_{12}, which are mainly in the liver, are generally large in comparison with daily intakes, so that the amount in the diet only affects circulating levels very slowly; i.e. it is a long term marker. When serum B_{12} concentrations fall below 90 pmol/l, the liver concentration is below the normal range[163] and serum B_{12} concentrations between 110 and 147 pmol/l (microbiological assay), are indicative of deficiency. In practice, this index seems incapable of defining individual intakes accurately and can only define group intakes in very broad categories relating to levels of deficiency. A marker for the full range of dietary intakes has yet to be described.

7.3.11 Vitamin C

Of all the vitamins, vitamin C exhibits possibly the strongest and most significant correlation between intake and biochemical indices, so that its intake can be predicted with moderate precision from the wide range of biochemical values that are encountered within the population of a Western country, e.g. the UK. Bioavailability of food sources of vitamin C is similar to that of the pure vitamin.[252] Basu and Schorah[168] reviewed the quantitative relationships between vitamin C intakes, plasma vitamin C, and leucocyte vitamin C. Plasma levels exhibit a characteristic S-shaped curve, with the steepest change in plasma levels between about 30 and 90 mg intake per day for adults (Fig. 7.2). Below 20 mg/day intake, most of the vitamin enters the tissues, and little is

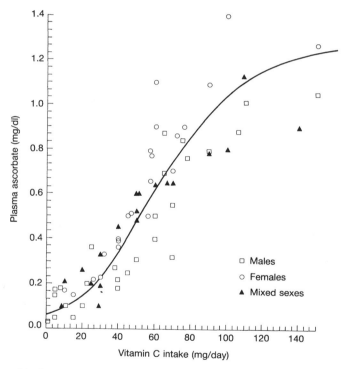

Fig. 7.2 Relationship between group mean values of plasma ascorbate and levels of vitamin C intake, from published studies. Data have been compiled from Basu and Schorah[168] and some more recently published studies; each data point represents a group of individuals of varying magnitude and composition, and assay procedures have also varied between different studies, so that the composite picture obtained is intended to give a generalized overview of the published data, not a precise relationship. There is a clear tendency for women to exhibit higher plasma ascorbate levels for a given intake, than men. Individual studies have explored this relationship[21,169–173] [0.2 mg/dl ≡ 11.4 µmol/l].

therefore available to circulate. Above 60–70 mg/day there is a marked renal threshold effect, with the excess of the circulating vitamin then being excreted in the urine. Thus, urine vitamin C is a potential marker for high intakes, although chemical instability is a potential problem, as well as the individual variability of the renal threshold. At even higher intakes, above 200 mg/d and into the multi-gram region intestinal absorption becomes the limiting factor.[174] Amounts in the buffy coat do not exhibit the lower threshold effect that plasma and urine levels do, and hence provide a more sensitive measure of lower intakes (Table 7.11, but the assays require more blood, are time-consuming, and are sometimes difficult to interpret for other reasons (e.g. leucocytosis during infection or surgery[175–177]). The long-term study of elderly men and women living at home in the UK[21] demonstrated a reasonably close relationship between vitamin C intakes and plasma or buffy coat levels. The confounding non-dietary influences here included a clear gender difference and an effect of smoking, both of which are well established influences on vitamin C status.[168,178] The closest temporal correlation was between the biochemical index value and the seven days of intake (estimate) immediately preceding the blood sample (Fig. 7.3). Longer periods of estimation were less relevant because of periodic fluctuation, both in intake and in

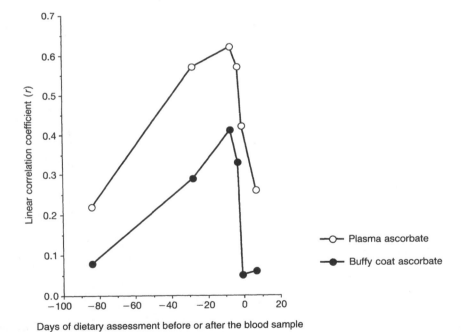

Days of dietary assessment before or after the blood sample

Fig. 7.3 Within-subject correlations between intake and plasma or buffy coat vitamin C levels in healthy, elderly men and women. Tabulated values from Table 7.4 of Bates *et al.*[21] are here presented graphically to illustrate the observation that maximum values for the positive correlation between estimated vitamin C intakes and either of the two biochemical index values were obtained when the dietary estimates extended for 7 days before the blood sample collection in each case.

status; shorter periods were less well correlated, probably because of inaccuracies in the short-term dietary measurements and medium-term buffering of plasma levels by the tissue pools. This analysis provided an indication of the time scale over which such biochemical markers of intake might be validated in the future.

A study of controlled vitamin C supplementation in Gambian lactating women[179] has further illustrated the strength of association between biochemical indices of vitamin C and its intake. This study provided a 'calibration curve' whereby the intake in a group of subjects could be predicted from the biochemical index values. Breast milk vitamin C was also found to be a potentially useful index in the low to moderate range of intakes, a conclusion that confirms that of other published studies.[92]

Brubacher[180] has shown that children exhibit a steeper relationship between their vitamin C indices and their dietary intake than adults. Thus age effects, plus the effects of gender, smoking,[181] and of infection[182,183] and other metabolic stresses on the intake:marker relationship, imply that any 'calibration curve' will be valid for only one particular population group; therefore the group (as well as the assay and diet assessment procedures) must be precisely specified. With this proviso, estimate of vitamin C intakes or of status indices can often provide a useful categorization of individuals into risk categories (either within a country such as the UK, or within a region such as Europe) that are strongly predictive of certain types of disease susceptibility. In a nutrition survey of the elderly in the UK[184], a comparison between one week of intake data and a single leucocyte ascorbate measurement yielded correlation coefficients $r = +0.49$ for men and $+0.36$ for women; both were significant at $P < 0.001$.

The measurement of vitamin C presents certain problems because of its instability. The most common substances used to stabilize ascorbate are trichloracetic acid and metaphosphoric acid and, in the writers' experience, plasma metaphosphoric acid-stabilized extracts stored at $-20°C$ are stable for several weeks, and for a year $-80°C$. It was shown that dithiothreitol (DTT) is an effective stabilizing reagent over a wide pH range.[185,186] If samples cannot be processed immediately, then whole blood stored up to 8 hours at $4°C$ in the dark before processing shows minimal changes in plasma ascorbate.[187]

Until recently, the commonest methods for measuring ascorbate have been colorimetric[188] or fluorimetric.[189] Liquid chromatography in conjunction with electrochemical detection improves selectivity and sensitivity by at least two orders of magnitude in comparison with colorimetric methods[190] making the measurement of ascorbate in 50 µl plasma easily attainable.

7.4 Markers of dietary intake: lipids, protein, dietary fibre, and energy

7.4.1 Lipids

Lipids are broadly defined as substances that can be extracted from biological materials with fat solvents, consisting primarily of esters or potential esters of fatty acids. There are many different types of lipids that can be described in animals and plants. They may be divided into (i) simple lipids such as fatty acids, neutral fats (mono-, di-, and triacylglycerols), and waxes (esters of fatty acids); and (ii) complex lipids such as ceramides, phosphoglycerides, plasmalogens, sphingolipids, glycolipids, sterols, and sterol esters.

The main lipids in human plasma are cholesterol, cholesteryl esters, triglycerides (triacylglycerol), phospholipids, and non-esterified fatty acids. Lipids are also structural components of cell membranes; here they are found in a molar ratio of 1:1 between phospholipid and free cholesterol. Short-chain fatty acids are water-soluble, but other lipids are insoluble in water, and to be carried in the bloodstream they need to be coated with a hydrophilic layer, made of phospholipids and proteins. The protein moiety is composed of several specific proteins (apolipoproteins). These complexes are termed lipoproteins and may be subdivided on the basis of their particle size and density (Table 7.12). The lipid composition of these lipoproteins differs substantially: chylomicrons are mainly triglyceride; VLDL is mainly triglyceride with phospholipid, cholesteryl esters and protein; the most common lipid in LDL is cholesteryl esters; and the major component in HDL is protein.

The vast majority of fat in the diet is triglyceride (TG), which is made up of glycerol and three fatty acids. In the process of digestion, fats are emulsified by bile salts in the small intestine and hydrolysed by intestinal and pancreatic lipases into di- (10%) and monoglycerides (40%) and fatty acids and glycerol (50%). About 70% are immediately resynthesized to TG, enter the lacteals as chylomicrons, pass into the lymphatic system and eventually enter the general circulation. Short-chain fatty acids are absorbed via the hepatic portal system. The rate of absorption is affected by transit time. When split from the glycerol moiety in the liver and other tissues, fatty acids enter the bloodstream as components of lipoproteins, and are oxidized, incorporated into membranes and other structures, or stored in adipose tissues via albumin.

Because lipids are found in all cell membranes, it is theoretically possible to measure lipid levels in any of these membranes. However, lipids are commonly measured in serum, plasma, or components of blood (red cells and white cells such as neutrophils, eosinophils, basophils, lymphocytes, and monocytes and platelets). Individual fatty acids can be measured in the cholesteryl ester, phospholipid or TG fractions of plasma or serum, or as free fatty acids. The turnover of the different cells from which the fatty acids are derived may reflect different time frames of dietary intake: platelets may reflect days and red cells months, although there is some exchange between membranes and plasma lipids throughout the life of the cell. It is probably desirable to assess fatty acids in specific compartments of the plasma rather than using a total plasma estimate. However, van Houwelinger et al.[193] showed that the per cent linoleic acid in total plasma lipid was as good an indicator of dietary intake as the proportion in phospholipid and cholesteryl esters. The measurement of total serum fatty acid composition is far less time consuming and can be applied to a large number of samples.[194]

The composition of fats can also be measured in adipose tissue and these levels probably reflect usual intake over several years. Adipose tissue fatty acid composition is a good indicator of linoleic acid intake but not of n-3 fatty acids.

In many studies, lipids and lipoprotein fractions are studied as outcome variables in their own right. For example, there is a vast literature on the dietary influences on cholesterol and fatty acid levels. In this chapter we are only focusing on the

Table 7.12 Properties and composition of human serum lipoproteins. (Modified from Edelstein,[191] ND, no data.)

	Chylomicrons	VLDL	LDL	HDL$_2$	HDL$_3$
Density (g/ml)	0.93–1.006	0.95–1.006	1.019–1.063*	1.063–1.125†	1.125–1.21†
Molecular weight	0.4–30×10^6	5–10×10^6	2–3×10^6	3.6×10^5	1.75×10^5
Diameter (Å)	750–6000	250–750	170–260	60–140	40–100
Components (% wt of total lipoprotein)					
Phospholipids	6–9	16–20	24–30	24–30	22–25
Free cholesterol	1–3	4–8	9–12	2–5	2–3
Cholesteryl ester	3–6	9–13	28–30	16–20	10–13
Triglycerides	82–86	50–60	7–11	4–5	4–5
Protein	1–2	8–11	20–22	41–50	55–58
Apoprotein (g/100g)					
A-I	33.0	0.9	0.8	58.7	64.9
A-II	Trace	0.2	0.4	10.0	25.6
A-IV	14.0	ND	ND	ND	Trace
B-48	5.0	Absent	Absent	Absent	Absent
B-100	Absent	25.0	95.0	3.0	Absent
C	32.0	55.0	2.0	13.0	5.0
D	ND	ND	Trace	2.0	4.0
E‡	10.0	15.0	3.2	3.0	1.0

* Subclasses I, II, III from reference 192.
† Subclass 2a, 2b; 3a, 3b; from reference 192.
‡ There are four phenotypes which may influence concentrations.

measurement of lipids as markers of dietary intakes, although much of the evidence for the relationship between dietary intake and tissue levels comes from studies that have sought to modify tissue levels by dietary modification. It is worth noting that, within a population, variations in plasma cholesterol may reflect genetic variation more than differences in fat intake, which show a real but small influence.[195]

Depending on the purpose of the study, different lipid fractions will be appropriate. The principle of a marker is that it is just that, a marker of intake. As with any measurement, the objective will be to measure that marker with required validity. In experimental studies the objective is to use the marker to confirm the dietary intake and to check compliance during the study. For example, in studies looking at the effects of changing the type or amount of fat in the diet on blood pressure, dietary intake can be assessed and related to levels in various plasma and blood cells or sampled in tissues depending on the time frame of the study. The marker needs to be sensitive to change within the time frame of the study. There is little point measuring change in adipose tissue fatty acids in a study lasting only several weeks. It may also be important that the marker does not change too much. For example, free fatty acids in plasma will be affected by what has just been eaten, and may not reflect the levels of fat incorporated in cell membranes. Platelets will be appropriate for short-term trials (e.g. for assessing eicosapentaenoic acid,[196]) whereas red cells may not be (although red cells may be better for docosahexaenoic acid). Fat biopsies may provide the most appropriate measure for very long studies.

Assessment of lipids (fatty acids in particular) is most commonly undertaken in experimental studies where the investigator aims to modify dietary fat intake and assess the effects on either short or long-term outcome measures predictive of heart disease, for example, blood pressure and serum lipids (total cholesterol or lipoproteins).

Non-functional tests of fatty acid and cholesterol status are most commonly used, such as concentrations in blood or cell membranes. At the lower limits of intake (i.e. to assess essential fatty acid status) it is also necessary to measure the derivatives of linoleic and alpha-linolenic acid, and plasma phospholipids are favoured because of the high rate of turnover.[197] While there are functional tests of lipid turnover and balance, these are not widely used in epidemiological studies and will not be discussed here. However, it is likely that, in metabolic ward studies, these functional tests will become more common.

Factors affecting lipid levels in general   Many factors influence blood lipid levels in general. Apart from the obvious dietary factors, intakes of carbohydrates (including non-starch polysaccharides), energy, alcohol, and smoking may alter lipid levels. Obesity, exercise, stress, sex hormones, and pregnancy have all been reported to affect lipid levels, given an unaltered dietary intake. It has been well demonstrated that, in malnourished children, cholesterol, triglycerides, and free fatty acid levels are affected in different ways depending on the degree of fatty liver change. In children with kwashiorkor, cholesterol and TG levels may be lowered, whereas in marasmic children levels may be lowered, normal or raised. Other disease states also affect lipid levels (see Table 7.6) and lipid levels may be lowered for several months after an acute myocardial infarction.

This list is not exhaustive and the main point is to consider the effect that the health of the subject could have on their lipid levels and also on the way they may respond to change.

It is important to consider the other factors in the diet and lifestyle of the subjects that may affect the lipid levels measured in the body. And it is necessary to consider the possibility of the effects of *de novo* synthesis when assessing the relationship between intake and tissue levels.

Applicability of lipid measurements in epidemiological studies   To date there are no markers of total fat intake. Work by Weinberg *et al*[198] demonstrates that apoA-IV levels change rapidly with changes in dietary fat intake and can be used to monitor *changes* in fat intake in the short term (days or weeks). In the long term, apoA-IV stabilizes in relation to the new dietary fat intake level and loses its value as a measure of total fat intake until a new change is introduced.

Measuring fatty acids in various cell compartments represents a very useful way to check on dietary compliance, provided that the tissue being used has been shown to be sensitively related to dietary levels and that the within-subject variability is within reasonable bounds (5%). It is often assumed that a level of fat derived from a tissue is a more reliable marker of intake than a level derived from a dietary questionnaire or recording technique. This may not always be the case, although the assertion either way is quite difficult to assess.

From an epidemiological point of view, in terms of measuring lipids as markers of intake, it is important to consider how the fatty acids and cholesterol that are taken into the body are handled by the body, and to consider how the availability of substrates necessary to transport the lipids (proteins, etc.) may influence the levels measured in the blood or in tissues. It is beyond the scope of this section to discuss all these issues, but they should be borne in mind when the relationship between dietary intake and tissue levels are being assessed.

Fatty acids   The simplest division of fatty acids is on the basis of whether they are saturated or unsaturated. Unsaturated acids have one or more double bond in the carbon chain, whereas saturated fatty acids have no double bond. Most naturally occurring fatty acids are straight-chain saturated or unsaturated acids containing an even number of carbon atoms. However, certain fish oils have an odd number of carbon atoms. Animal cells cannot form linoleic acid or linolenic acid, and these, together with oleic acid, are precursors for the biosynthesis of individual families of polyunsaturated fatty acids.

Fatty acids can be further classified on the basis of the number and location of the double bonds in the chain. For example, linolenic acid is designated 18;3n–3, which means that it has 18 carbons in the chain, three double bonds and that the first double bond is three carbons from the terminal methyl carbon. This basic structure is given for the main fatty acids in the diet in Table 7.13. Broadly, there are four groups of fatty acids in terms of the position of the first double bond, n3 (for example, 18:3n–3), n6 (18:2n–6 linoleic acid), n7 (16:1n–7 palmitoleic) and n9 (18:1n–9 oleic). Because of the double bonds in the molecule it is possible that unsaturated fatty acids can exist as either the cis or trans isomer. They have different properties, and changes from cis (the most common isomer) to trans in food processing may influence the metabolic activity and fate of the fatty acid.

The composition of the fatty acid profile is usually expressed as a relative percentage of the total (although a measure that reflected absolute levels of intake would obviously be preferred). Using relative levels, if one fatty acid increases, logically, others must go down, and it is therefore not possible to differentiate the absolute effect from the relative effect.

Up to 400 individual peaks representing different fatty acids on a chromatograph have been identified. However, in the human diet the major fatty acids are oleic (about 36%), palmitic (22%), linoleic (16%), stearic (10%), and linolenic (1%) (Table 7.13).

Fatty acids may be extracted from a large variety of cells, membranes, or tissues in the body. The levels measured in different tissues may be used to indicate dietary intakes in the short term (hours, e.g. plasma triglycerides), medium term (several days, e.g. cholesteryl esters and phospholipids in red cells), slightly longer (weeks, e.g. red cell membranes or platelets) or longer term (months or years, e.g. adipose tissue), depending on the nature of the study proposed.

Across the range of fatty acids in the diet (including longer chain fatty acids from fish oils) and in studies that aim to modify fatty acid intake by dietary manipulation, fatty acid levels measured in blood and other tissues reflect the dietary levels. For example, studies in the USA[199] and Holland[200,201] have shown good agreement between fat intake estimated from dietary surveys and levels of fatty acids measured in adipose tissue and in plasma. Kardinaal et al.[200] have also shown that there is good agreement between the ranking of subjects using adipose tissue and dietary estimates of linoleic acids. However, as Table 7.13 shows, in subjects following typical unchanged diets, the relative percentage of fatty acids varies from tissue to tissue, because there is competition between the n-3 and n-6 fatty acids. It is therefore important to have baseline assessments in each tissue level against which to compare change, and not to assume that levels will be comparable across tissues.

Despite differences in laboratories and methods used, there seems to be reasonably good agreement between studies in the relative proportions of fatty acids measured within the same tissue or plasma lipid fraction. As mentioned elsewhere, there should always be a strict protocol for the collection of samples to minimize bias. The prime concern should be on internal validity in experimental studies that modify diet. It is recommended that blanks and an internal reference standard are always used to check on quality control.

The methods used for measuring fatty acids (Table 7.14) are reasonably standardized (see Christie[214] for details). The methods listed in Table 7.14 are those that are cited most commonly in the recently published literature. At present, most centres following extraction of samples use gas liquid chromatography (GC or GLC) with a column. The HPLC system appears to work well for more simple fatty acid mixtures and can separate geometric isomers. It also has advantages in analysing polymeric, oxidized, less volatile, very polar, and heat labile components that cannot be separated by GLC. At the present time, for complex mixtures of fatty acids from animal organs and marine oils, the separation of the more polyunsaturated fatty acids is more difficult with HPLC than with GLC. Sample collection and storage needs careful attention (see Thompson[215]).

Table 7.13 Composition of fatty acids in various tissues.

Level of fatty acid (%)	Fatty acid							
	Palmitic (16:0)*	Palmitoleic (16:1n-7)	Stearic (18:0)	Oleic (18:1n-9)	Linoleic (18:2n-6)	Linolenic (18:3n-6)	Arachidonic (20:4n-6)	Docosahexaenoic (22:6n-3)
Usual diet	22	3	10	36	16	1	1	Trace
Total Serum Lipids	17–21	3	6–8	18–22	30–34	0.3–0.5	6–9	1–2
Serum Lipid Fractions								
Cholesteryl esters	12	4	1	20	50–54	7	8	0.5
Phospholipids	27	1	11–15	9–11	23	0.2	9	1–4
Triglycerides	24	6	3	38	20	1.2	2	0.4
Diglycerides	29	3	6	36	13	0.7	0.7	NS
Phosphotidylcholine	27	1	18	9	31	0.2	10	3
Free fatty acids	25	5	10	39	1.6	0.7	1	0.3
Red Blood Cells								
Phospholipid	21–25	NS	14–23	13–20	6–9	NS	13–15	NS
Phosphatidylcholine	39	NS	11	15	24	NS	5	NS
Phosphatidylethanolamine	19	NS	8	17	7	NS	19	NS
Platelets	NS	NS	NS	NS	9	NS	21	NS
Adipose tissue	19	8	4	47	12–16	NS	NS	NS
Cheek cells	23	7	20	37	8	NS	NS	NS

* Number of carbon atoms:number of bonds; n, position of first double bond from terminal methyl carbon; NS, not stated. Compiled from references 191, 192, 200, 202–213.

Table 7.14　Summary of methods used to measure lipids.*

Lipid	Methods
Fatty acids	Separate lipid fractions by
	i　　Thin layer chromatography (TLC)
	ii　 Tubular thin layer chromatography
	iii　TLC, flame ionization detector
	iv　 Silica cartridges
	Once in separate fractions measure fatty acid methyl esters
	i　　Gas–Liquid chromatography (with column) (GC or GLC)
	ii　 High performance liquid chromatography (HPLC)
	iii　Mass spectrometry (usually with GC) (MS/GC) analysed by electron impact ionization mode or soft ionization technique
Cholesterol	i　　Enzymatically (directly in plasma, H_2O_2 formed is measured spectrophotometrically)
	ii　 Colorimetrically (hydrolysis then extraction)
Triglycerides	i　　Enzymatically (NADH measured spectrophotometrically)
	ii　 Chemical (isolated by chromatography after extraction)
Lipoproteins	i　　ELISA kit
	ii　 Ultracentrifugation
	iii　Precipitation
	iv　 Adsorption
	v　　Gel filtration
	vi　 Affinity chromatography
	vii　Electrophoresis
	viii Immunochemical
	Subfractions sometimes calculated by subtraction using formula
	LDL = Total cholesterol (Serum TG/2.2–HDL)
	or LDL = Total cholesterol–HDL + VLDL. VLDL = Plasma TG/5
Phospholipids	i　　Colorimetrically (after lipid extraction and oxidation)
Apolipoproteins	i　　Immunoassay (radio, electro, radial)
	ii　 Immunonephelometry
	iii　Enzyme-linked and fluorescence immunoassays

* Method mentioned first is the most commonly cited at time of writing.

Cholesterol　The cholesterol that is taken into the body, together with endogenous production (up to twice the dietary intake), is carried in various lipoproteins. It is possible, therefore, to measure a total cholesterol level ignoring the distribution within lipoproteins, or to measure lipoprotein specific levels. The relationship between dietary cholesterol and total and lipoprotein levels of cholesterol is complex and appears to vary across the range of cholesterol intake. Because the low density lipoproteins contain the most cholesterol, LDL levels correlate most closely with total cholesterol levels. As indicated in Table 7.14, various formulae have been proposed to describe the relationship between fat intake and serum cholesterol levels. It is clear that dietary cholesterol is not the only determinant of serum cholesterol, and consideration must be given as to the effects of the type of fat in the diet and intakes of other nutrients or factors, such as dietary fibre. There is a vast literature on the effects of diet on serum cholesterol and a discussion of these data is beyond the scope of this chapter.

A summary of the methods most commonly used to measure serum cholesterol and the lipoproteins is given in Table 7.14. Fasting blood samples are not required, but consideration needs to be given as to how the samples are processed and stored.[215] Blood samples should be collected and processed in the same way for all subjects in the study. Total cholesterol is stable once frozen for a reasonably long time, however HDL is more susceptible to degradation and for this assay, serum should be stored at $-70°C$.

7.4.2 Protein

24-hour urine nitrogen

24-hour urine nitrogen is the most well known biological marker, with individual results from published metabolic studies where dietary intake is kept constant over prolonged periods of time showing a fair correlation between daily nitrogen intake and daily urine nitrogen excretion. Its use depends on the assumption that subjects are in nitrogen balance, there being no accumulation due to growth or repair of lost muscle tissue, or loss due to starvation, slimming, or injury. This was appreciated as early as 1924, when it was suggested that actual protein intake, as assessed from 24-hour urine excretion, was far lower than the recommended level.[216]

The apparent accuracy of 24-hour urine nitrogen as a biological marker has led to the suggestion that it be used to validate estimates of protein intake from various dietary survey methods.[217] In 1980, Isaksson summarized a number of studies carried out by his group and showed that estimates of protein intake obtained from 24-hour recalls of food intake were low when compared with the urine nitrogen, but those estimated from diet histories and records were in good agreement with the urine values.[217] Van Staveren also found good agreement between 24-hour urine and diet history estimates of protein intake.[218] However, these comparisons were only investigated on a group basis because each individual contributed only single or two 24-hour urine collections. Other early comparisons between average urine nitrogen and dietary intake have been summarized.[19,219]

To investigate the applicability of using 24-hour N to validate estimates of protein intake on an individual basis, four men and four women were given their usual varying diet over a 28-day period whilst living in a metabolic suite.[220] Duplicates of diets were made up each day for each individual and 24-hour urine and faecal collections were also made over this period, and diets, urines, faeces, and skin losses measured for their nitrogen content.[220] Table 7.15 shows the comparison between 28 days diet and urine estimation; there was almost complete agreement. Urine nitrogen underestimated intake at higher levels of protein intake and overestimated at lower levels but a constant factor for faecal and skin losses can be used to counteract this, and output from urine can be expressed as a percentage of intake, 0.81.[220] However, less good correlations between individual estimates of usual protein intake, and the 24-hour urine nitrogen output will be obtained if fewer observations on each individual are made, and if the collections are not verified for their completeness.

Verification of the completeness of 24-hour collections

Earlier studies used creatinine to check on the completeness of urinary collection. Creatinine excretion is dependent upon both creatinine intake, primarily from meat in

Table 7.15 Comparison of 24-hour* urine N output and dietary N intake with different numbers of observations.[220]

	Single day diet and urine	8 days urine 18 days diet	28 days urine 28 days diet
Correlation coefficient	0.47	0.95	0.99
Urine N as percentage of diet N average	81	81	81
Coefficient of variation	24	5	2

* All 24-hour urine colections verified for completeness.

the diet, and creatinine production, which is proportional to fat-free mass. Where diets vary considerably within individuals especially in their meat content, creatinine excretion is not a reliable marker of completeness. Where collections are known to be complete, within-subject variability of urinary creatinine has been shown to be of the order of 10%, similar to that for urinary nitrogen.[26,220] Between subject variation in creatinine excretion is about 23% in a mixed population, again similar to total nitrogen.[26] Two external makers are in use to verify the completeness of 24-hour urine collections. Lithium is completely absorbed and excreted and has been used for example to assess sodium consumption added as cooking or table salt.[221] Lithium can also be used to assess the completeness of 24-hour urine collections, although the salt does have to be given to subjects every day some days before the intended 24-hour urine collection in order that equilibrium can be achieved.

Para-amino benzoic acid (PABA) is actively absorbed and excreted, so that it can be used to check on the day of the 24-hour collection to verify completeness.[222] The method consists of three tablets of 80 mg PABA, taken with meals, which is quantitatively excreted within 24 hours so that single 24-hour collections containing less than 85% of the PABA marker can be classified as unsatisfactory, either because the tablets have not been taken, or because one or more specimens were omitted from the collection. Table 7.16 shows that there is a systematic difference, particularly in urea and total nitrogen between collections that are deemed complete by the PABA method and ones that contain less than 85% of the PABA marker. Omission of such a marker will, therefore, cause underestimation of 24-hour urine nitrogen or urea output, and contributes to the poor agreement between estimates of usual intake, diet, and estimates of 24-hour urine output. PABA has been used extensively in methodological studies carried out in the UK,[30,32,223–225] Italy,[226] France,[227] the USA,[228,229] and Denmark.[230]

Too few days of recording intake or excretion to be able to characterize an individual

The estimation of the relationship between intake and output depends partly on the variability of the measures used. Daily variation is such that on any one day an individual is not likely to be in balance, therefore measurements of intake and output are required over several days to characterize the relationship within an individual with reasonable reliability. Table 7.15 shows that expected correlations between daily intake

Table 7.16 Comparison of mean recoveries of analyses in incomplete and complete 24-hour urine samples colected from 156 women (Bingham *et al.*).[30]

	Mean	SD	Range	P, complete v incomplete
Complete (n = 125)				
PABA % recovery	94	6	85–128	–
Nitrogen g	10.1	2.2	5.0–17.7	0.001
Potassium mmol	74	22	27–198	0.001
Sodium mmol	114	39	14–328	0.001
Volume ml	1958	664	669–5440	0.001
Hours of collection	24.1	0.8	21.0–29.2	0.001
% reporting losses	13	33	–	0.01
Incomplete (n = 31)				
PABA % recovery	72	14	16–84	
Nitrogen g	8.8	2.3	2.4–15.6	
Potassium mmol	60	20	16–134	
Sodium mmol	101	36	25–217	
Volume ml	1568	617	340–3850	
Hours of collection	23.9	0.9	19.2–28.0	
% reporting losses	21	41	—	

and output are in the region of 0.5 when a single day's data are used, with a low estimate of precision giving a coefficient of variation of 24%. When 8 days of urine collections and 18 days of dietary observation are available, the correlation improves to 0.95, and the coefficient of variation falls to 5%. Several 24-hour collections, validated for their completeness are therefore required to make accurate comparisons with dietary intake data, the exact number depending on the reliability required. With an average coefficient of variation of 13% in urine nitrogen excretion, 8 days of collections will estimate nitrogen output to within 5%. In this case the expected ratio of urine to dietary N is 0.81 ± 0.05 for valid estimates of dietary intake.[220]

The use of 24-hour urine nitrogen to assess validity of dietary assessments

Depending on the assumption that subjects are in nitrogen balance, with no loss due to starvation or injury and with no gain, and providing sufficient complete 24-hour urines are obtained (see above), dietary estimates can be compared with urine excretion on an individual basis. When this is done, results agree with another validation measure, the doubly-labelled water technique (see Section 7.4.4), at least in a small group of post-obese subjects.[223] Using this technique, specific individuals who under-report their food intake have been documented.[30,223] Single urines have also been used; for example, reported protein intake in obese subjects (from a diet history) was only 46 g but on the basis of 24-hour urine collections it was 87 g. In another study, subjects who were overweight or diabetic seemed to report their prescribed diet rather than what they were actually eating as judged by the urine N excretion.[231,232] Surveillance measures in use by the UK government have also been validated with single urines.[225]

The extent to which methods are able to place individuals in the correct part of the distribution of intake can also be examined using correlation coefficients between individual estimates of nitrogen intake from different methods and estimates of output from repeat 24-hour urine collections. Table 7.17 summarizes results from studies which have used two or more methods to assess intake and compared results with 24-hour urine N excretion. Correlations are greater between the biomarker and estimates of intake from records, than from estimates of intake using food frequency questionnaires.

The close agreement (see Table 7.17) with intake from weighed records when sufficient observations are obtained and collections are verified for completeness suggests that 24-hour urine potassium could be used as a validation measure.[29] This has an advantage because potassium is found in a greater variety of foods than protein, for example vegetables. Urea has also been used (see below).

Partial 24-hour urine collections

Due to the difficulty of obtaining complete 24-hour collections, and the lack of reliability using one collection, replacement with partial collections has been investigated. Yamori *et al.*[41] obtained 24-hour collections split into four time periods from 16 volunteer medical students and the variation of urea and creatinine in relation to the full 24-hour period is shown in Table 7.18 together with the correlation coefficients between separate samples and the complete 24-hour urine collections. Values for overnight collections in relation to full 24-hour collections obtained from 21 men and women aged 19 to 65 years from the study of Ogawa[39] are also shown.

From this, it would seem that overnight collections contain both less urea and a lower urea to creatinine ratio than other collections, whereas afternoon values are higher. Correlation coefficients are of the same order for both evening and overnight collections. It is possible that the proportion of constituents in partial collections varies, as indicated by the relatively large standard deviations in Table 7.18, probably

Table 7.17 Correlations between estimates of intake using different methods and 24-hour urine N output in different studies.

Number of urine collections	Number of individuals	Correlation between 24-hour urine N and N from dietary methods				Reference
		Weighed records	Records	FFQ	24-hour recalls	
8	153	0.69	0.65	0.24	0.10	30
4	52	0.41	–	0.11	–	32
3	38	0.77	–	0.45	–	33
4	134	–	–	0.45	0.51	233
4	76	–	0.54	0.27	–	234

Table 7.18 Partial collections in relation to 24-hour urine collections.

Time of urine collection	Daily variation in 24-hour*		Correlation with 24-hour	
	Urea N	Urea/creatinine ratio[41]	Urea N	Urea/creatinine ratio[39,41]
Morning	101 (34)	103 (33)	0.63	0.72
Afternoon	122 (36)	111 (39)	0.72	0.50
Evening	114 (44)	106 (44)	0.78	0.81
Overnight	74 (27)	86 (29)	0.76	0.81
24-hour	100 (26)	100 (23)		

* Mean (SD) of all samples, converted so that the mean values in the 24-hour samples equals 100.[41]

depending on the timing of diet and main meal consumption. This is probably also true of different populations, so that it is not possible to make general statements of the utility of partial collections, other than that they are less accurate than full 24-hour collections for estimating protein intake.

To investigate the possibility that repeat overnight collections would improve comparisons between dietary N intake and N from partial urine collections, 39 men were asked to collect an overnight urine collection immediately prior to making a 24-hour collection on eight occasions. The correlation between the mean N excretion from eight collections and the excretion from a single 24-hour collection was 0.692, whereas the correlation between eight 24-hour collections and a single overnight was 0.285, and with repeat overnight 0.297.[38] Even repeat overnight collections cannot replace the necessity for full 24-hour urine collections, and a single 24-hour collection is better than none if several cannot be obtained from each individual in validation studies.

Urea and other markers of protein intake

Urine urea is a constant proportion (85%) of total nitrogen excretion when individuals are consuming normal mixed Western diets and are in overall nitrogen balance.[26] It can therefore replace the estimation of total nitrogen in these circumstances and is considerably easier to analyse. As a proportion of total nitrogen intake, 24-hour urine urea nitrogen is $70 \pm 7\%$ and urea plus creatinine nitrogen is $73 \pm 7\%$ of the habitual diet when eight 24-hour collections are obtained.[220] Other validation studies have used urine urea as a marker of protein intake.[33,235]

As a marker of sulphur amino acid intake, urinary sulphate was also measured by Yamori and colleagues.[41] Correlation coefficients ranged from 0.28 for morning urines versus 24-hour, to 0.72 for evening urine, with no improvement from adjustment for creatinine. Correlation coefficients were 0.84 for urinary sulphate to creatinine ratio in overnight versus 24-hour urines in the study of Ogawa.[39] Ogawa also measured 3-methyl histidine as a marker of muscle protein and found a correlation coefficient of 0.76 between overnight and 24-hour collections. Although 3-methyl histidine is specific for muscle protein,[236], it is comparatively difficult to analyse and is not specific for diet because it is also released from lean body tissue and endogenous variations occur from factors such as body size and the amount of exercise taken. Creatinine and 3-methyl histidine have been used in experimental studies as checks on dietary compliance. In this situation the objective is not to relate intake precisely to output, as in a metabolic ward study, but as a rather crude check on whether the subjects have followed dietary instructions. In this situation both of these markers have been shown to be useful in, for example, checking on compliance in subjects changing from an omnivore diet to a vegetarian diet.[237]

7.4.3   Dietary fibre (non-starch polysaccharides)

Faecal weight is known to increase in response to an increase in dietary fibre consumption, there being a linear response of an average 5 g increase in faecal weight for every 1 g of non-starch polysaccharides (NSP) consumed.[238] However, the measurement of faecal weight is fraught with problems and is unacceptable to the general public, particularly when an attempt is made to gain valid estimates. Valid estimates require observations of at least 5-day collections on individuals because there is great day to day variation in stool size and frequency. For accurate work, the collections also need to be validated for completeness using inert markers, such as radio-opaque plastic pellets taken by mouth.[239] Even when this is done, the relationship on an individual basis is poor, due largely to unexplained individual biological variation in both transit time and stool weight, even when constant diets are consumed.[239] On a group basis, collection of a single stool from each individual may either over or under estimate 24-hour faecal weight, depending on the frequency of daily bowel habit.

Other suggested markers for NSP consumption include faecal neutral detergent fibre (NDF)[240], but quantitative estimates again require stool collections. Also, the estimate is unlikely to represent total dietary NSP because the majority of NSP is fermented in the large bowel, and little NDF remains in faeces.[239] The indices of fermentation, breath methane and hydrogen, have been studied as markers of NSP and fermentable carbohydrate intake. There was no relationship if early morning fasting breath samples were obtained[30], but evening samples may be better predictors of dietary intake of fermentable carbohydrate.[241,242]

7.4.4   Total energy

The doubly-labelled water method is an important advance in the measurement of energy expenditure and it can be used on free-living individuals with virtually no interference with everyday life, in contrast to previous procedures. Subjects are given a carefully weighed oral dose of $^2H_2^{18}O$ and are then required only to donate timed urine samples over the next 15 days. Carbon dioxide production is measured as the difference in the water pool (measured by $^2H_2$) and the bicarbonate plus water pool (measured as ^{18}O) changes in body weight and the water pool can be used to correct measured energy intake in relation to energy expenditure from the doubly-labelled water method. When this is done, energy expenditure should equal energy intake.[244] This method has been used to validate dietary assessment methods intended for surveillance of UK population samples.[244]

In early reports, energy expenditure assessed from this method was unexpectedly low, 1.4 times the basal metabolic rate (BMR) on average in a small group of sedentary women. In women of normal weight, energy intake from weighed dietary records agreed with energy expenditure data but in obese women, energy intake assessed from 7-day weighed records was about 2 MJ (465 kcal) lower than expenditure, suggesting that overweight women do not report their habitual food intake.[245]

In a later study, energy expenditure also exceeded energy intake measured from 7-day records in 31 normal individuals, on average by 20%. As a ratio to BMR, energy intake was 1.46 ± 0.31, and energy expenditure was 1.82 ± 0.24, greater than reported previously.[246] These and other studies have been summarized and show that in general, self-reported energy intake tends to be less than energy expenditure as measured by the doubly-labelled water method.[247] Published results from dietary surveys show that, using the ratio of energy intake to calculated basal metabolic rate (see below), 24-hour recalls tend to give low results (many below limits compatible with normal energy expenditure with no loss in weight) whereas diet histories give higher, and records, intermediate values.[248]

The doubly-labelled water method is too expensive for routine use by most investigators, costing about £350 per subject for the isotope alone. For validation studies, 24-hour N and K can be used, and in addition, basal metabolic rate (BMR) can be calculated from body weight, using the equations shown in Table 7.19. The BMR then

Table 7.19 Equations for estimated basal metabolic rate from weight and correlation (r) between measured and calculated BMR.

Ages of subjects	n	r	SE
Under 3 years			
m BMR = 0.249 wt − 0.127	162	0.95	0.2925
f BMR = 0.244 wt − 0.130	137	0.96	0.2456
3–10 years			
m BMR = 0.095 wt + 2.110	338	0.83	0.2803
f BMR = 0.085 wt + 2.033	413	0.81	0.2924
10–18 years			
m BMR = 0.074 wt + 2.754	734	0.93	0.4404
f BMR = 0.056 wt + 2.898	575	0.80	0.4661
18–30 years			
m BMR = 0.063 wt + 2.896	2879	0.65	0.6407
f BMR = 0.062 wt + 2.036	829	0.73	0.4967
30–60 years			
m BMR = 0.048 wt + 3.653	646	0.60	0.6997
f BMR = 0.034 wt + 3.538	372	0.68	0.4653
Over 60 years			
m BMR = 0.049 wt + 2.459	50	0.71	0.6865
f BMR = 0.038 wt + 2.755	38	0.68	0.4511

From Schofield *et al.*[251] m, male; f, female; n, sample size; r, correlation coefficient; SE, standard error. BMR is expressed in MJ/24 h; weight (wt) is expressed in kg.

has to be multiplied by a factor to allow for total energy expenditure, which has been derived from the difference between total energy expenditure and BMR in different population samples and ranges from 1.2–4.5. In sedentary men and women, the factor to allow for physical activity is about 1.6.[249] Due to imprecision in measurement of both energy intake, and the calculated estimate of BMR and total energy expenditure, 'cut off' limits for under-reporting, when reports of intake using various methods are too low, are less than this, for example 0.90 if a single 24-hour recall is used, and 1.35 for 'normal circumstances'.[250]

7.5　Concluding remarks

Validation of biochemical markers as predictors of dietary intake of nutrients (as distinct from the development of biochemical indices for the estimation of status) is currently at an early and rather unsatisfactory stage of evolution. There are many interlocking factors to be taken into account and different conclusions for different nutrients.

For the minerals, there exists a small group of alkali metals and halide ions whose short-term intakes appear to be quite well predicted by the measurements of urinary excretion levels, provided that the completeness of urinary collections can be properly validated. For another group of minerals (alkaline earth metals, phosphate, probably sulphur and selenium) urinary excretion rates can provide a fairly good general estimate of intakes when other dietary factors are reasonably constant, but a number of interactions may affect the relationship, especially in free-living people. For the remaining minerals, especially the transition elements, urinary excretion is a minor route that does not reflect dietary intakes, and the best that can be hoped for is a very broad classification of long-term population group intakes, obtainable from a variety of markers in the bloodstream. For most purposes, their predictive power would be considered inadequate.

There are few instances of very close agreement between intake and biochemical markers for the vitamins, although broad categories of intake for population groups and sometimes for individuals can be achieved in certain cases. However, each vitamin must be considered separately, as few generalizations can be made about this entire category, or even about the subgroupings, such as fat-soluble vitamins, B-vitamins, etc.

For those vitamins for which urinary excretion is a major route of excess-disposal, e.g. vitamin C and certain B-group vitamins, the level of intake in the short term can be assessed moderately well in the moderate to high intake range by the level of urinary excretion, even though absorption is not quantitative. At the other end of the time and intake scale, red cell enzyme activation coefficients generally reflect long-term intakes in the low to medium, but not the high, intake range. The same tends to be true of red or white cell concentrations of vitamins, in those cases where measurement is both feasible and sensitive to intake. Plasma nutrient levels usually have a complex relationship with intakes, comprising both a short-term turnover component reflecting recent dietary intake and one or more long-term components, reflecting body stores and the flux between them. They can, in some instances, provide a useful reflection of intake over a limited range (e.g. plasma vitamin C), but in other cases they are so heavily influenced by controlled production of binding proteins (e.g. for plasma retinol), that the intake:marker relationship is limited to a narrow band within the deficient range. Where vitamins arise from a variety of dietary or non-dietary sources (e.g. niacin, vitamins A and D), the amount present in all the internal compartments will reflect the total amount that is made available from all sources, not just the preformed vitamin in the food. Variations in bioavailability are especially important, as much for the vitamins as for trace elements, and this may be affected by speciation (e.g. folate polyglutamates that are incompletely available), by specific interactions (e.g. vitamin B_{12} with intrinsic factor), by conversion during absorption (e.g. carotenoids to vitamin A) and many other processes. Thus, the amounts entering the body are seldom a simple reflection of the amount present in the diet. In addition, some of the vitamin content of the food may be destroyed by the gut flora or by other (chemical) processes in the gut. In contrast, vitamin K and certain B-vitamins may be produced and made available in useful amounts by the gut flora. Disease processes, drugs and xenobiotics, and physiological variations between individuals, will inevitably alter the 'normal' diet–marker relationships. It is probably for these reasons that biochemical indices have only infrequently been used as markers of dietary intake. However, if intake cannot be estimated directly, or if bioavailability rather than total nutrient intake is required, then biochemical markers may give very valuable information.

For lipids, markers of usual intake are limited to the analysis of the proportions of fatty acids in serum or plasma, in cell membranes, and in adipose tissue. While the blood compartments offer opportunities to examine these proportions over several time periods, ranging from hours to months, and adipose tissue may reflect diet over even long periods, there are no biochemical markers available at the moment that allow for an assessment of absolute intakes. Such markers would need to be widely distributed in known concentrations in all forms of dietary fat and to be excreted or stored quantitatively without major metabolic change. Alternatively, a functional metabolic marker that is associated with the quantity of fat either absorbed or metabolized is required. Additionally, there are numerous factors (e.g. dietary fibre intake, alcohol consumption, smoking) that are likely to influence the way in which fat is absorbed or metabolized, and these will be reflected in the measures that are used to distinguish one subject from another and should, in theory, be taken into account when attempting to rank or categorize individuals. At the moment, all that is available are markers that indicate the proportions, but not the absolute intakes, of dietary fats. For the longer-term markers, such as per cent linoleic acid in adipose tissue, little is known about how metabolic processes that differ between individuals influence the dietary time period reflected by the measurement.

For protein, the relationship between intake and urinary excretion of the marker is closer than for virtually all other nutrients (except perhaps sodium), assuming that the subject is in balance. The principal drawback from the epidemiological point of view is the necessity to collect multiple 24-hour urine samples, the completeness of which has to be verified. The use of shorter (e.g. overnight or casual) repeat specimens requires further investigation. Pursuance of these objectives opens the possibility of having a marker for the completeness of diet recording or reporting generally, as the level of agreement between validated urinary excretion of nitrogen and estimates of intake based on food composition tables (corroborated by duplicate diet analysis) is good.

This approach to assessing the completeness of records underlies some of the recent work comparing energy intake and expenditure using doubly-labelled water, but the high costs of this technique make it unsuitable for widespread use in nutritional epidemiological studies. A low-cost technique based on nitrogen excretion from short term urine specimens offers an attractive alternative. There is a need to develop low-cost biochemical markers for the assessment of dietary fibre and energy intake for use in epidemiological studies.

References

1. Quian, G., Ross, K., Yu, M., Yuan, J., Gao, Y., Henderson, B., *et al.* (1994) A follow-up study of urinary markers of aflatoxin exposure and liver cancer risk in Shanghai, People's Republic of China. *Cancer Epid. Biomarkers and Preven.* **3**: 3–10.
2. Whitehead, T. P. (1977) *Quality control in clinical chemistry.* Wiley, New York.
3. Glatzle, D., Weber, F. and Wiss, O. (1968) Enzymatic test for the detection of riboflavin deficiency. NADPH-dependent glutathione reductase of red blood cells and its activation by FAD *in vitro. Experimentia.* **24**: 1122.
4. Beutler, E. (1969) Effect of flavin compounds on glutathione reductase activity; *in vivo* and *in vitro* studies. *J. Clin. Invest.* **48**: 1957–66.
5. Garry, P. J. and Owen, G. M. (1976) An automated flavin adenine dinucleotide-dependent glutathione reductase assay for assessing riboflavin nutriture. *Am. J. Clin. Nutr.* **29**: 663–74.
6. Thurnham, D. I. and Rathakette, P. (1982) Incubation of NAD(P)H$_2$: glutathione oxidoreductase (EC.1.6.4.2) with flavin adenine dinucleotide for maximal stimulation in the measurement of riboflavin status. *Br. J. Nutr.* **48**: 459–66.
7. Thurnham, D. I. and Flora, P. S. (1988) Stability of individual carotenoids, retinol, and tocopherol in stored plasma. *Clin. Chem.* **34**: 1947.
8. Matthews-Roth, M. M. and Stampher, M. T. (1984) Some factors affecting the determination of carotenoids in serum. *Clin. Chem.* **30**: 459–61
9. Craft, N. E., Brown, E. D. and Smith, J. C. (1988) Effects of storage and handling conditions on concentrations of individual carotenoids, retinol, and tocopherol in plasma. *Clin. Chem.* **34**: 44–8.
10. Bro-Rasmussen, F. (1958) The riboflavin requirement of animals and man and associated metabolic relations (parts 1 and 2). *Nutr. Abstr. Rev.* **28**: 1–23, 369–86.
11. Horwitt, M. K. (1986) Interpretations of requirements for thiamin, riboflavin, niacin, tryptophan and vitamin E plus comments on balance studies and vitamin B$_6$. *Am. J. Clin. Nutr.* **44**: 973–85.
12. Bates, C. J. (1987) Human riboflavin requirements, and metabolic consequences of deficiency in man and animals. *Wld. Rev. Nutr. Diet.* **50**: 216–65.
13. Whitehead, C. C. (1981) The assessment of biotin status in man and animals. *Proc. Nutr. Soc.* **40**: 165–72.
14. Velazquez, A., Teran, M., Baez, A., Gutierrez, J. and Rodriguez, R. (1995) Biotin supplementation affects lymphocyte carboxylases and plasma biotin in severe protein-energy malnutrition. *Am. J. Clin. Nutr.* **61**: 385–91.
15. Fisher, M., Levin, P. H., Weiner, B. H., Johnson, M. H., Doyle, E. M., Ellis, P. A., *et al.* (1990) Dietary n-3 fatty acid supplementation reduces superoxide production and chemiluminescence in a monocyte-enriched preparation of leukocytes. *Am. J. Clin. Nutr.* **51**: 804–8.
16. Keys, A., Anderson, J. T. and Grande, F. (1965) Serum cholesterol response to changes in the diet. IV. Particular saturated fats in the diet. *Metabolism.* **14**: 376–87.

17. Hegsted, D. M., McGandy, R. B., Myers, M. L. and Stare, F. J. (1965) Quantitative effects of dietary fat on serum cholesterol in man. *Am. J. Clin. Nutr.* **17**: 281–95.
18. Boyd, N. F., Cousins, M., Benton, M., Krivkov, V., Lockwood, G. and Tritchler, D. (1990) Quantitative changes in dietary fat intake and serum cholesterol in women: results from a randomized, controlled trial. *Am. J. Clin. Nutr.* **52**: 470–6.
19. Bingham, S. A. (1987) The dietary assessment of individuals; methods, accuracy, new techniques and recommendations. *Nutr. Abstr. Rev.* **57**: 705–42.
20. Rutishauser, I. H. E., Bates, C. J., Paul, A. A. and Black. A. E. (1979) Long-term vitamin status and dietary intake of healthy elderly subjects: 1. Riboflavin. *Br. J. Nutr.* **42**: 33–42.
21. Bates, C. J., Rutihauser, I. H. E., Black, A. E., Paul, A. A., Mandal, A. R., and Patnaik, B. K. (1977) Long-term vitamin status and dietary intake of healthy elderly subjects. 2. Vitamin C. *Br. J. Nutr.* **42**: 43–56.
22. Thurnham, D. I. (1989) Vitamin A deficiency and its role in infection. *Trans. Roy. Soc. Trop. Med. Hyg.* **83**: 721–3.
23. Schachter, J., Harper, P. H., Radin, M. E., Caggiula, A. Q., McDonald, R. H. and Diven, W. F. (1980) Comparison of sodium and potassium intake with excretion. *Hypertension.* **2**: 695–9.
24. Holbrook, J. T., Patterson, K. Y., Bodner, J. E., Douglas, L. W., Veillon, C., Kelsay, J. L., Mertz, W. and Smith, C. (1984) Sodium and potassium intake in adults consuming self selected diets. *Am. J. Clin. Nutr.* **40**: 786–93.
25. Barlow, R. J., Connell, M. A. and Milne, F. J. (1986) A study of 48 h faecal and urinary electrolyte excretion in normotensive black and white South African males. *J. Hypertension.* **4**: 197–200.
26. Bingham, S., Williams, R., Cole, T. J., Price, C. P. and Cummings, J. H. (1988) Reference values for analytes of 24 h urine collections known to be complete. *Ann. Clin. Chem.* **25**: 610–19.
27. Liu, K. and Stamler, J. (1984) Assessment of sodium intake in epidemiological studies on blood pressure. *Ann. Clin. Res.* **16**: 49–54.
28. Bingham, S., Goldberg, G., Coward, W. A., Prentice, A. M. and Cummings, J. H. (1989) The effect of improved physical fitness on basal metabolic rate. *Br. J. Nutr.* **61**: 155–173.
29. Bingham, S. (1991) Validation of dietary assessment through biomarkers. In: Kok, F. J. and van't Veer, P. (ed.) *Biomarkers of dietary exposure.* Smith-Gordon, London.
30. Bingham, S., Cassidy, A., Cole, T., Welch, A., Runswick, S., Black, A. E., *et al.* (1995) Validation of weighed records and other methods of dietary assessment using the 24 h urine nitrogen technique and other biological markers. *Br. J. Nutr.* **73**: 531–50.
31. Clark, A. J. and Mossholder, S. (1986) Sodium and potassium intake measurements. *Am. J. Clin. Nutr.* **43**: 470–6.
32. O'Donnell, M. G., Nelson, M., Wise, P. H. and Walker, D. M. (1991) A computerised diet questionnaire for use in health education. *Br. J. Nutr.* **66**: 3–15.
33. Porrini, M., Gentile, M. G. and Fidanza, F. (1995) Biochemical validation of a self-administered food frequency questionnaire. *Br. J. Nutr.* **74**: 323–33.
34. Caggiula, A. W., Wing, R. R., Nowalk, M. P., Milas, N. C., Lee, S. and Langford, H. (1985) The measurement of sodium and potassium intake. *Am. J. Clin. Nutr.* **42**: 391–8.
35. Gregory, J., Foster, K., Tyler, H. and Wiseman, M. (1990) *The Dietary and Nutritional Survey of British Adults.* HMSO, London.
36. Elliot, P., Forrest, R. D., Jackson, C. A. and Yudkin, J. S. (1988) Sodium and blood pressure. *J. Hum. Hypertension.* **2**: 89–95.
37. Forster, J. I., Jeffery, R. W., Van Natta, M. and Pirie, P. (1980) Hypertension trial. *Am. J. Clin. Nutr.* **51**: 253–7.
38. Kehoe, C. (1993) *Comparison of some urinary analytes excreted in over night and 24h urine collections.* Industrial placement report for the University of Ulster at Coleraine; Supervisor's Drs. S. Bingham, and B. Livingstone.

39. Ogawa, M. (1986) Feasibility of overnight urine for assessing dietary intakes of sodium, potassium, protein in field studies. *Jap. Circ. J.* **50**: 595–600.
40. He, J., Klag, M., Whelton, P., Chen, J., Mo, J-P., Quian, M., *et al.* (1993) Agreement between overnight and 24-h urinary cation excretions in southern Chinese men. *Am. J. Epid.* **137**: 1212–20.
41. Yamori, Y., Kihara, M., Fujikawa, J., Soh, Y., Nara, Y., Ohtaka, M., *et al.* (1982) Dietary risk factors for stroke and hypertension in Japan. *Jap. Circ. J.* **46**: 933–8.
42. Khalaf, A. N., Bocker, J., Kerp, L. and Petersen, K. (1991) Urine screening in outdoor volunteers. *Eur. J. Clin. Chem. Clin. Biochem.* **29**: 185–8.
43. Nordin, B. E. C. and Marshall, D. H. (1988) Dietary requirements for calcium. In: Nordin, B. E. C. (ed.). *Calcium in human biology*. ISLI Human Nutrition Reviews, Springer-Verlag, London. 447–71.
44. Lowenstein, F. W. and Stanton, M. F. (1986) Serum magnesium levels in the United States 1971–1974. *J. Am. Coll. Nutr.* **5**: 399–414.
45. Quamme, G. A. (1980) Renal handling of magnesium: drug and hormone interactions. *Magnesium.* **5**: 248–72.
46. Life Sciences Research Office. (1981) Effects of dietary factors on skeletal integrity in adults: calcium, phosphorus, vitamin D and protein. *Fed. Am. Soc. Exp. Bio.*, Bethesda, MD.
47. FAO (1988) *Requirements of vitamin A, iron, folate and vitamin B₁₂*. Report of a joint FAO/WHO expert consultation. FAO Food and Nutrition Series, No. 23. Rome.
48. King, J. C. and Turnlund, J. R. (1989) Human zinc requirements. In Mills, C. F. (ed.). *Zinc in human biology*. ILSI Human Nutrition Reviews, Springer-Verlag, London. 335–50.
49. Sandstrom, B. (1989) Dietary pattern and zinc supply. In: Mills, C. F. (ed.). *Zinc in human biology*. ISLI Human Nutrition Reviews, Springer-Verlag, London. 351–63.
50. Gallagher, S. K., Johnson, L. K. and Milne, D. B. (1989) Short-term and long-term variability of indices related to nutritional status I: Ca, Cu, Fe, Mg and Zn. *Clin. Chem.* **35**: 369–73.
51. Varry, R., Castillo-Duran, R., Fisberg, M., Fernandez, N. and Valenzuela, A. (1985) Red cell superoxide dismutase activity on an index of human copper nutrition. *J. Nutr.* **115**: 1650–5.
52. Delves, H. T. (1976) The microdetermination of copper in plasma protein fractions. *Clin. Chim. Acta.***71**: 495–500.
53. Solomons, N. W. (1985) Biochemical, metabolic, and clinical role of copper in human nutrition. *J. Am. Coll. Nutr.* **4**: 83–105.
54. Nève, J. (1995) Human selenium supplementation as assessed by changes in blood selenium concentration and glutathione peroxidase activity. *J. Trace Elements Med. Biol.* **9**: 65–73.
55. Robinson, J. R., Robinson, M. E., Levander, O. A. and Thomson, C. D. (1985) Urinary excretion of selenium by New Zealand and North American human subjects on differing intakes. *Am. J. Clin. Nutr.* **41**: 1023–31.
56. WHO. (1967) *Technical Report Series No. 362. Requirements of Vitamin A, Thiamine, Riboflavin and Niacin.* Report of a Joint FAO/WHO Expert Group. Geneva.
57. Flores, H., Campos, F., Aranjo, C. R. A. and Underwood, B A. (1984) Assessment of marginal vitamin A deficiency in Brazilian children using the relative dose response procedure. *Am. J. Clin. Nutr.* **40**: 1281–9.
58. Duitsman, P. K., Cook, L. R., Tanumihardjo, S. A. and Olson, J. A. (1995) Vitamin inadequacy in socio–economically disadvantaged pregnant Iowan women as assessed by the modified relative dose response (MRDR) test. *Nutr. Res.* **15**: 1263–76.
59. Wahed, M. A., Alvarez, J. O., Khalad, M. A., Mahalanabis, D., Rahman, M. M. and Habte, D. (1995) Comparison of the modified relative dose response (MRDR) and the relative dose response (RDR) in the assessment of vitamin A status in malnourished children. *Am. J. Clin. Nutr.* **61**: 1253–6.

60. Gregory, J. R., Collins, D. L., Davies, P. S. W., Hughes, J. M. and Clarke, P. C. (1995) *National diet and nutrition survey: children aged 1.5 to 4.5 years.* Vol. 1. Report of the diet and nutrition survey. HMSO, London.

61. Olson, J. A. (1984) Serum levels of vitamin A and carotenoids as reflectors of nutritional status. *J. Nat. Cancer. Inst.* **73**: 1439–44.

62. World Health Organization. (1976) *Vitamin A deficiency and xerophthalmia.* WHO Technical Series No. 590. Geneva.

63. Sauberlich, H. E., Dowdy, R. P. and Skala, J. H. (ed.). (1974) *Laboratory tests for the assessment of nutritional status.* CRC Press, Florida.

64. Thurnham, D. I. (1985) Interpretation of biochemical measurements of vitamin status in the elderly. In: Kemm, J. (ed.). *Vitamin deficiency in the elderly.* Pergamon Press, London. 46–67.

65. Lawson, D. E. M., Paul, A. A., Black, A. E., Cole, T. J., Mandal, A. R. and Davie, M. (1979) Relative contributions of diet and sunlight to vitamin D state in the elderly. *Br. Med. J.* **2**: 303–5.

66. Thurnham, D. I., Davies, J. A., Crump, B. J., Situnayake, R. D. and Davis, M. (1986) The use of different lipids to express serum tocopherol: lipid ratios for the measurement of vitamin E status. *Ann. Clin. Biochem.* **23**: 514–20.

67. Horwitt, M. K., Harvey, C. C., Dahm, C. H. and Searcy, M. T. (1972) Relationships between tocopherol and serum lipid levels for the determination of nutritional adequacy. *Ann. N. Y. Acad. Sci.* **203**: 223–36.

68. Quick, A. J. (1970) *Bleeding problems in clinical medicine.* WB Saunders & Co., Philadelphia.

69. Greer, F. R. (1995) The importance of vitamin K as a nutrient during the first year of life. *Nutr. Res.* **15**: 289–310.

70. Thurnham, D. I., Singkamani, R., Kaewichit, R. and Wongworapat, K. (1990) Influence of malaria infection on peroxyl-radical trapping capacity in plasma from rural and urban Thai adults. *Br. J. Nutr.* **64**: 257–71.

71. Thurnham, D. I., Kwiatkowsky, D., Hill, A. V. S. and Greenwood, B. M. (1990) The influence of malaria on plasma retinol. *Int. J. Vit. Nutr. Res.* **60**: 184.

72. Reddy, V., Bhaskaram, P., Raghuramulu, N., Milton, R. C., Rao, V., Madhusudan, J,. *et al.* (1986) Relationship between measles, malnutrition and blindness: a prospective study in Indian children. *Am. J. Clin. Nutr.* **44**: 924–30.

73. Bieri, J. G., Brown, E. D. and Smith, J. C. Jr. (1985) Determination of individual carotenoids in human plasma. *J. Liq. Chromatogr.* **8**: 473–84.

74. Milne, D. B. and Botnen, J. (1986) Retinol, α-tocopherol, lycopene, and α- and β-carotene simultaneously determined by isocratic liquid chromatography. *Clin. Chem.* **32**: 874–6.

75. Thurnham, D. I., Smith, E. and Flora, P. S. (1988) Concurrent liquid-chromatographic assay for retinol, α-tocopherol, β-carotene, α-carotene, lycopene and β-cryptoxanthin in plasma, with tocopherol acetate as internal standard. *Clin. Chem.* **34**: 377–81.

76. Thurnham, D. I. and Flora, P. S. (1988) Stability of individual carotenoids, retinol, and tocopherol in stored plasma. *Clin. Chem.* **34**: 1947.

77. Tanum Ihardjo, S. A., Furr, H. C., Erdman, J. W. Jr. and Olson, J. A. (1990) Use of the modified relative dose response (MRDR) in rats and its application to humans for the measurement of vitamin A status. *Eur. J. Clin. Nutr.* **44**: 219–24.

78. Fuchs, G. J., Ausayakhun, S., Ruckphaopunt, S., Tansuhaj, A. and Suskind, R. M. (1994) Relationship between vitamin A deficiency, malnutrition and conjunctival impression cytology. *Am. J. Clin. Nutr.* **60**: 293–8.

79. Rahman, M. M., Mahalanabis, D., Wahed, M. A., Islam, M., Habte, D., Khaled, M. A., *et al.* (1995) Conjunctival impression cytology fails to detect subclinical vitamin A deficiency in young children. *J. Nutr.* **125**: 1869–74.

80. Bauernfeind, J. C. (1984) *The safe use of vitamin A. A report of the International Vitamin A Consultative Group (IVACG).* The Nutrition Foundation, New York.

81. Wallingford, J. C. and Underwood, B. A. (1986) Vitamin A deficiency in pregnancy, lactation and the nursing child. In: Bauernfeind, J. C. (ed.) *Vitamin A deficiency and its control.* Academic Press, London. 101–52.

82. Dimitrov, N. V., Meyer, C., Ullrey, D. E., Chenoweth, W., Michelakis, A., Malone, W., *et al.* (1988) Bioavailability of β-carotene in humans. *Am. J. Clin. Nutr.* **48**: 298–304.

83. Romieu, I., Stampfer, M. J., Stryker, W. S., Herandez, M., Kaplan, L., Sober, A., *et al.* (1990) Food predictors of plasma β-carotene and α-tocopherol: validation of a food frequency questionnaire. *Am. J. Epid.* **131**: 864–76.

84. Tangney, C. C., Shebelle, R. B., Raynor, W., Gale, M. and Betz, E. P. (1987) Intra- and inter-individual variation in measurements of β-carotene, retinol and tocopherols in diet and plasma. *Am. J. Clin. Nutr.* **45**: 764–9.

85. Thurnham, D. I. (1989) Lutein, cholesterol and risk of cancer. *Lancet.* **ii**: 441-2.

86. Heinonen, M. I., Ollilainen, V., Linkola, E. K., Varo, P. T. and Koivistoinen, P. E. (1989) Carotenoids in Finnish foods: vegetables, fruits and berries. *J. Agric. Food Chem.* **37**: 655–9.

87. Thurnham, D. I. and Flora, P. S. (1988) Do higher vitamin A requirements in men explain the difference between the sexes in plasma provitamin A carotenoids and retinol. *Proc. Nutr. Soc.* **47**: 181A.

88. Ito, Y., Ochiai, J., Sasaki, R., Otani, M. and Aoki, K. (1990) *Serum concentrations of carotenoids in healthy persons aged 7–86 years.* Ninth International Symposium on Carotenoids, Abstract 151.

89. Kostic, D., White, W. A. and Olson, J. A. (1995) Intestinal absorption, serum clearance and interactions between lutein and β-carotene when administered to human adults in separate or combined oral doses. *Am. J. Clin. Nutr.* **62**: 604–10.

90. Haddad, J. G. and Chyu, K. J. (1971) Competitive protein binding radioassay for 25-hydroxycholecalciferol. *J. Clin. Endocrinol.* **33**: 992–5.

91. Clements, M. R. (1989) The problem of rickets in UK Asians. *J. Hum. Nutr. Dietet.* **2**: 105–16.

92. Bates, C. J. and Prentice, A. (1988) Vitamins, minerals and essential trace elements. In: Bennett, P. N. (ed.). *Drugs and human lactation.* Elsevier, London. 433–93.

93. Bauernfeind, J. (1980) Tocopherols in foods. In: Machlin, L. J. (ed.) *Vitamin E, a comprehensive treatise.* Dekker, New York. 99–169.

94. Desai, I. D. (1980) Assay methods. In: Machlin, L. J. (ed.). *Vitamin E, a comprehensive treatise.* Dekker, New York. 67–98.

95. Lehmann, J., Rao, D. D., Canary, J. J. and Judd, J. T. (1988) Vitamin E and relationships among tocopherols in human plasma, platelets, lymphocytes and red blood cells. *Am. J. Clin. Nutr.* **47**: 470–4.

96. Diplock, A. T. (1985) Vitamin E. In: Diplock, A. T. (ed.). *Fat-soluble vitamins, their biochemistry and applications.* Technomic Publications Co., Lancaster, PA. 154–224.

97. Thurnham, D. I. (1990) Antioxidants and pro-oxidants in malnourished populations. *Proc. Nutr. Soc.* **49**: 247–59.

98. Fukuzawa, K., Tokumura, A., Ouchi, S. and Tsuka, H. (1982) Antioxidant activities of tocopherols in Fe^{2+}-ascorbate-induced lipid peroxidation in pecithin liposomes. *Lipids.* **17**: 511–13.

99. Gey, K. F. (1986) On the antioxidant hypothesis with regard to arteriosclerosis. *Bibliotheca. Nutritio. et Dieta (Basle).* **37**: 53–91.

100. Per Haga, M. D., Ek, J. and Kran, S. (1982) Plasma tocopherol levels and vitamin E/β-lipoprotein relationships during pregnancy and cord blood. *Am. J. Clin. Nutr.* **36**: 1200–4.

101. Horwitt, M. K., Harvey, C. C., Duncan, G. D. and Wilson, W. C. (1956) Effects of limited tocopherol intake in man with relationship to erythrocyte haemolysis and lipid oxidation. *Am. J. Clin. Nutr.* **4**: 408–19.

102. Cynamon, H. A. and Isenberg, J. N. (1987) Characterization of vitamin E status in cholestatic children by conventional laboratory standards and a new functional assay. *J. Ped. Gastroenterol. Nutr.* **6**: 46–50.

103. Vatassery, G. T., Krezowski, A. M. and Eckfeldt, J. H. (1983) Vitamin E concentrations in human blood plasma and platelets. *Am. J. Clin. Nutr.* **37**: 1020–4.

104. Kaempf, D. E., Miki, M., Ogihara, T., Okamoto, R., Konishi, K. and Mino, M. (1994) Assessment of vitamin E nutritional status in neonates, infants and children on the basis of α-tocopherol levels in blood components and buccal mucosal cells. *Int. J. Vit. Nutr. Res.* **64**: 185–91.

105. Shearer, M. J., McBurney, A. and Barkham, P. (1974) Studies on the absorption and metabolism of phylloquinone (vitamin K) in man. *Vit. Horm.* **32**: 513–42.

106. Mummah-Schendel, L. L. and Suttie, J. W. (1986) Serum phylloquinone concentrations in a normal adult population. *Am. J. Clin. Nutr.* **44**: 686–9.

107. Suttie, J. W., Mummah-Schendel, L. L., Shah, D. V., Lyle, B. J. and Greger, J. L. (1988) Vitamin K deficiency from dietary vitamin K restriction in humans. *Am. J. Clin. Nutr.* **47**: 475–80.

108. Booth, S. L., Sokoll, L. J., O'Brien, M. E., Tucker, K., Dawson-Hughes, B. and Sadowski, J. A. (1995) Assessment of dietary phylloquinone intake and vitamin K status in postmenopausal women. *Eur. J. Clin. Nutr.* **49**: 832–41.

109. Shearer, M. J. (1995) Vitamin K. *Lancet.* **345**: 229–34.

110. Blanchard, R. A., Furie, B. C., Kruger, S. F., Waneck, G., Jorgensen, M. J. and Furie, B. (1983) Immunoassay of human prothrombin species which correlate with functional coagulation activities. *J. Lab. Clin. Med.* **101**: 242–55.

111. Olson, J. A. (1987) Recommended dietary intakes (RDI) of vitamin K in humans. *Am. J. Clin. Nutr.* **45**: 687–92.

112. Krasinski, S. D., Russell, R. M., Furie, B. C., Kruger, S. F., Jacques, P. F. and Furie, B. (1985) The prevalence of vitamin K deficiency in chronic gastrointestinal disorder. *Am. J. Clin. Nutr.* **41**: 639–43.

113. Hazell, K. and Baloch, K. H. (1970) Vitamin K deficiency in the elderly. *Gerontol. Clin. (Basel).* **12**: 10–17.

114. Golding, J., Paterson, M. and Kinlen, L. J. (1990) Factors associated with childhood cancer in a national cohort study. *Br. J. Cancer.* **62**: 304–8.

115. Von Kries, R., Shearer, M., McCarthy, P. T., Haug, M., Harzer, G. and Gobel, U. (1987) Vitamin K_1 content of maternal milk: influence of the stage of lactation, lipid composition and vitamin K supplementation given to the mother. *Paed. Res.* **22**: 513–17.

116. Gibson, R. S. (1990) *Principles of nutritional assessment.* Oxford University Press, Oxford.

117. Reinhold, J. G., Nicholson, J. T. L. and Elsom, K. O. (1944) The utilization of thiamin in the human subject: the effect of high intake of carbohydrate or of fat. *J. Nutr.* **28**: 51–62.

118. Consolazio, C. F., Johnson, H. L., Krzywicki, H. J., Daws, T. A. and Barnhart, R. A. (1971) Thiamin, riboflavin, and pyridoxine excretion during acute starvation and calorie restriction. *Am. J. Clin. Nutr.* **24**: 1060–7.

119. Ziporin, Z. Z., Nunes, W. T., Powell, R. C., Waring, P. P. and Sauberlich, H. E. (1965) Excretion of thiamine and its metabolites in the urine of young adult males receiving restricted intakes of the vitamin. *J. Nutr.* **85**: 287–96.

120. Interdepartmental Committee on Nutrition for Defence. (1963) *Manual for nutrition surveys.* US Government Printing Office, Washington.

121. Baines, M. (1985) Improved high performance chromatographic determination of erythrocyte transketolase activity and the thiamine pyrophosphate effect during storage of blood. *Ann. Clin. Biochem.* **22**: 423–7.

122. Burch, H. B., Bessey, O. A., Love, R. H. and Lowry, O. H. (1952) The determination of thiamine and thiamine phosphates in small quantities of blood and blood cells. *J. Biol. Chem.* **198**: 477.

123. Bender, D. A. and Bender, A. E. (1986) Niacin and tryptophan metabolism: the biochemical basis of niacin requirements and recommendations. *Nutr. Abs. Rev. (Ser. A)*. **56**: 695–719.

124. Thurnham, D. I., Singkamani, R., Situnayake, R. D. and Davis, M. (1986) Vitamin B₆ concentrations in patients with chronic liver disease and hepatocellular carcinoma. *Br. Med. J.* **293**: 695.

125. Li, A. and Lumeng, L. (1981) Plasma PLP as an indicator of nutritional status: relationship to tissue vitamin B_6 content and hepatic metabolism. In: Leklem, J. E. and Reynolds, R. D. (ed.). *Methods in vitamin B_6 nutrition*. Plenum, New York. 289–96.

126. Herbert, V. (1967) Biochemical and haematological lesions in folic acid deficiency. *Am. J. Clin. Nutr.* **20**: 562–9.

127. Hodges, R. E., Hood, J., Canham, J. E., Sauberlich, H. E. and Baker, E. M. (1971) Clinical manifestation of ascorbic acid deficiency in man. *Am. J. Clin. Nutr.* **24**: 432–43.

128. Windsor, A. C. W. and Williams, C. B. (1970) Urinary hydroxyproline in the elderly with low leucocyte ascorbic acid levels. *Br. Med. J.* **1**: 732–3.

129. Dutra de Oliveira, J. E., Pearson, W. N. and Darby, W. J. (1959) Clinical usefulness of the oral ascorbic acid tolerance test in scurvy. *Am. J. Clin. Nutr.* **7**: 630–3.

130. Iber, F. L., Blass, J. P., Brin, M. and Leevy, C. M. (1982) Thiamin in the elderly – relation to alcoholism and to neurological degenerative disease. *Am. J. Clin. Nutr.* **36**: 1067–82.

131. Vir, S. C. and Love, A. H. G. (1979) Nutritional status of institutionalised and non-institutionalised aged in Belfast, Northern Ireland. *Am. J. Clin. Nutr.* **32**: 1934–47.

132. Vir, S. C., Love, A. H. G. and Thompson, W. (1980) Thiamin status during pregnancy. *Int. J. Vit. Nutr. Res.* **50**: 131–40.

133. Puxty, J. A. H., Haskew, A. E., Ratcliffe, J. G. and McMurrey, J. (1985) Changes in erythrocyte transketolase activity and the thiamine pyrophosphate effect during storage of blood. *Ann. Clin. Biochem.* **22**: 423–7.

134. Anderson, S. H. and Nicol, A. D. (1986) A fluorimetric method for measurement of erythrocyte transketolase activity. *Ann. Clin. Biochem.* **23**: 180–9.

135. Thurnham, D. I., Migasena, P. and Pavapootanon, N. (1970) The ultramicro glutathione reductase assay for riboflavin status: its use in field studies in Thailand. *Mikrochim. Acta.* **5**: 988–93.

136. Bamji, M. S., Bhaskaram, P. and Jacob, C. M. (1987) Urinary riboflavin excretion and erythrocyte glutathione reductase activity in preschool children suffering from upper respiratory tract infections and measles. *Ann. Nutr. Metab.* **31**: 191–6.

137. Horwitt, M. K., Hills, O. W., Harvey, C. C., Liebert, E. and Steinberg, D. L. (1949) Effects of dietary depletion of riboflavin. *J. Nutr.* **39**: 357–73.

138. Horwitt, M. K., Harvey, C. C., Hills, O. W. and Liebert, E. (1950) Correlation of urinary excretion of riboflavin with dietary intake and symptoms of ariboflavinosis. *J. Nutr.* **41**: 247.

139. Bates, C. J., Prentice, A. M., Paul, A. A., Sutcliffe, B. A., Watkinson, M. and Whitehead, R. G. (1981) Riboflavin status in Gambian pregnant and lactating women and its implications for recommended daily allowances. *Am. J. Clin. Nutr.* **34**: 928–35.

140. Thurnham, D. I., Migasena, P., Vudhivai, N. and Supawan, V. (1972) The effect of riboflavin supplementation on the urinary hydroxyproline index in a resettlement village in rural Tahiland. *Br. J. Nutr.* **28**: 99–104.

141. Glatzle, D., Korner, W. F., Christellar, F. and Wiss, O. (1969) Method for the detection of biochemical riboflavin deficiency. *Int. J. Vit. Nutr. Res.* **40**: 166–83.

142. Tillotson, J. A. and Baker, E. M. (1972) An enzymatic measurement of the riboflavin status in man. *Am. J. Clin. Nutr.* **25**: 425–31.

143. Belko, A. Z., Obarzanek, E., Kalkwarf, H. J., Rotter, M. A., Bogusz, S., Miller, D., *et al.* (1982) Effects of exercise on riboflavin requirements of young women. *Am. J. Clin. Nutr.* **37**: 509–17.

144. Boisvert, W. A., Mendoza, I., Castenada, C., De Portocarrero, L., Solomons, N. W., Geshoff, S. N., *et al.* (1993) Riboflavin requirement of healthy elderly humans and its relationship to macronutrient composition of the diet. *J. Nutr.* **123**: 915–25.

145. Thurnham, D. I., Rathakette, P., Hambidge, K. M., Munoz, N. and Crespi, M. (1982) Riboflavin, vitamin A. and zinc status in Chinese subjects in a high-risk area for oesophageal cancer in China. *Hum. Nutr.: Clin. Nutr.* **36C**: 337–49.

146. Low, C. S. (1985) Riboflavin status of adolescent southern Chinese: riboflavin saturation studies. *Hum. Nutr.: Clin. Nutr.* **39C**: 297–301.

147. Gopalan, C. and Srikantia, S. G. (1960) Leucine and pellagra. *Lancet.* **i**: 954–7.

148. Bender, D. A. (1983) Effects of dietary excess of leucine on the metabolism of tryptophan in the rat: a mechanism for the pellagrogenic action of leucine. *Br. J. Nutr.* **50**: 25–32.

149. Hankes, L. V. (1984) Nicotinic acid and nicotinamide. In: Machlin, L. J. (ed.). *Handbook of vitamins*. Dekker, New York. 329–77.

150. Fu, C. S., Swendseid, M. E., Jacob, R. A. and McKee, R. W. (1989) Biochemical markers for assessment of niacin status in young men: Levels of erythrocyte niacin coenzymes and plasma tryptophan. *J. Nutr.* **119**: 1949–55.

151. Pelletier, O. and Brassard, R. (1977) Automated and manual determinations of N^1-methylnicotinamide in urine. *Am. J. Clin. Nutr.* **30**: 2108–16.

152. De Lange, D. J. and Joubert, C. P. (1964) Assessment of nicotininc acid status of population groups. *Am. J. Clin. Nutr.* **15**: 169–74.

153. Shibata, K. and Matsuo, H. (1989) Correlation between niacin equivalent intake and urinary excretion of its metabolites, N^1-methyl nicotinamide, N^1-methyl-2-pyridone-5-carboxamide and N^1-methyl-4-pyridone-3-carboxamide in humans consuming a self-selected food. *Am. J. Clin. Nutr.* **50**: 114–19.

154. Manore, M. M., Vaughan, L. A., Carroll, S. S. and Leklem, J. E. (1989) Plasma pyridoxal 5-phosphate concentration and dietary vitamin B_6 intake in free-living, low-income elderly people. *Am. J. Clin. Nutr.* **50**: 339–45.

155. Vermaak, W. J. H., Ubbink, J. B., Barnard, H. C.., Potgieter, G. M., Jaarsveld, H. V. and Groenewald, A. J. (1990) Vitamin B_6 nutrition status and cigarette smoking. *Am. J. Clin. Nutr.* **51**: 1058–61.

156. Black, A. L., Guirard, B. M. and Snell, E. E. (1978) The behaviour of muscle phosphorylase as a reservoir for vitamin B_6 in the rat. *J. Nutr.* **108**: 670–7.

157. Thurnham, D. I. (1981) Red cell enzyme tests of vitamin status: do marginal deficiencies have any physiological significance? *Proc. Nutr. Soc.* **40**: 155–63.

158. Bender, D. A. (1987) Oestrogens and vitamin B_6: actions and interactions. *Wld. Rev. Nutr. Diet.* **51**: 140–88.

159. Park, Y. H. and Linkswiler, H. (1970) Effect of vitamin B_6 depletion in adult man on the excretion of cystathionine and other methionine metabolites. *J. Nutr.* **100**: 110–16.

160. Lui, A., Lumeng, L., Aronoff, G. R. and Li, T. K. (1985) Relationship between body store of vitamin B_6 and plasma phosphate clearance: metabolic balance studies in humans. *J. Lab. Clin. Med.* **106**: 491–7.

161. Kretsch, M. J., Sauberlich, H. E., Skala, J. H. and Johnson, H. L. (1995) Vitamin B_6 requirement and status assessment: young women fed a depletion diet followed by a plant or animal-protein diet with graded amounts of vitamin B_6. *Am. J. Clin. Nutr.* **61**: 1091–101.

162. Bates. C. J., Fleming, M., Paul, A. A., Black, A. E. and Mandal, A. R. (1980) Folate status and its relation to vitamin C in healthy elderly men and women. *Age Ageing.* **9**: 241–8.

163. Rothenburg, S. P. and Cotter, R. (1978) Nutrient deficiencies in man: vitamin B_{12}. In: Rechcigl, M. Jr. (ed.). *CRC handbook series in nutrition and food. Section E: nutritional disorders.* Vol. III. CRC Press, Florida. 474–97.

164. Chanarin, I. (1990) *The megaloblastic anaemias.* 3rd edn. Blackwell Scientific Publications, Oxford.

165. Shane, B., Tamura, T. and Stokstad, E. L. R. (1980) A comparison of radioassay and microbiological methods. *Clin. Chim. Acta.* **100**: 13–19.
166. Vanden Berg, H., Finglas, P. M. and Bates, C. (1994) FLAIR intercomparisons on serum and red cell folate. *Int. J. Vit. Nutr. Res.* **64**: 288–93.
167. Luhby, A. L., Cooperman, J. M., Teller, N. and Donnenfeld, A. M. (1958) Excretion of formimine glutamic acid in folic acid deficiency states. *J. Clin. Invest.* **37**: 915.
168. Basu, T. K. and Schorah, C. J. (1982) *Vitamin C in health and disease.* Croom Helm, London.
169. Garry, P. J., Goodwin, J. S., Hunt, W. C. and Gilbert, B. A. (1982) Nutritional status in a healthy elderly population: vitamin C. *Am. J. Clin. Nutr.* **36**: 332–9.
170. Newton, H. M. V., Morgan, D. B., Schorah, C. J. and Hulli, R. P. (1983) Relation between intake and plasma concentration of vitamin C in elderly women. *Br. Med. J.* **287**: 1429.
171. Newton, H. M. V., Schorah, C. J., Habibzadeh, N., Morgan, D. B. and Hullin, R. P. (1985) The cause and correction of low blood vitamin C concentrations in the elderly. *Am. J. Clin. Nutr.* **42**: 656–9.
172. Van der Jagt, D. J., Garry, P. J. and Bhagavan, H. N. (1987) Ascorbic acid intake and plasma levels in healthy elderly people. *Am. J. Clin. Nutr.* **46**: 290–4.
173. Jacob, R. A., Otradovec, C. L., Russell, R. M., Munro, H. N., Hartz, S. C., McGandy, R. B., *et al.* (1988) Vitamin C status and nutrient interactions in a healthy elderly population. *Am. J. Clin. Nutr.* **48**: 1436–42.
174. Hornig, D., Vuilleumier, J-P. and Hartmann, D. (1980) Absorption of large, single, oral intakes of ascorbic acid. *Int. J. Vit. Nutr. Res.* **50**: 309–14.
175. MacLennen, W. J. and Hamilton, J. C. (1977) The effect of acute illness on leucocyte and plasma ascorbic acid levels. *Br. J. Nutr.* **38**: 217–23.
176. Schorah, C. J., Habibzadeh, N., Hancock, M. and King, R. F. G. T. (1986) Changes in plasma and buffy layer vitamin C concentrations following major surgery: what do they reflect? *Ann. Clin. Biochem.* **23**: 566–70.
177. Vallance, S. (1988) Changes in plasma and buffy layer vitamin C following surgery. *Br. J. Surg.* **75**: 366–70.
178. Kallner, A. B., Hartman, D. and Hornig, D. H. (1981) On the requirements of ascorbic acid in man: steady state turnover and body pool in smokers. *Am. J. Clin. Nutr.* **34**: 1347–55.
179. Bates, C. J., Prentice, A. M., Prentice, A., Lamb, W. H. and Whitehead, R. G. (1983) The effect of vitamin C supplementation on lactating women in Keneba, a West African rural community. *Int. J. Vit. Nutr. Res.* **53**: 68–76.
180. Brubacher, G. (1979) Relevance of a borderline vitamin deficiency in relation to the question of vitamin requirement. *Bib. Nutr. Diet.* **28**: 176–83.
181. Pelletier, O. (1968) Vitamin C status in cigarette smokers and nonsmokers. *Am. J. Clin. Nutr.* **23**: 520–4.
182. Sahud, M. A. and Cohen, R. J. (1971) Effect of aspirin ingestion on ascorbic acid levels in rheumatoid arthritis. *Lancet.* **i**: 937–8.
183. Manchanda, S. S., Khanna, S. and Lal, H. (1971) Plasma ascorbic acid as an index of vitamin C nutrition. *Ind. Paediatr.* **8**: 184–8.
184. DHSS. (1972) *A nutrition survey of the elderly.* Report on health and social subjects No. 3. HMSO, London.
185. Okamura, M. (1980) Improved method for determination for L-ascorbic and L-dehydro-ascorbic acid in blood plasma. *Clin. Chim. Acta.* **103**: 259–68.
186. Margolis, S. A. and Davis, T. P. (1988) Stabilization of ascorbic acid in human plasma, and its liquid-chromatographic measurement. *Clin. Chem.* **34**: 2217–23.
187. Galan, P. Hercberg, S., Keller, H. E., Bellio, J. P., Bourgeois, C. F. and Fourlon, C. H. (1988) Plasma ascorbic acid determination: is it necessary to centrifuge and stabilize blood samples immediately in the field? *Int. J. Vit. Nutr. Res..* **58**: 473–4.

188. Roe, J. H. and Keuther, C. A. (1943) The determination of ascorbic acid in whole blood and urine through the 2,4-dinitrophenyl hydrazine derivative of dehydroascorbic acid. *J. Biol. Chem.* **147**: 399–407.

189. Deutsch, M. J. and Weeks, C. E. (1965) Microfluorimetric assay for vitamin C. *J. Assoc. Off. An. Chem.* **48**: 1248–56.

190. Washko, P. W., Welch, R. W., Dharwal, K. R., Wang, Y. and Levine, M. (1992) Ascorbic acid and dehydroascorbic acid analyses in biological samples. *Anal. Biochem.* **204**: 1–14.

191. Edelstein, C. (1986) General Properties of Plasma Lipoproteins and Apolipoproteins. In: Scanu, A. M. and Spector, A. A. (ed.) *Biochemistry and biology of plasma lipoproteins.* Marcel Dekker, New York. 495–504.

192. Griffen, B. A. and Zampelas, A. (1995) Influence of dietary fatty acids on the atherogenic lipoprotein phenotype. *Nutr. Res. Rev.* **8**: 1–26.

193. Van Houwelinger, A. C., Kester, A. D. M. and Hornstra, F. (1989) Comparison between habitual intake of polyunsaturated fatty acids from fish and their concentrations in serum lipid fractions. *Eur. J. Clin. Nutr.* **43**: 11–20.

194. Lepage, G. and Roy, C. C. (1986) Direct transesterification of all lipid classes in a one step reaction. *J. Lipid Res.* **27**: 114–20.

195. Sanders, T. A. B. and Roshanai, F. (1983) The influence of different types of n-3 polyunsaturated fatty acids on blood lipids and platelet function in healthy volunteers. *Clin. Sci.* **64**: 91–9.

196. Sanders, T. A. B., Hinds, A. and Pereira, C. C. (1989) Influence of n-3 fatty acids on blood lipids in normal subjects. *J. Int. Med.* **225**(Suppl. 1): 99–104.

197. Sanders, T. A. B. (1988) Essential and trans-fatty acids in nutrition. *Nutr. Res. Rev.* **1**: 57–78.

198. Weinburg, R. B., Dantzker, C. and Patton, C. S. (1990) Sensitivity of serum apolipoprotein A-IV levels to changes in dietary fat content. *Gastroenterology.* **98**: 17–24.

199. Hunter, D. J., Rimm, E. B., Sacks, F. M., *et al.* (1991) Comparison of measures of fatty acid intake by subcutaneous fat aspirate, food frequency questionnaire and diet records in a free living population of US men. *Am. J. Epid.* **135**: 418–27.

200. Kardinaal, A. F. M. van't Veer, P., Brants, H. A. B., van den Berg, H., van Schoonhoven, J. and Hermus, R. J. J. (1995) Relations between antioxidant vitamins in adipose tissue, plasma, and diet. *Am. J. Epid.* **141**: 440–50.

201. Van Staveren, W. A., Deurenberg, P. ,Katan, M. B., *et al.* (1986) Validity of the fatty acid composition of subcutaneous fat tissue micro-biopsies as an estimate of the long-term average fatty acid composition of the diet of separate individuals. *Am. J. Epid.* **123**: 455–63.

202. Sacks, F. M., Rouse, I. L., Stampfer, M. J., Bishop, L. M., Lenherr, C. F. and Walther, R. J. (1987) Effect of dietary fats and carbohydrate on blood pressure of mildly hypertensive patients. *Hypertension.* **10**: 452–60.

203. Melchert, H-U., Limasathayouat, N., Mihajlovic, H., Eichberg, J., Thefeld, W. and Rottka, H. (1987) Fatty acid patterns in triglycerides, olig1ycerides, free fatty acids, cholesteryl esters and phosphatidylcholine in serum from vegetarians and non-vegetarians. *Atherosclerosis.* **65**: 159–66.

204. Heagerty, A. M., Ollerenshaw, J. D., Robertson, D. I., Bing, R. F. and Swales, J. D. (1986) Influences of dietary linoleic acid on leucocyte sodium transport and blood pressure. *Br. Med. J.* **293**: 295–7.

205. Berry, E. M., Hirsch, J., Most, J., McNamara, D. J. and Thornton, J. (1986) The relationship of dietary fat to plasma lipid levels as studied by factor analysis of adipose tissue fatty acid composition in a free-living population of middle-aged American men. *Am. J. Clin. Nutr.* **44**: 220–31.

206. Kestin, M., Clifton, P., Belling, G. B. and Nestel, P. J. (1990) n-3 fatty acids of marine origin lower systolic blood pressure and triglycerides but raise LDL cholesterol compared with n-3 and n-6 fatty acids from plants. *Am. J. Clin. Nutr.* **51**: 1028–34.

207. Heine, R. J., Mulder, C., Popp-Snijders, C., van der Meer, J. and van der Veen, E. A. (1989) Linoleic acid-enriched diet: long term effects on serum lipoprotein and apolipoprotein concentrations and insulin sensitivity in non-insulin dependent diabetic patients. *Am. J. Clin. Nutr.* **49**: 448–56.

208. Delany, J. P., Vivian, V. M., Snook, J. Y. and Anderson, P. A. (1990) Effects of fish oil on serum lipids in man during a controlled feeding trial. *Am. J. Clin. Nutr.* **5**: 477–85.

209. Phinney, S. D., Odin, R. S., Johnson, S. B. and Holman, R. T. (1990) Reduced arachidonate in serum phospholipids and cholesteryl esters associated with vegetarian diets in humans. *Am. J. Clin. Nutr.* **51**: 385–92.

210. Glatz, J. F. C., Soffers, A. E. M. F. and Katan, M. B. (1989) Fatty acid composition of serum cholesteryl esters and erythrocyte membranes as indicators of linoleic acid intake in man. *Am. J. Clin. Nutr.* **49**: 209–16.

211. Schafer, L. and Overvad, K. (1990) Subcutaneous adipose-tissue fatty acids and vitamin E in humans: relation to diet and sample site. *Am. J. Clin. Nutr.* **52**: 486–90.

212. McMurchie, E. J., Margetts, B. M., Beilin, L. J., Croft, K. D., Vandongen, R. and Armstrong, B. K. (1984) Dietary-induced changes in the fatty acid composition of human cheek cell phospholipids: correlation with changes in the dietary polyunsaturated/saturated fat ratio. *Am. J. Clin. Nutr.* **39**: 975–80.

213. Simon, J. A., Hodgkins, M. L., Bronwer, N. S., *et al.* (1995) Serum fatty acids and the risk of coronary heart disease. *Am. J. Epid.* **142**: 409–16.

214. Christie, W. W. (1989) *Gas chromatography and lipids*. The Oily Press, Ayr.

215. Thompson, G. R. (1990) *A handbook of hyperlipidaemia*. Current Science, Philadelphia.

216. Denis, W. and Borgstrom, P. (1924) A study of the effect of temperature on protein intake. *J. Biol. Chem.* **61**: 109–16.

217. Isaksson, B. (1980) Urinary nitrogen as a validity test in dietary surveys. *Am. J. Clin. Nutr.* **33**: 4–12.

218. Van Staveren, W. A., de Boer, J. A. and Burema, J. (1985) Validity of the dietary history method. *Am. J. Clin. Nutr.* **42**: 554–9.

219. Baghurst, K. I. and Baghurst, P. A. (1981) The measurement of usual dietary intake in individuals and groups. *Transactions of Menzies Foundation.* **3**: 139–60.

220. Bingham, S. A. and Cummings, J. H. (1985) Urine nitrogen as an independent validatory measure of dietary intake: a study of nitrogen balance in individuals consuming their normal diet. *Am. J. Clin. Nutr.* **42**: 1276–89.

221. Sanchez-Castillo, C. P., Branch, W. J. and James, W. P. T. (1987) A test of the validity of the lithium-marker technique for monitoring dietary sources of salt in man. *Clin. Sci.* **72**: 87–94.

222. Bingham, S. and Cummings, J. H. (1983) The use of 4-amino benzoic acid to validate the completeness of 24 h urine collections in man. *Clin. Sci.* **64**: 629–35.

223. Black, A. E., Jebb, S. A., Bingham, S. A., Runswick, S. and Poppitt, S. (1994) The validation of energy and protein intakes in post-obese subjects. *J. Hum. Nutr. Diet.* **8**: 51–64.

224. Vorster, H., Jerling, J., Oosthuisen, W., Cummings, J., Bingham, S., Magee, L., *et al.* (1995) Tea drinking and haemostasis. *Haemostasis.* **26**: 58–64.

225. Hughes, J. M., Smithers, G., Gay, C., Clarke, P., Smith, P., Lowe, C., *et al.* (1995) The British national diet and nutrition survey of people aged 65 years and over: protocol and feasibility study. *Proc. Nutr. Soc.* **54**: 631–43.

226. Leclerq, C., Maiani, G., Polito, A. and Ferro-Luzzi, A. (1991) Use of the PABA test to check completeness of 24-h urine collections in elderly subjects. *Nutrition.* **7**: 350–4.

227. Gerber, M., Hubert, A., Dolques, V., Teisson, C., Astre, C., Segala, C., *et al.* (1993) Quality control in nutritional epidemiology. *Eur. J. Clin. Nutr.* **47**(Suppl. 2): [abstract].

228. Fong, A. and Kretch, M. (1994) Urinary nitrogen as a reliable indicator of usual dietary nitrogen intake. *Am. J. Clin. Nutr.* **57**: 300S.

229. Roberts, S. B., Morrow, F. D,. Evans, W. J., Shepard, D. C., Dallas, G. E., Meredith, C. N., *et al.* (1990) Use of p-aminobenzoic acid to monitor compliance with prescribed dietary regimens during metabolic balance studies in man. *Am. J. Clin. Nutr.* **51**: 485–8.

230. Heitman, B. L. and Lissner, L. (1995) Dietary under-reporting by obese individuals – is it specific or non-specific? *Br. Med. J.* **31**: 986–9.

231. Steen, B., Isaksson, B. and Svanborg, A. (1977) Intake of energy and nutrients and meal habits in 70-year-old males and females in Gothenburg, Sweden: a population study. *Acta. Med. Scand.* **611**(Suppl.): 39–86.

232. Warnold, I., Carlgren, G. and Krotkiewski, M. (1978) Energy expenditure and body composition during weight reduction in hyperplastic obese women. *Am. J. Clin. Nutr.* **31**: 750–63.

233. Ocke, M. (1996) *Assessment of vegetable, fruit, and antioxidant vitamin intake in cancer epidemiology.* PhD Thesis. University of Wageningen, The Netherlands.

234. Rothenberg, E. (1994) Validation of the FFQ with the 4-day record method and analysis of 24-h urinary nitrogen. *Eur. J. Clin. Nutr.* **48**: 725–35.

235. Vissner, M., de Groot, L. C. P. G., Deurenburg, P. and van Staveren, W. A. (1995) Validation of dietary history method in a group of elderly women using measurements of total energy expenditure. *Br. J. Nutr.* **74**: 775–85.

236. Young, V., Alexis, S., Balige, B., Munroe, H. and Muecke, W. (1972) Metabolism of administered 3 methyl histidine. *J. Biol. Chem.* **247**: 3592–8.

237. Prescott, S. L., Jenner, D. A., Beilin, L. J., Margetts, B. M. and Vandongen, R. (1988) A randomised controlled trial of the effect on blood pressure of dietary non-meat protein versus meat protein in normotensive omnivores. *Clin. Sci.* **74**: 665–72.

238. Cummings, J. H. (1986) The effect of dietary fibre on faecal weight and composition. In: Spiller, G. A. (ed.) *CRC handbook of dietary fibre in nutrition.* CRC Press, Florida. 211–80.

239. Cummings, J. H., Jenkins, D. J. A. and Wiggins, H. S. (1976) Measurement of mean transit time of dietary residue through the human gut. *Gut.* **17**: 219–15.

240. Jacobsen, A., Newmark, H., Bright-See, E., McKeown Eyssen, G. and Bruce, W. R. (1984) Biochemical changes as a result of increased fibre consumption. *Nutr. Rep. Int.* **30**: 1049–59

241. McKeown, A. (1992) *Hydrogen and methane production in man.* Industrial project report, Coleraine University.

242. Le Marchand, L., Wilkens, I. R., Harwood, P. and Cooney, R. V. (1992) Use of breath hydrogen and methane as markers of colonic fermentation. *Epid. Stud. Environ. Hlth. Perspect.* **98**: 199–202.

243. Davies, P. S. W., Coward, W. A., Gregory, J., White, A. and Mills, A. (1994) Total energy expenditure and energy intake in the preschool child: a comparison. *Br. J. Nutr.* **72**: 13–20.

244. Prentice, A. M,. Coward, W. A., Davies, H., Murgatroyd, P., Black, A., Goldberg, G., *et al.* (1985) Unexpectedly low levels of energy expenditure in healthy women. *Lancet.* **i**: 1419–22.

245. Prentice, A. M., Black, A. E., Coward, W. A., Davies, H. L., Goldberg, G. R., Murgatroyd, P. E., *et al.* (1986) High levels of energy expenditure in obese women. *Br. Med. J.* **292**: 983–7.

246. Livingstone, M. B. E., Prentice, A. M., Strain, J. J., Coward, W. A., Black, A. E., Barker, M. E., *et al.* (1990) Accuracy of weighed dietary records in studies of diet and health. *Br. Med. J.* **300**: 708–12.

247. Schoeller, D. A. (1990) How accurate is self-reported dietary energy intake? *Nutr. Rev.* **48**: 373–9.

248. Black, A. E., Goldberg, G. R., Jebb, S. A., Livingstone, M. B. E., Cole, T. J. and Prentice, A. M. (1991) Evaluating the results of published surveys. *Eur. J. Clin. Nutr.* **45**: 583–99.

249. Black, A. E., Coward, W. A., Cole, T. J. and Prentice, A. M. (1996) Human energy expenditure in affluent societies: an anlysis of 574 doubly-labelled water measurements. *Eur. J. Clin. Nutr.* **50**: 72–92.

250. Goldberg, G. R., Black, A. E., Jebb, S. A., Cole, T. J., Murgatroyd, P. R., Coward, W. A., *et al.* (1991) Derivation of cut-off limits to identify under-reporting. *Eur. J. Clin. Nutr.* **45**: 569–81.

251. Schofield, W. N., Schofield, C. and James, W. P. T. (1985) Basal metabolic rate. *Hum. Nutr.: Clin. Nutr.* **39C**(Suppl. 1): 1–96.

252. Mangels, A. R., Block, G., Frey, C. M., Pattison, B. H., Taylor, P. R., Norkus, E. P. *et al.* (1993) The bioavailability to humans of ascorbic acid from oranges, orange juice and cooked broccoli is similar to that of synthetic ascorbic acid. *J. Nutr.* **123**: 1054–61.

8. The validation of dietary assessment

Michael Nelson

8.1 Introduction

Ever since records of diet were first kept, we have had an unerring but misguided confidence in our ability to measure our own food consumption – until, that is, nutritional epidemiology revealed to us the error of our ways. The battle of the 7-day weighed record (in the British corner) versus the diet history/24-hour recall/food frequency questionnaire (Rest of the World) is over. We now recognize that errors are inherent in any assessment of dietary status, and that no measure of diet will convey the truth about an individual's, household's, or nation's food consumption or nutrient intake. The consequence of this new awareness is an appreciation of the need for validation studies which help us to understand the relationship between what we have measured and the truth. The matter of questionnaire design is discussed further in Chapter 2 (Appendix I), Chapter 6, and Section 8.4.2.

Epidemiological studies require techniques of dietary assessment which are rapid and not labour intensive. At the same time, measurements of dietary variables must be as accurate as possible at the level of assessment (which may be a nation, household, or individual). Measures are usually devised in an attempt to strike a compromise between these conflicting demands and are often regarded as an effective 'short-cut' between speed and accuracy. To discover whether or not the measurements made are accurate, however, it is essential to compare them with measurements made using other techniques of dietary assessment. As no single measure is entirely valid, a knowledge of the relationships between measures can help to establish the likely relationship with the truth. The activity which determines this knowledge is known as 'validation'. The validation process relates to the measurement, not the method from which the measurement is derived. Validation therefore considers the context within which the method is being used.

The process is a necessary step in the understanding of diet-related disease risk. It is essential in the development of instruments for assessing diet (particularly food frequency and amount questionnaires (FFQs)), and provides evidence of the likely misclassification of individuals based on dietary measures. Poor measures will obscure diet–disease relationships which would become evident using more accurate techniques of dietary assessment. Using an unvalidated dietary assessment instrument in nutritional epidemiology is equivalent to using uncalibrated equipment in the laboratory. A general discussion on the design of validation studies is given by Burema *et al.*[1]

The purpose of this chapter is to outline the general principles that should be applied in the design of validation studies of dietary measurements, and to consider some of the statistical techniques that have been developed to overcome the problem which arises from the absence of a measure of 'true' dietary intake. These principles apply equally to all forms of dietary assessment, but are particularly important in relation to the validation of FFQs which feature in many nutritional epidemiological studies. Descriptions of dietary assessment methods are given in Chapter 6.

8.2 Definitions

8.2.1 Validity

Validity is an expression of the degree to which a measurement is a true and accurate measure of what it purports to measure. Establishing validity requires a true external reference measure (an absolute standard) against which the measurement can be compared. In nutrition, no such reference measure exists. Because every measurement of dietary intake includes an element of bias (see Chapters 4 and 6), one can assess only the 'relative' or 'congruent' validity of measurements, comparing the results obtained with what are believed to be more accurate measures of food or nutrient intake, or energy expenditure. Selection of appropriate reference measures for comparison and how to construct and interpret the measures of agreement are the two principle themes of this chapter.

8.2.2 Reproducibility (repeatability, reliability)

Reproducibility indicates the extent to which a tool is capable of producing the same result when used repeatedly in the same circumstances. The terms 'repeatability' and 'reliability', although often used synonymously with 'reproducibility', imply slightly different aspects of measurement: repeatability is part of the process of establishing reproducibility, while reliability is a quality of a measure that has reproducibility. A measurement may have good reproducibility and yet have poor validity, but a measurement which has good validity cannot have poor reproducibility.

Because the diet of every individual varies on a daily, weekly, and seasonal basis, the concept of 'the same circumstances' does not exist when trying to assess the reproducibility of a dietary measure. Indeed, because many measures seek to assess 'usual' intake, part of the variation in observations collected will relate to genuine variability of diet, and part will relate to biases associated with the method. If due consideration is given to these time-related factors when devising a validation study, the variability associated with reproducibility can in theory be separated from that associated with genuine biological variation. This is an important step in identifying likely subject misclassification when assessing diet–disease risks.

8.3 The context of validation

When deciding on the best method for validating a measure, the purpose of the dietary assessment and its frame of reference (e.g. time-scale, type of study) must be clearly defined. The stated purpose will dictate the techniques which are suitable for validation, and a clearly demarcated frame of reference will help to identify the important confounders of the validation process.

The aims of dietary assessments are as myriad as the questions posed by nutritional epidemiology, but the key aspects can be summarized under four major headings:

(1) current or past intake (8.3.1);
(2) food consumption or nutrient intake (8.3.2);
(3) determination of absolute or relative intakes of individuals (8.3.3);
(4) determination of group averages versus individual intakes (8.3.4).

8.3.1   Current or past intake

The majority of validation studies have compared estimates of food consumption or nutrient intake assessed using the 'test' method with more rigorous assessments of current or very recent diet. If the main purpose of the epidemiological study is to examine the relationship between current diet and disease, then such an approach to validation is satisfactory. Often, however, investigations of diet–disease relationships predicate an aetiological role for diet at some period in the past (e.g. in case-control studies). The validation process then becomes much more difficult. If the dietary assessment (usually a questionnaire) asks about food consumption in the distant past, then in theory validation requires a reference measure which was measured at the time to which the assessment relates. In practice, such standards are rare. Investigators are then faced with an unhappy choice: either to question subjects about past diet with no validation of the method, or to ask about current diet using a method which can be validated, and be forced to make a number of untestable assumptions about the way in which current and past diet are related. The latter is a particular problem in case-control studies, where the relationships between current and past diet may be different in the two groups due to the influence of the disease process on diet.

'Current or past intake' also begs the question about the time frame within which the validation process takes place. Questionnaires, for example, are often used to assess 'usual' intake over some specified period ('last month', 'over the last year', etc.). In theory, if the measure is a true measure of 'usual' diet over the period specified, such questionnaire responses should be free of error attributable to within-subject variance. If questionnaire results are then compared with short-term records of diet (e.g. seven-day weighed intakes), the lack of agreement (in ranking, for instance) can be attributed in part to the within-subject variance which is inherent in the shorter but more accurate reference measure. Alternatively, if the questionnaire is compared with a diet history (another measure of 'usual' intake), then some of the common characteristics of the methods of assessment (e.g. conceptualization of portion sizes) may lead to an over-estimate of the validity of the test measure. This problem relating to the independence of the sources of error in the two measures is discussed further in Section 8.6.

8.3.2   Food consumption and nutrient intake

Abramson et al.[2], in a study of the effect of diet on anaemia in pregnancy, validated a food frequency list (for assessing frequency of consumption of foods per week) by comparing the results with frequency data from a 30-minute interview. While the interview itself may have been biased, the comparison was appropriate in that both techniques were addressing the question of usual frequency of consumption. The authors concluded that food frequency data were best suited to generating hypotheses, provided the sample under investigation was sufficiently heterogeneous.

Mojonnier and Hall[3] were interested in assessing adherence to prescribed diets in the National Diet–Heart study. The test measure was a 'subjective' interviewer rating which classified patients into four categories of adherence – excellent, good, fair, and poor – based on her total knowledge of each patient's performance. These ratings were compared with 'semi-objective' ratings of adherence (the reference measures) based on 7-day recall and 7-day records of diet. All the ratings reflected frequency of consumption of prescribed foods but not amounts consumed. There was better agreement of the 'subjective' ratings independently with the two 'objective' ratings than there was between the 'objective' ratings themselves. The poorer agreement between the 'objective' ratings can be attributed in part to the shortness of the two assessments, neither of which was sufficient to characterize 'usual' frequency. This illustrates the importance, particularly in food frequency validation studies, of the need to have reference measures which cover a sufficient time span to give results which are representative of the habits being assessed by the test measure. This also applies to measures of patterns of food consumption (meal frequency, interval of consumption between meals or items, etc.).

Frequency data alone are too weak for many epidemiological purposes where quantity consumed is important in estimating exposure. Questionnaires which use frequency data with fixed portion sizes to estimate food consumption may 'over-standardize' consumption[4], denying subjects the opportunity to describe their true diet and reducing apparent variability. The agreement between questionnaire and reference measure is thus likely to be poor unless frequency itself is the overriding factor in estimating consumption. More on the estimate of portion sizes is discussed below under 'Validation techniques' (Section 8.4).

Where test and reference measures both rely upon food composition tables to estimate nutrient intake, differences in the nutrient databases may contribute to differences between measures (e.g. comparing household budget data with individual intake data – see Table 6.1). Conversely, using the same nutrient database may overstate the true level of agreement between methods (see Chapter 5). Because the day-to-day variation in the intake of many nutrients will be less than for many foods, fewer days of data are generally needed to classify individuals correctly according to level of nutrient intake than for food consumption. There are, of course, exceptions (e.g. assessing vitamin C intake may take 14 days (see Table 6.5), whereas consumption of table sugar for regular users may take only a few days).

8.3.3   Absolute or relative intakes

In some circumstances, it may be sufficient simply to rank subjects according to food consumption or nutrient intake without having an absolute measure. For example, if the risk of heart disease were being assessed in relation to fifths of linoleic acid intake, then a questionnaire which ranked people correctly but consistently measured only

75% of linoleic acid sources in the diet would fit the purpose. On the other hand, if the aim was to identify a dietary threshold for the intake of linoleic acid above which risk of heart disease decreased, then this type of relative measure of intake would not suffice, and the validation process would need to address both ranking and agreement with a reference measure which gave the best possible estimate of absolute intake. The different statistical techniques appropriate for these two types of analysis are discussed in Section 8.6.

8.3.4 Group versus individual intakes

For ecological studies or other comparisons between groups of people, a mean value for food consumption or nutrient intake will be sufficient. The key issue is therefore to establish agreement between mean values based on test and reference measures. It may be adequate for purposes of validation to demonstrate that the test and reference measures rank groups similarly (using an inter-class correlation coefficient, for example). If, however, an absolute measure of intake or consumption is needed, then statistical demonstration of the comparability of the means will require an estimate of the standard errors of the two methods. For example, results from a questionnaire administered within a group of subjects could be validated against any measure which provides an accurate mean value, such as one day records. A further advantage of individual records for the evaluation of group means is the subsequent ability to control for dietary confounding factors in the analysis of disease risk. Repeat measures of the reference values allow an analysis of variance which will identify the component which within-subject variability contributes to the group mean error. Over a sufficient number of observations, this contribution is likely to be very small.

8.4 Validation techniques

8.4.1 Choosing a reference measure

A key issue in designing a validation study is the choice of reference measure against which to assess the test measurement. Box 8.1 shows the kinds of problems likely to be associated with each of the potential choices. All of these measures relate to recent intakes. Each of them applies to only one or a very limited range of nutrients. Although one could argue, for example, that repeat 24-hour recalls used to validate a dietary questionnaire could be regarded as appropriate to validate a number of nutrients, in practice, the within-subject variability in intakes will render the validation process more thorough for those nutrients which vary little in intake from day to day than for other nutrients which vary more widely.

Current intakes

The choice of the reference measure is a difficult one, and depends on the validity of the measure itself. Two methods widely adopted for many years were the weighed inventory[6] and the full Burke diet history.[7] Both techniques can be used (with appropriate attention to length of record or period of recall) to assess both food

Box 8.1 Limitations of reference methods appropriate for validation of dietary assessment measures.

Reference method	Limitations
Doubly-labelled water	– energy only – assumptions of model regarding water partitioning may not apply in cases of gross obesity or high alcohol intake – very expensive
Urinary nitrogen (completeness of samples confirmed using PABA)	– protein only – PABA analysis affected by paracetamol and related products
Urinary nitrogen only	– protein only – danger of incomplete samples
Weighed records or Household measures	– under-reporting – unrepresentative of 'usual' diet over insufficient number of days – distortion of food habits due to recording process
Diet history	– interviewer bias – inaccuracy of portion size reporting due to conceptualization and memory errors – errors in reporting of frequency, especially over-reporting of related foods listed separately (e.g. individual fruits and vegetables) – requires regular eating habits
Repeat 24-hour recalls	– under- or over-reporting of foods due to reporting process (e.g. alcohol and fruit) – unrepresentative of 'usual' diet over insufficient number of days – inaccuracy of portion size reporting due to conceptualization and memory errors
Biochemical measurements of nutrients in blood or other tissues	– complex relationship with intake mediated by digestion, absorption, uptake, utilization, metabolism, excretion, and homeostatic mechanisms – cost and precision of assays – invasive

consumption (frequency and amounts) and nutrient intakes for a wide variety of foods and nutrients. Neither of these techniques is able to measure diet without error, however. Recent studies have used techniques such as doubly-labelled water and urinary nitrogen excretion to establish the validity of the reference measures themselves (see Sections 6.7.2 and 6.7.4). These techniques help to exclude from the validation comparisons those subjects whose reference measures are believed to be flawed. When subjects are excluded in this way, however, the group upon which the validation is based may no longer be representative of the population in which the test method is to be used. The validity of the diet–disease risk assessments may then be suspect.

Repeat 24 hour recalls may also provide the basis for reference measures, behaving similarly to independent days from dietary records. But errors relating to memory, conceptualization or portion sizes, and distortion of reported diet will contribute to loss of validity in the reference measure, and some form of independent confirmation (e.g. urinary nitrogen excretion) will be necessary.

An unusual standard used by Jain and co-workers[8] was a quantitative record of husband's food consumption kept over 30 days by their wives, but this technique limits validation to married couples, and it is not clear that husbands would be as effective recorders as wives if the women's intakes were under scrutiny. Moreover, the accuracy of the spouses recording is not itself open to validation. Items which may be outside the purview of the partner (e.g. secret drinking or chocolate consumption) would be likely to be absent from both sets of observations, giving apparent agreement but hiding the truth.

Isotope and biochemical techniques

Methods such as the doubly-labelled water technique[9], balance studies[10], urinary nitrogen excretion, adipose tissue fatty acid composition, or leukocyte ascorbic acid content (see Chapter 7) all have a role to play in validation. They are often very expensive, however, can be used to validate only one nutrient at a time, and may be far more time-consuming and/or invasive than weighed inventory or history techniques. They are needed, however, to ensure that the reference measures themselves are robust.

With biochemical techniques, there is a fine line to be drawn between validation of dietary assessment and the need to establish the relationship between consumption and tissue levels of nutrients for purposes of public health policy (i.e. to assess risk in relation to exposure). Doubly-labelled water and urinary nitrogen relate directly to energy intake and nitrogen intake, respectively. Differences between estimated energy intake and measured energy expenditure, or between estimated nitrogen intake and measured nitrogen excretion, are likely to reflect real problems with the completeness of dietary reporting (see Section 6.9.4). Other biochemical measures and their relationships to intake (e.g. serum vitamin C levels and dietary intake of vitamin C) are far less direct. In some instances, homeostatic mechanisms may render biochemical measures wholly inappropriate as reference standards (see Chapter 7).

There are three sources of error when comparing results of dietary assessments with biochemical reference standards:

(1) the difference between the dietary assessment and the true intake;
(2) the effects of digestion, absorption, uptake, utilization, metabolism, excretion, and homeostatic mechanisms, all of which bear on the relationship between the amount ingested and the biochemical measurement;
(3) the error associated with the biochemical assay itself.

These errors are likely to attenuate the observed strength of association between estimated intake and biochemical measurement. They will not help to identify the component of error in estimating intake associated with the method of dietary assessment (e.g. errors in reporting of frequency on a questionnaire). Poor agreement between a biochemical reference measure and estimated intake does not necessarily indicate that the dietary measure has failed to assess intake correctly. Thus, such techniques can justify statements about a strong association between consumption and biochemical end-points, but not about lack of association.

In some circumstances, biochemical validation may be the only technique available. For example, salt intake is poorly assessed using reference measures which rely on food composition tables, and comparison of questionnaire scores on consumption of salty foods with seven consecutive measurements of urinary sodium excretion has proved useful.[11] The validity of a questionnaire on iodine intake, where again food composition data may be scanty, has been assessed against urinary iodine excretion.[12]

Past intakes

Selection of reference standards for past intakes involves identification of past dietary assessments which have used techniques sufficiently robust to provide valid data. None of the published studies on past intakes has undertaken reference measures which accord with the requirements set out above regarding the identification of poor reporters. Bakkum et al.[13] identified a group of subjects who had completed full diet histories 12–14 years earlier, against which they compared retrospective assessments of diet again based on diet histories. Byers and co-workers[14], similarly, compared past diet histories with an abbreviated (47 food item) retrospective questionnaire. Van Leeuwen et al.[15] identified 7-day weighed inventories completed four years earlier for comparison with retrospective diet histories. In each of these studies, the interval of retrospective assessment was dictated by circumstances, but they all demonstrated that for selected food items or nutrients, the ranking of subjects based on retrospective histories was closer to that recorded in the past than to ranking based on current intakes. Two other studies[16,17], using less rigorous past assessments of intake based on limited FFQs collected up to 25 years earlier, came to similar conclusions concerning retrospective assessments. In each of these studies, however, the range of correlation coefficients was very wide, and the values for 'r' for similar food groups or nutrients vary widely between studies (Table 8.1). For example, recall of bread consumption amongst controls in Study 5 correlated only moderately with past intake ($r = 0.32$), whereas in Study 2, assessed over a similar time interval, the correlation was -0.04. In these particular studies, the ability to assess nutrient intake in the past was better than the ability to assess food consumption, due probably to the 'cancelling out' of errors when calculating nutrient intakes. It is of interest in Study 5 to note that cases and controls seemed to be able to recall foods with similar levels of accuracy.

All these findings suggest that retrospective assessments are of value, but the investigator who chooses to use them without an appropriate past standard opens him or herself to the dangers inherent in using any questionnaire which has not been properly validated, i.e. the true ranking of subjects may not be reflected in the observed rankings and the extent of the error in ranking remains unknown.

Table 8.1 Comparison of dietary assessments in the past with recalls of past diet. Correlation coefficients for foods and nutrients.

	Study number					
	1	2	3	4	5	
	r_s	r	r	r_s	r_s	
					Cases	Controls
	(79)	(175)	(323)	(46)	(117)	(99)
Food						
Meat	0.47	0.07	0.39	0.22	0.75	0.74
Vegetables	0.34	−0.01 to 0.36	0.41	0.41	0.20	0.25
Fruit	–	–	0.41	–	0.26	0.23
Milk	0.35	0.47	0.58	0.14	0.28	0.54
Bread	0.68	−0.04	0.51	0.44	0.22	0.32
Eggs	–	–	0.42	–	0.35	0.46
Tea	–	0.44	0.64	–	0.12	0.50
Coffee	0.67	0.52	0.71	–	0.60	0.61
Nutrient						
Energy	0.68	–	–	0.69	–	–
Protein	0.47	–	–	0.50	–	–
Fat	0.68	–	0.50	0.64	–	–
Dietary fibre	0.54	–	0.61	–	–	–
Vitamin A	–	–	0.61	–	–	–

1. Van Leeuwen et al.[15]   79 M+F, 25–65, 7-d WI 1977 vs. DH 1981
2. Byers et al.[16]   63 M, 112 F, 50–74, FFQ 1957–65 vs. FFQ 1982
3. Byers et al.[14]   323 M+F, FFQ 1975–79, vs. short FFQ 1984
4. Bakkum et al.[13]   46 M+F, elderly, DH 1971–72 vs. DH 1984–85
5. Lindsted & Kuzma[17]   216 M+F, <82, FFQ 1960 vs. short FFQ 1984

8.4.2 Validation procedures

The basic model of validation involves the comparison of a test method against a reference measure of known validity. It is important to consider as a separate issue the design of the validation study, in particular, the sequence of administration of measuring instruments, and the basis for the design of questionnaires.

Sequence of administration

Ideally, the test instrument being validated should be administered prior to the assessment of the reference measure, for two reasons. The first is that subjects would normally, in the course of the main investigation in which the test measure was to be used, encounter it independent of any other dietary assessment, and the validation procedure should mimic this. Secondly, the act of completing the work for the assessment of the reference measure may in itself draw respondents' attention to their diets. If the test measure were to be completed after the standard, subjects might attempt to recreate in their responses the pattern of diet assessed for the reference. This might explain, for example, very high levels of agreement in the reported frequencies of food consumption between 7-day records and questionnaires completed either during or immediately after the recording period.[18]

Stigglebout et al.[19] designed a questionnaire to assess 'usual' retinol and carotene intake over the previous year, and tested the effect of order of administration on questionnaire response when validating it against a full diet history (average interval between assessments was 25 days). The questionnaire responses agreed better with the diet history when the diet history was administered first (although the differences in response failed to reach statistical significance, possibly because of poor power at moderate sample size). A separate problem may be that a period of dietary assessment prior to completion of the test measure may draw respondents' attention to aspects of their diet which they wish to modify, and there is the danger that an expression of the desired modification would find itself reflected in their reporting of diet.

Frame of reference

Theoretically, the period of assessment should be the same for both test and reference measure, i.e. one should compare like with like. Because FFQs, for example, are by their nature retrospective, it would therefore seem sensible in a validation study to administer the FFQ *after* the reference measure (e.g. multiple days of diet record over the period covered by the FFQ). The assumption has to be that when a sufficient time after the last reference measurement has elapsed (say one month), further dietary measures will not be influenced by previous measurement procedures. In practice, this may not be justified, and it is appropriate to administer a test measure both before *and* after the reference measure. Willett et al.[20] addressed these problems in a study in which 173 nurses recorded diet by weighed inventory for one week four times during the course of a year, and compared the results with an FFQ administered once at the beginning and once at the end of the study. The second FFQ correlated better with the records than the first FFQ (correlations ranged from 0.33 to 0.73 compared with 0.18 to 0.53), suggesting that a learning process may have influenced the second set of responses.

In general, the frame of reference for validation should be dictated by the purpose of the test measure. If 'usual' diet is to be assessed, and seasonal influences are either not important or are taken into account when determining responses, then the test measure should be administered prior to the standard. Epstein and co-workers[21] administered a short questionnaire (for use in the Israel Ischaemic Heart Disease Study) using lay interviewers, and compared the results with Burke type diet histories obtained by trained nutritionists between 4 and 30 days later. They reported good correlations between the two methods in a wide variety of samples when assessing intakes of energy, carbohydrate, protein, and fat (Table 8.2). The results were not consistent between subgroups, however, and an important finding was that the strength of the correlation was directly proportional to the number of foods consumed (see Section 8.5.9).

Table 8.2 Correlation coefficients (Pearson r) between short and long FFQ estimates of nutrient intake (from Epstein et al.[21])

| | Study group | | | | | |
	A	B	D	E	L	M
Calories	0.65	0.50	0.58	0.82	0.62	0.73
Carbohydrate	0.70	0.31	0.48	0.81	0.49	0.57
Protein	0.52	0.42	0.69	0.80	0.53	0.57
Fat	0.63	0.46	0.24	0.66	0.56	0.81

A   25 M, 20–39, North African
B   18 M, 20–39, European
D   22 M, 40+,   North African, <5 yr of school
E   24 M, 40+,   North African, ≥5 yr of school
L   25 F, 40+,   North African
M   25 F, 40+,   European

Basis for questionnaire design

A difficulty arises when information derived from the reference measurements is used in designing the test instrument. Numerous workers have, very sensibly, obtained detailed records or histories of diet from samples in the populations in which the intended questionnaire is to be used, in order to determine the key foods which contribute to nutrient intakes or which feature regularly in the diet. These foods have then been used as the backbone of an FFQ, for example. The investigators have then administered the FFQ to the same group of subjects, and determined the validity (usually in terms of correlation coefficients) by comparing the questionnaire results with the standard. This procedure leads inevitably to an overstatement of validity. When questionnaires designed in this way have been re-evaluated in similar but independent samples drawn from the same population, the resulting correlation coefficients have always, disappointingly, been lower.[22,23]

The questionnaire design, therefore, should be based upon as complete an assessment of usual diet in the population as is available, but the validation procedure should always be carried out in a sample which is representative of the population and independent of the samples used to provide the initial dietary profile.

8.5 Factors affecting the design of validation studies

When validating a test measure, there are many factors which potentially undermine the validation process, some of which have been alluded to in the previous section. Jacobs et al.[24] suggests that the influence of these factors can be so great as to obscure completely any relationship between the test and reference measures. Their potential influence must therefore be addressed comprehensively if the value of a validation study is not to be lost. It is equally important to remember that a test measure which has been validated in one setting may not have the same validity in another. The list of potential factors is long, and it may be necessary to undertake a new validation study to establish how the test measure performs in the new setting.

8.5.1 Gender

There is good reason to believe that women respond to dietary assessment differently from men. If a measure validated in one gender is then used in the other, one cannot say that the relationship between the test and reference measures is necessarily the same in both groups. This may in part explain the failure in some studies to detect similar diet–disease relationships in both sexes.[25,26] The corollary of this notion is that a validation study which includes both men and women must be analysed separately by gender. The range of values across both sexes may yield a correlation coefficient which is significant, but when the data are analysed by gender separately, one or the other may fail to reach statistical significance. For example, Fig. 8.1 shows that the correlation coefficient for zinc intake assessed by questionnaire and by 16-day weighed inventory is $r=0.43$ ($n=52$, $P<0.01$), but when the results are analysed separately by gender, women show a much higher correlation ($r=0.69$, $n=28$, $P<0.001$) than men ($r=0.33$, $n=24$, $P<0.05$).[27] The number of subjects in this example is small, and the 95% confidence intervals around the values for r for the two sexes in fact overlap (i.e. there is no statistically significant difference in r between the sexes), but the point is clearly illustrated. Statistical techniques for determining 95% confidence intervals around correlation coefficients are given in the Appendix.

8.5.2 Age

Adults between the ages of 18 and 64 do not generally show any consistent differences according to age in their ability to complete questionnaires satisfactorily. Outside this range, however, factors such as memory and conceptualization skills may have

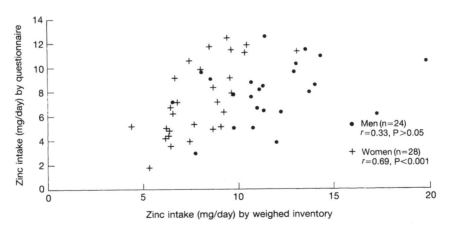

Fig. 8.1 Zinc intake (mg/day) estimated by questionnaire and by 16-day weighed inventory in 24 men and 28 women aged 25–64 years, by gender.

important influences on subjects' abilities to complete dietary assessments success-fully[28], and validity in these groups should be assessed separately.

8.5.3 Region, country

A test measure validated in one region or country may perform quite differently in another. This is a particular problem in multi-centre studies (especially between countries and if more than one language is involved), as differences in the observed diet–disease relationships between centres may be in part due to differences in the way in which the test measures assess intake.

Multi-centre trials have raised the issue of 'calibration'. Calibration refers to a process of scaling, ensuring that the differences in the biases in test measures between centres are properly taken into account (see Section 8.6).

8.5.4 Disease process

Many diseases, including vascular diseases and those of the gastro-intestinal tract, may have a profound influence on food consumption, either through patients' awareness of dietary risk factors or changes in appetite and digestion. Dietary assessment by questionnaire in a case-control study, for example, may be substantially biased by the disease process in the cases. A questionnaire which has been validated only in subjects who are representative of the controls[29] may not therefore perform in the same way in the cases, and an attempt should be made to ensure that the quality of the responses is the same in both groups. This may only be feasible for hospitalized patients by comparing questionnaire results with those from a full diet history, as prospective techniques may not be an option. In these circumstances, care must be taken not to confound 'usual' diet with recall of the hospital diet.

8.5.5 Recency and lag time

The difference in time between the relevant dietary exposure and the appearance of disease is the lag time. In cohort studies, lag time can be measured prospectively, but in case-control studies it must be estimated, and subjects may be asked to recall relevant diet in some period before the interview (often months or years). Several authors have reported a 'recency' effect, that is, the tendency for the recall of past diet to be influenced by recent consumption.[8,30,14,16] If the disease process has had a profound effect on diet, clearly this influence will be greater in cases than in controls.[8] This is very difficult to address as part of the validation process, because it is unlikely that the necessary standards for comparison, measured at the appropriate time period in the past, will exist for both cases and controls (except, perhaps, as part of a nested case-control study). An assessment of case-control differences in current diet may shed light on the ways in which recall of past diet may have been biased, but it does not assist in the assessment of the past diet *per se* nor necessarily reflect the way in which past diet may have influenced the disease process. One way around this problem is to assess the case-control comparison in different strata within the study (e.g. social class groups). If the same *pattern* of differences between cases and controls can be seen in the different strata, this supports the credibility of the observed diet–disease relationship.

8.5.6 Socio-economic group, education, language, and culture

Validation studies are characteristically completed in groups of intelligent, highly motivated volunteers from non-manual occupational groups. When the test measure is used in subjects from the general population, however, important but unmeasured biases may influence estimates of consumption. Clearly, the sample in a validation study should, wherever possible, include a broad cross-section of the population, and analysis should control for social class or education.

Language may be a problem in relation to regional dialects or between-country comparisons, and cultural differences may influence the way in which subjects respond to a dietary assessment (e.g. perceptions about 'healthy' and 'unhealthy' foods differ between cultures and may influence reported levels of consumption). A study which proposes to compare dietary risk factors for heart disease in white and non-white populations, for example, must ensure that observed differences are not due to language or cultural differences.

8.5.7 Sequence and proximity of test and reference measurements

These factors have been discussed above under *Frame of reference* (Section 8.4.2). It is worth reiterating that the learning process associated with the measurement of the reference measure is likely to have an influence on the way in which subjects complete test measures. The errors associated with the two measures are then more likely to be correlated, raising the apparent level of agreement between the two measures (see Section 8.6). Test measures should therefore be administered first, and the reference measure subsequently.

8.5.8 Auto-correlation

This has been discussed above under *Basis for questionnaire design* (8.4.2). If a validation study is carried out in the same sample in which the food profile which provided the basis for an FFQ was initially measured, then the agreement between the FFQ and the reference measure will be substantially greater than if the two measures had been measured independently in another sample drawn from the same population.[23,31] This type of overstatement of agreement is analogous to that in which estimated intakes based on three days of diet record are correlated with the entire week's data from which the three days are drawn.[32] The same kind of error can occur (as illustrated by Romieu et al.[33]) if questionnaire responses are weighted to reflect multiple regression prediction of measurements of serum β-carotene and α-tocopherol, and the weighted values are then used to calculate a revised correlation coefficient within the same sample.

8.5.9 Number of foods listed

In the same way that auto-correlation will lead to an overstatement of validity, the *omission* from an FFQ of foods which are frequently eaten or which are major contributors of nutrient will naturally reduce the accuracy of a questionnaire assessment and limit its validity.[34] Nomura et al.[35] also observed that it was more difficult to demonstrate agreement between repeat questionnaires (at six months and at two years) for items which were reportedly eaten less frequently than for those which were eaten frequently, although Kuzma and Lindsted[36] observed that the frequency of consumption of rarely eaten foods was also recalled accurately. Thus, one is more likely to select foods which are eaten frequently or very infrequently for inclusion in a questionnaire. In populations where the total number of foods eaten is small, it is probable that all of the major sources of nutrients for most subjects will be included. As the number of foods eaten increases and the variation in sources of nutrients between subjects becomes greater, the likelihood of misclassifying certain subjects because their food profile is different from the majority becomes greater and greater. This is reflected in Epstein et al.'s[21] observation that agreement between short questionnaires and reference measures (comprehensive FFQs) improved with an increasing number of foods reportedly consumed. Thus, those whose diets were similar to the selected profile were seen to have good agreement with the reference measure, while those whose diets differed and were presumably unable to find listed in the short questionnaire the foods which contributed to their intakes, showed poorer agreement with the reference measure.

Thus, it may be worthwhile to include in the questionnaire some foods which are eaten less frequently but which may be important contributors to nutrient intake in the diets of relatively few individuals, resulting in fewer misclassifications. Choosing the foods to include may therefore involve assessing the range of contribution that foods can make to the diets of individuals rather than looking simply at the average contribution in the population as a whole. This is particularly important in multiracial societies in which the breadth of food choice may be especially wide[37–39], but it can of course lead to exceptionally long lists of foods.[40]

8.5.10 Portion size

Two problems regarding estimates of portion size are particularly important. First, if the intention is to assess intake based on 'standard' portion sizes, allowing the respondent little or no opportunity to describe the amounts actually consumed, it is possible to inadvertently 'standardize out' the true variation in intake.[41] This will naturally reduce the observed level of agreement between test and reference measures. Second, where portion size is to be assessed in several groups whose dietary habits differ, a single set of standard portions may not reflect the true variation in portion size, as Tillotson et al.[42] observed in their study of Japanese men living in Japan, Hawaii, and California. Recent studies on errors associated with the use of photographs to assess portion size show systematic biases in the perceptions of subjects who are elderly (they tend to overestimate portion size) or overweight (they tend to underestimate portion size)[28], as well as a general tendency amongst all subjects to overestimate small portion sizes and underestimate large portion sizes.[43]

8.5.11 Dietary supplements

Dietary supplements are contributing to the nutrient intakes of an increasing proportion of the population. The main consequence is a small but significant proportion of the population with exceptionally high intakes. How they are handled in a validation study depends on the purpose of the validation. If the aim is to assess the validity of a test instrument in assessing food consumption or the nutrient intake based on foods alone, then supplements should be excluded from calculations. If the aim is to compare nutrient intakes across the entire range of intakes, then supplements should be included. If the agreement between test and reference measures is based on correlation coefficients, however, this will have a magnifying effect on the goodness of agreement between measures (even if non-parametric correlation coefficients are calculated). A more effective comparison would be in terms of classification by quantiles. One might expect to see good agreement at the upper end of the distribution of intakes, but not necessarily in the middle or bottom of the distribution.

8.6 Statistical techniques and interpretation

There is no reference measure which gives a true measure of diet against which to assess the validity of test measures used in epidemiological studies. The problem in validation studies is therefore to devise comparisons of results between methods that take us further toward an understanding of the relationship between the test measure and the truth.

In any comparison, there is usually one method which is regarded as 'better' than the other, and this is the method which provides the 'reference' measure (e.g. FFQ (test measure) vs. 16 days of weighed record (reference measure); 7 days of weighed record (test measure) vs. urinary nitrogen excretion (reference measure)). The usefulness of the test measure in determining dietary intake can be assessed by looking at the extent to which the test measure and the reference measure agree, and the extent to which it is believed that the reference measure approaches the truth.

The simplest model which describes the relationship between disease risk and dietary exposure is given by the equation:

$$\log(\text{disease risk}) = \lambda + \theta T$$

where λ is a constant which describes underlying risk of disease in the population when $T = 0$ (when there is no exposure), and θT describes the change (θ) in risk in relation to true exposure (T).[50] Because we cannot measure T directly, but we can measure Q (the observed or test measure), it is necessary to establish the relationship between Q and T. The simplest expression of the relationship between Q and T can be described as:

$$Q = T + e_Q$$

where e_Q is the error associated with the measure of Q. The error may be due to a number of causes, and the expansion of the error term is described fully in Chapter 4.

In a validation study, the main aim is to establish the relationship between Q and T. This can be done by describing the correlation between Q and T (ρ_{QT}); by determining a proportional scaling factor (slope of a regression line) which relates Q and T (β_Q); and by finding the variance of T (σ_T^2). These three measures help to define the relationship between the test measure and the truth. Calibration studies, in contrast, focus on finding a value for λ. This is particularly important in multi-centre studies (such as EPIC), in which the value of λ may differ between centres.[51]

Because ρ_{QT} cannot be measured directly, but can only be approximated by assessing ρ_{QR} (the correlation between the test measure and the reference measure), the practical aim of a validation study, therefore, is to find the correlation between the test measure and the reference measure, and to describe the likely relationship between the reference measure and the truth.

Independence of errors

A key issue in validation studies is the independence of errors between and within methods.[50] The effect of the independence of errors is shown in Fig. 8.2. Say the aim is to establish a valid estimate of ρ_{QT}. An assumption will be made concerning the usefulness of the reference measure as an approximation of the truth, but there will of course be errors in the reference measure itself. If the errors in the reference measurement in relation to the truth are in the same direction as the errors in the test measure, then the reference measure and the test measure will appear to be more similar than they are in reality. For example, if a diet history (reference measure) is used to validate an FFQ (test measure), and the errors in the estimate of food portion size are similar in both methods (that is, subjects tend to overestimate small portion sizes and underestimate large portion sizes), then the observed correlation between the two methods may be greater than the true correlation between the test measure and the truth.

In contrast, if the test measure is based on a series of repeat observations (say repeat 24-hour recalls), and the errors between repeat measures are not independent (say, for example, that the consumption of fruit is always overstated), then the real variation in the subject's consumption may be underestimated. The underestimate of the variation in a subject's test measure may exaggerate the difference between the test measure and

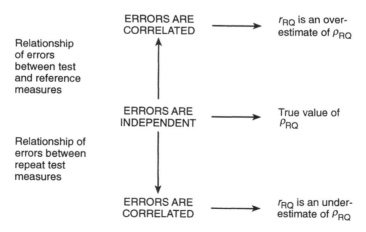

Fig. 8.2 The effects of the independence of measurement errors on apparent agreement between methods in validation studies.

the reference measure. The consequence is that the observed correlation between the test and reference measures is likely to be less than the true correlation between the test measure and the truth.

It is therefore important to try and maintain independence of errors between the test and reference measures. The comparison between an FFQ and 16 days of weighed diet recording might be assumed to have independent errors: in the FFQ, errors would relate to memory and conceptualization of frequency and portion size, while in the weighed records, errors would relate to dietary distortions caused by the recording process and errors in recording itself. It may be, however, that a subject under-reports diet in a similar way in the two methods, and for this reason biochemical checks on the completeness of recording (e.g. urinary nitrogen with PABA) or as an independent measure (e.g. serum vitamin C) are attractive. The use of several measures to examine the relationship between the test measure and the truth is discussed below (Section 8.6.2). Some authors also assume that the memory and conceptualization errors are different between FFQs (long-term) and repeat 24-hour recall (short-term).[52] Equally, it is important to take into account the correlation of errors in repeat measurements of the test measure (the within-subject variance, s_w^2), and for this reason it is always desirable to have repeat measurements of the test measure in at least a subsample of the study group.

Deviations of the test measure from the reference measure can be expressed in a number of ways:

(1) comparison of group means (or medians) (unpaired comparisons);
(2) differences between measurements within individuals (paired comparisons);
(3) ranking by thirds, fourths, fifths, etc.;
(4) correlation analysis (Pearson, Spearman, intra-class, method of triads);
(5) regression analysis;
(6) Bland-Altman analysis.

8.6.1 Comparisons between means

In studies in which differences between groups are important (e.g. geographical correlation studies between estimated intake and disease prevalence in different regions[53], validation should assess the ability of the test measure to reflect the group mean. Comparisons between test and reference measures of nutrient intake are best examined using t-tests (undertaking log-transformations where appropriate). For foods, the distributions are less likely to be parametric, and not necessarily amenable to transformation, so non-parametric tests are more likely to be appropriate. Yarnell et al.[45] compared the results of a short questionnaire to assess a wide variety of nutrient intakes against 7-day weighed records, and showed that in 119 men the questionnaire significantly underestimated the group mean for every nutrient except alcohol, in spite of the fact that the portion sizes used in the questionnaire were derived from the weighed intake data. The studies by Willett et al.[20] in nurses and by O'Donnell et al.[27] in adult men and women show similar findings (although the Willett questionnaire significantly overestimated some nutrients). If, however, the biases between group means are constant between the groups whose diet–disease status is being assessed, then the observed ranking of groups will be consistent with their true ranking.

8.6.2 Ranking and regression

The most common method of assessing the validity of questionnaires is to test the agreement in ranking of subjects between questionnaire and standard. Consistency of ranking is usually measured using the Pearson product–moment correlation coefficient (often on $\log_e$ transformed data to improve approximation to the normal distribution), although other correlation coefficients (Spearmans, intra-class) are also used.

The correlation coefficient, however, describes only one aspect of agreement that relates to ranking. A number of authors[54–58] have noted that poor agreement can exist between test and reference values even when correlation coefficients are high. There may be a significant difference between means (constant bias between methods). The slope of the regression line may be significantly different from unity, either because the test measure increases as a proportion of the reference measure (proportional bias), or because there is a regression to the mean or regression dilution effect (over-reporting of low intakes and under-reporting of high intakes). Validity cannot therefore be described using correlation coefficients alone, and requires other measures of agreement to characterize the relationship between the test and reference measures.

As the correlation coefficient between the test and reference measures falls, the number of people misclassified in the top or bottom of the distribution of intakes increases. A bivariate normal model can be used to show the level of agreement between r and the correct ranking of subjects in the extreme thirds (Table 4.1, Chapter 4). The number of subjects correctly classified in the extremes of the distribution falls substantially as the value for r drops from 0.9 (over 80% correctly classified) to 0.5 (60%) to 0.1 (43%). Few correlations in questionnaire validation studies reach 0.9, and many are below 0.5. The sensitivity of many questionnaires may thus be so low as to fail to demonstrate a diet–disease association (assuming one exists) because so many subjects are incorrectly classified. Statistical significance of a correlation coefficient ($p < 0.05$) merely indicates that it is unlikely to be equal to zero, and not the extent of agreement between the two measures.

Part of this problem relates to the inherent variability in both test and reference measures. In a study of three towns in which 438 men and women aged 35–54 completed 24-hour records of diet, followed three years later by a food frequency and amount questionnaire[5], statistically significant Spearman correlation coefficients (r_s) varied from 0.15 ($p < 0.002$) for vitamin A to 0.36 ($p < 0.001$) for energy. Mathematical modelling techniques were used to calculate the maximum correlation coefficient likely to be detected, accounting for diet record measurement error, FFQ measurement error, change in diet over time, and the likely within- to between-subject variance ratio. If one were to assume that there were no errors in either measurement and no change in diet, then given the within- to between-subject variance ratio (taken from the literature), the highest detectable values for r_s would have been 0.34 for vitamin A and 0.6 for energy. Allowing for a 23% measurement error in the diet record, 18% error in the FFQ, and a 6% average change in diet over time, the calculated correlations agreed well with those observed. Thus, the questionnaire seemed to be performing as well as might be expected. Correctness of classification by fifths showed that almost two-thirds of subjects were classified by the questionnaire to within ± one fifth of their recorded intake. This gives a better impression of the value of the questionnaire for separating subjects into classes of intake than the correlation coefficient. Neither of these measures of agreement, however, may be adequate for assessment of diet–disease risks.

The value for the correlation coefficient reflects the agreement between test and reference measures. It is likely that the relationship between the test measure and the truth is better than it first appears because the reference measure itself is not a perfect measure (Fig. 8.3). In theory, if the relationship between the reference measure and the truth could be estimated as a correlation coefficient, and if the errors in the test and reference measures were independent, it would be possible to estimate the relationship between the test measure and the truth using the simple relationship:

$$r_{RQ} = r_{QT} \times r_{RT} \tag{8.1}$$

Freudenheim and Marshall[59] have demonstrated using mathematical modelling the extent to which the problem of misclassification (expressed in terms of correlation coefficients) can be addressed. If $_{RQ}$ is the observed correlation between test and reference measure, r_{QT} is the correlation between test measure and the truth, and r_{RT} is the correlation between the reference measure and the truth, then from (8.1) $r_{QT} = r_{RQ}/r_{RT}$. If one assumes that the correlation between the reference measure and the truth is modest (say $r_{RT} = 0.6$), then for the observed value for energy and vitamin A quoted above, r_{QT} would equal 0.6 and 0.25 respectively. The ratio of true to total variance for energy is $(r_{RQ})^2/(r_{RT})^2 = 0.36^2/0.6^2 = 0.36$, and for vitamin A, $0.25^2/0.6^2 = 0.17$, that is, 36% of the variation in true energy intake and 17% of the variation in true vitamin A intake is explained by the questionnaire. This may be too small to be effective when trying to assess diet–disease relationships. Freudenheim and Marshall have shown that a true median relative risk of 2.41 between lowest and highest fifths of intake is attenuated to 1.40 when the variance ratio is 0.18. Thus, in this example, one would be

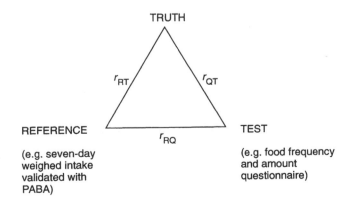

Fig. 8.3 The relationship between test and reference measures and the truth.

unlikely to detect an association of risk between diet and vitamin A intake at a level which would be regarded as important even though a relationship might exist.

Table 8.3 shows correlation coefficients for a number of nutrients based on a variety of questionnaires. Several features stand out. First, there is no consistency in the strength of correlation for a given nutrient, except for alcohol, which is well correlated. There is more consistency in results *within* studies, suggesting that a questionnaire tends to be generally good or generally poor. Study 1 shows exceptionally good results, while Studies 5 and 6 seem generally poorer than the others, yet the standard was based on weighed records in each case (7, 7, and 28 days respectively), and there is no reason to believe why one group of subjects should perform so much better than another. The range of foodstuffs assessed was greater in Studies 5 and 6 than in Study 1, and the range of diets was probably much narrower in the former compared with the latter study. But in circumstances not dissimilar to Study 6, Pietinen et al.[47,48] (Studies 8 and 9) showed much better correlations, with the suggestion that the use of photographs is of some benefit in improving subjects' estimates of portion size and hence correlation with the standard. An excellent result was obtained by Willett et al.[46] (Study 7) when questionnaire results were compared with a standard obtained from food records kept over an entire year, but one must then consider carefully the nature of subjects who would be willing to undertake such a study and that their ability to describe their food habits was perhaps better than most. Women do not seem generally better at describing their habits than men (as has often been stated), and the differences in Study 11, although striking, do not reach statistical significance. The diversity of these results emphasizes even more strongly the need to validate questionnaires in the population in which they are to be used.

More recently, Ocké and Kaaks[60] have used the method of triads to estimate the level of agreement between a test measure and the truth (Fig. 8.4). This is an extension of Fig. 8.3 which does not require an estimate of r_{RT} (the correlation between the reference measure and the truth), but relies instead on the correlations between three measures to estimate the likely relationships between the observed measures and the truth. An advantage of this method is that it does not require an assumption regarding a reference measure. Weaknesses of the model include assumptions regarding independence of

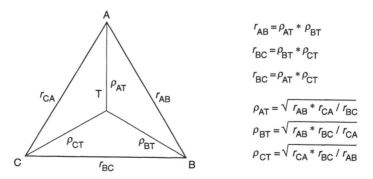

$$r_{AB} = \rho_{AT} * \rho_{BT}$$

$$r_{BC} = \rho_{BT} * \rho_{CT}$$

$$r_{BC} = \rho_{AT} * \rho_{CT}$$

$$\rho_{AT} = \sqrt{r_{AB} * r_{CA} / r_{BC}}$$

$$\rho_{BT} = \sqrt{r_{AB} * r_{BC} / r_{CA}}$$

$$\rho_{CT} = \sqrt{r_{CA} * r_{BC} / r_{AB}}$$

Fig. 8.4 Graphical representation of the method of triads (source: Ocké and Kaaks[60]).

Table 8.3 Correlation coefficients between FFQ and 'standard' estimates of nutrient intake.

	Study number 1	2	3	4	5	6	7	8	9	10 (a)	10 (b)	11	12
	(14)	(87)	(16)	(50)	(119)	(173)	(27)	(168)	(190)	(20)	(20)	(52)	(29)
Energy	0.74	0.34	0.43	0.63	0.30	–	0.67	0.57	0.45	0.56	0.29	0.35	0.50
Protein	0.80	–	0.32	0.60	0.41	0.18	0.60	0.53	–	0.42	0.42	0.43	–
Fat: total	0.94	0.36	0.53	0.58	0.34	0.27	0.76	0.51	0.56	0.59	0.08	0.39	0.59
SFA	0.85	0.40	0.50	0.51	0.31	0.31	0.74	0.56	0.60	0.60	0.12	–	0.58
PUFA	0.69	0.38[a]	0.27[a]	0.60[a]	–	0.31	0.74[a]	0.65	0.60	0.45	0.06	–	–
Cholesterol	–	0.42	0.61	0.47	–	0.46	0.67	0.54	–	–	–	–	–
Carbohydrate	–	–	–	–	0.27	0.48	0.60	0.60	–	0.55	0.48	0.35	–
Sugar	–	–	–	–	0.45	0.52	–	0.54	–	0.31	0.18	0.31	–
Dietary fibre	–	–	0.24	0.70	0.37	–	–	0.71	0.61	0.40	0.37	0.67	–
Alcohol	–	–	–	–	0.75	–	–	0.80	–	0.90	0.46	0.74	–
Vitamin A	–	–	–	–	–	0.21	0.63	0.41	0.40	–	–	0.31[b]	0.54[b]
Vitamin C	–	–	0.63	0.64	0.36	0.46	0.38	0.58	0.44	–	–	0.33	0.48
Vitamin D	–	–	–	–	–	–	–	0.47	–	–	–	0.27	–
Vitamin E	–	–	–	–	–	–	–	0.64	0.53	–	–	0.39	0.45
Calcium	–	–	–	–	–	–	0.63	0.61	–	–	–	0.53	–
Iron	–	–	–	–	–	–	0.47	–	0.38	–	–	0.66	–
Percent energy from fat	–	–	–	–	–	–	–	0.38	–	–	–	–	–
P/S ratio	–	–	–	–	–	–	–	0.76	0.81	–	–	–	–

a. based on loge transformed values
b. retinol

1. Balogh et al.[44] 14 M, 40–59   FFQ vs. 7-day WI
2. Morgan et al.[29] 87 F   DHQ vs. 4-day diet record
3. Jain et al.[8] 16 M, 25–59   DHQ vs. 30-day record by spouse
4. Jain et al.[34] 50 F, 40–59   DHQ vs. DH interview at home
5. Yarnell et al.[45] 119 M   FFQ vs. 7-day WI
6. Willett et al.[20] 173 F, 34–59   FFQ vs. 28-day WI
7. Willett et al.[46] 27 M+F, 20–54   FFQ vs. 1-year diet record
8. Pietinen et al.[47] 168 M, 55–69   Food Use Quest. vs. 24-day WI
9. Pietinen et al.[48] 190 M, 55–69   FFQ vs. 24-day WI
10. (a) Boutron et al.[49] 20 M+F, 30–79   FFQ (meals) vs. 14-day WI
   (b) Boutron et al.[49] 20 M+F, 30–79   FFQ (foods) vs. 14-day WI
11. O'Donnell et al.[27] 52 M+F, 25–64   FFQ vs. 16-day WI
12. O'Brien and Nelson (unpublished) 29 M+F, 50–70   FFQ vs. 7-day WI

errors between methods, and, particularly in circumstances where this assumption may be violated, the generation of values of ρ which are greater than unity (so-called Heywood cases).[61]

Multivariate regression models allow for an explicit measure of change in the test measure in relation to the change in the reference measure. This may be more helpful than a simple correlation coefficient in understanding the relationship between the test measure and disease outcome. Such models also make possible control for covariance of factors in which the assumptions regarding independence of errors may not apply. This may be particularly important in relation to energy when assessing the quality of assessment of energy-related nutrients such as fat and carbohydrate. Appropriate techniques for energy adjustment have been described by Willett and Stampfer[62], Palmgren[63], and Martin-Moreno[64], and are discussed in Section 6.10.

8.6.3 Other measures of agreement

An argument against using Pearson or Spearman correlation coefficients is that the null hypothesis assumes that there is *no* association between the two measures, but this seems unlikely when two techniques are used to measure the same variable. Lee[65] suggests that a better measure of association is the intra-class correlation r_I for interval measurements, or the Kappa statistic k for nominal (ordinal) measurements. This allows for a degree of association between two related measures which is likely to arise by chance, and tends to give lower values than r.

Table 8.4 gives the results for a validation study of anti-oxidant vitamins carried out in 29 men and women aged 50–70 years (O'Brien and Nelson, unpublished). The table shows mean intakes assessed by 7-day weighed record and by questionnaire, the within-to between-subject variance ratio (based on analysis of variance of the weighed records), Pearson (r_{RQ}), and intra-class (r_I) correlation coefficients, and correction of the correlation coefficients for attenuation (loss of precision) because the 7-day record itself does not measure true intake (i.e. $r_{RT} \neq 1$). One observes immediately that the questionnaire gives higher mean values for nutrient intake than the weighed records, the average difference for all nutrients except retinol being significantly greater than zero. The scale of the difference in relation to the mean is similar for energy and fat, and substantially greater for the vitamins, suggesting that there may be a bias in the over-reporting of fruits and vegetables compared to other food groups. The Pearson correlation coefficients compare favourably with those shown in Table 8.3.

The intra-class correlation coefficient takes into account both the degree of correlation and the size of disagreement within pairs, and is calculated as $(s_b^2 - s_w^2)/(s_b^2 + s_w^2)$, where s_b^2 is the variance of the sum of the pairs of observations, and s_w^2 is the variance of the differences between pairs. As expected, all of the values for r_I are less than those for r. Those above 0.4 show what is regarded as good agreement, while values less than zero suggest that the differences within pairs are so great as to confound any meaningful ranking of subjects. The interpretation of r_I is sometimes difficult, as it is possible to have a questionnaire which correlates perfectly with the standard using Pearson's r, but which has a large variance of differences within pairs (s_w^2). Thus, if the assessment of *ranking* is the primary objective of the validation, then Pearson's r is a better measure, whereas if the aim is to assess the level of *agreement* between the

Table 8.4 Analysis of agreement between FFQ and seven-day weighed inventory (WI) estimates of energy and nutrient intake in 14 men and 15 women aged 50–70 years.

| | WI | FFQ | Mean difference (FFQ-WI) | s_w^2/s_b^2 | Correlation coefficients | | | | |
					Pearson r_{RQ}	Intra-class r_I	Attenuation r_{RT}	Adjusted r_{QT}
Energy kcal	1762	2163	400**	0.83	0.50	0.29	0.94	0.53
Fat: total g	76.3	94.1	17.8**	1.29	0.59	0.41	0.92	0.64
SFA g	25.9	31.9	6.0*	1.35	0.58	0.42	0.92	0.64
Retinol µg	912	1405	493	3.92[a]	0.54[a]	0.51[a]	0.80[a]	0.67[a]
β-Carotene µg	2150	3223	1073**	4.28[a]	0.56[a]	0.39[a]	0.79[a]	0.71[a]
Vitamin A equivalents µg	1270	1943	673*	5.07[a]	0.49[a]	0.45[a]	0.76[a]	0.64[a]
Vitamin C mg	56	94	38***	2.43	0.48	0.16	0.86	0.55
Vitamin E mg	4.0	6.1	2.1***	1.44	0.45	0.05	0.91	0.49

a – based on log$_e$ transformed values

* p<0.05
** p<0.01
*** p<0.001

measures, then the intra-class correlation is more helpful. Neither, however, indicates the degree of attenuation to be expected when assessing diet–disease relationships.

Because neither the questionnaire nor the 7-day record assesses true intake, the correlation of the two measures is inevitably an underestimate of the correlation of the questionnaire with the truth (see Fig. 8.3). The values for r_{RT} are the unobservable correlations between the 7-day weighed record data and the truth, calculated from the formula given in Nelson et al.[66], $r = (d/(d + s_w^2/s_b^2))^{0.5}$, where d is the number of days for which records were kept, s_w^2 is the within-subject variance, and s_b^2 the between-subject variance. This calculation addresses only the question of imprecision in the estimate of intake based on 7 days of record, and ignores any bias which may be present. r_{RQ} divided by r_{RT} gives the likely minimum correlation of the questionnaire with the truth (r_{QT}). This correction suggests that up to 10% more subjects would be correctly classified by thirds. The value for r_{QT} is the same as that obtained using the method suggested by Borrelli[67], based on Liu et al.[68]

An alternative method for assessing the extent of differences is to use the approach suggested by Bland and Altman[57] to plot the difference against the sum of each pair of observations. Like the intra-class correlation, this makes no assumption about which of the measures is the better measure (this is left open to interpretation by the investigator) and assesses only the level of agreement. Fig. 8.5 shows the plot for energy from the study by O'Brien and Nelson (unpublished). It can be seen that the variation around the mean difference is wide, and that as a method for determining an individual's intake the questionnaire would be likely to give rise to substantial error. Moreover, there appears to be a trend suggesting that as intake increases, the size of the difference between the measurements increases also. The two methods could not be regarded as interchangeable for the assessment of an individual's intake. Again, however, if the aim

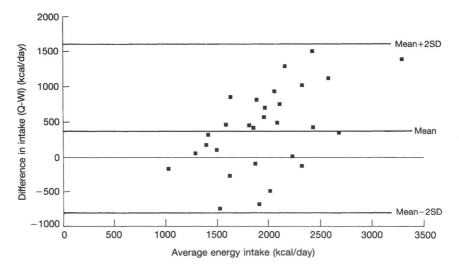

Fig. 8.5 Difference against mean of energy intake estimated by questionnaire and 7-day weighed inventory in 14 men and 15 women aged 50–70 years.

is to be able to distinguish those in the bottom part of the distribution of intakes from those in the top, then the confidence interval around individual values of intake based on the questionnaire would allow approximately 60% of subjects to be correctly classified in the extreme thirds. This will naturally lead to an attenuation of the odds ratio calculation in a case-control study, and the true odds ratio will in all likelihood be higher (see Fig. 4.5, Chapter 4). Similar examples have been published using data relating to smokers[69] and to adolescents (based on medians and Spearman correlation coefficients.[70]

Finally, subjects can be classified according to their position in the distribution of a measurement (thirds, fourths, fifths, etc.). Validation can then take the form of a comparison between classifications according to the test and reference measures. If there were perfect agreement between methods, every subject would be classified in the same fraction of the distribution (top, middle, or bottom third, for example) according to both measures.

Perfect agreement between methods would be indicated by 100% of subjects falling into the same category by both methods, and 0% in adjacent or opposite thirds. Even if there were no agreement between the two methods, however, one third (33.3%) of subjects would fall in the same third of the distribution, 44.4% would be in adjacent thirds, and 22.2% in opposite thirds, just by chance. Garrow[71] has suggested that it would be helpful to present *all* comparisons of methods by reporting the percentage that fell in the same categories of the distribution and the percentage that fell into the extreme opposite categories. The closer the results were to the situation indicated by perfect agreement, the greater the validity the test method could be assumed to have.

Helpful as this approach may be, there are many limitations. First, a great deal of information is discarded when categorizing subjects rather than using the original measures on which the categorization is based. Second, the level of disagreement between the two measures within a category may be larger than the level of disagreement between measures whose results fall into different categories. Burema *et al.*[72] argue in favour of correlation coefficients, especially Spearman's (for non-normally distributed variables), intraclass, and Cohen's *kappa* statistic, the latter two of which take into account associations likely to occur by chance. They suggest that some measure of the dispersal of differences is necessary, and a visual representation (such as the Bland-Altman approach outlined above) is helpful, or a measure of the percentage of the differences falling within a given level (10% disagreement, 20% disagreement, etc.). Ultimately, as Margetts and Thompson[73] indicate, the crucial issue is the effect that the measurement error is likely to have on the estimate of the association between diet and disease.

8.7 Concluding remarks

The validity of measures of dietary exposure must be assessed:

(1) to ensure that the measuring instrument used in nutritional epidemiological studies will allow the detection of diet–disease relationships, should they exist;
(2) to determine the error associated with their use to facilitate the correct interpretation of disease risk in relation to diet.

Inadequate attention paid to validation may result in a substantial waste of resources and, more serious, the failure to observe the true relationship between diet and disease. The amount of resource which needs to be devoted to the validation process should not be underestimated at the initial design stages, and a model for finding the most cost-efficient design has been put forward by Stram et al.[74] A summary of the basic principles of design of validation studies has been published by the BGA Commission on Nutritional Epidemiology.[75]

At the end of a validation study, there is always the (sometimes difficult) decision as to whether or not the test measure is felt to be satisfactory as a measuring instrument. There are no hard and fast rules as to what constitutes 'satisfactory', as it is usually dependent on the size and power of the study. Most investigators continue to use the test measure in the main study in the form used in the validation study, as the extent of the errors associated with its use are defined. To change the questionnaire could mean that the observed agreement between test and reference measure is altered, and the extent of the error is then unknown. Often, there is a difficult point of decision when, having evaluated the test measure, it is felt to be too insensitive to be of use. Three options are available: abandon the measure and find an alternative method to assess the nutritional exposure; modify the test measure in order to overcome its apparent defects without re-evaluation; or repeat the entire validation process with a revised test measure.

If the performance of the test measure in relation to the reference measure is really very poor, then the first option may be the most practicable. If no satisfactory alternative exists, then it may be better to cut one's losses at an early point and abandon the study until an appropriate measuring device can be found. Choosing the second option is a matter of judgement. If the flaws in the test measure which are responsible for the lack of agreement with the reference measure are very obvious, then it may be possible to modify the test measure in the likelihood that the changes will produce a better measuring instrument. The error associated with its use will then have to be estimated, however, as the error based on the original validation study will no longer apply. It is worth bearing in mind, also, that disagreement between test and reference measures may not be due to a design fault in the test measure but to some factor in the calculation of nutrient intake (e.g. a faulty value in the food table which biases the results for test and reference measures in different directions). This option is safe only when design errors are obvious, however, and should be adopted with great caution (and fully acknowledgement in the final write-up!). The final option is usually outside the scope of the resources which have been allocated to the study, but in some circumstances (e.g. when there has already been a substantial investment in the project) may be a viable choice.

Appendix: Calculation of the 95% confidence interval around a correlation coefficient (from Snedecor and Cochran).[76]

The correlation coefficient r is transformed to the variable z with a nearly normal distribution by the equation:

$$z = 0.5 \times [\log_e(1+r) - \log_e(1-r)]$$

and with the standard error given by:

$$\sigma_z = \frac{1}{\sqrt{n-3}}$$

Since z is nearly normally distributed, the upper and lower 95% confidence limits are given as:

Upper limit $= z + 1.96$ SE
Lower limit $= z - 1.96$ SE

These values for the upper and lower confidence limits can then be transformed back to the corresponding values of r using the equation:

$$r = \frac{e^{2z}-1}{e^{2z}+1}$$

so permitting the determination of the confidence interval. When the number of observations is small, the standard error is large in relation to z, and the confidence interval is wide. But if the validation study includes both sexes and is sufficiently large, then there is a greater likelihood of detecting significant differences in the correlation coefficient between sexes, which in turn may enhance the analysis of the disease risk in relation to diet.

References

1. Burema, J., van Staveren, W. A. and van den Brandt, P. A. (1988) Validity and reproducibility. In: Cameron, M. E. and van Staveren, W. A. (ed.). *Manual on methodology for food consumption studies*. Oxford University Press, Oxford. 171–81
2. Abramson, J. H., Slome, C. and Kosovsky, C. (1963) Food frequency interview as an epidemiological tool. *Am. J. Publ. Hlth.* **53**: 1093–101.
3. Mojonnier, L. and Hall, Y. (1968) The national diet–heart study – assessment of dietary adherence. *J. Am. Diet. Assoc.* **52**: 288–92.
4. Hankin, J. H., Reynolds, W. E. and Margen, S. (1967) A short dietary method for epidemiologic studies. II. Variability of measured nutrient intakes. *Am. J. Clin. Nutr.* **20**: 935–45.
5. Margetts, B. M., Cade, J. E. and Osmond, C. (1989) Comparison of a food frequency questionnaire with a diet record. *Int. J. Epid.* **18**: 868–73.
6. Widdowson, E. M. (1936) A study of English diets by the individual method. Part I. Men. *J. Hyg.* **36**: 269–92.
7. Burke, B. S. (1947) The dietary history as a tool in research. *J. Am. Diet. Assoc.* **23**: 1041–6.
8. Jain, M., Howe, G. R., Johnson, K. C. and Miller, A. B. (1980) Evaluation of a diet history questionnaire for epidemiologic studies. *Am. J. Epid.* **111**: 212–19.
9. Prentice, A. M., Coward, W. A., Davies, H. L., Murgatroyd, P. R., Black, A. E., Goldberg, G. R., *et al.* (1985) Unexpectedly low levels of energy expenditure in healthy women. *Lancet.* i: 1419–22.
10. Fairweather-Tait, S. J., Johnson, A., Eagles, J., Ganatra, S., Kennedy, H. and Gurr, M. I. (1989) Studies on calcium absorption from milk using a double-label stable isotope technique. *Br. J. Nutr.* **62**: 379–88.
11. Shepherd, R., Farleigh, C. A. and Land, D. G. (1985) Estimation of salt intake by questionnaire. *Appetite.* **6**: 219–33.
12. Nelson, M., Quayle, A. and Phillips, D. I. W. (1987) Iodine intake and excretion in two British towns: aspects of questionnaire validation. *Hum. Nutr.: Appl. Nutr.* **41A**: 187–92.
13. Bakkum, A., Bloemberg, B., van Staveren, W. A., Verschuren, M. and West, C. E. (1988) The relative validity of a retrospective estimate of food consumption based on a current dietary history and a food frequency list. *Nutr. Cancer.* **11**: 41–53.
14. Byers, T., Marshall, J., Anthony, E., Fiedler, R. and Zielezny, M. (1987) The reliability of dietary history from the distant past. *Am. J. Epid.* **125**: 999–1011.
15. Van Leeuwen, F. E., de Vet, H. C. W., Hayes, R. B., van Staveren, W. A., West, C. A. and Hautvast, J. G. A. J. (1983) An assessment of the relative validity of retrospective interviewing for measuring dietary intake. *Am. J. Epid.* **118**: 752–8.
16. Byers, T. E., Rosenthal, R., Marshall, J. R., Rzepka, T. F., Cummings, K. M. and Graham, S. (1983) Diet history from the distant past: a methodological approach. *Nutr. Cancer.* **5**: 69–77.
17. Lindsted, K. D. and Kuzma, J. W. (1989) Long-term (24 years) recall reliability in cancer cases and controls using a 21-item food frequency questionnaire. *Nutr. Cancer.* **12**: 135–49.
18. Stefanik, P. A. and Trulson, M. F. (1962) Determining the frequency intakes of foods in large group studies. *Am. J. Clin. Nutr.* **11**: 335–43.
19. Stigglebout, A. M., van der Giezen, A. M., Blauw, Y. H., Blok, E., van Staveren, W. A. and West, C. E. (1989) Development and relative validity of a food frequency questionnaire for the estimation of retinol and beta-carotene. *Nutr. Cancer.* **12**: 289–99.
20. Willett, W. C., Sampson, L., Stampfer, M. J., Rosner, B., Bain, C., Witschi, J., *et al.* (1985) Reproducibility and validity of a semi-quantitative food frequency questionnaire. *Am. J. Epid.* **122**: 51–65.

21. Epstein, L. M., Reshef, A., Abrahamson, J. H. and Biacik, O. (1970) Validity of a short dietary questionnaire. *Israel. J. Med. Sci.* **6**: 589–97.

22. Marr, J. W., Heady, J. A. and Morris, J. N. (1961) *Towards a method for large-scale individual diet surveys*. Proceedings of the 3rd International Congress of Dietetics, London, 10–14th July, 1961. Newman Books, London. 85–91.

23. Hankin, J. H., Messinger, H. B. and Stallones, R. A. (1970) A short dietary method for epidemiologic studies. IV. Evaluation of questionnaire. *Am. J. Epid.* **91**: 562–7.

24. Jacobs, D. R. Jr, Anderson, J. T. and Blackburn, H. (1979) Diet and serum cholesterol: do zero correlations negate the relationship? *Am. J. Epid.* **110**: 77–87.

25. Kune, S., Kune, G. A. and Watson, L. F. (1987) Observations on the reliability and validity of the design and diet history method in the Melbourne colorectal cancer study. *Nutr. Cancer.* **9**: 5–20.

26. Kune, S., Kune, G. A. and Watson, L. F. (1987) Case-control study of dietary etiological factors: the Melbourne colorectal cancer study. *Nutr. Cancer.* **9**: 21–42.

27. O'Donnell, M. G., Nelson, M. and Wise, P. H. (1991) A computerised diet questionnaire for use in health education. I. Development and validation. *Br. J. Nutr.* **66**: 3–15.

28. Nelson, M., Atkinson, M. and Darbyshire, S. (1994) Food photography 1. The perception of food portion size from photographs. *Br. J. Nutr.* **72**: 649–63.

29. Morgan, R. W., Jain, M., Miller, A. B., Choi, N. W., Matthews, V., Munan, L.,*et al.* (1978) A comparison of dietary methods in epidemiologic studies. *Am. J. Epid.* **107**: 488–98.

30. Rohan, T. E. and Potter, J. D. (1984) Retrospective assessment of dietary intake. *Am. J. Epid.* **107**: 876–87.

31. Hankin, J. H., Rhoads, G. G. and Glober, G. A. (1975) A dietary method for an epidemiologic study of gastrointestinal cancer. *Am. J. Clin. Nutr.* **28**: 1055–61.

32. Stuff, J. E., Garza, C., O'Brian-Smith, E., Nichols, B. L. and Montandon, C. M. (1983) A comparison of dietary methods in nutritional studies. *Am. J. Clin. Nutr.* **37**: 300–6.

33. Romieu, I., Stampfer, M. J., Stryker, W. S., Hernandez, M., Kaplan, L., Sober, A., *et al.* (1990) Food predictors of plasma beta-carotene and alpha-tocopherol: validation of a food frequency questionnaire. *Am. J. Epid.* **131**: 864–76.

34. Jain, M. G., Harrison, L., Howe, G. R. and Miller, A. B. (1982) Evaluation of a self-administered dietary questionnaire for use in a cohort study. *Am. J. Clin. Nutr.* **36**: 931–5.

35. Nomura, A., Hankin, J. H. and Rhoads, G. G. (1976) The reproducibility of dietary intake data in a prospective study of gastrointestinal cancer. *Am. J. Clin. Nutr.* **29**: 1432–6.

36. Kuzma, J. W. and Lindsted, K. D. (1989) Determinants of long-term (24 year) diet recall ability using a 21-item food frequency questionnaire. *Nutr. Cancer.* **12**: 151–60.

37. Pickle, L. W. (1985) A comparison of frequency and quantitative dietary methods for epidemiologic studies of diet and disease. [letter]. *Am. J. Epid.* **121**: 776–8.

38. Block, G. (1982) A review of validation of dietary assessment methods. *Am. J. Epid.* **115**: 492–505.

39. Borrud, L. G., McPherson, S., Nichaman, M. Z.,, Pillow, P. C. and Newell, G. R. (1989) Development of a food frequency instrument: ethnic differences in food source. *Nutr. Cancer.* **12**: 201–12.

40. Mullen, B. J., Krantzler, N. J., Grivetti, L. E., Schultz, H. G. and Meiselman, H. L. (1984) Validity of a food frequency questionnaire for the determination of individual food intake. *Am. J. Clin. Nutr.* **39**: 136–43.

41. Hankin, J. H., Rawlings, V. and Nomura, A. (1978) Assessment of a short dietary method for a prospective study on cancer. *Am. J. Clin. Nutr.* **31**: 355–9.

42. Tillotson, J. L., Kato, H., Nichaman, M. Z., Miller, D. C., Gay, M. L., Johnson, K. G. and Rhoads, G. G.(1973) Epidemiology of coronary heart disease and stroke in Japanese men living in Japan, Hawaii and California: methodology for comparison of diet. *Am. J. Clin. Nutr.* **26**: 177–84.

43. Nelson, M., Atkinson, M. and Darbyshire, S. (1996) Food photography 2. Use of food photographs for estimating portion size and the nutrient content of meals. *Br. J. Nutr.* **76**: 31–49.

44. Balogh, M., Medalie, J. N., Smith, H. and Groen, J. J. (1968) The development of a dietary questionnaire for an ischaemic heart disease survey.. *Israel. J. Med. Sci.* **4**: 195–203.

45. Yarnell, J. W. G., Fehily, A. M., Millbank, J. E., Sweetnam, P. M. and Walker, C. L. (1983) A short questionnaire for use in epidemiological surveys: comparison with weighed dietary records. *Hum. Nutr.: Appl. Nutr.* **37A**: 103–12.

46. Willett, W. C., Reynolds, R. D., Cottrell-Hoehner, S., Sampson, L. and Browne, M. L. (1987) Validation of a semi-quantitative food frequency questionnaire: comparison with a 1-year diet record. *J. Am. Diet. Assoc.* **87**: 43–7.

47. Pietinen, P., Hartman, A. M., Haapa, E., Rasanen, L., Haapakoski, J., Palmgren, J., *et al.*(1988a) Reproducibility and validity of dietary assessment instruments. I. A self-administered food use questionnaire with a portion size picture booklet. *Am. J. Epid.* **128**: 655–66.

48. Pietinen, P., Hartman, A. M., Haapa, E., Rasanen, L., Haapakoski, J., Palmgren, J., *et al.* (1988b) Reproducibility and validity of dietary assessment instruments. II. A quantitative food frequency questionnaire. *Am. J. Epid.* **128**: 667–76.

49. Boutron, M. C., Faivre, J., Milan, C., Gorcerie, B. and Esteve, J. (1989) A comparison of two diet history questionnaires that measure usual food intake. *Nutr. Cancer.* **12**: 833–91.

50. Kaaks, R., Riboli, E. and van Staveren, W. (1995) Calibration of dietary intake measurements in prospective cohort studies. *Am. J. Epid.* **142**: 548–56.

51. Kaaks, R. (1996) Validation and calibration of dietary intake measurements in the EPIC study: methodological considerations. *Int. J. Epid.* (In press.)

52. Cameron, M. E. and van Staveren, W. A. (ed.) (1988) *Manual on methodology for consumption studies.* Oxford University Press, Oxford.

53. Barker, D. J. P., Morris, J. A. and Nelson, M. (1986) Vegetable consumption and acute appendicitis in 59 areas in England and Wales. *Br. Med. J.* **292**: 927–30.

54. Hebert, J. R. and Miller, D. R. (1991) The inappropriateness of conventional use of the correlation coefficient in assessing validity and reliability of dietary assessment methods. *Eur. J. Epid.* **7**: 339–43.

55. Bellach, B. (1993) Remarks on the use of Pearson's correlation coefficient and other association measures in assessing validity and reliability of dietary assessment methods. *Eur. J. Clin. Nutr.* **47**(Suppl. 2): S42–S45.

56. Delcourt, C., Cubeau, J., Balkau, B., Papoz, L., and the CODIAB-INSERM-ZENECA Pharma Study Group. (1994) Limitations of the correlation coefficient in the validation of diet assessment methods. *Epidemiology.* **5**: 518–24.

57. Bland, J.M. and Altman, D. G. (1986) Statistical methods for assessing agreement between two methods of clinical measurement. *Lancet.* **i**: 307–10.

58. Bland, J. M. and Altman, D. G. (1995) Comparing two methods of clinical measurement: a personal history. *Int. J. Epid.* **24**(Suppl 1): S7–S14.

59. Freudenheim, J. L. and Marshall, J. R. (1988) The problem of profound mismeasurement and the power of epidemiological studies of diet and cancer. *Nutr. Cancer.* **11**: 243–50.

60. Ocké, M. and Kaaks, R. (1996) Biochemical markers as an additional measurement in dietary validity studies: application of the method of triads with examples from the European Prospective Investigation into Cancer and Nutrition. *Am. J. Clin. Nutr.* (In press.)

61. Dunn, G. (1989) *Design and analysis of reliability studies.* Edward Arnold, London.

62. Willett, W. and Stampfer, M. J. (1988) Total energy intake: implications for epidemiological analyses. *Am. J. Epid.* **124**: 17–27.

63. Palmgren, J. (1993) Controlling for total energy intake in regression models for assessment of macronutrient effects on disease. *Eur. J. Clin. Nutr.* **47**(Suppl 2): S46–S50.

64. Martin-Moreno, J. M. (1993) Adjustment for total caloric intake in nutritional studies: an epidemiological perspective. *Eur. J. Clin. Nutr.*. **47**:(Suppl 2): S51–S52.

65. Lee, J. (1980) Alternative approaches for quantifying aggregate and individual agreements between two methods for assessing dietary intakes. *Am. J. Clin. Nutr.* **33**: 956–8.

66. Nelson, M., Black, A. E., Morris, J. A. and Cole, T. J. (1989) Between-and within-subject variation in nutrient intake from infancy to old age: estimating the number of days required to rank dietary intakes with desired precision. *Am. J. Clin. Nutr.* **50**: 155–67.

67. Borrelli, R. (1990) Collection of food intake data: a reappraisal of criteria for judging the methods. *Br. J. Nutr.* **63**: 411–17.

68. Liu, K., Stamler, J., Dyer, A., McKeever, J. and McKeever, P. (1978) Statistical methods to assess and minimize the role of intra-individual variability in obscuring the relationship between dietary lipids and serum cholesterol. *J. Chron. Dis.* **31**: 399–418.

69. Thompson, R. L. and Margetts, B. M. (1993) Comparison of a food frequency questionnaire with a 10-day weighed record in cigarette smokers. *Int. J. Epid.* **22**: 824–33.

70. Andersen, L. F., Ness, M., Lillegaard, I. T., Sandstad, B., Bjørneboe, G. E. and Drevon, C. A. (1995) Evaluation of a quantitative food frequency questionnaire used in a group of Norwegian adolescents. *Eur. J. Clin. Nutr.* **49**: 543–54.

71. Garrow, J. S. (1995) Validation of methods for estimating habitual diet: proposed guidelines. [editorial]. *Eur. J. Clin. Nutr.* **49**: 231–2.

72. Burema, J., van Staveren, W. A. and Feunekes, G. I. J. (1995) Guidelines for reports on validation studies. [letter]. *Eur. J. Clin. Nutr.* **49**: 932–3.

73. Margetts, B. M. and Thompson, R. L. (1995) Validation of dietary intake estimation. [letter]. *Eur. J. Clin. Nutr.* **49**: 934.

74. Stram, D. O., Longnecker, M. P., Shames, L., Kolonel, L. N., Wilkens, L. R., Pike, M. C., *et al.* (1995) Cost-efficient design of a diet validation study. *Am. J. Epid.* **142**: 353–62.

75. BGA Commission on Nutritional Epidemiology. (1993) Recommendations for the design and analysis of nutritional epidemiologic studies with measurement errors in the exposure variables. *Eur. J. Clin. Nutr.* **47**(Suppl 2): S53–S57.

76. Snedecor, G. W. and Cochran, W. G. (1967) *Statistical methods.* 6th edn. Iowa State University Press, Iowa.

9. Socio-demographic and psycho-social variables

Sally Macintyre and Annie Anderson

9.1 Socio–demographic variables

There is an old joke that everything in epidemiology is 'broken down by age and sex' (including epidemiologists). In most forms of epidemiology the populations of interest are described in terms of their socio–demographic characteristics (age, gender, ethnicity, etc.); data are usually presented separately for different age or gender groups; and socio–demographic variables are used in the analysis either as the main focus of interest (does age influence this nutritional exposure?) or as controls in the analysis of the relationship between other variables (does the observed relationship between nutritional exposure and health outcome hold for all age/gender groups? Is it confounded by age or gender?)

Box 9.1   Socio–demographic and psycho–social variables

Main 'facesheet' socio–demographic variables:

- age
- gender
- ethnicity

Other major socio–demographic variables:

- social class/occupation
- residential area
- marital status
- household composition

Psycho–social and intervening variables:

- knowledge/beliefs
- attitudes/norms/values
- role obligations
- social pressures
- income/health
- psycho–social properties
- behaviours

The most common socio–demographic variables used in British epidemiology are age, gender, and social class (Box 9.1). These are sometimes called 'facesheet' variables because they are routinely recorded on the front page, or 'facesheet', of questionnaires, interview schedules, and medical or other records They are commonly used not only because they serve to identify people, but also because they are closely related to virtually every imaginable exposure or outcome variable of interest. An investigator who presents the results of an analysis of the relationship between, say, eating chips and blood pressure, without either describing the age, gender, or social class composition of the sample of subjects, or controlling for age, gender, and social class, would be subject to criticism in epidemiological circles because 'we all know' that both the consumption of chips and blood pressure are patterned by age, gender, and social class.[1,2] We also know that other behaviours or personal characteristics which might be related both to chip consumption and to blood pressure are also patterned by these same socio–demographic variables, and might be spuriously producing an apparent association between chip consumption and blood pressure. For example, men may be more likely to eat chips than women (see Table 9.1). Women might have lower blood pressure than men, either for biological reasons, or because their blood pressure may be better controlled as a result of more frequent blood pressure checks associated with contraceptive, obstetric, or well-women visits to doctors. An apparent association between chip eating and high blood pressure might thus be concealing what is really a gender effect. Higher social class groups tend to eat less chips and to have lower blood pressure, so here too a real, social class effect on blood pressure might spuriously appear as a chip-eating effect. Furthermore, high levels of chip consumption tend to be associated with high intakes of salt, sausages and meat pies, and low intakes of green vegetables, and may be associated with a low level of physical exercise, and these correlated exposures may be more relevant to blood pressure than chips *per se*. This type of dietary pattern is also associated with higher body mass index, which is an independent risk factor for blood pressure.

Table 9.1 Percentage of respondents reporting never eating shop-bought chips; 38 and 58-year-olds in the west of Scotland. (Source: Finnegan, F., Hunt, K. and Ford, G. (1992) *Dietary patterns and distribution of nutrient intakes among adults living in the central Clydeside conurbation.* MRC Medical Sociology Unit Working Paper No. 38.)

Gender		Age		
	38		58	
	%	n	%	n
Male	47	(166/379)	62	(224/399)
Female	62 ***	(276/473)	70 **	(386/459)

*** Gender difference significant at $p < .001$
** Gender difference significant at $p < .01$

Despite the fact that 'we all know' that these socio–demographic variables are associated with so many aspects of life and health, investigators are often remarkably incurious about the reasons for these associations. For example, data on all sorts of topics are often presented separately for men and women, but without there being any discussion of the differences (or lack of them) between the sexes, or the reasons for the differences. As a consequence researchers may not notice that male/female differences in the outcomes of interest may vary over time, or by age, or by other characteristics.[3] It has been shown recently, for example, that gender differences in health may be rather less than has often been asserted, and that rather than there being a universal female excess in ill health and disability, there may be a male excess in some conditions. It has been argued that a picture of marked and substantial female excess in ill health may have persisted for a considerable length of time because investigators have tended to explore differences within each gender rather than between them.[4]

9.1.1 Age

The meaning and significance for nutritional epidemiology of even apparently straightforward and unambiguous variables such as age and gender may not be as obvious as they might first appear. The variable 'age' for example may be an indicator of *biological* states and processes (e.g. growth, development, maturation, metabolism, repair); of *historical* processes and contexts (e.g. the Dutch hunger famine may have marked out particular age cohorts affected by it[5]); and of *psychological* and *social* processes (e.g. role obligations or patterns of activity may be more common at certain ages for social or psychological reasons; a woman of 60 is no longer likely to be the primary food provider for young children and infants, and a woman of 80 may not be expected to have a fit, trim figure).

The social significance of chronological age may vary over time and by gender.[6] The age at which one can legally leave school, or at which one is eligible for a state pension, for example, has varied historically. The social status of school-leaving at 14 in the 1930s might be equivalent to school-leaving at 16 in the 1980s, and consequently in an all-age sample it would not be sensible to treat 'chronological age at leaving school' as a simple, continuous variable with the same meaning for respondents of all ages. If there is an interest in the effects of retirement from paid work it might be sensible to group women into those aged under and over 60, and to group men into those under or over 65, since these are the ages at which people in Britain currently become eligible for state or occupational pensions and are expected to retire. However, it would not be appropriate in the USA, where it is illegal for employers to enforce a compulsory retirement age, and it will soon be no longer appropriate in Britain because European Community rulings have rendered different mandatory retirement ages for men and women illegal. Moreover, such bureaucratic distinctions between working and re-tirement ages may be unrelated to actual employment patterns; for example, a study in the west of Scotland found that 55% of a cohort of 55-year-olds were already no longer in the labour market in 1988.[7]

The relationship between chronological and social or physiological age may vary historically and culturally. An affluent 60-year-old woman in Florida, USA, may consider herself, and be considered by others, to be merely middle-aged, while a

60-year-old woman in many Third World countries would be considered elderly. Socio–economically deprived people may age faster than their more advantaged counterparts. Comparison of mortality rates at specific ages in Glasgow and Edinburgh led to the observation that: 'For the same chronological age, Glaswegians are physiologically about four years older than people in Edinburgh. At any given age, Glaswegians have more miles on the clock'.[8]

9.1.2 Gender

How someone's gender might relate to nutritional exposures and to the health outcomes of these exposures might similarly vary from the *biological* (e.g. body size and composition, reproductive state), through the *cultural* and *social* (e.g. conventional divisions of labour in most cultures prescribe that women have more responsibility than men for food preparation and cooking, and in many cultures men are given more to eat, and may be given different types of food, compared to women[9,10]); to the *behavioural* (e.g. women and men tend to engage in different types of physical recreation, and men to drink more alcohol) and *psychological* (e.g. women may be more concerned about body image, or may have lower self-esteem than men). Biological, social, psychological, and behavioural aspects of differences between genders may interact with each other, and vary historically and culturally, so that even something as apparently fixed and clear-cut as gender may differ considerably in its significance for nutritional exposures and outcomes.[11] The strength of each of these factors may vary between nutrients. For example, women may experience stronger psychological pressures than men to reduce energy intake in order to reduce body size[12], but may not experience any greater pressure than men to increase dietary iron when suffering from mild anaemia.

It may thus be reasonably easy to measure age and gender with accuracy, but harder to conceptualize what it is about age and gender which is related to the exposures and outcomes of interest, or to interpret observed associations or interactions with age and gender. When one moves from such apparently fixed, simple properties of individuals to more complex ones such as ethnicity, social class, and household composition, there are problems not only with conceptualization but also with the valid and reliable measurement of the underlying constructs.

9.1.3 Ethnicity

The term 'ethnicity' should be distinguished from 'race' in epidemiological and social research. 'Ethnicity' signifies shared and inherited cultural, linguistic, and religious traditions. It is not necessarily the same as nationality, migrant status, or skin colour (for example, people of Punjabi Sikh descent in Glasgow may be British citizens and have been born in Scotland; in the USA one can be categorized as 'black, Hispanic' or 'white, Hispanic'). 'Race' was a taxonomic classification used by biologists to refer to divisions of humans, below the level of species, based on physical characteristics such as skin colour. Its epidemiological utility has increasingly been questioned given that there is more genetic variability within than between races[13] and the genes responsible for characteristics such as skin colour are few and tend not to be associated with specific diseases.[14–16] The term 'race' is more commonly used in the USA than in Europe, and in the USA it is often used as a proxy indicator for socio–economic status, since in the United States race is a more commonly recorded item of information in vital statistics than is occupation.[17] It may be useful in some fields of epidemiology in which the interest is in the likelihood of certain diseases (such as sickle cell anaemia), or responses to environmental exposures (such as favism), which are related to geographical variation in gene frequency.[14]

It is important to distinguish between all the various elements of social and biological differentiation (such as minority status, economic position, cultural practices, country of origin, and genetic makeup) which can be inferred from ethnic or racial categorizations. Many conditions which at first sight are assumed to be genetic in origin may on further study appear to result from environmental exposures or to gene/environment interactions. There are, for example, marked international differences in the rates of coronary heart disease (CHD). Epidemiological studies of migrants have shown that people who have migrated from a low risk country (e.g. Japan or India) to a high risk country (e.g. USA or UK) tend to show similar CHD rates to the new host population[18,19]; the same has been shown for height, with mean height among people of Japanese origin being greater in the USA than in Hawaii or Japan.[18] This suggests that CHD risk and height are sensitive to environmental (including dietary) exposures rather than just to genetic factors (Wilkie has made a similar point in relation to the assumed genetic basis of the short stature of Scots[20]). Interactions between genes and environment have been found for several diet-related diseases such as diabetes; studies of the Pima Indians of North America have, for example, indicated that a combination of genetic susceptibility and exposure to Western lifestyle results in an increased tendency to develop diabetes.[21]

There are few instances in which 'racial' or 'ethnic' differences can unequivocally be associated with biological variation. One is the case of lactose intolerance. People from central and north-west Europe and from areas in Africa with a long history of dairy farming have the ability to digest lactose after weaning, but for much of the world's population, lactose (in amounts commonly consumed in Britain) will be malabsorbed with accompanying gastro-intestinal symptoms.

Ethnicity is increasingly used as a variable in social epidemiology in Britain but there are a number of problems with its usage. These mainly involve difficulties of measurement, the heterogeneity of the populations being studied, lack of clarity about research aims, and ethnocentric interpretations of data.[14] Most classifications are based on self-report, and, to an extent which may depend on the context and the classification scheme used, the same subjects may classify themselves differently on different occasions.[22] The ethnic classification used for the first time in the UK national decennial census in 1991 was based on pilot studies to ensure reliability and ease of comprehension, but is a conceptually muddled classification (it offered the options: 'white, black–Caribbean, black–African, black–(other, please describe), Indian, Pakistani, Bangladeshi, Chinese, and any other ethnic group (please specify)').

Because ethnicity is clearly a powerful predictor of life chances and behaviours in modern multi-cultural societies it may often offer important information about dietary exposures and the outcomes of these exposures, but care must be taken in nutritional epidemiology not to assume too high a correlation between self-reported ethnic group and other factors of interest (for example, place or diet of upbringing, genetic predisposition, attitudes or responses to food, etc.). It is particularly important to guard against the assumptions either that all ethnic differences are biological, or that they are all cultural. In fact, very few nutrition-related disorders can be so well differentiated as being either biological or cultural, and many more are likely to result from gene/environment interactions shaped by cultural and socio–economic factors.

Favism is a rare example of a true biological disorder within a particular ethnic group. This disease, a form of acute haemolytic anaemia caused by ingestion of Fava beans, is caused by an expression of a mutation of the glucose-6-phosphatase dehydrogenase (G-6PD) gene, and is found predominantly in the tropics and Mediterranean area (where heterozygotes suffer less from malarial infections). More typical in trying to untangle biological and cultural differences is the case of rickets and osteomalacia. These disorders arise from a deficiency of vitamin D due to inadequate dietary intake of the vitamin and inadequate exposure to sunlight. Studies of South Asians in Glasgow have shown that a lacto–vegetarian diet is more rachitogenic than an omnivore diet, but the development of rickets is also related to exposure to sunlight, which may be culturally and socially determined, and to the action of and response to ultra-violet radiation on the skin, which is likely to be biologically determined.[23] Further studies of South Asians in Glasgow show that nutrient intake varies across generations such that second and subsequent generation migrants have diets more similar to the ethnic majority than do first generation migrants[24], suggesting that the risk of rickets arising from dietary exposures may lessen in subsequent generations of South Asians as their diet approximates more to that of the host country.

9.1.4 Social class

Social class is also strongly predictive of life chances and therefore a key variable in nutritional epidemiology. Table 9.2 illustrates that a variety of measures of socio–economic status (their social class based on the occupation, income, housing tenure (whether the home is owned or rented), and completed education) are all associated with the likelihood of reported eating habits fitting or diverging from current dietary guidelines. Like ethnicity, 'social class' can be measured in a number of ways, lacks a gold standard against which to assess accuracy of measurement, and is subject to conceptual unclarities.

In the USA and Europe various scales of socio–economic position, most of which combine information about occupation, income, and education, have been developed and used in epidemiology.[25] In Britain, occupation has been used since 1923 as the basis for the Registrar General's classification of occupational social class.[26,27] This has six categories; three non-manual (I, professional, e.g. doctor; II, intermediate, e.g. teacher; III non-manual, e.g. typist); and three manual (III manual, e.g. miner; IV, semi-skilled manual, e.g. farmworker; V, unskilled manual, e.g. labourer).[28] It operates as a ranked scale embodying occupational skill and prestige, and is highly predictive of everything from height and life expectancy to the type of television programmes watched and examination results achieved; but it is not based on any conceptually tight theory about occupational or social stratification in modern industrial societies.[29] (It is worth noting that in some other countries, the higher the classifying number the higher the social

Table 9.2 Distribution of 'healthy eating' according to gender, occupational class, household income, housing tenure, educational qualifications, and marital status among 35-year-olds in the west of Scotland (n = 73). (Source: Anderson and Hunt[46])

Variable	'Healthy eaters'		'Less healthy eaters'		Significance[a]
	n	(row %)	n	(row %)	
Gender					
Female	218	(49)	222	(51)	
Male	112	(33)	231	(67)	P < 0.0001
HOH occupational class[b]					
Non-manual	210	(52)	191	(48)	
Manual	111	(32)	239	(68)	P < 0.0001
Missing	9		23		
Own occupational class[c]					
Non-manual	241	(50)	246	(50)	
Manual	83	(29)	203	(71)	P < 0.0001
Missing	6		4		
Household income (per week)					
<£100	46	(32)	97	(68)	
£100–£159	60	(31)	134	(69)	
£160–£249	126	(48)	135	(52)	P < 0.0001
£250 +	89	(55)	74	(45)	
Missing	9		13		
Housing tenure					
Owner occupied	245	(51)	239	(49)	
Other	85	(28)	214	(72)	P < 0.0001
Education					
Left school with qualifications	222	(50)	223	(50)	
no qualifications	108	(32)	229	(68)	P < 0.0001
Missing	0		1		

[a] Using Chi-Square test in SPSS X
[b] Defined by occupation of head of household (OPCS, 1980)[28]
[c] Defined by occupation of respondent (OPCS, 1980)[28]

class, unlike in the UK where the lower the classifying number the higher the social class).

There are a number of conceptual and measurement problems with this occupationally-based, socio–economic classification, including: what to do with people not in the labour market (children and young people, homemakers, the long-term sick, and retired); difficulties in comparisons over time because of changes in the skills and prestige of occupations or the appearance and disappearance of occupations; the specificity of some types of occupation to particular points in the life cycle (it's hard to achieve a social class I occupation at 20); and whether it is the individual's or the household's social position which is important.[29,30] A number of alternative classifications have been proposed or used in the UK. These include: socio–economic groups (17 groups based on employment, occupation, and industry); the Hope-Goldthorpe scale (based on the perceived social desirability of occupations); and the A, B, C1, C2 schemes used by the British market research industry.[31] In this last mentioned scheme grade A households are upper middle class (e.g. physician); grade B, middle class (e.g. pharmacist); C1, lower middle class (e.g. radiographer); C2, skilled working class (e.g. plumber); grade D, semi- and unskilled working class (e.g. fisherman); and grade E are those at the lowest level of subsistence (e.g. casual labourer).[31]

The postcode of an address can also be used, not only to provide an indication of the geographical location, but also of the socio–economic characteristics of the neighbourhood. There are a number of residentially based indices of social deprivation which use census data to classify the demographic and social characteristics of small areas such as postcode sectors or wards; for example, the Carstairs classification[32] and the Townsend classification[33], which were initially based on the 1981 census data and applied to Scotland, England, and Wales, respectively; and the classification based on the 1991 census produced by the Office of Population Censuses and Surveys.[34]

While all such socio–economic scales may be predictive of nutritional exposures and outcomes, which one is appropriate will depend on the specific research aims, and it should not be assumed that they are all measuring exactly the same thing. If a female doctor is married to a clerical officer and the census enumerator decides to treat the husband as the 'head of household' (see below), then she will be classified as social class III non-manual if the head of household classification is used, and social class I if classification by own occupation is used. Living in an area with a high concentration of deprived people in it (as measured by the Carstairs or Townsend indices) means that it is more likely that an individual or household has a low standard of living, but individual and area level deprivation do not always go together. At each extreme of area deprivation, localities are fairly socially homogeneous (suburbs with lots of big detached houses are unlikely to contain many very poor people, and run-down inner city areas are unlikely to contain many very rich people), but areas classified as of medium deprivation may include both rich and poor people, so living in one of these areas may not be highly predictive of a person's or family's personal circumstances.[35]

9.1.5 Marital status

Other variables commonly used in nutritional epidemiology relate to marital status or household composition. These are used to modify or expand other measures such as social class (for example, women are often given a social class classification based on husband's occupation if married, and on own occupation if not married). They can also be used as socio–demographic variables in their own right. Marital status, for example, is related to physical and mental and life expectancy, and to eating habits. Married persons tend to have better health than non-married persons, and to have better dietary habits[36], (the latter not necessarily being the reason for the former).

The social meaning and significance of marital statuses vary by age, cohort, and gender; being a widowed female at age 75 may be considered socially quite normal, but being a widowed man at 30 might have quite different epidemiological and social significance.[36] Marital status is a civil status which may increasingly bear little relationship to actual living arrangements or emotional commitments, so it may be less valid than it once was for observers to infer other characteristics (such as cohabitation, disposable income, or parenthood) from legal marital status.

9.1.6 Household composition

Households are defined for census purposes as being persons who usually live and eat together (commensality), so households have obvious relevance for nutritional epidemiology. However, this means that a 'household' may not be the same as 'a family' or 'co-residents' and may include or exclude those with unusual or complex living arrangements (for example, adult co-resident offspring who do their own cooking and shopping, or joint or extended families who share catering and cooking duties). A study in Glasgow of young women of South Asian origin found that their families might not share a front door, but might nevertheless share all cooking and shopping. In one example, residents of five flats off the same close (common stairwell) shopped jointly.[37] There are variations in household structures between ethnic groups in Britain. Among women aged 16–35 with children of their own, Asians were more likely than those from other ethnic groups to be living with their parents or parents in law; blacks were more likely than others to be living as lone parents, outside the parental home; and whites were more likely to be living with a husband or partner in their own home.[38]

There is some evidence that members of a household (for example, couples) may share similar dietary patterns[39], but this may not be constant throughout a given period and need not imply similar nutrient intake for the men and women involved.[40]

The concept of 'head of household' is used for official purposes (for example, the 'head of household' is responsible for completing census or council tax forms), and may be used by social scientists to allocate socio–economic classifications to people without occupations, but it may have little practical or symbolic meaning in people's everyday lives. It tends in practice to be assumed that the 'head of household' will be a man, although this is not an official requirement even in homes in which both men and women are present. There is variation between ethnic groups in the meaning and relevance of the concept of 'head of household'. Among Asian communities in Britain the 'household head' is likely to be defined as a man, but which man in an extended or joint household might depend on social circumstances (i.e. it might not necessarily be the oldest, if he does not speak English or is not in charge of the family business). Among black communities there are more lone mothers who will be defined as the 'head of household', and men may play a lesser role in the household economy than in white or Asian culture.[38] Caution should therefore be exercised in defining and using concepts such as 'head of household' across a range of cultures.

Household composition or size is important both as a predictor in its own right of nutritional exposures or outcomes, and as a control for other variables. For example, the meaning of a household income of £20000 per annum, or of living in a seven-bedroomed house, will differ between families with six children and families with none, and there are algorithms which have been devised to take account of family size and structure when using income or overcrowding in analysis. Typically these involve allocating weights to household members of different ages, sexes, and relationships to each other.[41–43]

9.1.7 Criteria for sound variables

It is important that the measurement of all the above variables be conducted in as standardized a way as possible in order to optimize comparability. A useful guide to standard ways of eliciting information out of which these variables can be constructed is *Harmonising questions asked in government surveys*, produced by the Government Statistical Service.[44]

It has been suggested that the attributes of a sound epidemiological variable are as follows:

(1) it should be measurable accurately;
(2) it should differentiate populations in some underlying characteristic relevant to health (such as income, childhood circumstances, hormonal status, genetic inheritance, and lifestyle);
(3) observed differences in patterns of disease should generate testable aetiological hypotheses or be applicable to the planning and delivery of health care.[14]

Socio–demographic variables such as age, gender, ethnicity, social class, and marital status certainly fulfil the second and the third criteria; they differentiate populations in ways which capture significant differences in nutritional exposures and/or outcomes of these exposures, and these significant differences can be used to generate testable hypotheses about the mechanisms likely to link socio–demographic characteristics with nutritional exposures and health outcomes. The first criterion is harder to fulfil since these variables are markers for complex social exposures and meanings, for which there is no gold standard against which the accuracy of their measurement can be assessed. The important goal in these circumstances is therefore appropriateness; the key question is not 'what is the most accurate measure of social class or ethnicity?', but 'what is the most appropriate measure for the particular research (or policy) purpose at hand?'. This relates to the third criterion listed above; documenting differences between different groups of the population is only of value if this suggests hypotheses about causal mechanisms which can then be tested in further studies. Knowing that people in lower social classes are less likely to adhere to current healthy diet guidelines[45–47], Table 9.2 is not enough in itself; one then needs to know what it is about social class position that explains these differences. Is it low disposable income, lack of information about the properties of foods and how to cook them, poor cooking facilities, unavailability of healthy foods, lack of time for food purchase and preparation, disbelief in the efficacy of any dietary change, or a combination of these?

Observing that some people of South Asian descent in Britain are more likely than others to develop rickets should be the beginning of an investigation rather than the end of it, since the observation does not of itself explain whether this is because of different nutritional exposures, different responses to similar nutritional exposures, or to other non-nutritional factors such as exposure to sunlight or amount of exercise taken.

However, the hypotheses generated by observations of associations with socio-demographic factors are frequently not explicitly developed and tested, but rather are left implicit, as if 'social class' or 'ethnicity' or 'gender' were in themselves sufficient explanations. In consequence one observer may assume that a social class, ethnic, or gender difference in some nutritional exposure is attributable to genetic or biological factors, while another may assume that the same association is attributable to cultural or behavioural factors. Without further research there is no evidence available to allow one to judge which of these competing (or interacting) hypotheses is correct.[48] It is thus important to consider moving on from observation of socio–demographic differences to testing hypotheses about the reasons for these differences.

9.2 Psycho–social and other intervening variables

Most investigators do not assume that class, ethnicity, gender, and so on directly influence nutritional exposures and their outcomes, but that these socio–demographic characteristics predict other intervening psycho–social, socio–economic, or cultural variables which influence exposures. In the nutrition field the following intervening mechanisms are often hypothesized or assumed:

(1) knowledge (e.g. understanding what a healthy diet is, knowing the vitamin or energy (caloric) content of different foods, awareness of correlations between diet and disease);
(2) beliefs (e.g. beliefs about appropriate foodstuffs, the applicability of dietary advice to oneself, the efficacy of exercise as a means of weight control);
(3) attitudes/norms/values (e.g. symbolic aspects of food such as the importance of 'a proper meal', ideas about families eating together, ideal body shape norms);
(4) role obligations (e.g. age or gender related expectations about who does the food purchase and preparation, or performs other tasks such as wage earning or educating children);
(5) social pressures (e.g. mass media or advertising influences, peer group or family pressures);
(6) income/wealth/other personal resources (e.g. money available to buy food, standard of cooking and food storage facilities, access to cars or other transport facilities);
(7) psycho–social properties (e.g. self-esteem, body image, stress, perceived self-efficacy, self control);
(8) other behaviours which may modify eating behaviours (e.g. smoking, alcohol consumption, work related or recreational exercise).

All these hypothesized intervening variables are complex and difficulty to measure, and interpretation of models which include them are liable to difficulties. All require simple and reliable indicators or scales as indicators of complex, underlying social constructs, with all the associated measurement problems this presents. Given the point made earlier, that the key question is 'what is the most accurate measure of the concept?', it is impossible in the space available here to list or discuss what might be the best scales for all the variables listed above. Many of the conceptual and measurement issues involved in choosing and validating measures for these variables are covered in textbooks of statistics, social psychology, sociology, and social survey methods, and those interested in selecting measures of these states or processes are advised to consult the many specialist works in the field. Particular problems include:

(1) imprecision of measurement;
(2) the intercorrelations between variables, and possible confounding between them;
(3) lack of conceptual clarity about what exactly is being measured and why;
(4) lack of formal validation;
(5) poor cross-disciplinary understanding.

Living in a household which owns one or more cars is, for example, associated with longer life expectancy[49,50], but may be an imprecise measure of an individual's access to and use of a car. Its meaning and significance may depend on one's gender and whether one lives in the country or a town or city. It may be associated with life expectancy because it is a marker for household income or wealth[51], but it may also be because car ownership is an indicator of psycho–social characteristics such as power or control, or because a car is a useful container for transporting food, children, medications, etc. Sometimes it is not clear which of these possible explanations for the observed association is being assumed (although living in a car-owning household often seems to be treated simply as a marker of wealth). Other possessions similarly used as indices of wealth could also be treated either as markers of material well-being or as conferring some direct health advantage. In a study in rural Uganda, for example, the number of cooking pots in a household was shown to be a good indicator of socio–economic status in a rural community, and was found to be inversely associated with the likelihood of HIV transmission.[52] While number of cooking pots may be a good marker of socio–economic status in this community, it is a rather indirect indicator, and its inverse association with HIV infection might arise not only because it is a measure of assets but also because of its association with other, possibly infection related, factors (such as propensity to use income on cooking utensils, the value put on food preparation, the quality and quantity of food provided, and standards of hygiene). One problem about the use of such indicators is that researchers or practitioners from different disciplines may be assuming, rather than making explicit, different underlying causal processes, and it is therefore important to be clear about the way in which one is conceptualizing such indicators and what one believes them to be measuring.

9.3 Concluding remarks

Socio–demographic and psycho–social variables pose problems of measurement and interpretation, but are important and need to be included in nutritional epidemiological studies.

Firstly, it is vital to report, and to control for, socio–demographic variables in order to check for the generalizability of the findings and to detect possible sources of bias or of spurious associations. Age, gender, social class, ethnicity, and marital status are such powerful influences on social behaviours and on health that findings relevant to one group cannot necessarily be extrapolated to other populations or subgroups (see Tables 9.1 and 9.2). Moreover, relationships observed between other explanatory variables and outcomes may differ according to socio–demographic characteristics. For example, an observed relationship between dietary improvements and changes in health or functioning among men or middle class populations may be weaker for women or for working class populations (for example it was observed in the British health and lifestyles survey that giving up smoking during the seven year interval between the two survey sweeps had a more beneficial effect on respiratory function among non-manual social class respondents than among manual class respondents).[47]

Secondly, taking these socio–demographic variables into account helps to refine the accuracy of estimates of the strength and direction of relationships between other variables. If an exposure of interest is highly correlated with some socio–demographic variable, then its relationship to an outcome may be overestimated. For example, it has been pointed out that because smoking is highly social class patterned, and both smoking and low social class are independently associated with mortality, the reduction in mortality that might be achieved through reductions in smoking rates may have been overestimated. Davey Smith and Shipley have argued that such estimates need to be based on comparisons between smokers, ex-smokers, and never smokers *in the same socio–economic groups*. Using data from the Whitehall study of civil servants, they showed that taking into account the employment grade led to reduced estimates of the contribution of smoking to mortality; they have suggested that confounding by socio–economic factors may be a common problem in observational designs in epidemiology.[53]

Thirdly, as noted earlier, observations of associations between socio–demographic variables and nutritional exposures and outcomes can help to generate and test hypotheses about causal mechanisms. The observation that coronary heart disease mortality is higher among people in Britain of South Asian descent generates hypotheses about the role of diet, physical activity, migrant status, experience of racism, stress, socio–economic position, domestic conditions, and genetic factors in the aetiology of CHD; the fact that it is not high among people in Britain of African Caribbean descent draws our attention to the danger of having oversimplified hypotheses about the role of some of these factors. Similarly, the fact that although high cholesterol levels are a risk factor for CHD, lower social class groups in the UK have higher CHD rates, but not higher cholesterol levels, than higher social class groups[54], should make us refine hypotheses about the role of cholesterol and its interaction with other factors in the genesis of CHD.

Fourthly, in order to clarify aetiological or causal processes and mechanisms it is important to move beyond socio–demographic, 'facesheet' variables and to test hypotheses about the role of the intervening variables through which these socio–demographic variables exert their influence. It is not social class or age or ethnicity which directly effect nutritional exposures and health; rather, these are markers for features of people's lives which influence nutritional exposures and health. These features of people's lives may range from macro level, environmental contexts (living in certain sorts of areas, such as inner city estates), through features of the household and workplace, to characteristics of individuals such as knowledge, attitude, and behaviours.

Fifthly, it is important to take into account social factors, and in particular the intervening variables described above, when trying to formulate or evaluate dietary/nutritional interventions or policies designed to improve health. Some interventions may be directed specifically at the types of variables listed; one might choose, for example, to target public knowledge about diet or health, or disposable income, or self efficacy, or mass media depictions of diet or health, according to whether one hypothesized that the main influence on the nutritional exposure in question was, respectively, cognitions, money, beliefs about control, or social pressures. Formulating policies or designing interventions on the basis of epidemiological research is a good means of forcing oneself to be very explicit about the underlying mechanisms one hypothesizes to be important, and about how to move from the underlying concepts firstly to items in a data collection instrument (how to measure the concept) and secondly to variables used in analysis (how to analyse and interpret the measure).

In this chapter we have shown three things: that socio–demographic factors are important in nutritional epidemiology and it is therefore important to include them in nutritional epidemiological studies; that it is important to be precise about what it is one is trying to measure; and that in aetiological and policy research it is important to move beyond documenting associations between socio–demographic factors and nutrition or health towards exploring the reasons for these associations. The fact that these variables are difficult to measure and conceptualize does not mean that they should not be used, just that one needs to be explicit (particularly for a multi-disciplinary audience) about the status and meaning of the variables in the particular context.

References

1. Gregory, J., Foster, K., Tyler, H. and Wiseman, M. (1990) *The dietary and nutritional survey of British adults*. HMSO, London.
2. Macintyre, S. (1988) A review of the social patterning and significance of measures of height, weight, blood pressure, and respiratory function. *Soc. Sci. Med.* **27**: 327–37.
3. Macintyre, S. (1993) Gender differences in longevity and health in Eastern and Western Europe. In: Platt, S., Thomas, H., Scott, S. and Williams, G. (ed.) *Locating health; sociological and historical explorations*. Avebury, Amersham. 57–73.
4. Macintyre, S., Hunt, K. and Sweeting, H. (1996) Gender differences in health: are things as simple as they seem? *Soc. Sci. Med..* (In press.)
5. Stein, Z., Susser, M. and Saenger, M. F. (1975) *Famine and human development; the Dutch hunger winter of 1944–5*. Oxford University Press, Oxford.
6. Finch, J. (1986) Age. In: Burgess, R. (ed.) *Key variables in social investigation*. Routledge and Kegan Paul, London. 12–30.
7. Ford, G. (1995) MRC Medical Sociology Unit, Glasgow. [personal communication].
8. Watt, G. C. M. (1993) Differences in expectations of life between Edinburgh and Glasgow: implications for health policy in Scotland. *Hlth. Bull.* **51**: 407–17.
9. Murcott, A. (1982) On the social significance of the 'cooked dinner' in South Wales. *Soc. Sci. Inf.* **21**: 677–96.
10. Murcott, A. (1983) 'Its a pleasure to cook for him': food, mealtimes and gender in some South Wales households. In: Garmarnikov, E. (ed.). *The public and private*. Heinemann, London. 78–90.

11. Morgan, D. (1986) Gender. In: Burgess, R. (ed.). *Key variables in social investigation*. Routledge and Kegan Paul, London. 31–53.

12. Department of Health. (1995) *Obesity. A report from the Nutrition and Physical Activity Task Forces*. HMSO, London.

13. Lewontin, R. C. (1991) *The doctrine of DNA: biology as ideology*. Penguin, Harmondsworth.

14. Senior, P. and Bhopal, R. (1994) Ethnicity as a variable in epidemiological research. *Br. Med. J.* **309**: 327–30.

15. Smaje, C. (1995) Health, 'race' and ethnicity: making sense of the evidence. Kings Fund Institute, London.

16. Smaje, C. (1996) The ethnic patterning of health; new directions for theory and research. *Sociol. Hlth. Illness.* **18**: 139–71.

17. Krieger, N., Rowley, D. L., Herman, A. A., Avery, B. and Phillips, M. T. (1993) Racism, sexism and social class: implications for studies of health, disease and well-being. *Am. J. Prev. Med.* **9**(Suppl.): 82–122.

18. Kagan, A., Marmot, M. G. and Kata, H. (1980) The Ni-Hon-San study of cardiovascular disease epidemiology. In: Kesteloot, H. and Joosens, J. V. (ed.). *The epidemiology of arterial blood pressure*. Martinus Nijhoff, The Hague. 423–36.

19. Balarajan, R. (1991) Ethnic differences in mortality from IHD and CVD in England and Wales. *Br. Med. J.* **302**: 560–4.

20. Wilkie, T. (1993) *Perilous knowledge: the human genome and its implications*. Faber and Faber, London. 184.

21. West, K. (1978) Epidemiology of diabetes and its vascular lesions. Elsevier, New York.

22. Storkey, M. (1994) *London's ethnic minorities: one city, many communities*. London Research Centre, London.

23. Henderson, J. B., Dunnigan, M. G., Mcintosh, W. B., Abdul-Motaal, A. and Hole, D. (1990) Asian osteomalacia is determined by dietary factors when exposure to UV radiation is restricted: a risk factor model. *Q. J. Med.* **76**: 923–34.

24. Anderson, A., Lean, M. E. J., Bush, H., Bradby, H. and Williams, R. (1995) Macro-nutrient intake in South Asian and Italian women in the West of Scotland. *Proc. Nutr. Soc.* **54**: 203A.

25. Liberators, P., Link, B. G. and Kelsey, J. L. (1988) The measurement of social class in epidemiology. *Epid. Rev.* **10**: 87–121.

26. Stevenson, T. H. C. (1923) The social distribution of mortality from different causes in England and Wales, 1910–12. *Biometrika.* **15**: 382–400.

27. Stevenson, T. H. C. (1928) The vital statistics of wealth and poverty. *J. R. Stat. Soc.* **XLI**: 207–30.

28. Office of Population Censuses and Survey. (1980) *Classification of occupations 1980*. HMSO, London.

29. Marsh, K. (1986) Social class and occupation. In: Burgess, R. (ed.). *Key variables in social investigation*. Routledge and Kegan Paul, London. 123–52.

30. Berkman, L. and Macintyre, S. (1996) The measurement of social class in health studies: old measures and new formulations. In: Susser, M., Kogevinas, M. and Pearce, N. (ed.). *Socio–economic factors and cancer*. IARC Scientific Publications, Lyons. (In press.)

31. Joint Industry Committee for National Readership Surveys. (1985) *Social grading on the national readership survey*. JICNARS, London.

32. Carstairs, V. and Morris, R. (1991) *Deprivation and health in Scotland*. Aberdeen University Press, Aberdeen.

33. Townsend, P., Philimore, P. and Beattie, A. (1987) *Health and deprivation: inequality and the North*. Croom Helm, London.

34. Wallace, M., Charlton, J. and Denham, C. (1995) The new OPCS area classification. *Pop Trends.* **79**: 15–30.

35. Mcloone, P. (1994) *Carstairs scores for Scottish postcode sectors for the 1991 census.* Public Health Research Unit, University of Glasgow, Glasgow.

36. Macintyre, S. (1992) The effects of family position and status on health. *Soc. Sci. Med.* **35**: 453–64.

37. Bradby, H. (1996) *Cultural strategies of young women of South Asian origin in Glasgow.* [dissertation]. University of Glasgow. (N).

38. Heath, S. and Dale, A. (1994) Household and family formation in Great Britain: the ethnic dimension. *Pop. Trends.* **77**: 5–13.

39. Garn, S. M., *et al.* (1980) Synchronous fatness changes in husbands and wives. *Am. J. Clin. Nutr.* **32**: 2375–7.

40. Kemmer, D., Anderson, A. S. and Marshall, D. (1995) Eating together for the rest of your life. *Appetite.* **24**: 270.

41. Department of Social Security. (1993) *Households below average income 1979–1990/91.* HMSO, London.

42. Goodman, A. and Webb, S. (1994) For richer for poorer. The changing distribution of income in the UK 1961–91. Institute of Fiscal Studies, London.

43. Dale, A. and Marsh, C. (ed.). (1993) *The 1991 census users guide.* HMSO, London.

44. Government Statistical Service. (1995) *Harmonising questions asked in government surveys.* HMSO, London.

45. Bolton-Smith, C., Smith, W. C. S., Woodward, M. and Tunstall-Pedoe, H. (1991) Nutrient intakes from different social class groups: results from the Scottish Heart Health Study. *Br. J. Nutr.* **65**: 321–35.

46. Anderson, A. and Hunt, K. (1992) Who are the healthy eaters? Eating patterns and health promotion in the west of Scotland. *Hlth. Ed. J.* **51**: 3–10.

47. Cox, B. D., Huppert, F. A. and Whichelow, M. J. (ed.). (1993) *The Health and Lifestyle Survey: seven years on.* Dartmouth, Aldershot.

48. Bhopal, R. S. (1995) Ethnicity, race, health, and research: black box, junk, or enlightened epidemiology? *J. Epid. Comm. Hlth.* **49**: 534.

49. Goldblatt, P. (1990) Mortality and alternative social classifications. In: Goldblatt, P. (ed.). *Longitudinal Study: mortality and social organisation.* HMSO, London. 163–92.

50. Filakti, H. and Fox, J. (1995) Differences in mortality by housing tenure and by car access from the Longitudinal Study. *Pop. Trends.* **81**: 27–30.

51. Davey-Smith, G., Shipley, M. J. and Rose, G. (1990) The magnitude and causes of socio–economic differentials in mortality: further evidence from the Whitehall study. *J. Epid. Comm. Hlth.* **44**: 265–70.

52. Seeley, J., Malamba, S. S., Nunn, A. J., Mulder, D. M., Kengaya-Kayondo, J. F. and Barton, T. G. (1994) Socio–economic status, gender and risk of HIV-1 infection in a rural community in South West Uganda. *Med. Anthr. Q.* **8**: 78–89.

53. Davey-Smith, G. and Shipley, M. J. (1991) Confounding of occupation and smoking: its magnitude and consequences. *Soc. Sci. Med.* **32**: 1297–300.

54. Office of Population Censuses and Surveys. (1994) *English health survey for England 1993.* HMSO, London.

10. Anthropometric measures

Stanley J. Ulijaszek

10.1 Introduction

Anthropometry has an important place in nutritional epidemiology in that it is a sensitive measure of nutritional status because growth and body size are influenced by dietary intake, energy expenditure, and general health[1], and because slowing or cessation of growth is an early response to nutritional inadequacy.[2] However, many anthropometic measures reflect more than the nutritional environment alone, and this can confuse its use and interpretation in epidemiological study. Moreover, the assessment of growth and body size must be made relative to some norm of adequate growth and appropriate body size presumed to be associated with optimal health and nutritional status. This is not straightforward. It is with these two points in mind that this chapter begins with factors which influence growth, body size, and composition, and the validity of the use of international growth references for nutritional assessment.

Although anthropometic measures such as height and weight have been used as broad measures of health status of industrialized populations, of military recruits, and of slaves to the New World going back over 200 years[3,4], it is only over the past 50 years that an emphasis on the correct identification of under-nutrition in less industrialized nations has become important. In industrialized nations, the screening and monitoring of populations prone to obesity has an equally long history. Most recently, there has been increased concern with the growing prevalence of obesity in the rapidly modernizing, less developed nations, as well as the growth of underprivileged groups within industrialized nations suffering from under-nutrition. This has added complexity to the anthropometric study of malnutrition. Further complexity has arisen with greater attention being paid to over-nutrition in children, and under-nutrition in adults: formerly the concern was with under-nutrition in small children (a less developed country problem) and over-nutrition in adults (an industrialized country problem). Now there is also concern with both under-nutrition and over-nutrition in adults in the less developed but modernizing countries as well as over-nutrition in children in both settings.

The use of anthropometric markers of nutritional exposure or outcome ought to be simple but is not. In this chapter, general problems associated with anthropometric measurement are discussed, and appropriate measurements and indices for the assessment of under-nutrition and over-nutrition in children and adults respectively, are considered. Although there are many sources of reference data, discussion of the appropriateness of one set against another is not to be entered, except when giving outline to general principles. A number of reviews: (i) concerned with the use of growth reference data[5–8]; (ii) of different sources of reference data[9–11]; and (iii) giving critiques of the National Center for Health Statistics (1977)[12] references in particular[13–16] have been published, to which readers can turn. Detailed descriptions of how to make anthropometic measurements are given elsewhere[9,11,17–23] and are not considered here.

10.2   Factors influencing growth, and the use of international growth references

The use of anthropometric measurement in public health surveillance arose in the western industrialized nations in the early part of the nineteenth century.[3] This has continued to the present day, in the form of school and community surveys, and is known as auxological epidemiology. From such large scale surveys, anthropometric data has been organized to generate a variety of growth curves, in many countries. Such curves are population based constructs which are used variously for growth monitoring of individuals, health surveillance at population level, as well as in nutritional assessment. The use of indigenously produced growth references for the monitoring of the growth performance of members of the same population is largely uncontroversial. However, the use of growth references developed in industrialized nations for the use of nutritional assessment of individuals in less developed nations is not.

In nutritional epidemiology, anthropometry can be used as a proxy for nutritional status, or as a measure of exposure to nutritional stress. The flaw with this is that poor growth is not the simple outcome of nutritional stress, but of combined stresses, some of which are in synergy with nutritional stress. One of the problems with the use of anthropometry in nutritional assessment is that the measured outcome is due to interactive processes, such as those between under-nutrition and infection, which are still poorly understood. Another is the extent to which deviations in growth are due to a genetic variation, environmental factors, or the interaction of the two.[24,25] Potential sources of variation for any anthropometric phenotype are given in Table 10.1. Genetic and non-genetic effects are not mutually exclusive, and any phenotype will have an interactive component in which, for example, non-additive genetic effects interact with environmental components such as nutrition, infection, and/or the interaction of the two. Given a high quality environment, segmental and body lengths are under a greater degree of genotypic control than any other morphological measurement[25,26], especially measures of fatness.[27] Thus, if it can be accepted conditionally that there is little variation in the genetic potential for pre-adolescent growth in stature between most of the world's populations apart from Asians[28,29], then reference data for skeletal measurements, including stature, are likely to be more reliable as non-pathological yardsticks than are those for soft tissue measurements, including composite measures such as weight.

A reference population may be used as a yardstick for internal comparison of a group or population, with the transformation of data relative to reference values, in the form of Z scores, allowing the pooling of data across a range of ages for data which is very much age-dependent, at least in childhood. Absolute values for the reference popu-lation are less important than the shape of the growth curve, since age-dependent errors can be made if the reference population is odd in some way, or poorly sampled, or the

Table 10.1 Potential sources of variation for an anthropometric phenotype measured at a given age. (Modified from Bouchard.[27])

	Source of variation
Genetic	Additive and non-additive genetic effects
	Paternal and maternal genetic effects
	Effects linked to X or Y chromosomes
	Major gene effect
	Sex-limited effect
	Pleiotropism
Non-genetic	Nutritional status
	Disease state
	Nutrition–infection interactions
	Age or maturity status
	Psychological stress
	Measurement error
	Other environmental factors, e.g. overcrowding

data are badly modelled. There are many sources of potential reference data, but according to Johnston and Ouyang[7], all must fit three criteria of appropriateness. These are that anthropometric reference data must be:

(1) based on a sound theoretical base;
(2) based on an adequate empirical set of observations;
(3) valid for the specific purpose of the evaluation being conducted.

Waterlow *et al.*[30] give more specific minimal criteria for anthropometric reference data, which are given in Box 10.1.

Johnston[31] argues for the use of a single set of references for the sake of international comparability. Pragmatically, this is the best approach in countries which do not have growth references which meet the criteria set in Box 10.1, and where a study requires data on children to be standardized for age. If children of very similar age are to be

Box 10.1 Minimal criteria for anthropometric reference data in nutritional evaluation.[30]

1. The population should be well-nourished.
2. Each age/sex group of the sample should contain at least 200 individuals.
3. The sample should be cross-sectional.
4. Sampling procedures should be defined and reproducible.
5. Measuring procedures should be optimal.
6. Measurements should include all variables used in nutritional evaluation.
7. Raw data and smoothing procedures should be available.

followed prospectively or where a study involves the measurement of adults, it may not be necessary to use growth references at all, merely to make within-group comparisons.

10.3 Raw measurements

Although a wide range of anthropometic measurements can be made[17,18,32], a rather more limited list is appropriate to nutritional anthropometry. These are summarized in Table 10.2. This includes the measures recommended by the WHO[33], but excludes measures giving more limited nutritional information, such as bicristal and biacromial diameters, stem length, and sitting length. Measures added to this list are waist and hip circumferences. All measurements are appropriate to the determination of under-nutrition, while waist and hip ratios are appropriate to the assessment of risk associated with over-nutrition.

The most basic measurements, height and weight, are fundamental to all nutritional anthropometric studies, since they give the simplest measures of attained size and tissue mass. Arm and calf circumferences are used as proxies for soft tissue mass, using the assumption that the cross-sectional area of bone in the upper arm and lower leg is standard across populations, and unaffected by acute under-nutrition. Skinfolds are used as proxies for body fatness although they are measures of subcutaneous fatness only; since body fatness is largely comprised of both subcutaneous and visceral fat, the use of skinfolds assumes that the partitioning of subcutaneous to visceral fat does not vary across nutritional states. The use of waist and hip circumferences give a composite measure of fatness, both subcutaneous and visceral. Lower limb skinfold and circum-ference measures are valuable, since it cannot be assumed that measures of the upper body are also representative of the lower body; upper body–lower body differences in

Table 10.2 Recommended measurements for nutritional anthropometric assessment. (Modified from Lohman et al.[32] and WHO.[33])

Age group (years)	Practical field observations	More detailed observations
0–1	Weight, length	Head and arm circumference; triceps and subscapular skinfolds
1–5	Weight, length (up to 3 yrs), height (over 3 yrs), arm circumference	Triceps and subscapular skinfolds
5–20	Weight, height, arm circumference	Triceps and subscapular skinfolds; medial calf skinfold; calf circumference
Over 20	Weight and height	Arm and calf circumference; triceps; biceps; subscapular, suprailiac, and medial calf skinfolds; waist and hip circumferences (over-nutrition only)

fatness and muscularity are possible in individuals performing hard work on a regular basis, and calf circumference is a useful measure of general muscle loss in response to a reduction in physical activity.[34,35]

10.3.1 Recumbent anthropometry

Brief mention needs to be made of anthropometric measurement of those not able to stand. These may include the elderly, the very sick, and the hospitalized. Recumbent anthropometry has been described by Chumlea[36] for the elderly. Measurements on an immobile sample vary in difficulty. Height and weight become difficult to measure, while it may be possible to measure skinfolds and limb circumferences in the usual way. Where height cannot be measured, knee height can serve as a useful proxy. It is highly correlated with height[37], and height for adults can be calculated using the formulae:[38]

$$\text{Men Stature (cm)} = (2.02 \times \text{knee height}) - (0.04 \times \text{age}) + 64.19 \qquad (10.1)$$
$$\text{Women Stature (cm)} = (1.83 \times \text{knee height}) - (0.24 \times \text{age}) + 84.88 \qquad (10.2)$$

Both sets of estimation equations (height and weight) were developed from a sample of United States elderly people, so caution is advised in their use. Knee height can also be used to predict body weight, in association with measures of calf circumference, mid upper arm circumference, and subscapular skinfold thickness, using the following equations:

$$\text{Men Weight (kg)} = (0.98 \times \text{CC}) + (1.16 \times \text{KH}) + (1.72 \times \text{AC}) \qquad (10.3)$$
$$+ (0.37 \times \text{SS}) - 81.69$$
$$\text{Women Weight (kg)} = (1.27 \times \text{CC}) + (0.87 \times \text{KH}) + (0.98 \times \text{AC}) \qquad (10.4)$$
$$+ (0.4 \times \text{SS}) - 62.35$$

where CC = calf circumference; KH = knee height; AC = arm circumference; and SS = subscapular skinfold.[39] These equations can give only rough estimates, since the 90% error bounds for estimates of stature are about 6.0cm for both men and women[36], while the 95% bounds for weight are 9.0kg for men, and 7.6kg for women, respectively.[39]

10.4 Training, and the accuracy and precision of measurement

It is important that measurements are made accurately. Possible errors are of three sorts: imprecision, undependability, and inaccuracy.[19] Imprecision is due to within- and between-observer measurement differences. Undependability is due to non-nutritional factors that influence the reproducibility of the measurement, such as differences in height of an individual across the day as a consequence of compression of the spinal column. Inaccuracy is a function of instrument error. Some anthropometric measurements are easier to do than other measures of nutritional exposure or outcome, and there is often a tendency to delegate measurement to less-qualified members of the research team. Although there is nothing wrong with this, all potential anthropometrists should receive adequate training from an expert or supervisor to reach a measurable level of expertise prior to survey, and maintain this level of expertise throughout.

Targets for anthropometric assessment have been put forward by Zerfas[40], using a repeat-measures protocol. The trainee and trainer measure the same subjects until the difference between the two of them is good, or at the very least, fair (Table 10.3). These values should not be used uncritically, since differences between trainee and trainer at the upper level of 'goodness' for height, weight, arm circumference, and skinfolds represent different proportions of the absolute measure according to the size of the measurement. Thus, although Zerfas[40] gives values for differences that are possible given the techniques available, a 5mm difference in height measurement is more accurate than the same difference in arm circumference.

Table 10.4 gives the proportion of the total measurement of a model young child and model adult which would be represented by measurement differences between trainee and trainer at the maximum level considered good in the Zerfas scheme.[40] Acceptable measurement difference in length, height, and weight is less than 1% of the measurement, while for arm circumference it is 3.2% and 1.7% for the model child and adult

Table 10.3 Evaluation of measurement error among trainees (after Zerfas, 1985).[40]

| Measurement | Difference between trainee and trainer | | | |
	Good	Fair	Poor	Gross error
Height/length (cm)	0–0.5	0.6–0.9	1.0–1.9	2.0 or >
Weight (kg)	0–0.1	0.2	0.3–0.4	0.5 or >
Arm circumference (cm)	0–0.5	0.6–0.9	1.0–1.9	2.0 or >
Skinfolds (any) (mm)	0–0.9	1.0–1.9	2.0–4.9	5.0 or >

Table 10.4 Proportion of total measurement represented by maximum acceptable measurement difference between trainer and trainee according to Zerfas (1985)[40], for a model young child and model adult

| | Real measurement | | Percentage of real measurement represented by maximum acceptable measurement difference | |
	Child	Adult	Child	Adult
Height/length (cm)	85	170	0.6	0.3
Weight (kg)	12	70	0.8	0.1
Arm circumference (cm)	16	30	3.2	1.7
Triceps skinfold (mm)	8	8	11.2	11.2
Subscapular skinfold (mm)	5	9	18.0	10.0

Table 10.5 Proportion of total measurement represented by maximum acceptable measurement difference between trainee and trainer according to Zerfas (1985)[40], for male children aged 1–1.9 years on the 5th, 50th, and 95th centiles of the combined National Health and Nutrition Examination Surveys I and II.[41]

	Percentage of total measurement due to maximum acceptable measurement difference		
	5th	50th	95th
Length	0.7	0.6	0.5
Weight	1.0	0.9	0.7
Arm circumference	3.5	3.1	2.7
Triceps skinfold	13.8	9.0	5.8
Subscapular skinfold	22.5	15.0	9.0

respectively, while for both triceps and subscapular skinfolds, it is in excess of 10% of the measurement. Thus the Zerfas recommendations[40] for acceptable measurement error are good for length, height, and weight, acceptable for arm circumference, but perhaps too high for skinfolds. This problem is greater in the youngest age groups, and among the smallest children within any age group. For example, Table 10.5 shows the proportion of total measurement represented by the maximum level of measurement difference considered good by Zerfas[40], in male children aged 1–1.9 years on the 5th, 50th, and 95th centiles of the combined National Health and Nutrition Examination Surveys I and II.[41] The proportion of total measurement represented by measurement difference is still 1% or less for length and weight, while for skinfolds, the value is vastly greater in the 5th centile child than in the 95th centile child. At this higher centile, this aspect of measurement error in skinfold measurement is lowest, but error due to correctly finding and measuring the site is greatest.[42] In summary, use of the Zerfas scheme[40] is appropriate for the training of anthropometrists, but should be used with care for measurements other than length, height, and weight. In addition to reducing measurement differences between trainee and trainer, the repeat measurement protocol should report on any systematic biases in measurement and should attempt to reduce these in the course of training, since such bias is likely to be due to differences in measuring technique between the two measurers.

As part of any study, anthropometric estimate of measurement error is needed; the most commonly used measures of this are the technical error of measurement (TEM) and reliability (R).[43] The TEM is obtained by carrying out a number of repeat measurements on the same subject, either by the same observer, or by two or more observers, taking the differences and entering them into an appropriate equation. For within-observer TEM, and between-observer TEM involving two measurers only, the equation is:

$$TEM = \sqrt{\frac{\Sigma D^2}{2N}} \tag{10.5}$$

where D is the difference between measurements, and N is the number of individuals measured. When more than two observers are involved, the equation is more complex:

$$TEM = \sqrt{\sum_{1}^{N} \frac{\left[\sum_{1}^{K} M(n)^2 - \frac{\left(\sum_{1}^{K} M(n) \right)^2}{K} \right]}{N(K-1)}} \tag{10.6}$$

where N is the number of subjects, K is the number of determinations of the variable taken on each subject, and M(n) is the nth replicate of the measurement, where n varies from 1 to K. The units of TEM are the same as the units of the anthropometric measurement in question. Although acceptable maximum TEMs have been recommended as reference values for a variety of measures by Frisancho[41], these ignore the age dependence of TEM[44], and fail to give values for height. The coefficient of reliability, R, ranges from 0–1, and can be calculated using the following equation:

$$R = 1 - \left[\frac{TEM^2}{SD^2} \right] \tag{10.7}$$

where SD is the total between-subject variance for the study, including measurement error. This coefficient reveals what proportion of the between-subject variance in a measured population is free from measurement error. In the case of a measurement with an R of 0.9, 90% of the variance is due to factors other than measurement error. Measures of R can be used to compare the relative reliability of different anthropometric measurements, and to estimate sample size requirements in anthropometric surveys.[43]

Although it might be expected that between-observer TEM should be larger than within-observer TEM, this is not consistently the case.[42] Based on calculations of TEM at set levels of R using published data from the combined NHANES I and II surveys,[41] Ulijaszek and Lourie[42] have put forward references for the upper limits for TEM at two levels of reliability, for males and females respectively. These use total TEM, which in the case of a single observer is equivalent to within-observer TEM. When more than one observer is involved, total TEM can be obtained thus:

$$Total\ TEM = \sqrt{TEM(within)^2 + TEM(between)^2} \tag{10.8}$$

In cross-sectional studies, a proportion of the total variance observed in a population is due to measurement error. The partitioning of the variance can be summarized thus:

$$V(t) = V(b) + V(e,1) + V(e,2) + V(e,3) \tag{10.9}$$

where $V(t)$ = total variance observed; $V(b)$ = biological, or true variance; $V(e,1)$ = variance due to within-observer measurement error; $V(e,2)$ = variance due to between-observer error; and $V(e,3)$ = variance due to instrument error.

Usually, anthropometric data are reported as though $V(t)$ were $V(b)$. Although the two are often so close that for all practical purposes the slight difference does not matter, this is not always the case. If the variances are large, they may mask true biological differences in anthropometric characteristics between groups.

10.5 Anthropometric indices

Anthropometric indices combine two or more raw measures to give more detailed information about nutritional status than single measurements. These include body mass index (BMI), arm muscle area (AMA), arm fat area (AFA), mid arm circumference to height ratio, waist-hip ratio, and triceps to subscapular skinfold ratio. Although the use of head circumference to chest circumference ratio as a measure of chronic energy deficiency was recommended by Jelliffe[45], empirical testing of this association showed the measure to be disappointing.[46] Most indices involving two measurements only can be calculated by dividing the first by the second. Indices involving more than two measurements or more than straightforward division can be calculated in the following way:

Body mass index

$$\text{weight (kg)/height (m)}^2 \tag{10.10}$$

Arm muscle area (AMA)

$$\text{AMA (cm}^2) = (\text{AC} - \pi((\text{BI} + \text{TRI})/2))^2/4\pi \tag{10.11}$$

where AC = arm circumference (cm); BI = biceps skinfold (cm); and TRI = triceps skinfold (cm). Alternatively, if only the triceps skinfold is used[41, 47]:

$$\text{AMA} = (\text{AC} - (\pi \times \text{TRI}))^2/4\pi \tag{10.12}$$

Arm fat area (AFA)[41]

$$\text{AFA} = (\text{AC}^2/4\pi) - \text{AMA} \tag{10.13}$$

Reference centile values exist for BMI[41,48–50], AMA, and AFA.[41] These can be used to calculate Z scores. If data are to be used as continuous variables, tests for skewness and possible transformation for normality of distribution are appropriate after the index has been derived, not before, even if the raw variables making up that index are skewed. Although simple logarithmic transformations should be tried first, an alternative transformation for BMI is $-1/x$.[51] The use of cut-offs for indices is usually only appropriate where the index itself is under test or calibration, such as in studies of BMI as a measure of chronic energy deficiency in adults[52–54], or where the functional significance of the cut-offs used is known.

Sometimes of value in nutritional studies is an estimate of percentage body fat, and of fat-free mass. The first of these can be calculated by estimating body density and subsequently body fat from regression equations of skinfold thicknesses against body density.[21] Such equations have been derived from studies in which the skinfolds of a large number of subjects have been correlated with their body density as estimated by a reference method, such as densitometry or isotope dilution. Although a number of prediction equations have been developed in this way[55–58], none has been extensively or systematically tested among non-European populations.[47] Perhaps the most rigorously tested are those of Durnin and Womersley.[56]

10.6 Treatment of data prior to analysis

When using raw values it is important to ensure that data are not skewed prior to analysis. Most nutritional anthropometric data are skewed, with the exception of height. However, this generalization may not hold true in extremely nutritionally homogeneous samples, population subsets, or in extremely undernourished populations where soft tissue values are not only low but show little variation between individuals. In most cases, the distribution of significantly skewed data can be normalized by a simple logarithmic transformation, either log(10) or log(e).[59] If this does not work, anthropometric alternative transformation for height and arm skinfold is $-1/sqrt(x)$, while for trunk skinfolds $-1/x$ is an alternative.[51] Raw values are usually useful only in the anthropometric characterization of adults, since measurements in growing individuals are extremely age-dependent.

Before age-dependent anthropometric measures can be used, they must be standardized for age. This can be done using centiles, Z scores, or percentage of median growth reference values. The first method is often inappropriate for nutritional assessment in many less developed countries, where the vast majority of children may fall below the lowest centile[14], and where the number of children at extreme degrees of risk cannot be quantified, since centiles below the 3rd are not available for the reference population.[60] Conversion to Z scores relative to a reference population is probably the most common method in current use, and a short review of available software for such conversion is given by Sullivan et al.[61] The choice of reference population depends on the type of study and analysis intended. Many nations have developed reference data for internal use. For studies involving internal comparisons either of the study group or the study group with other groups or populations within the same country, these are perfectly good if the reference data meet the criteria stipulated in Box 10.1. For international comparisons, the growth references adopted by the WHO for international use[12] are the most appropriate[6,7,30], acknowledging the problems associated with them.[10,13–16,29] However, these do not provide a comprehensive set of reference data for a variety of measures, and for investigators wishing to examine or use more than weight and height or length in children, or make comparisons of adult and child anthropometric status, there is a choice of data from a variety of sources, samples, and populations[9,11], including the United States.

The use of percentage of median values for weight, length, and height[9] is another way in which children who are far below the lowest centile of reference values can be counted and categorized. However, this method does not take into account the variability in the relative width of distributions of the growth reference.[14] Thus, a given per cent of median is not constant across ages and does not have the same meaning for different indices.[30,62] However, despite the finding that the classification of nutritional status as per cent of reference median or Z score gives very similar results in predicting death in undernourished children with diarrhoea in young Indian children[63], further studies are needed to determine whether this result generalizes to other populations and conditions.

10.7 Anthropometry and nutritional status

10.7.1 Under-nutrition in children

The most common measures of under-nutrition in children are weight and height, either individually or combined, relative to reference values. Relationships between these measures and morbidity and mortality have been studied in a number of countries, and the functional meanings of low height for age, weight for age, and weight for height are now reasonably understood.[64-66] The two preferred indices are height for age and weight for height, since they can be used to discriminate between acute and chronic under-nutrition.[30,60] In some studies weight measurement is all that is possible, and the use of weight for age is acceptable. Table 10.6 summarizes the usefulness of weight for age, height for age, and weight for height in nutritional assessment in children. Weight for height is useful in populations where date of birth is not recorded or age is not known, and in identifying wasted children, and acutely undernourished children, but cannot identify nutritional stunting. The reverse is true of height for age, which can identify stunting, but not wasting, is insensitive to short term weight change, and is reliant upon reasonable age estimations of the children. Weight for age is also reliant upon reasonable age ascertainment, but is intermediate in its usefulness in identifying stunting, wasting, and acute under-nutrition. Although references for BMI in childhood exist[41,48-50], they have been little used in the assessment of under-nutrition. The likelihood that low BMI is a perfectly good measure of under-nutrition has not been tested prospectively, although a retrospective demographic and anthropometric analysis of 602 populations worldwide has shown BMI to have poor associations with life expectancy at birth for children between 5–10 years, compared with height and weight alone.[1]

Table 10.6 The usefulness of weight and height measures relative to reference data (after Gorstein *et al.* 1994).[15]

	Weight for age	Height for age	Weight for heigh
Usefulness in populations where age is unknown or inaccurate	4	4	1
Usefulness in identifying wasted children	3	4	1
Usefulness in identifying stunted children	2	1	4
Sensitivity to weight change over a short time frame	2	4	1

Arm circumference is a composite measure of muscle, fat, and bone. It is particularly useful for the assessment of under-nutrition in the age group 1–5 years, where in well-nourished children, the age related increase in arm muscle is more or less compensated for by an age-related decline in arm subcutaneous fat, making it a roughly age-independent measure of nutritional status for this age group.[69] Age-independent cut-offs have been recommended and used for the rapid assessment of under-nutrition under emergency situations, or where the ages of children are uncertain. An alternative is to use Z scores of arm circumference, using reference values of Frisancho[41] for children above the age of one year. In this way, it is possible to assess nutritional status with arm circumference beyond the age of five years. Skinfolds are useful in more detailed studies, but investigators should be aware of the high degree of inaccuracy in measurement and the difficulty of estimating differences in skinfold values in longitudinal studies, and use them only when any of these criteria are met: (i) where skinfolds are likely to give useful information above that of weight, length/height, and arm circumference; (ii) when the expected change in values or sample size is large enough for statistical treatment. A way in which anthropometric measurement error can be removed from data for use in cross-sectional analysis is given in Ulijaszek and Lourie.[42]

Other measures of under-nutrition in children include medial calf skinfold and calf circumference. Although calf circumference has been shown to be better associated with clinical signs of protein—energy malnutrition than arm circumference in young Indian children[68], this has not been widely used. However, the use of calf measures in older children may be appropriate for more detailed investigations and where children are engaged in some type of productive physical work, as is common in various parts of the developing world[69], where upper body measurements alone may not be representative of the whole body. Head circumference is commonly used in paediatric practice to detect pathological conditions such as hydrocephalus or microcephaly.[9] It can also be used as a measure of chronic under-nutrition during the first two years of life[11], relative to reference data such as those created using measurements of healthy United States children.[70] Head circumference for age is not sensitive to acute under-nutrition.[71] Large head circumference at birth, relative to length[70] or arm circumference[72] is suggestive of intra-uterine growth retardation, if it is known that the child was born neither pre- or post-mature. Indices such as AMA, AFA from arm circumference, and skinfold measures can also be used to assess nutritional status in children.[11,41]

10.7.2 Under-nutrition in adults

The most common anthropometric measures of under-nutrition in adults are weight, and weight for height. Of indices of weight for height, the most commonly used is BMI, although a retrospective demographic and anthropometric study of 602 populations showed adult BMI to have weaker associations with life expectancy at birth than either height or weight alone.[1] Degrees of underweight have been defined as 'chronic energy deficiency' (CED) according to level of BMI, and cut-offs of 18.5, 17, and 16 have been put forward as defining mild, moderate and severe chronic energy deficiency, respectively.[73,74] It is perhaps premature to use cut-offs of low BMI in any definitive sense, since the relationships between the recommended cut-offs of BMI and aspects of function such as physical work capacity and morbidity are at an early stage of evaluation, and results are not clear-cut. For example, the BMI below cut-off of 18.5 is associated with higher morbidity in Pakistan, but not in the Philippines and Ghana[53] while in Calcutta, a cut-off below 16 is associated with higher morbidity.[52] Furthermore, BMI below 18.5 shows little systematic association with lactation performance across 41 study populations.[75] Some of the challenges associated with the use of BMI for classifying CED are summarized in Box 10.2.

It is unclear whether the normal range of BMI varies with age, but this might well be so.[76] The health risk associated with low BMI is also likely to vary with the type of environmental hazard, be it type of, and exposure to, the disease environment, and the extent and duration of under-nutrition. In Western populations, for example, low BMI is most commonly associated with higher lung cancer risk, and smoking[77-79], while high mortality at low BMI among African Americans is strongly associated with smoking.[80] In the rapidly modernizing, less developed countries where life expectancy at birth is increasing, it is likely that nutritional anthropometry will become important in the study of lung cancer in adult populations where the prevalence of both under-nutrition and smoking is high. The functional meaning of any given level of BMI is also likely to vary with gender[1,54] and population type, inasmuch as there are some population-specific differences in body proportion and composition.[81] However, these are unlikely to be important in epidemiological studies in the range 20—25.[81] Although pragmatically BMI may be the most useful measure for assessing the extent of chronic energy deficiency in adults[82], its use in epidemiological studies should still be circumspect.

AMA is a more sensitive index of health than BMI in Sarawaki adults[54], while in Calcutta, a logistic regression model showed BMI to be a more sensitive index of morbidity than either AFA, percent body fat, or AMA.[52] Furthermore, to discriminate between the body composition changes in some epidemiological studies it is probably important to incorporate at least one other measurement, such as triceps skinfold, or

---

Box 10.2 Problems associated with the use of BMI for classifying chronic energy deficiency in adults, in epidemiological studies (modified from James, 1994).[129]

Suitability of cut-offs:
- gender-specific cut-offs?
- age dependency?
- thresholds vary with environmental hazards?
- between-population differences in body composition?
- additional anthropometric criteria needed for refining specificity (e.g. arm circumference)?

Suitability for use:
- in identifying and categorizing populations and groups at risk
- according to type of risk, morbidity, type of morbidity, mortality
- in predicting pregnancy outcome
- in studies of work and economic performance indicators associated with nutritional status

better, triceps skinfold and arm circumference. In populations where hard physical work is the norm, upper body measurements of fatness and muscularity may not be typical of the whole body, and measurements of medial calf skinfold and calf circumference may be appropriate.

10.7.3 Over-nutrition in children

Anthropometric indices of over-nutrition in childhood include weight, height, as well as various circumferences and skinfolds. Weight, unadjusted for height, gives limited information about the extent of adiposity, and is useful only when used longitudinally. Many weight-for-height indices have been used to assess obesity in childhood, most having a height bias.[83] BMI reference data can be used to identify and categorize individuals with high values. Body fat is better correlated with BMI than other weight–height indices at all ages in childhood[84], while children with a tendency to early rebound in increasing BMI also have a tendency to remain obese into adult life.[85] Furthermore, BMI has been shown to be a better index than weight over height, weight over height cubed, and weight over height to the power of π from birth to 20 years of age, on the basis of best correlations with weight and skinfolds, but poorest correlations, with height.[51] Thus, BMI is the best weight–height index for the assessment of over-nutrition in childhood[84], after transformation into Z scores.

In a similar way, Z scores of triceps and/or subscapular skinfolds, or AFA using reference data[41], can be used to define individuals or groups of children according to relative fatness. The triceps skinfold is the site most frequently chosen for a single indirect measure of body fat[11], and gives a good estimate of percentage body fat in children[86], and the most representative measure of subcutaneous fat for boys up to the age of 16 years.[87] However, distribution of subcutaneous fatness varies by ethnicity[88] as well as gender and age, and it is not clear whether the above finding, which is based on data collected on Europeans, generalizes to non-European populations. Thus it cannot be assumed that a single skinfold taken at the triceps site is representative of general subcutaneous fatness in all populations.

10.7.4 Over-nutrition in adults

Weight and height are the most common measures of nutritional status in adults, often combined as weight-for-height indices such as BMI. In Western populations, various studies have reported an inverse relationship between height and risk of cardiovascular morbidity and mortality in men[89–93] as well as women.[94,95] Furthermore, various studies show positive relationships between height and breast cancer, and negative associations between BMI and breast cancer in pre-menopausal women.[96] More generally, the association of mortality risk with BMI follows a J-shaped curve, with increased mortality for those with very low BMI, and for those with high BMI.[97,98] Similar relationships are also likely to hold for populations in less developed countries, although the causes of increased mortality at low BMI and relative weight (weight/ desirable weight) were found to be the best indices of fatness in men, with lowest correlations with height and highest correlations with percentage body weight as fat and fat mass in adult males.[99] Furthermore, BMI was shown to have the highest correlation with skinfolds in both men and women in the United States Health and Nutrition Examination Survey.[100] Although the BMI is easy to use, and in adults a simple range of values can be used to define the range of normality, this has changed with time. In 1985, this range was set at 18.6–23.9 for men and 20.0–24.9 for women.[101] In 1988, cut-offs of 18.5–24.9 for both men and women were put forward.[73] Furthermore, different cut-offs defining levels of obesity have been put forward in Britain[102], the United States[103], and Canada.[104] Since such cut-offs are meant for clinical or public health screening and are usually based on curvilinear relationships between BMI and mortality risk, their exact values are to some extent arbitrary, may not generalize across populations, and may be of limited utility in epidemiological studies, unless the aim is to test the cut-offs in different populations or circumstances. If it is important to classify a population according to fatness as assessed by this index, it is more appropriate to use Z scores of BMI against one of the references available, to divide the group into low, moderate, and high subgroups; or to use the index as a continuous variable in a multifactorial model. If the data are to be used with parametric statistics, then they should be tested for skewness and transformed if necessary. Although useful, BMI, and all weight—height indices should be used cautiously, since they cannot distinguish between overweight due to muscle, bone, water, or fat.[99] The precise relationship between BMI and percentage body fat is not clearly established[11], BMI being significantly correlated with lean body mass, frame size, and sitting height as well as body fat.[105,106]

In conjunction with measures of height and weight, skinfolds[109], and waist and hip circumference[107], measurements have been recommended for the assessment of obesity in adults. Fat distribution across the body in association with obesity has been shown to be related to risk of non-insulin dependent diabetes mellitus[108–111], hypertension[112–115], cardiovascular disease[116–120], and breast cancer.[121] Skinfolds are useful additional measures in cancer epidemiology as more specific measures of fatness[122], measuring a different dimension of fat distribution to circumference indices.[123] Table 10.7 gives

Table 10.7 Applied considerations for the use of skinfold measurements in cancer epidemiology studies (after Micozzi).[122]

Skinfold	Representative of:	Ease[a]	Frequency[b]	Coefficient of reliability[c]
Triceps	Upper extremity	1	1	>0.95
Subscapular	Upper trunk	2	1	0.90–0.95
Midaxillary	Upper trunk	2	3	0.90–0.95
Suprailiac	Lower trunk	3	2	<0.90
Medial calf	Lower extremity	3	3	>0.95

[a] Ease of measurement: (1) good, involving minimal amount of undressing, short time to make measurement, limited technical difficulty, little discomfort for subject or observer; (2) intermediate for all factors; (3) maximum amount of undressing, long time required for measurement, significant technical difficulty, greatest discomfort for subject or observer.

[b] Relative frequency of usage in epidemiological studies: (1) commonly used, popular; (2) less commonly used; (3) rarely used, uncommon.

[c] Coefficeint of reliability: usual error as a proportion of total variance subtracted from 1. A value of less than 0.90 is poor.

applied considerations for the selection of skinfold measurements for such studies. These vary in their ease of measurement and reliability, the most common measures being triceps and subscapular skinfold. These two measures are useful in combination for assessing the relationship between truncal and peripheral fatness and hypertension[112] and cardiovascular disease.[120,124,125] On the basis of Blair et al.'s study[112], it has been recommended that triceps and subscapular skinfolds should be used above all others in the study of ischaemic heart disease.[126]

The waist–hip ratio appears to be little influenced by genetics[123,127] and has been shown to be associated with the incidence of stroke[117], NIDDM[110,113] and coronary heart disease[117], although relationships with blood pressure vary between studies, ranging from good to non-existent.[115] In general, where relationships have been found, greater waist fatness relative to the hips is associated with disease risk.[126] The value of waist—hip ratio associated with increased morbidity risk varies with gender, age, and type of morbidity[126], and centiles defining low, moderate, high, and very high risk are given in Gray and Bray.[128]

10.8 Concluding remarks

There are good reasons for incorporating anthropometric measures in studies of nutritional epidemiology. Anthropometry is usually portable, cheap, quick, and easy to do. However, this ease is deceptive and often a source of error, if the measurer is poorly chosen and/or trained. Care is needed to determine:

(1) the anthropometric measurements to be made;
(2) whether or not measurements are combined as indices;
(3) where necessary, the way in which data are compared with the growth references;
(4) which growth references are used for comparison, again where necessary;
(5) whether variables are to be used categorically (e.g. defining subgroups as under or overnourished) or as continuous variables;
(6) if they are to be used as continuous variables, whether they require normalization.

The combination of choices depends on the nature of the study; whether the research question involves anthropometric estimation of:

(1) undernutrition, overnutrition, or both;
(2) fat patterning;
(3) children or adults;
(4) men, women, or both.

There is no one right answer, nor is it likely that there ever will be. As nutritional epidemiological studies must be shaped to take into consideration changing nutritional circumstances globally, including the nutritional and health transition currently taking place in many less developed nations, so must the anthropometric methods employed.

References

1. Gage, T. B. and Zansky, S. M. (1995) Anthropometric indicators of nutritional status and level of mortality. *Am. J. Hum. Biol.* **7**: 679–91.
2. Martorell, R. (1985) Child growth retardation: a discussion of its causes and its relationship to health. In: Blaxter, K. and Waterlow, J. C. (ed.). *Nutritional adaptation in man.* John Libbey, London. 13–30.
3. Tanner, J. M. (1981) *A history of the study of human growth.* Cambridge University Press, Cambridge.
4. Floud, R., Wachter, K. and Gregory, A. (1990) *Height, health and history. Nutritional status in the United Kingdom, 1750–1980.* Cambridge University Press, Cambridge.
5. Stephenson, L. S., Latham, M. C., and Jansen, A. (1983) *A comparison of growth standards. Similarities between NCHS, Harvard, Denver and privileged African children and differences with Kenyan rural children.* Cornell International Nutrition Monograph Series No. 12 Cornell University, Ithaca, New York.
6. Sullivan, K., Trowbridge, F., Gorstein, J. and Pradilla, A. (1991) Growth references. *Lancet.* **337**: 1420–1.
7. Johnston, F. E. and Ouyang, Z. (1991) Choosing appropriate reference data for the anthropometric assessment of nutritional status. In: Himes, J. H. (ed.). *Anthropometric assessment of nutritional status.* Wiley-Liss, New York. 337–46.
8. Cole, T. J. (1993) The use and construction of anthropometric growth reference standards. *Nutr. Res. Rev.* **6**: 19–50.
9. Jelliffe, D. B. and Jelliffe, E. F. P. (1989) *Community nutritional assessment.* Oxford University Press, Oxford.
10. Cole, T. J. (1989) The British, American NCHS, and Dutch weight standards compared using the LMS method. *Am. J. Hum. Biol.* **1**: 397–408.
11. Gibson R. S. (1990) *Principles of nutritional assessment.* Oxford University Press, Oxford.
12. National Center for Health Statistics. (1977) *NCHS Growth curves for children. Birth–18 years.* US Department of Health, Education and Welfare Publication No. (PHS) 78–1650. National Center for Health Statistics, Hyattsville, Maryland.
13. Cole, T. J. (1985) A critique of the NCHS weight for height standard. *Hum. Biol.* **57**: 183–96.
14. Dibley, M. J., Goldsby, J. B., Staehling, N. W. and Trowbridge, F. L. (1987) Development of normalised curves for the international growth reference: historical and technical considerations. *Am. J. Clin. Nutr.* **46**: 736–48.
15. Gorstein, J., Sullivan, K., Yip, R., de Onis, M., Trowbridge, F., Fajans, P. and et al. (1994) Issues in the assessment of nutritional status using anthropometry. *Bull. WHO.* **72**: 273–83.
16. Macfarlane, S. B. J. (1994) A universal growth reference or fool's gold? *Eur. J. Clin. Nutr.* **49**: 745–53.
17. Weiner, J. S. and Lourie, J. A. (1969) *Practical human biology.* Blackwell Scientific Publications, Oxford.
18. Weiner, J. S. and Lourie, J. A. (1981) *Practical human biology.* Academic Press, London.
19. Heymsfield, S. B., McManus, C. B., Seitz, S. B., Nixon, D. W. and Andrews, J. S. (1984) Anthropometric assessment of adult protein–energy malnutrition. In: Wright, R. A., Heymsfield, S. and McManus, C. B. (ed.) *Nutritional assessment.* Blackwell Scientific Publications, Inc., Boston. 27–81.
20. Cameron, N. (1986) The methods of auxological anthropometry. In: Falkner, F. and Tanner, J. M. (ed.) *Human growth. A comprehensive treatise.* Vol. 3. Plenum Press, New York. 3–46.
21. Lohman, T. G. (1988) Anthropometry and body composition. In: Lohman, T. G., Roche, A. F. and Martorell, R. (ed.) *Anthropometric standardization reference manual.* Human Kinetics Books, Champaign, Illinois. 125–9.

22. Fidanza, F. I. (ed.) (1991) *Nutritional status assessment*. Chapman and Hall, London.
23. Malina, R. M., and Bouchard, C. (1991) *Growth, maturation, and physical activity*. Human Kinetics Books, Champaign, Illinois.
24. Mora, J. O. (1986) The pitfalls of anthropometry. In: Taylor, T. G., and Jenkins, N. K. (ed.) *Proceedings of the XIII International Congress of Nutrition*. John Libbey, London 270–3.
25. Bouchard, C.. (1991) Genetic aspects of anthropometric dimensions relevant to assessment of nutritional status. In: Himes, J. H. (ed.) *Anthropometric assessment of nutritional status*. Wiley Liss, Inc., New York. 213–31.
26. Howells, W. W. (1953) Correlations of brothers in factor scores. *Am. J. Phys. Anthropol.* **11**: 121–40.
27. Bouchard, C. and Perusse, L. (1988) Heredity and body fat. *Ann. Rev. Nutr.* **8**: 259–77.
28. Martorell, R., Mendoza F. and Castillo, R. (1988) Poverty and stature in children. In: Waterlow, J. C. (ed.) *Linear growth retardation in less developed countries*. Nestle Foundation Nutrition Workshop Series Vol 14. Raven Press, New York. 57–73.
29. Ulijaszek, S. J. (1994) Between-population variation in pre-adolescent growth. *Eur. J. Clin. Nutr.* **48** (Suppl. 1): S5–S14.
30. Waterlow, J. C., Buzina, A., Keller, W., Lane, J. M., Nichaman, M. Z. and Tanner, J. M. (1977) The presentation and use of height and weight data for comparing the nutritional status of groups of children under the age of 10 years. *Bull. WHO.* **55**: 489–98.
31. Johnston, F. E. (1986) Reference data for physical growth in nutritional anthropology. In: Quandt, S. A. and Ritenbaugh, C. (ed.) *Training manual in nutritional anthropology*. American Anthropological Association, Washington, DC 60–5.
32. Lohman, T. G., Roche, A. F. and Martorell, R. (ed.) (1988) *Anthropometric standardization reference manual*. Human Kinetics Books, Champaign, Illinois.
33. World Health Organization (1970) *Nutritional status of populations A manual on anthropometric appraisal of trends*. Document No. Nutr./70.129. World Health Organization, Geneva.
34. Fentem, P. H., Jones, P. R. M., MacDonald, I. C. and Scriven, P. M. (1976) Changes in the body composition of elderly men following retirement from the steel industry. *J. Physiol.* **258**: 29P—30P.
35. Patrick, J. M., Bassey, E. .J and Fentem, P. H. (1982) Changes in body fat and muscle in manual workers at the retirement. *Eur. J. Appl. Physiol.* **49**: 187–96.
36. Chumlea, W. C. (1991) Anthropometric assessment of nutritional status in the elderly. In: Himes, J. H. (ed.) *Anthropometric assessment of nutritional status*. Wiley-Liss, New York 399–418.
37. Zoreb, P. A., Prime, F. J. and Harrison, A. (1963) Estimation of height from tibial length. *Lancet.* **1**: 195–6.
38. Chumlea, W. C., Roche, A. F. and Steinbaugh, M. L. (1985) Estimating stature from knee height for persons 60 to 90 years of age. *J. Am. Geriatr. Soc.* **33**: 116–20.
39. Chumlea, W. C., Guo, S. Roche, A. F. and Steinbaugh, M. L. (1988) Prediction of body weight for the non-ambulatory elderly. *J. Am. Diet. Assoc.* **88**: 564–88.
40. Zerfas, A. J. (1985) *Checking continuous measures: Manual for anthropometry*. Division of Epidemiology, School of Public Health, University of California, Los Angeles.
41. Frisancho, A. R. (1990) *Anthropometric standards for the assessment of growth and nutritional status*. University of Michigan Press, Ann Arbor.
42. Ulijaszek, S. J. and Lourie, J. A. (1994) Intra-and inter-observer error in anthropometric measurement. In: Ulijaszek, S. J. and Mascie-Taylor, C. G. N. (ed.) *Anthropometry: the individual and the population*. Cambridge University Press, Cambridge 30–55.
43. Mueller W. H., and Martorell R. (1988) Reliability and accuracy of measurement. In: Lohman, T. G., Roche, A. F. and Martorell, R. (ed.) *Anthropometric standardization reference manual*. Human Kinetics Books, Champaign, Illinois 83–6.

44. Lourie, J. A. and Ulijaszek, S. J. (1992) Observer error in anthropometry: age dependence of technical error of measurement. *Am. J. Phys. Anthropol.* **14**(Suppl): 113.
45. Jelliffe, D. B. (1966) *The assessment of nutritional status of the community*. World Health Organization Monograph Series No 53 WHO, Geneva.
46. Martorell, R., Yarbrough, C., Malina, R. M., Habicht, J-P., Lechtig, A. and Klein, R. E. (1975) The head circumference/chest circumference ratio in mild-to-moderate protein-calorie malnutrition. *Environ. Child. Hlth.* **21**: 203–7.
47. Norgan, N. G. and Jones, P. R. M. (1990) Anthropometry and body composition. In: Collins, K. J. (ed.) *Handbook of methods for the measurement of work performance, physical fitness and energy expenditure in tropical populations*. International Union of Biological Sciences, Paris. 95–115.
48. Cronk, C. E., Roche, A. F., Kent, R., Berkey, C., Reed, R. B., Valadian, I., *et al.* (1982) Longitudinal trends and continuity in weight/stature from 3 months to 18 years. *Hum. Biol.* **54**: 729–49.
49. Rolland-Cachera, M. F., Sempe, M., Guilloud-Bataille, M., Patois, E., Pequignot-Guggenbuhl, F. and Fautrad, V. (1982) Adiposity indices in children. *Am. J. Clin. Nutr.* **36**: 178–84.
50. Rolland-Cachera, M. F., Cole, T. J., Sempe, M., Tichet, J., Rossignol, C. and Charraud, A (1991) Body mass index variations: centiles from birth to 87 years. *Eur. J. Clin. Nutr.* **45**: 13–21.
51. Gasser, T. H., Ziegler, P., Seifert, B., Prader, A., Molinar, L., and Largo, R. (1994) Measures of body mass and of obesity from infancy to adulthood and their appropriate transformation. *Ann. Hum. Biol.* **21**: 111–25.
52. Campbell, P. and Ulijaszek, S. J. (1994) Relationships between anthropometry and retrospective morbidity in poor men in Calcutta, India. *Eur. J. Clin. Nutr.* **48**: 507–12.
53. Kennedy, E. and Garcia, M. (1994) BMI and economic productivity. *Eur. J. Clin. Nutr.* **48** (Suppl. 3): S45–S53.
54. Strickland, S. S. and Ulijaszek, S. J. (1994) Body mass index and illness in Sarawak. *Eur. J. Clin. Nutr.* **48** (Suppl. 3): S98–S109.
55. Sloan, A. W. (1967) Estimation of body fat in young men. *J. Appl. Physiol.* **23**: 311–15.
56. Durnin, J. V. G. A. and Womersley, J. (1974) Body fat assessed from total body density and its estimation from skinfold thickness: measurements on 481 men and women aged from 16 to 72 years. *Br. J. Nutr.* **32**: 77–97.
57. Jackson, A. S. and Pollock, M. L. (1974) Generalised equations for predicting body density of men. *Br. J. Nutr.* **40**: 497–504.
58. Jackson, A. S., Pollock, M. L. and Ward, A. (1980) Generalised equations for predicting body density of women. *Med. Sci. in Sports and Exercise* **12**: 175–82.
59. Mascie-Taylor, C. G. N. (1994) Statistical issues in anthropometry. In: Ulijaszek, S. J. and Mascie-Taylor, C. G. N. I.(ed.) *Anthropometry: the individual and the population*. Cambridge University Press, Cambridge. 56–77.
60. World Health Organization Working Group. (1986) Use and interpretation of anthropometric indicators of nutritional status. *Bull. WHO.* **64**: 929–41.
61. Sullivan, K. M., Garstein, J., Dean, A. G. and Fichtner, R. R. (1990) The use and availability of anthropometric software. *Food Nutr. Bull.* **12**: 116–19.
62. Keller, W. and Fillmore, C. M. (1983) Prevalence of protein energy malnutrition. *World Health Stat Q* **36**: 129–67.
63. Sachdev, H. P. S., Satyanarayana, L., Shiv Kumar, and Puri, R. K. (1992) Classification of nutritional status as 'Z score' or per cent of reference median – does it alter mortality prediction in malnourished children? *Int. J. Epid.* **21**: 916–21.
64. Pelletier, D. L. (1991) *Relationships between child anthropometry and mortality in developing countries: implications for policy, programs and future research*. Cornell Food and Nutrition Policy Program Monograph No 12. Cornell University, Ithaca, New York.

65. Vella, V., Tomkins, A., Borghesi, A., Migliori, G. B., Adriko, B. C. and Crevatin, E. (1992) Determinants of child nutrition and mortality in north-west Uganda. *Bull. WHO.* **70**: 637–43.
66. Schroeder, D. G. and Brown, K. H. (1994) Nutritional status as a predictor of child survival: summarizing the association and quantifying its global impact. *Bull. WHO.* **72**: 569–79.
67. Burgess, H. J. L. and Burgess, A. P. (1969) A modified standard for mid-upper arm circumference in young children. *J. Trop. Pediat.* **15**: 189.
68. Visweswara Rae, K., Reddy, P. J. and Narayan, T. P. (1978) A comparison of arm and calf circumferences as indicators of protein–calorie malnutrition in early childhood. *Ind. J. Nutr. Diet.* **17**: 25.
69. Strickland, S. S. (1990) Traditional economies and patterns of nutritional disease. In: Harrison, G. A. and Waterlow, J. C. (ed.) *Diet and disease in traditional and developing societies.* Cambridge University Press, Cambridge 209–39.
70. Hamill, P. V. V., Drizd, T. A., Johnson, C. L., Reed, R. B., Roche, A. F. and Moore, W. M. (1979) Physical growth: National Center for Health Statistics percentiles. *Am. J. Clin. Nutr.* **32**: 607–29.
71. Yarbrough, C., Habicht, J-P., Martorell, R. and Klein, R. E .(1974) Anthropometry as an index of nutritional status. In: Roche, A. F. and Falkner, R. (ed.) *Nutrition and malnutrition: identification and measurement* Plenum Press, New York 15–26.
72. Sasanow, S. R., Georgieff, M. K. and Periera, G. R. (1986) Mid-arm circumference and mid-arm/head circumference ratios: standard curves for anthropometric assessment of neonatal nutritional status. *J. Pediat.* **109**: 311–15.
73. James, W. P. T., Ferro-Luzzi, A. and Waterlow, J. C. (1988) Definition of chronic energy deficiency in adults. *Eur. J. Clin. Nutr.* **42**: 969–81.
74. Ferro-Luzzi, A., Sette, S., Franklin, M. F. and James, W. P. T. (1992) A simplified approach to assessing adult chronic energy deficiency. *Eur. J. Clin. Nutr.* **46**: 173–86.
75. Prentice, A. M., Goldberg, G. R. and Prentice, A. (1994) Body mass index and lactation performance. *Eur. J. Clin. Nutr.* **48** (Suppl 3): S78–S86.
76. James, W. P. T. and Francois, P. (1994) The choice of cut-off point for distinguishing normal body weights from underweight or 'chronic energy deficiency' in adults. *Eur. J. Clin. Nutr.* **48**(Suppl 3): S179–S184.
77. Knekt, P., Heliovaara, M., Rissanen, A., *et al.* (1991) Leanness and lung-cancer risk. *Int. J. Cancer* **49**: 208–13.
78. Kabat, G. C. and Wynder, E. L. (1992) Body mass index and lung cancer risk. *Am. J. Epid.* **135**: 769–86.
79. Goodman, M. T. and Wilkens, L. R. (1993) Relation of body size and the risk of lung cancer. *Nutr. Cancer* **20**: 179–86.
80. Stevens, J., Keil, J. E., Rust, P. F., Verdugo, R. R., Davis, C. E., Tyroler, H. A., *et al.* (1992) Body mass index and body girths as predictors of mortality in black and white men. *Am. J. Epid.* **135**: 1137–46.
81. Norgan, N. G. (1994) Population differences in body composition in relation to the body mass index. *Eur. J. Clin. Nutr.* **48** (Suppl. 3): S10–S27.
82. Shetty, P. S. and James, W. P. T. (1994) *Body mass index. A measure of chronic energy deficiency in adults.* FAO Food and Nutrition Paper No 56. Food and Agriculture Organization of the United Nations, Rome.
83. Poskitt, E. M. E. (1995) Assessment of body composition in the obese. In: Davies, P. S. W. and Cole, T. J. (ed.) *Body composition techniques in health and disease.* Cambridge University Press, Cambridge 146–65.
84. Cole, T. J. (1991) Weight-stature indices to measure underweight, overweight and obesity. In: Himes, J. H. (ed.) *Anthropometric assessment of nutritional status.* Wiley-Liss, New York 83–111.

85. Rolland-Chachera, M-F., Deheeger, M., Bellisle, F., Sempe, M., Guilloud-Bataille, M. and Patois, E. (1984) Adiposity rebound in children: a simple indicator for predicting obesity. *Am. J. Clin. Nutr.* **39**: 129–35.

86. Roche, A. F., Siervogel, R. M., Chumlea, W. C. and Webb, P. (1981) Grading body fatness from limited anthropometric data. *Am. J. Clin. Nutr.* **34**: 2831–8.

87. Seirvogel, R. M., Roche, A. F., Himes, J. H., Chumlea, W. C. and McCammon, R. (1982) Subcutaneous fat distribution in males and females from 1 to 39 years of age. *Am. J. Clin. Nutr.* **36**: 162–71.

88. Eveleth, P. B. and Tanner, J. M. (1976) *Worldwide variation in human growth.* Cambridge University Press, Cambridge

89. Paffenbarger, R. S., Wolf, P. A., Notkin, J. and Thorne, M. C. (1966) Chronic disease in former college students. I. Early precursors of fatal coronary heart disease. *Am. J. Epid.* **83**: 314–28.

90. Morris, J. N., Kagan, A., Pattison, D. C. and Gardner, M. J. (1966) Incidence and prediction of ischaemic heart disease in London busmen. *Lancet* **2**: 553–9.

91. Marmot, M. G., Rose, G., Shipley, M., *et al.* (1978) Employment grade and coronary heart disease in British civil servants *J. Epid. Comm. Hlth.* **32**:244–9.

92. Davey Smith, G., Shipley, M. J. and Rose, G. (1990) Magnitude and causes of socio–economic differentials in mortality: further evidence from the Whitehall Study. *J. Epid. Community Hlth.* **44**: 265–70.

93. Rimm, E. R., Stampfer, M. J., Giovannucci, E., Ascherio, A., Spiegelman, D., Colditz, G. A., *et al.* (1995) Body size and fat distribution as predictors of coronary heart disease among middle-aged and older US men. *Am. J. Epid.* **141**: 1117–27.

94. Palmer, J. R., Rosenberg, L. and Shapiro, S. (1990) Stature and the risk of myocardial infarction in women. *Am. J. Epid.* **132**: 27–32.

95. Rich-Edwards, J. W., Manson, J. A. E., Stampfer, M .J., Colditz, G. A., Willett, W. C., Rosner, B., *et al.* (1995) Height and the risk of cardiovascular disease in women. *Am. J. Epid.* **142**: 909–17.

96. Hunter, D. J. and Willett, W. C. (1993) Diet, body size, and breast cancer. *Epid. Rev.* **15**: 110–32.

97. Waaler, H. T. (1984) Height, weight and mortality. The Norwegian experience. *Acta. Med. Scand.* **215**(Suppl.679): 1–56.

98. Bray, G. A. (1987) Overweight is risking fate. Definition, classification, prevalence, and risks. *Ann. NY Acad. Sci.* **499**: 14–28.

99. Norgan, N. G. and Ferro-Luzzi, A. (1982) Weight–height indices as estimators of fatness in men. *Hum. Nutr.: Clin. Nutr.* **36C**: 363–72.

100. Frisancho, A. R. and Flegal, P. N. (1982) Relative merits of old and new indices of body mass with reference to skinfold thickness *Am. J. Clin. Nutr.* **36**: 697–9.

101. FAO/WHO/UNU (1985) *Energy and protein requirements.* World Health Organization Technical Report Series 724. World Health Organization, Geneva.

102. Garrow, J. S. (1983) Indices of adiposity. *Nutr. Abs. Rev.* **53**: 697–708.

103. Kuczmarski, R. J. and Johnson, C. (1991) National nutritional surveys assessing anthropometric status. In: Himes, J H (ed). *Anthropometric assessment of nutritional status.* Wiley-Liss, New York 319–35.

104. Health and Welfare Canada (1988) *Canadian guidelines for healthy weights.* Report of an Expert Committee convened by Health Promotion Directorate, Health Services and Promotion Branch, Health and Welfare, Ottawa.

105. Micozzi, M. S., Albanes, D., Jones, D. Y. and Chumlea, W. C. (1986) Correlations of body mass indices with weight, stature, and body composition in men and women NHANES I and II. *Am. J. Clin. Nutr.* **44**: 725–31.

106. Micozzi, M. S. and Albanes, D. (1987) Expanding on the three limitations of body mass indices. *Am. J. Clin. Nutr.* **46**: 376–7.

107. Bjorntorp, P. (1987) Classification of obese patients and complications related to the distribution of surplus fat. *Am. J. Clin. Nutr.* **45**: 1120–5.

108. Evans, D. J., Hoffman, R. G., Kalkoff, R. K. and Kissebah, A. H. (1984) Relationships of body fat topography to insulin sensitivity and metabolic profiles in pre-menopausal women. *Metabol.* **33**: 68–75.

109. Lev-Ran, A. and Hill, L. R. (1987) Different body-fat distributions in IDDM and NIDDM. *Diabetes Care* **10**: 491–4.

110. Dowse, G. K., Zimmet, P. Z., Gareeboo, H., Alberti, K. G. M. M., Toumilehto, J., Finch, C. F., *et al.* (1991) Abdominal obesity and physical inactivity are risk factors for NIDDM and impaired glucose tolerance in Indian, Creole, and Chinese Mauritians. *Diabetes Care* **14**: 271–82.

111. Colman, E., Toth, M. J., Katzel, L. I., Fonong, T., Gardener, A. W. and Poehlman, E. T. (1995) Body fatness and waist circumference are independent predictors of the age-associated increase in fasting insulin levels in healthy men and women. *Int. J. Obes.* **19**: 798–803.

112. Blair, D., Habicht, J-P., Simms, E. A. H., Sylvester, D. and Abraham, S. (1984) Evidence for an increased risk for hypertension with centrally located body fat and the effect of race and sex on this risk. *Am. J. Epid.* **119**: 526–40.

113. Hartz, A. J., Rupley, D. C. and Rimm, A. A. (1984) The association of girth measurements with disease in 32,856 women. *Am. J. Epid.* **119**: 71–80.

114. Gerber, L. M., Schnall, P. L. and Pickering, T. G. (1990) Body fat and its distribution in relation to casual and ambulatory blood pressure. *Hypertension* **15**: 508–13.

115. Gerber, L. M., Schwartz, J. E., Schnall, P. L. and Pickering, T. G. (1995) Body fat distribution in relation to sex differences in blood pressure. *Am. J. Hum. Biol.* **7**: 173–82.

116. Lapidus, L., Bengtsson, C., Larsson, B., Pennert, K., Rybo, E. and Sjostrom, L. (1984) Distribution of adipose tissue and risk of cardiovascular disease and death: a 12-year follow-up of participants in the population study of women in Gothenburg, Sweden. *Br. Med. J.* **289**:1257–61.

117. Larsson, B., Svardsudd, K., Welin, L., Wilhelmsen, L., Bjorntorp, P. and Tibblin, G. (1984) Abdominal adipose tissue distribution, obesity, and risk of cardiovascular disease and death: 13-year follow-up of participants in the study of men born in 1913. *Br. Med. J.* **288**: 1401–4.

118. Yao, C-H., Slattery, M. L., Jacobs, D. R., Folsom, A. R. and Nelson, E. T. (1991) Anthropometric predictors of coronary heart disease and total mortality: findings from the US Railroad Study. *Am. J. Epid.* **134**: 1278–89.

119. Folsom, A. R., Kaye, S. A., Sellers, T. A., Hong, C. P., Cerhan, J. R., Potter, J. D,. *et al.* (1993) Body fat distribution and 5-year risk of death in older women *J. Am. Med. Assoc.* **269**: 483–7.

120. Freedman, D. S., Williamson, D. F., Croft, J. B., Ballew, C. and Byers, T. (1995) Relation of body fat distribution to ischemic heart disease. *Am. J. Epid.* **142**: 53–63.

121. Sellers, T. A., Gapstur, S. M., Potter, J. D., Kushi, .L H., Bostick, R. M. and Folsom, A. R. (1993) Association of body fat distribution and family histories of breast and ovarian cancer with risk of post-menopausal breast cancer *Am. J. Epid.* **138**: 799–803.

122. Micozzi, M. S. (1990) Applications of anthropometry to epidemiologic studies of nutrition and cancer. *Am. J. Hum. Biol.* **2**: 727–39.

123. Selby, J. V., Newman, B., Queensberry, C. P., Fabsitz, R. R., Carmelli, D., Meaney, F. J., *et al.* (1990) Genetic and behavioural influences on body fat distribution. *Int. J. Obes.* **14**: 593–602.

124. Ducimetiere, P., Richard, J. and Cambien, F. (1986) The pattern of subcutaneous fat distribution in middle-aged men and the risk of coronary heart disease: the Paris Prospective Study. *Int. J. Obes.* **10**:229–40.

125. Kannel, W. B., Cupples, L. A., Ramaswami, R., Stokes, J. 3rd, Kreger, B. E. and Higgins, M. (1991) Regional obesity and risk of cardiovascular disease: the Framingham Study. *J. Clin. Epid.* **44**: 183–90.

126. Van Itallie, T. B. (1988) Topography of body fat relationship to risk of cardiovascular and other diseases. In: Lohman, T. G., Roche, A. F. and Martorell, R. (ed.) *Anthropometric standardization reference manual.* Human Kinetics Books, Champaign, Illinois. 143–9.

127. Kaye, S. A., Folsom, A. R., Prineas, R. J., Potter, J. D. and Gapstur, S. M. (1990) The association of body fat distribution with lifestyle and reproductive factors in a population study of post-menopausal women. *Int. J. Obes.* **14**: 583–91.

128. Gray, D. S. and Bray, G. A. (1991) Anthropometric assessment in an adult obesity clinic. In: Himes, J. H. (ed.) *Anthropometric assessment of nutritional status.* Wiley-Liss, New York. 383–98.

129. James, W. P. T. (1994) Introduction: the challenge of adult chronic energy deficiency. *Eur. J. Clin. Nutr.* **48** (Suppl. 3): S1–S9.

Further reading

Bjorntorp, P. (1985) Regional patterns of fat distribution. *Ann. Int. Med.* **103**: 994–5.

Kannam, J. P., Levy, D., Larson, M.G. and Wilson, P. W. (1994) Short stature and risk for cardiovascular disease morbidity and mortality: the Framingham Heart Study. *Circulation* **90**: 224–7.

11. Gene–nutrient interactions in nutritional epidemiology

Lenore Kohlmeier, David DeMarini and Walter Piegorsch

11.1 Introduction

Traditionally, dietary measures of exposure have related to food consumption and nutrient intake on the one hand, and characteristics of tissue exposure to nutrients on the other. It is now becoming clear that the ways in which we handle nutrients metabolically are, in part, genetically determined. This chapter concerns the extent to which genetic characteristics influence diet–disease relationships and interact with dietary exposures.

11.2 Gene–nutrient interactions in the context of molecular and genetic epidemiology

Molecular and genetic epidemiology are two relatively new fields that are changing the profile of epidemiological research. Molecular epidemiology should enhance our ability to detect and quantify disease–exposure relationships with objective and quantitative markers of either exposure or effects of the exposures within the organism. Molecular epidemiology depends on the molecular dosimetry of exposures at some organ level such that the biological marker relates quantitatively to exposure levels. Genetic epidemiology, on the other hand, uses genetic markers as indicators or modulators of disease risk. These can be either markers of germline DNA differences between individuals that can result in differences in the coding and subsequent production of metabolically important proteins, or markers of somatic mutations. Proteins may influence total metabolic processes, whereas mutation markers can influence the onset of disease, starting with an alteration in a single cell and resulting in devastating consequences for the individual (cancer). The relationships of biomarkers to exposure and disease have been categorized at the level of the environment, the organism, and the organ. A review of types of biomarkers is beyond the scope of this text (see [1]). For the purposes of this chapter, it is important to distinguish between biomarkers of exposure, intermediary markers of effect or early disease, markers of genetic integrity, and markers of genetic susceptibility to disease.[2]

The incorporation of information of this nature in the study of relationships between dietary intakes and disease may revolutionize nutritional epidemiology. Molecular and genetic epidemiology have the potential for linking dietary exposures with current knowledge of disease mechanisms in a more objective manner. In the area of nutritional epidemiology, this refers to new and, in some cases, classic approaches for studying the impact of the four types of gene–nutrient interactions. This chapter provides an overview of gene–nutrient interactions as we currently understand them, reviews available measures for studying them, and discusses how these mechanisms can enhance traditional and new epidemiological study design and improve the analysis of exposure–disease relationships.

11.3 The four types of gene–nutrient interactions

Gene–nutrient interactions can affect disease risk in four ways. Three of these involve direct effects of food-borne substances on DNA, and the fourth involves effects of genetic differences on diet-related susceptibility to specific diseases. A review of carcinogenesis with a number of the pathways of dietary influences on carcinogenesis is presented in Fig. 11.1. The various types of interaction are outlined in Box 11.1.

11.3.1 Nutrient regulation of gene transcription

The science of nutrition is founded on the knowledge that nutrients affect growth, reproduction, and immune function. More recently, molecular biology has demon-

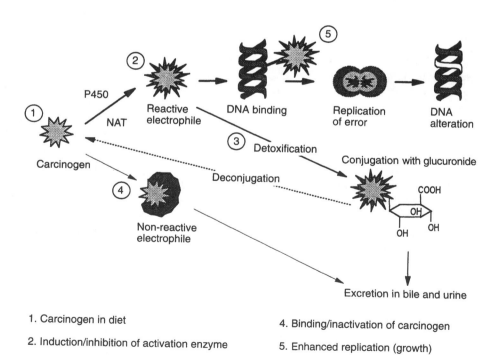

1. Carcinogen in diet
2. Induction/inhibition of activation enzyme
3. Induction/inhibition of detoxification enzyme
4. Binding/inactivation of carcinogen
5. Enhanced replication (growth)

Fig. 11.1 Dietary influences on carcinogenesis.

> **Box 11.1** Types of gene–nutrient interaction.
>
> 1. Nutrient affects DNA
>   1.1 Nutrient regulation of transcription (vitamin D_3 and calbindin)
>   1.2 Food induced DNA damage (Aflatoxin B1 adducts)
>   1.3 Phytochemical enhancement of DNA integrity (anti-oxidants)
>
> 2. Gene affects nutrient activity
>   2.1 Genetic susceptibility to nutrient-related diseases (NAT genotype and colon cancer)

strated that some nutrients influence gene transcription. Most nutritionists have this in mind when they conceptualize gene–nutrient interactions.

Nutrient regulation of transcription is poorly understood. The basic model operates under two premises:

(1) in order to serve a metabolic or information function, the presence of a nutrient has to be recognized;
(2) for a nutrient to influence gene transcription, it must trigger a regulatory change in the nucleus.

A general model would involve the interaction of a nutrient or its metabolite with a receptor or its movement directly into the cytosol. For the receptor interaction to be regulatory, it is believed that a high specificity is required. Nutrient binding to a receptor protein may alter the conformation of the receptor, triggering a signal to a second messenger within the cytoplasm. A DNA-binding protein would then move from the cytoplasm to the nucleus. Binding of the nuclear receptor to the regulatory portion of a gene then stimulates or reduces gene transcription.[3] The consequence of this is the production of more or less product. Amino acids, some polyunsaturated fatty acids, and the fat-soluble vitamins A and D alter transcription. The $1,25(OH)_2$ vitamin D_3 metabolite is the active form that binds to intracellular receptors, forming a steroid receptor complex that binds to DNA and results in enhanced synthesis in the intestines and kidney of regulatory proteins such as calbindin.[4]

Enzymes that regulate carcinogen metabolism are also inducible by diet. Cytochrome P450 enzymes (enzymes that activate carcinogens through oxidation) can be either induced or inhibited by diet. Diets high in protein can increase the ability of cytochrome P450 to catalyze oxidation reactions[5] and, for example, the metabolism of theophyline.[6] Protein-deficient diets reduce the rate of drug metabolism.[5] Experimental diets rich in heterocyclic amines increase CYP1A2 (a gene coding for the cytochrome P450 1A2 enzyme) activity.[7] Thiols in garlic, believed to be antimutagenic and anticarcinogenic against nitrosamines[8], induce cytochrome P450 2B1 and lower the concentration of cytochromes P450 3A and P450 2E1.[9]

Few studies have incorporated these mechanisms to study disease occurrence using epidemiological methods. For this we need indicators of change in transcription rates for use as an outcome or a modifier of the effect of the exposure of interest. These might be measures of the product levels before and after exposure, measurement of mRNA, metabolites of the enzyme products or indirect measures of enzyme levels. This can be accomplished by loading individuals with a particular substrate for the enzyme of interest and measuring the rate of substrate metabolism as the expression of some of these genes (phenotypic variation).[10] CYP1A2 activity can be measured in humans by determining the amount of caffeine metabolites excreted in the urine after caffeine consumption.[11] None of these methods lends itself to the study of large populations. Circulating enzyme levels might be useful but few of the enzymes of interest are currently measurable directly in serum. In addition, the transcription level of interest may be tissue specific, and access to target-organ tissue is rarely possible in epidemiological studies. Nonetheless, changes in transcription by dietary components may presage important health effects and, thus, merit measurement.

11.3.2 Dietary damage to DNA integrity

A wide range of compounds in our diet are mutagens and/or carcinogens.[12–14] These include mycotoxins, plant-derived alkaloids, hydrazines, flavonoids, precursors for nitrosamine formation, and cooked-food mutagens. Food-borne mutagens interact with DNA, causing DNA damage such as DNA adducts (an agent bound covalently to DNA) or DNA-strand breaks. If not properly repaired or removed, damaged DNA may be processed by the cell in ways that result in a mutation (a change in the sequence of nucleotides in the DNA).

Some food mutagens require no modification by metabolism, whereas others are not mutagenic as consumed. The latter require activation before they can induce damage. A brief discussion of some of the mutagens/carcinogens on the food, in the diet, and that result from food preparation will serve to illustrate how food can cause DNA damage.

Among the first group of mutagens/carcinogens recognized on foods were mycotoxins, secondary metabolites of fungi. Most notable among these are the aflatoxins, such as aflatoxin B1(AFB1). Members of the genus *Aspergillus* produce aflatoxins on mouldy corn and legumes. Although efforts are being made to prevent or reduce exposure to AFB1-contaminated food, AFB1-associated liver cancer is still endemic in parts of China and Africa.[15]

People exposed to aflatoxin B1 have detectable AFB1-DNA adducts in their liver, AFB1-albumin adducts in their serum, and AFB1 metabolites in their urine.[14] These adducts presumably lead to specific mutations in the p53 tumor-suppresser gene in human tumors.[16] A resulting G to T base substitution, preferentially at the third position of codon249 in the p53 tumor-suppresser gene, is found in AFB1-associated liver tumours and in the normal liver of AFB1-exposed people.[15] To date, AFB1 is the best documented example of cause-and-effect between a dietary component, a specific mutation in a specific gene in a specific organ, and the production of cancer in that organ.

Pyrolysis products of cooked meats and fish, such as polycyclic aromatic hydrocarbons (PAHs) and heterocyclic amines (HAs) are also known mutagens in Ames assays, and are created during food preparation. The presence of mutagenic PAHs, such as benzo[a]pyrene on broiled steak, was first reported over 30 years ago[17], and more identifications in broiled or grilled meats and fish have followed.[18] HAs resulting from the pyrolysis of amino acids were first reported nearly 20 years ago.[19] Thirteen such compounds have now been characterized chemically from fried meats and evaluated for mutagenicity and carcinogenicity in animal studies.[20–21] Consumption of fried meats results in the production of mutagenic PAH metabolites that are detectable in the urine and HA DNA adducts that are detectable in various tissues.[10] The relevance to humans of the rodent studies demonstrating the carcinogenicity of HAs has yet to be established. These laboratory models are useful in the development of a mechanistic understanding of HA-induced colon cancer and potential biomarkers of HA exposure and effect. Although a direct link to human cancer has not been established, epidemiological studies have reported associations between red meat consumption and colon cancer.[22–23]

Although not as well studied as AFB1, PAHs, and HAs, many mutagens/carcinogens are produced by plants, especially herbs and spices, and consumed in levels in these plant foods capable of expressing measurable activity.[24] An example of these compounds is estragole, present in tarragon and basil. Estragole induces liver cancer in mice. These exposed mice have DNA adducts at the N2-position of guanine in their livers.[14] Such 'nature's pesticides' are mutagenic and carcinogenic in experimental systems at human exposure levels. The presence of anticarcinogens in the same foods and our inherent DNA repair capacity may limit their role as human carcinogens.

Nutrients such as iron and ascorbic acid can play a dual role at different levels of tissue exposure and may interact with other factors. Although these are essential for growth and meeting physiological requirements against risk of tissue damage, and may protect against the free radical load of smokers, they may also act as mutagens in the diet. For example, Fe(II) induces mutants in Chinese hamster ovary cells in culture[25] and in human peripheral blood T-lymphocytes.[26] Vitamin C produces DNA breaks in human lymphocytes exposed in vitro.[27]

The diet may also cause DNA damage by increasing metabolic rates. In animals, energy restriction reduces cancer rates and increases longevity substantially. The mechanism of action is not known. One theory is that increased mitochondrial activity produces more free radicals that are released into the cell.[28]

Epidemiology can contribute to knowledge of dietary mutagens through studies in which DNA damage is assessed by the presence of DNA adducts or strand breaks (as measured by P32 post-labelling or single-cell gel electrophoresis assays, respectively), or mutations of the gene or chromosome (as measured by the salmonella or micronucleus assays, respectively). These assay results are used as measures of DNA integrity or indicators of dietary exposure. Presence of DNA (or protein) adducts of a specific type (i.e. heterocyclic amine adducts) is indicative of exposure to grilled meats. Other adducts may, however, be relatively non-specific. PAH adducts can, for example, originate from dietary or other environmental sources. Recent studies reporting higher adduct levels among cancer cases than controls are difficult to interpret because the adducts leading to the detected cancer occurred many years prior to these measurements.[29,30] Experimental feeding studies using adduct levels as outcomes, and cohort studies that collect tissue for adduct measurement in a nested case-control design (because they apply the appropriate temporality) would best utilize these measures. Alternatively, detection of mutation would be a marker of effect, because the presumptive exposure has resulted in a change in the DNA sequence and potentially, the function of the protein coded by the mutated gene.

Genetic markers of preclinical disease or disease risk provide outcome estimates that are not biased by their dependency on the subject going to a doctor for diagnosis or differential recall of prior exposures between cases and controls. Early genetic markers of disease risk can reduce the potentially long delays between exposures and chronic disease development. Few such disease markers exist. Examples of these that do include the genetic alterations seen with colon cancer (p53, H-ras). These markers are used in analyses as alternative outcome measures.

11.3.3   Dietary enhancement of DNA integrity

DNA integrity can also be protected by components of the diet. Antimutagens and anticarcinogens have been recognized in laboratory systems since the 1950s.[31] Many food-borne antimutagens and anticarcinogens have been identified over the years[32,33] including carotenoids, indole-3-carbinol, vitamin E, soybean extracts, polyphenols from green tea, isoflavones, chlorophyllin, and vanillin.[34] These agents can exert anti-mutagenic and/or anticarcinogenic effects through a variety of mechanisms.[31] Some agents inactivate mutagens directly by preventing oxidative damage to DNA. Dietary antioxidants are examples of direct-acting agents. Vitamins C and E and carotenoids may reduce or prevent oxidative attack of DNA by donating electrons and, thereby, stabilizing free radicals and electrophiles.[31] Others act indirectly, by binding to mutagens and preventing their activation to electrophilic moieties.* A good example of this is chlorophyllin. This water-soluble salt of chlorophyll, present in all plant leaves, binds non-specifically to a wide range of carcinogens.

Thus, the diet is a mixture of mutagenic/carcinogenic agents in combination with antimutagenic/anticarcinogenic agents. This mixture of compounds complicates the study of gene–nutrient interactions in epidemiological studies. Studies of food mutagens, as well as environmental epidemiological studies, may need to consider not only the activation enzymes (such as cytochrome P450s and N-acetyl transferases) but also the factors affecting levels of detoxification enzymes and the possible consumption of direct-acting antimutagens. These preventive factors need to be quantified and considered either as primary determinants of disease or effect modifying covariates of disease risk in epidemiological studies. Co-linearity needs to be examined before models are developed, including multiple diet-related parameters.

11.3.4   Genetic susceptibility to nutrient-moderated disease

The study of genetic susceptibility has been enhanced in recent years by the development of molecular techniques for amplifying, cloning, and sequencing DNA that are fast, inexpensive, and accurate.[35] In addition, the list of genes known to be involved in disease susceptibility is growing dramatically. For example, multiple genes are involved in cancer susceptibility, including carcinogen metabolizing genes, genes involved in DNA repair and stability, tumour suppressor genes and proto-oncogenes,

---

* Others act by induction of enzymes that inactivate mutagens or by inhibiting enzymes that activate promutagens. These can have either a protective or a risk enhancing effect. They have been discussed in Section 11.3.1 on nutrient effects on transcription.

genes that regulate receptor sites, and those involved in senescence. The carcinogen metabolizing genes have been among the first to receive intense study.

Many of the genes coding for enzymes activating or inactivating carcinogens (phase I and phase II metabolism genes) are polymorphic in the human population, i.e. are present in various mutant forms or may be completely absent in subgroups.[36] Consequently, the interaction of food mutagens with the human genome varies among people, resulting in a range of effects and potential health outcomes.[37,38] The ability to measure these genetic differences and to incorporate such information into study designs may enhance the value of nutritional epidemiological studies. It can allow identification of risks previously concealed by mixtures of people under study who were heterogeneous in their susceptibility to a diet-related disease. For example, the combined rapid CYP1A2-rapid NAT-2 phenotype was found in 35% of a group of 75 cancer/polyp cases and in only 16% of a group of 205 controls.[36] Univariate analysis of a questionnaire indicated that age, rapid–rapid phenotype, and consumption of well-done red meat were associated with increased risk of colorectal neoplasia. The odds ratios for cooked meat preference and phenotype combinations ranged from 1.00 for rare-medium preference with slow–slow phenotype to 6.45 for well-done preference with rapid–rapid NAT-2/CYP1A2 phenotype. This study suggests that metabolic phenotype combined with a measure of exposure to food-borne heterocyclic amine carcinogens are important risk factors in human colorectal cancer.[36]

Genotypic variation for various cytochrome P450 genes and other genes involved in phase I and phase II metabolism can now be determined by relatively simple, PCR-based methods. More than 30 human cytochrome P450 enzymes have been characterized thus far, and many are polymorphic, presenting a diversity of reactions to xenobiotic exposures.[37] NAT (N-acetyl transferase), one of the primary enzymes responsible for acetylation of arylamines, is coded by 2 distinct genes (NAT1 and NAT2), each of which has at least five known alleles. There is evidence that individuals who are rapid metabolizers, ie acetylate more quickly, have increased susceptibility to colon cancer. This suggests that they respond to carcinogens in the colon in a more dangerous fashion.[39]

The natures of the relationships between genotype–dietary exposures and disease risk are still poorly understood. Figure 11.2 presents a theoretical model of this interplay. In the absence of exposure, no one has an additional risk of the disease resulting from this exposure. At moderate exposure levels the risk ratios scissor apart such that the normal (wild-type) individuals have subdued risks compared with the homo-and heterozygotes carrying the altered allele.[40] Extremely high levels of a carcinogen may be saturating the system, making genotype and, thus, individual susceptibility, less important a factor in the risk differential.

This concept is based on the observation that levels of adducts were higher among NAT2 slow acetylators exposed to moderate levels of 4-aminobiphenyl, than in NAT2 rapid acetylators. Little difference in adduct levels exist however between slow and rapid acetylators at high exposure levels. It has also been observed that all 15 (100%) of workers engaged in 2-naphthylamine manufacturing and exposed to very high levels of the carcinogen, developed bladder cancer.[41] Although these are not dietary studies, they suggests that the levels of a particular biomarker (e.g., DNA adducts) are

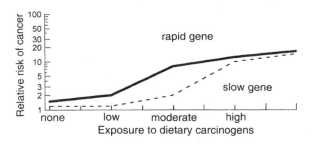

Fig. 11.2 Gene–nutrient relationships.

influenced by the genotype at moderate levels of exposure to a dietary component but not at high levels.

Gene-gene interactions may also complicate gene–nutrient interactions. Many biochemical pathways are complex cascades with multiple critical enzymes. Combinations of activities of metabolizing genes and those responsible for receptors may be of critical importance. If polymorphisms arise at various levels, their interplay will also be important in epidemiological analyses. For example, alleles of the NAT1 gene (NAT1*10) produce a two-fold higher NAT1 enzyme activity relative to the putative wild-type gene.[42] In combination with NAT2 rapid acetylation, this allele appears to impart a 3.8-fold risk for colorectal cancer.[43] In another example, individuals who inherit a slow NAT2 combined with a rapid NAT1 (NAT1*10) genotype have an elevated risk of bladder cancer and a high level of DNA adducts in urinary bladder mucosa.[44] The presence of both genetic factors seems to impart an elevated risk. Thus, determination of these genotypes may provide useful information in evaluating the role of diet-related factors in colon carcinogenesis.

Genetic markers of susceptibility will be particularly useful in epidemiological research if their incidence in the population is high.[45] The prevalences of rapid and slow NAT acetylators is close to 50:50, making this a particularly attractive genetic susceptibility maker. One does not have to go to the expense and trouble of searching large populations of individuals for a sample size large enough to be meaningful. The breakdown of populations by NAT1 and 2 alleles allows testing for stronger dietary interactions with one group than the other. Genetic polymorphisms (altered forms of a gene) are most valuable in an epidemiological context if they are present in at least 10% of the population under study. Theoretically, to be effective, these altered genes should be functional. However, non-functional markers of functional polymorphisms will be equally useful in identifying risk groups and interactions. Currently, research is focused more on the identification of polymorphisms of enzymes that may have important functional roles in carcinogenesis, cardiovascular disease, or metabolic disorders and their distributions in the population.

The incorporation of information on previously hidden genetic polymorphisms should strengthen the risks measured in a study. The study of vulnerable subgroups should reduce dilution of effect from inclusion of these not at risk through this pathway.[46]

Susceptibility markers can generally be considered effect modifiers in epidemiological analysis. They may be dichotomous (screening for phenylketonuria), continuous (the use of circulating LDL-cholesterol levels as an indicator of cardiovascular disease risk), or categorical (apolipoprotein E genotypes 2, 3, and 4 in the study of Alzheimer or cardiovascular disease).

Under a few basic assumptions, studies of interactions between genes and environment can be vastly simplified by using case-only studies.[47] Case-only studies involve the use of cases but no controls for analysis of interaction. The lack of need for controls saves time and resources and decreases concerns about selection bias and comparability with the baseline populations. Genetic analyses allow analyses of germ-line DNA at the time of diagnosis without concern that the biomarker in question has been influenced by the disease state. Therefore, given that the exposure can be assessed retroactively, there remains little reason for focusing on cohort studies. The critical assumption is that exposure levels and genetic susceptibility are independent of one another. This may not be true if there are ethnic differences in the allele frequency and also ethnic differences in eating behaviour. Details of these and other design considerations are presented in the following section.

11.3.5 Design and analytical implications for gene–nutrient interactions

As this chapter has emphasized, molecular genetic biomarkers can be meaningful indicators of disease risk, and their interaction with nutritional factors is important. As such, assessing gene–nutrient interactions must become a key consideration in epidemiological studies. Fundamental to this endeavour is proper statistical design and data analysis, in order to ensure that inferences made about the interaction(s) are accurate.[48–51] In this section, we discuss basic implications for proper design and analysis of nutritional epidemiological studies, with emphasis on identifying gene–nutrient interactions. Our goal is not to survey methods in study design and data analysis; other chapters in this volume direct greater attention to these issues. Rather, we will emphasize the complexities brought on when studying interactions, by describing statistical tests for gene–nutrient interaction in some simple retrospective and prospective sampling scenarios, and by using these tests as the basis for calculating minimum samples sizes necessary to achieve reasonable levels of power to detect the interaction.

Retrospective sampling: Case-control studies

Statistical models for gene–nutrient interactions in case-control studies   The ability to study indices of genetic susceptibility lends itself well to applications in retrospective epidemiological studies[47], with the case-control study a popular design for assessing genetic susceptibility.[52–55] Standard statistical methodology is available for analyzing case-control data, including the popular form of logistic regression[56] and other generalizations of linear regression models.[47,57,58] For testing gene–nutrient (or any other form of) interactions, these methods may be extended in a straightforward fashion, although in some cases the interactions may lead to additional complexities in the model structure.[59,60]

To illustrate, consider the simple case of one binary nutritional factor interacting with one binary genetic factor. That is, individuals are exposed or in some other way subjected to a nutritional factor, E, or not, $\overline{E}$, and they fall into either a genetic 'susceptible' group, G, or a non-susceptible group, $\overline{G}$. This produces a pair of 2×2 tables of counts, one 2×2 table for the cases and one 2×2 table for the controls. Since sampling in such a case-control study is conditioned on disease status, the case-series total N and the control-series total M are fixed by the design. Our interest is in specifying the number of cases, N, and the number of controls, M, needed to ascertain the underlying relative risks of disease in the populations under study. The pertinent relative risks are those associated with exposure, r_E, genetic susceptible state, r_G, or their interaction r_{EG}.

To establish a baseline, non-interactive model, we consider a multiplicative interaction that is expressed in terms of the log of the ratio of relative risks. That is, equate r_{EG} with the product of the two separate relative risks $r_E r_G$:[62]

$$H_0 : log \{r_{EG} / r_E r_G\} = 0 \tag{11.1}$$

Recall that under a rare disease assumption, odds ratios approximate relative risks, so that (11.1) implies that the odds ratio of the interaction equals the products of the odds ratios of the individual components; see Appendix equation (11.5). For simplicity, we write $\psi = log \{r_{EG} / r_E r_G\}$. Departures from the null hypothesis (11.1) suggest interactive departures from a simple multiplicative relationship between exposure and genetic susceptibility.

Statistical tests for gene-nutrient interactions in case-control studies   As we detail in the Appendix, the interaction parameter associated with (11.1) can be written as a ratio of odds ratios, which in turn leads to a fairly simple form for its maximum likelihood estimator (MLE) $\hat{\psi}$, a ratio of the observed odds ratios.[62,63] (Details for the construction are given in the Appendix.) For testing H_0 in (11.1), we take the MLE and divide it by its standard error, $\sigma[\hat{\psi}]$. The resulting test statistic is distributed under H_0 as standard normal (approximately), and rejection occurs when the ratio $|\hat{\psi}|/\sigma[\hat{\psi}] > z_{\alpha/2}$ where $z_{\alpha/2}$ is the upper-$(\alpha/2)$ critical point from a standard normal distribution. This methodology is known as a *Wald test*, after Wald's[64] derivation of the general approach; the associated ratio of the MLE to its standard error is the *Wald statistic*.

Other methodologies for testing H_0 besides the Wald test are possible, of course, including likelihood-ratio and score-based tests.[63] The Wald statistic is one of the simplest forms of test statistic available for testing interactions in a case-control study, however, and it lends itself readily to calculation of minimal sample sizes for testing ExG interaction.[65] Since this latter concern is one of our primary goals, we limit our consideration to the Wald test as a basis for determining sample size for retrospective studies of gene–nutrient interaction.

Sample sizes for testing gene–nutrient interactions in case-control studies   An important design consideration when planning a case-control study is determination of a minimal number of subjects (*sample sizes*) to ensure that the study has sufficient power to detect an interaction, if it exists. Accurate sample size determinations for case-control studies contribute to design economy, by identifying minimum number(s) of subjects for use, or, in settings with restricted resources, by suggesting that low sample sizes may not have a reasonable chance to detect an important effect.[48,66-68]

In a certain sense, however, gene–nutrient interactions represent effects of a higher order than those associated with either of the separate main effects. As such, greater numbers of subjects are required for assessing interactions than those typical for studying a single disease factor.[65,69]

Use of the Wald test statistic allows for straightforward computation of sample sizes for testing the no-interaction null hypothesis in (11.1). One starts by specifying a significance level, α, corresponding to the false positive error rate. A common value is $\alpha = 0.05$. Next, select the power desired to detect a true departure from H_0, denoted herein by $\bar{\beta}$; that is, the probability of detecting values of ψ that differ from zero. (This is also 1 minus the false negative error rate, β, motivating our notation: $\bar{\beta} = 1-\beta$.) Below we will set $\bar{\beta} = 80\%$. Then, if the investigator has some good knowledge of the individual relative risks, the large-sample power associated with use of the Wald test is found to be a function of ψ

$$\bar{\beta}(\psi) = 1 - \Phi\left(z_{\alpha/2} + \frac{\psi}{\sigma[\hat{\psi}]}\right) + \Phi\left(-z_{\alpha/2} + \frac{\psi}{\sigma[\hat{\psi}]}\right) \tag{11.2}$$

where $\Phi(z)$ is the standard normal cumulative distribution function, available in many tabulated sources or computer packages. As we show in the Appendix, under the assumption that the exposure and genetic factors are independent in the population under study, which is not unreasonable when studying ExG interactions[45,47], $\sigma[\hat{\psi}]$ is a function of the relative risks, N and $\rho = M/N$. The latter quantity is the ratio of number of controls to number of cases. Additionally, one must specify the individual prevalences of exposure and of genetic susceptibility, and the spontaneous disease rate $\Pr\{D|\overline{EG}\}$. Then, solving equation (11.2) for N leads to specification of the sample sizes. We have computed solutions for (11.2) for the specific case of $\alpha = 0.05$, $\bar{\beta} = 0.8$, and $\rho = 2$; over a range of different values of r_E, r_G, r_{EG}, the prevalence probabilities, and $\Pr\{D|\overline{EG}\}$. The results are minimum sample sizes required to yield power of 80% at 5% significance when twice as many observations are desired in the control-series as in the case-series; they appear in Table 11.1 in the Appendix. (To aid in comparisons, the table also lists e^ψ, which at 1.0 would indicate no departure from H_0.) For example, suppose the exposure and genetic susceptibility population prevalences both equal 10%, and one expects the relative risk of exposure or of genetics to be 1.0 (i.e. no increase in disease risk due to either factor singly). If the relative risk of exposure *and* genetic susceptibility doubles the risk, so that $e^\psi = 2$, and if we take $\Pr\{D|\overline{EG}\} = 0.001$, then to use the Wald test we require a minimum of N = 2215 cases and (since $\rho = 2$) M = 4430 control subjects. If we felt instead that $\Pr\{D|\overline{EG}\}$ were in fact as high as 0.010, then the required number of cases drops to N = 2165, and the number of controls drops to M = 4330. The table displays similar computations for a variety of relative risk and spontaneous disease probabilities.

Retrospective sampling: case-only studies

The assumption made for the case-control scenario that the exposure and genetic factors are independent in the population under study generates interesting and important sequelae. Under this assumption the interaction parameter simplifies into a sum of two components, the first we denote as γ, and the second is identically zero. (That is $\psi = \gamma + 0$ under exposure-genetics independence.) The corresponding MLE of the interactive effect and its standard error may be determined in a straightforward fashion, as described in the Appendix. The null hypothesis of a simple multiplicative effect between the genetic and exposure factors, corresponding to (11.1), is now $H_0: \gamma = 0$. To test this against some form of non-multiplicative interaction between the genetic and exposure factors, we apply again a Wald test. Here, the test rejects H_0 when the statistic $|\hat{\gamma}|/\sigma[\hat{\gamma}]$ exceeds $z_{\alpha/2}$.

An important consequence of this case-only formulation is that the case-series standard error $\sigma[\hat{\gamma}]$ is always less than or equal to the associated case-control standard error $\sigma[\hat{\psi}]$, under full case-control sampling.[47,70] Thus, greater precision is possible for estimating the interaction parameter under the assumption of independence between the exposure and genetic factors. Translated into a design consideration, this suggests that lower sample sizes are necessary to achieve the same level of statistical power using the case-only design.

To illustrate this effect, we recalculated the minimum sample sizes in Table 11.1 using the case-only statistics above. The required case-series total, N, is found by solving a straightforward analogue of the power function in (11.2); see equation (11.7) in the Appendix. As above, one can solve this equation for N given a fixed significance level, α, the desired power, $\bar{\beta}$, the relative risks r_E, r_G, r_{EG}, and the individual exposure and genetic susceptibility prevalence probabilities. (Notice that since there is no interest in identifying control subjects for analysis, values for M, or alternatively, $\rho = M/N$, are not required.)

We have computed solutions for (11.7) for the specific case $\alpha = 0.05$ and $\bar{\beta} = 0.8$ over a range of values corresponding to those employed in Table 11.1. The results are minimum case-series sample sizes need to yield (approximate) power of 80% at 5% significance when only the case-series is used to assess the gene–nutrient interaction; they appear in Table 11.2 in the Appendix. (Again, for simplicity of comparison, the table lists e^γ, which at 1.0 would indicate no departure from H_0.) To emphasize the possible reductions available, Table 11.2 also lists for each parameter configuration the per cent reduction from the (smallest) comparable case-series sample size from Table 11.1. For example, suppose in Table 11.2 that the exposure and genetic susceptibility population prevalences are both equal to 10%, and one expects the relative risk of exposure or genetics to be 1.0 (ie no increase in disease risk due to either factor singly). If the relative risk of exposure *and* genetic susceptibility doubles the risk, so that $e^\gamma = 2$, then to use the Wald statistic in a case-only analysis, we require a minimum of $N = 1213$ case subjects. This compares with $N = 2165$ subjects for the full case-control study (from Table 11.1), a 44% reduction in the case-series. Similar sorts of reductions are seen throughout the table.

We emphasize that the case-only design is useful for assessing interactions in retrospective data only when the assumption is valid that the genetic and exposure factors are independent in the population under study. Depending on the application, this may be a fairly straightforward assumption to verify or presuppose, but in other studies it may be patently untrue. In the latter setting, the case-only methods are contraindicated.

Even when independence between exposure and genetic factors is valid, some invest-igators may be unwilling to undertake a study when design does not include control information. Indeed, although the assumption leads to greater efficiency for testing interaction, it does possess drawbacks: (i) there is no way to assess the independence assumption with only the case-series, so it must be accepted based on previous data or on basic principles; and (ii) certain main effect parameters, such as the odds ratio for genetic susceptibility, cannot be estimated from just the case-series data. In some settings, therefore, the case-only design may be most useful as a *preliminary screen*[71] – where limited information is gathered only on cases in order to test for potential gene–nutrient interactions – from which a larger study that includes control-series data is designed. Since the sample size requirements for testing interaction in a case-only design can be much lower than those for a full case-control study, this strategy can lead to efficient management of limited resources, yet still provide investigators with good power to detect gene–nutrient interactions.

Prospective sampling: cohort studies

Statistical tests for gene–nutrient interactions in cohort studies   For those invest-igators wishing to undertake a prospective study of the interaction between a genetic and a nutritional factor, the simple cohort study may be considered.[72] (Other altern-atives include a case-cohort design[73,74], or some form of experimental study.[75]) The prospective nature of the sampling changes the basic statistical model, which in turn leads to different forms of test statistics[76], and different requirements for minimum sample sizes.[48,66,68,77] As with retrospective sampling, however, it remains the case that larger numbers of subjects are required to test for interactive effects, compared to that for testing the main effect of either factor.

To illustrate, suppose as in the preceding sections that we study the interaction between a binary genetic factor (susceptible, G, or non-susceptible, $\overline{G}$) and a binary nutritional/exposure factor (E or $\overline{E}$). Under prospective sampling the cell totals are fixed in advance, and these become the sample sizes of interest. We denote them as $N_{ij}(i=1,0;j=0,1)$. As we detail in the Appendix, attention again centres on the relative risks of disease for each main effect (E and G), and also on the relative risk of disease for the joint condition, $E \times G$. These are, respectively, r_E, r_G, and r_{EG}. We take as the null effect the simple multiplicative model $r_E r_G = r_{EG}$ corresponding to (11.1).

Under prospective sampling, the binomial model yields a straightforward MLE for the interaction parameter, $\psi = log\{r_{EG}/(r_E r_G)\}$, given in Appendix equation (11.8). A large-sample standard error, $\sigma[\hat{\psi}]$, is also available, as detailed in the Appendix. To test H_0: $\psi = 0$ against some form of interactive departure, we calculate the Wald statistic $|\hat{\psi}|/\sigma[\hat{\psi}]$. As above, this ratio is distributed under H_0 as standard normal. Rejection occurs when $|\hat{\psi}|/\sigma[\hat{\psi}] > z_{\alpha/2}$.

Sample sizes for testing gene–nutrient interactions in cohort studies   Under the prospective sampling model, the power function of the Wald test is again analogous to (11.2):

$$\bar{\beta}(\psi) = 1 - \Phi\left(z_{\alpha/2} + \frac{\psi}{\sigma[\hat{\psi}]}\right) + \Phi\left(-z_{\alpha/2} + \frac{\psi}{\sigma[\hat{\psi}]}\right) \tag{11.3}$$

Consider the special case of *balanced* sampling, $N_{00} = N_{01} = N_{10} = N_{11} = N$ (say). Given a fixed significance level, α, a value for the desired power, $\bar{\beta}$, the three relative risks r_E, r_G, r_{EG}, and any single disease probability, such as $\pi_{00} = Pr\{D|\overline{EG}\}$, we can solve (11.3) for the common sample size N. The total sample size is then 4N. (The disease probabilities π_{ij} are the probabilities that a subject in the $(i,j)^{th}$ cell is diseased by the end of the prospective study period.)

We have computed solutions for (11.3) for the specific case of $\alpha = 0.05$, and $\bar{\beta} = 0.8$ over a range of different values of r_E, r_G, r_{EG}, and π_{00}. The results are minimum per-group sample sizes needed to yield (approximate) power of 80% at 5% significance to assess the gene–nutrient interaction; they appear in Table 11.3 in the Appendix. (Again, for simplicity of comparison, the table lists e^{ψ}, which at 1.0 would indicate no departure from H_0.) For example, suppose in Table 11.3 that the spontaneous disease probability $\pi_{00} = Pr\{D|\overline{EG}\}$ equals 0.1%, and one expects the relative risk of exposure or of genetics to be 1.0 (i.e. no increase in disease risk due to either factor singly). If the relative risk of exposure *and* genetic susceptibility doubles the risk, so that $e^{\psi} = 2$, then to use the Wald statistic in a cohort analysis, we require a minimum of N = 57 112 subjects *per cell*. The total sample size is four times this, or 228 448. (Clearly, a very large value to require in practice!) If one felt that the spontaneous disease probability was much greater, say $\pi_{00} = 10\%$, then the per-cell sample size requirement drops radically, to N = 507 subjects; the associated total sample size is 2028.

These calculations help illustrate the well-known feature that a cohort study often requires many more observations than a similarly targeted case-control (or case-only) study.[48,78] When interactions are of interest, however, the differences in required sample sizes can be even more dramatic than might be seen when studying only a single effect or factor.

In closing, we note that more elaborate calculations are necessary when the study design is more complex than the simple 2×2 structures studied herein, whether it be a case-control, case-only, or cohort design under consideration.[79] Assessing interactions in such settings is not always an elementary endeavour, and research on how to exploit features such as the case-only design with molecular genetic biomarkers is still in its infancy.[47,70]

11.4 Ethical issues

Any treatise on gene–nutrient interactions would not be complete without a word about the ethical issues underlying this type of epidemiological research. As scientists, we are obligated to inform all human subjects of the risk involved in participation in our studies and to receive their consent before participation. Measurement of genetic components, particularly genetic polymorphisms, can reveal risks to individuals and their groups. However, such measurements may potentially benefit the subjects and their groups. Risk occurs, for example, when employers or insurers require disclosure of any information on health status and disease risk. Disclosure can result in higher premiums, or nonacceptance into the health plan or the job in question. Identification of higher incidences of risk-carrying polymorphisms in certain ethnic groups can expose them to discrimination. At the other extreme, this knowledge can direct individuals to lifestyle choices that reduce exposures and therefore risks. It can also stimulate direct research that may result in long-term reductions in disease rates in these groups. The benefits and risks are detailed in a recent consensus statement.[80]

Nationally representative surveys that collect blood samples and preserve DNA have tremendous potential for providing information on genetic polymorphisms at a low cost. Follow up studies can quantify the risk of specific diseases as a function of the presence of specific alleles. As a consequence of the ethical concerns, this potential is being severely limited. So, for example, no DNA testing has begun on the NHANES III biological samples, which have been available for a number of years. The intention is to prevent the individuals from being identifiable when DNA analyses are conducted. This also means that the information will not be cross-linked to other personal characteristics and will not be useful for follow-up studies of future disease occurrence.

Informed consent is needed to protect individuals' right to determine how their samples will be used. Legislation is also needed to protect them against misuse of this important knowledge.

Appendix: Technical formulae for sample size determinations

We provide in this technical Appendix greater statistical and mathematical detail for specifying sample sizes in retrospective and prospective studies of gene–nutrient interaction.

Retrospective sample: case-control studies   In the full case-control setting we observe counts Y_{ij} (cases) and W_{ij} (controls), where $i = 0,1$ and $j = 0,1$ correspond to E, $\overline{E}$ and G $\overline{G}$, respectively. For example, Y_{01} is the number of cases observed at the non-exposed ($\overline{E}$), genetic susceptible (G) combination; W_{01} is the corresponding number of controls. The data quadruples $\{Y_{ij}\}$ and $\{W_{ij}\}$ represent observations from the case-series and control-series, respectively. Statistically, the retrospective study design induces independent multinomial distributions on each of these quadruples, with probabilities of response $\{P_{ij}\}$ and $\{Q_{ij}\}$, respectively. Note that the sums $\Sigma\Sigma P_{ij}$ and $\Sigma\Sigma Q_{ij}$ both must equal 1.0 under this statistical model, but in general $P_{ij} + Q_{ij} \neq 1$.

Of interest are the relative risks of disease corresponding to exposure (E), genetic susceptible state (G), or their interaction (E × G). These are $r_E = \Pr\{D|EG\}/\Pr\{D|\overline{E}G\}$, $r_G = \Pr\{D|\overline{E}G\}/\Pr\{D|\overline{E}\overline{G}\}$, and $r_{EG} = \Pr\{D|EG\}/\Pr\{D|\overline{E}\overline{G}\}$, where, e.g., $\Pr\{D|EG\}$ is the probability of disease for exposed, genetically susceptible individuals; the other disease probabilities are interpreted similarly. The underlying multinomial probabilities P_{ij} and Q_{ij} may be written in a similar notation; e.g. $P_{01} = \Pr\{G|D\}$ or $Q_{01} = \Pr\{G|\overline{D}\}$, etc. The interaction parameter, $\psi = log\{r_{EG}/r_E r_G\}$, from (11.1) may be written in terms of these disease probabilities:

$$\psi = log\left(\frac{\Pr\{D|EG\}\Pr\{D|\overline{E}\overline{G}\}}{\Pr\{D|\overline{E}G\}\Pr\{D|E\overline{G}\}}\right)$$

Unfortunately, the retrospective nature of the case-control design does not allow for direct estimation of the disease probabilities. Careful application of Bayes rule leads, however, to an expression for ψ that is estimable under the multinomial model:[56]

$$\psi = log\left(\frac{\Pr\{EG|D\}\Pr\{\overline{E}\overline{G}|D\}}{\Pr\{\overline{E}G|D\}\Pr\{E\overline{G}|D\}}\right) + log\left(\frac{\Pr\{\overline{E}G\}\Pr\{E\overline{G}\}}{\Pr\{EG\}\Pr\{\overline{E}\overline{G}\}}\right) \tag{11.4}$$

In Equation (11.4), the first term in the sum is simply $log\{P_{00}P_{11}/P_{01}P_{10}\}$, which we will see below may be estimated directly from the multinomial data. We denote this as $\gamma = log\{P_{11}P_{00}/P_{01}P_{10}\}$. The second additive term in (11.4) is a log-ratio of joint prevalence rates. Under the common assumption that the disease is rare in the population under study, this latter quantity is, approximately, $log\{Q_{01}Q_{10}/Q_{11}Q_{00}\}$. Combining this with γ produces

$$\psi \approx log\left(\frac{P_{00}P_{11}Q_{01}Q_{10}}{P_{01}P_{10}Q_{11}Q_{00}}\right) \tag{11.5}$$

a ratio of *odds ratios*. Of interest is assessing whether ψ as given in (11.4) or (11.5) is equal to zero.

Under the multinomial sampling model, the maximum likelihood estimator (MLE) of (11.5) is simply a ratio of the observed odds ratios[62,63] simplifying to the form

$$\hat{\psi} = log\left(\frac{Y_{00}Y_{11}W_{01}W_{10}}{Y_{01}Y_{10}W_{11}W_{00}}\right)$$

Associated with this estimator, we construct a test of $H_0: \psi = 0$ by dividing the MLE by its standard error,

$$\sigma[\hat{\psi}] = \sqrt{\Sigma\Sigma\{(1/P_{ij}) + (\rho/Q_{ij})\}/N} \tag{11.6}$$

where $\rho = M/N$ is the ratio of number of controls to number of cases. Since the Wald statistic $\hat{\psi}/\sigma[\hat{\psi}]$ is distributed under H_0 as standard normal (approximately), rejection corresponds to $|\hat{\psi}|/\sigma[\hat{\psi}] > z_{\alpha/2}$. In practice, the values of P_{ij} and Q_{ij} are not known, and these must be replaced in $\sigma[\hat{\psi}]$ by their sample estimates, Y_{ij}/N and W_{ij}/M, respectively.

Use of the Wald test statistic allows for straightforward computation of sample sizes for testing the no-interaction null hypothesis $H_0: \psi = 0$. If the investigator can specify values for the eight multinomial probabilities P_{ij} and Q_{ij}, the value of ψ can be approximated using (11.5), and the standard error of $\hat{\psi}$ in (11.6) can be determined. From these, it is straightforward to show that the large-sample power associated with use of (11.6) may be written as a function of $\hat{\psi}$ (and, implicitly, the P_{ij} and Q_{ij} values). This is given in equation (11.2). Given values for α, $\bar{\beta}$, the case-to-control ratio ρ, and assuming knowledge of the P_{ij} and Q_{ij} values, (11.2) is an expression with only one unknown: the number of cases N. Solving it for N leads to specification of the sample sizes, N and $M = \rho N$.

In practice, it is uncommon for an investigator to have good knowledge of the individual multinomial probabilities P_{ij} and Q_{ij}. Using various rules of probability, however, it is possible to reformulate $\sigma[\hat{\psi}]$ in (11.6). One additional assumption that is required is for the exposure and genetic factors to be independent in the population under study, which is not unreasonable when studying $E \times G$ interactions.[45,47] Then, one can define the four multinomial case-series probabilities P_{ij} as functions only of the relative risks, r_E, r_G, r_{EG}, and of the individual prevalences $Pr(E)$, $Pr(G)$:

$$P_{00} = \frac{[1-Pr(E)][1-Pr(G)]}{r_{EG}Pr(E)Pr(G) + r_E Pr(E)[1-Pr(G)] + r_G[1-Pr(E)]Pr(G) + [1-Pr(E)][1-Pr(G)]}$$

$$P_{01} = r_G P_{00}\frac{Pr(G)}{[1-Pr(G)]}$$

$$P_{10} = r_E P_{00}\frac{Pr(E)}{[1-Pr(E)]}$$

$$P_{11} = r_{EG}P_{00}\frac{Pr(G)}{[1-Pr(G)]}\frac{Pr(E)}{[1-Pr(E)]}$$

If, in addition, one can specify the spontaneous disease probability $\Pr\{D|\overline{EG}\}$, the multinomial control-series probabilities are available as:

$$Q_{00} = \frac{[1-\Pr(E)][1-\Pr(G)]}{\Pr(\overline{D})} \left\{1-\Pr\{D|\overline{EG}\}\right\}$$

$$Q_{01} = \frac{[1-\Pr(E)]\Pr(G)}{\Pr(\overline{D})} \left\{1-r_G\Pr\{D|\overline{EG}\}\right\}$$

$$Q_{10} = \frac{\Pr(E)[1-\Pr(G)]}{\Pr(\overline{D})} \left\{1-r_E\Pr\{D|\overline{EG}\}\right\}$$

$$Q_{11} = \frac{\Pr(E)\Pr(G)}{\Pr(\overline{D})} \left\{1-r_{EG}\Pr\{D|\overline{EG}\}\right\}$$

Note that under a rare disease assumption, $\Pr(\overline{D}) \approx 1$ and $\Pr\{D|\overline{EG}\} \approx 0$. This approximation simplifies the Q_{ij}s, and if employed, it does away with the need to specify $\Pr\{D|\overline{EG}\}$. Such a simplification appears to underlie the sample sizes calculations made by Hwang et al.[45] in their study of $E \times G$ interactions.

To set a minimum case-series sample size, N, all that is required is specification of the relative risks r_E, r_G, r_{EG}, the individual prevalences $\Pr(E)$, $\Pr(G)$, and the spontaneous disease rate $\Pr\{D|\overline{EG}\}$. Along with α, $\bar{\beta}$, and ρ, these values may be used to solve for N in (11.2). Selected results appear in Table 11.1.

Retrospective sampling: case–only studies   Under the assumption made for the case-control scenario that the exposure and genetic factors are independent in the population under study, the joint population prevalences factor into their single components parts: e.g. $\Pr\{EG\} = \Pr(E)\Pr(G)$, $\Pr\{\overline{EG}\} = \Pr(\overline{E})\Pr(G)$, etc. As a result, the second term in equation (11.4) simplifies to $log\{1\}$, which is always zero. Thus the interaction parameter becomes

$$\psi = log\left(\frac{\Pr\{EG|D\}\Pr\{\overline{EG}|D\}}{\Pr\{E\overline{G}|D\}\Pr\{\overline{E}G|D\}}\right)$$

i.e. a function of only the case-series probabilities: $log\{P_{11}P_{00}/P_{01}P_{10}\}$. Above, we denoted this term as γ, so that now we may write $\psi = \gamma$. Clearly, only case-series data are required to estimate this value under the assumption of independence between exposure and genetic factors.

The MLE for γ under this *case-only* formulation is $\hat{\gamma} = log\{Y_{00}Y_{11}/Y_{01}Y_{10}\}$ with large-sample standard error $\sigma[\hat{\gamma}] = \sqrt{\Sigma\Sigma[1/(NP_{ij})]}$. Under the assumption that the exposure and genetic factors are independent in the population, the null hypothesis of a simple multiplicative effect between the genetic and exposure factors, corresponding to (11.1), is now $H_0:\gamma = 0$. To test this against some form of non-multiplicative interaction between the genetic and exposure factors, the Wald test rejects H_0 when the statistic $|\hat{\gamma}|/\sigma[\hat{\gamma}]$ exceeds $z_{\alpha/2}$. As above, when the P_{ij}s are unknown (as is common), we replace them in $\sigma[\hat{\gamma}]$ with their estimated values, Y_{ij}/N.

Table 11.1 Minimum sample sizes required for case-control study to identify true E × G interaction with power = 80%, at significance level $\alpha = 0.05$. Ratio of number of controls (M) to number of case (N) set at M/N = 2.

Pr(E)*	Pr(G)	r_E	r_G	r_{EG}	Pr{D|$\overline{EG}$}	e^{ψ}	N	M
0.1	0.1	1.0	1.0	2.0	0.001	2.0	2215	4430
0.1	0.1	1.0	1.0	2.0	0.010	2.0	2165	4330
0.1	0.1	1.0	1.0	4.0	0.001	4.0	455	910
0.1	0.1	1.0	1.0	4.0	0.010	4.0	443	886
0.1	0.1	1.0	2.0	4.0	0.001	2.0	1786	3572
0.1	0.1	1.0	2.0	4.0	0.010	2.0	1716	3432
0.1	0.1	1.0	2.0	8.0	0.001	4.0	395	790
0.1	0.1	1.0	2.0	8.0	0.010	4.0	377	754
0.1	0.1	2.0	1.0	4.0	0.001	2.0	1786	3572
0.1	0.1	2.0	1.0	4.0	0.010	2.0	1716	3432
0.1	0.1	2.0	1.0	8.0	0.001	4.0	395	790
0.1	0.1	2.0	1.0	8.0	0.010	4.0	377	754
0.1	0.1	2.0	2.0	8.0	0.001	2.0	1500	3000
0.1	0.1	2.0	2.0	8.0	0.010	2.0	1361	2722
0.1	0.1	2.0	2.0	16.0	0.001	4.0	350	700
0.1	0.1	2.0	2.0	16.0	0.010	4.0	320	640
0.1	0.3	1.0	1.0	2.0	0.001	2.0	1040	2080
0.1	0.3	1.0	1.0	2.0	0.010	2.0	1015	2030
0.1	0.3	1.0	1.0	4.0	0.001	4.0	232	464
0.1	0.3	1.0	1.0	4.0	0.010	4.0	225	450
0.1	0.3	1.0	2.0	4.0	0.001	2.0	1006	2012
0.1	0.3	1.0	2.0	4.0	0.010	2.0	961	1922
0.1	0.3	1.0	2.0	8.0	0.001	4.0	239	478
0.1	0.3	1.0	2.0	8.0	0.010	4.0	225	450
0.1	0.3	2.0	1.0	4.0	0.001	2.0	822	1644
0.1	0.3	2.0	1.0	4.0	0.010	2.0	788	1576
0.1	0.3	2.0	1.0	8.0	0.001	4.0	194	388
0.1	0.3	2.0	1.0	8.0	0.010	4.0	183	366
0.1	0.3	2.0	2.0	8.0	0.001	2.0	796	1592
0.1	0.3	2.0	2.0	8.0	0.010	2.0	713	1426
0.1	0.3	2.0	2.0	16.0	0.001	4.0	198	396
0.1	0.3	2.0	2.0	16.0	0.010	4.0	175	350
0.3	0.3	1.0	1.0	2.0	0.001	2.0	489	978
0.3	0.3	1.0	1.0	2.0	0.010	2.0	477	954
0.3	0.3	1.0	1.0	4.0	0.001	4.0	121	242
0.3	0.3	1.0	1.0	4.0	0.010	4.0	117	234
0.3	0.3	1.0	2.0	4.0	0.001	2.0	472	944
0.3	0.3	1.0	2.0	4.0	0.010	2.0	450	900
0.3	0.3	1.0	2.0	8.0	0.001	4.0	125	250
0.3	0.3	1.0	2.0	8.0	0.010	4.0	117	234
0.3	0.3	2.0	1.0	4.0	0.001	2.0	472	944
0.3	0.3	2.0	1.0	4.0	0.010	2.0	450	900
0.3	0.3	2.0	1.0	8.0	0.001	4.0	125	250
0.3	0.3	2.0	1.0	8.0	0.010	4.0	117	234
0.3	0.3	2.0	2.0	8.0	0.001	2.0	454	908
0.3	0.3	2.0	2.0	8.0	0.010	2.0	402	804
0.3	0.3	2.0	2.0	16.0	0.001	4.0	129	258
0.3	0.3	2.0	2.0	16.0	0.010	4.0	111	222

* Input Parameters: Pr(E), Pr(G) are individual prevalence rates for exposure and genetic susceptibility, respectively; r_E, r_G, and r_{EG} are population relative risks of disease due to exposure effect, genetic effect, and joint E × G effect, respectively; Pr{D|$\overline{EG}$} is the population spontaneous disease probability; and e^{ψ} is the ratio $r_{EG}/r_E r_G$.

The associated power function is an analogue of (11.2):

$$\bar{\beta}(\gamma) = 1 - \Phi\left(z_{\alpha/2} + \frac{\gamma}{\sigma[\hat{\gamma}]}\right) + \Phi\left(-z_{\alpha/2} + \frac{\gamma}{\sigma[\hat{\gamma}]}\right) \tag{11.7}$$

We solve this for N given a fixed significance level, α, a value for the desired power, $\bar{\beta}$, and the four multinomial case probabilities P_{ij}. If the P_{ij} values are not available, then we use the relationships given above between P_{ij} and the relative risks r_E, r_G, r_{EG}, and individual prevalences $Pr(E)$, $Pr(G)$. As functions of r_E, r_G, r_{EG}, $Pr(E)$, and $Pr(G)$, selected solutions for N using (11.7) appear in Table 11.2.

Prospective sampling: cohort studies   Under prospective sampling, as would occur, e.g., in a simple cohort study, we denote the observed counts among cases again as Y_{ij}, where $i = 0,1$ and $j = 0,1$ correspond to $\bar{E}$, E and $\bar{G}$, G, respectively. In this sampling scheme, the cell totals, $N_{ij}(i = 1,0; j = 0,1)$, are fixed in advance, and the associated control observations are simply the differences $N_{ij} - Y_{ij}$. The corresponding statistical

Table 11.2 Minimum sample sizes required for case-only study to identify true E × G interaction with power = 80%, at significance level $\alpha = 0.05$.

Pr(E)*	Pr(G)	r_E	r_G	r_{EG}	e^γ	N	% reduce†
0.1	0.1	1.0	1.0	2.0	2.0	1213	44.0
0.1	0.1	1.0	1.0	4.0	4.0	204	54.0
0.1	0.1	1.0	2.0	4.0	2.0	785	54.3
0.1	0.1	1.0	2.0	8.0	4.0	145	61.5
0.1	0.1	2.0	1.0	4.0	2.0	785	54.3
0.1	0.1	2.0	1.0	8.0	4.0	145	61.5
0.1	0.1	2.0	2.0	8.0	2.0	508	62.7
0.1	0.1	2.0	2.0	16.0	4.0	102	68.1
0.1	0.3	1.0	1.0	2.0	2.0	610	39.9
0.1	0.3	1.0	1.0	4.0	4.0	125	44.4
0.1	0.3	1.0	2.0	4.0	2.0	579	39.8
0.1	0.3	1.0	2.0	8.0	4.0	133	40.9
0.1	0.3	2.0	1.0	4.0	2.0	394	50.0
0.1	0.3	2.0	1.0	8.0	4.0	87	52.5
0.1	0.3	2.0	2.0	8.0	2.0	374	47.5
0.1	0.3	2.0	2.0	16.0	4.0	93	46.9
0.3	0.3	1.0	1.0	2.0	2.0	305	36.1
0.3	0.3	1.0	1.0	4.0	4.0	75	35.9
0.3	0.3	1.0	2.0	4.0	2.0	290	35.6
0.3	0.3	1.0	2.0	8.0	4.0	80	31.6
0.3	0.3	2.0	1.0	4.0	2.0	290	35.6
0.3	0.3	2.0	1.0	8.0	4.0	80	31.6
0.3	0.3	2.0	2.0	8.0	2.0	275	31.6
0.3	0.3	2.0	2.0	16.0	4.0	85	23.4

* Input Parameters: Pr(E), Pr(G) are individual prevalence rates for exposure and genetic susceptibility, respectively; r_E, r_G, and r_{EG} are population relative risks of disease due to exposure effect, genetic effect, and joint E × G effect, respectively; and e^γ is the ratio $r_{EG}/r_E r_G$.
† Percent reduction from minimum comparable case sample size (N) from Table 11.1.

model is a binomial distribution for the Y_{ij}'s, with sample size parameters N_{ij}, and with response probabilities π_{ij} ($i=0,1$; $j=0,1$). The π_{ij} values are the probabilities that a subject in the $(i,j)^{th}$ cell is diseased by the end of the prospective study period; e.g., $\pi_{01}=\Pr\{D|G\}$. Of interest are the relative risks of disease for each main effect (E and G), and also the relative risk of disease for the joint condition, $E \times G$. These are respectively, $r_E=\pi_{10}/\pi_{00}$, $r_G=\pi_{01}/\pi_{00}$, and $r_{EG}=\pi_{11}/\pi_{00}$. Once again, we take as the null effect a simple multiplicative model $r_E r_G = r_{EG}$ corresponding to (11.1). In terms of the π_{ij}'s, this is $\psi = log\{(\pi_{00}\pi_{11})/(\pi_{01}\pi_{10})\}$, in $H_0:\psi=0$.

Under prospective sampling, the bionomial model yields straightforward MLEs for the disease probabilities: $\hat{\pi}_{ij}=Y_{ij}/N_{ij}$. The corresponding MLE for ψ is

$$\hat{\psi} = log\left\{\frac{Y_{00}Y_{11}N_{01}N_{10}}{Y_{01}Y_{10}N_{11}N_{00}}\right\} \tag{11.8}$$

In the balanced case where all the cell sizes are taken to be equal, i.e., $N_{00}=N_{01}=N_{10}=N_{11}=N$ (say), (11.8) simplifies to $\hat{\psi}=log\{Y_{11}Y_{00}/Y_{01}Y_{10}\}$.

The large-sample standard error of the MLE in (11.8) is given by $\sigma[\hat{\psi}] = \sqrt{\Sigma\Sigma\{(1-\pi_{ij})/(N_{ij}\pi_{ij})\}}$. To test $H_0:\psi=0$ against some form of interactive departure, we reject H_0 when $|\hat{\psi}|/\sigma[\hat{\psi}]>z_{\alpha/2}$. When the values of π_{ij} are not known, they are replaced in $\sigma[\hat{\psi}]$ by their sample estimates, Y_{ij}/N_{ij}.

The corresponding power function is again analogous to (11.2), and is given in equation (11.3) above. For the special case of balanced sampling, and given a fixed significance level, α, a value for the desired power, $\bar{\beta}$, and the four disease probabilities π_{ij}, one can solve this equation for the common sample size N. (The total sample size is then 4N.) If all the π_{ij} values are not immediately available, we use instead the three relative risks r_E, r_G, r_{EG}, and any single disease probability, such as π_{00}. Then, for example, in the balanced case an alternative expression for $\sigma[\hat{\psi}]$ is

$$\sigma[\hat{\psi}] = \sqrt{\left(\frac{1+(1/r_E)+(1/r_G)+(1/r_{EG})}{N\pi_{00}} - \frac{4}{N}\right)}$$

We have computed solutions for N in (11.3) using this special case with $\alpha=0.05$ and $\bar{\beta}=0.8$, over a range of different values of r_E, r_G, r_{EG}, and π_{00}. The results appear in Table 11.3

Table 11.3   Minimum sample sizes required for cohort study to identify true $E \times G$ interaction with power = 80%, at significance level $\alpha = 0.05$. Number of subjects per group is constant (N), so that total sample size is 4N.

π_{00}*	r_E	r_G	r_{EG}	e^ψ	N
0.001	1.0	1.0	2.0	2.0	57112
0.01	1.0	1.0	2.0	2.0	5653
0.1	1.0	1.0	2.0	2.0	507
0.001	1.0	1.0	4.0	4.0	13257
0.01	1.0	1.0	4.0	4.0	1311
0.1	1.0	1.0	4.0	4.0	117
0.001	1.0	2.0	4.0	2.0	44860
0.01	1.0	2.0	4.0	2.0	4428
0.1	1.0	2.0	4.0	2.0	384
0.001	1.0	2.0	8.0	4.0	10705
0.01	1.0	2.0	8.0	4.0	1056
0.1	1.0	2.0	8.0	4.0	91
0.001	2.0	2.0	8.0	2.0	34650
0.01	2.0	2.0	8.0	2.0	3407
0.1	2.0	2.0	8.0	2.0	282
0.001	2.0	2.0	16.0	4.0	8408
0.01	2.0	2.0	16.0	4.0	827
0.1	2.0	2.0	16.0	4.0	68

* Input Parameters: π_{00} is spontaneous disease probability; r_E, r_G, and r_{EG} are population relative risks of disease due to exposure effect, genetic effect, and joint $E \times G$ effect, respectively; and e^ψ is the ratio $r_{EG}/r_E r_G$.

References

1. Sexton K., Callahan, M. A. and Bryan, E. R. (1995) Estimating exposure and dose to characterize health risks: the role of human tissue monitoring in exposure assessment. *Environ Hlth. Persp.* **103**: 13–29.
2. Kohlmeier, L. (1991) What you should know about your marker. In: Kok, F., van't Veer, P. (ed.). *Biomarkers of dietary exposure. Proceedings of the 3rd meeting on Nutritional epidemiology.* Smith-Gordon, London, 15–25.
3. Hargrov, J. L. and Berdainer, C. D. (1993) Nutrient receptors and gene expression. In: Berdanier, C. D. and Hargrove, J. L. (ed.). *Nutrition and gene expression.* CRC Press, Boca Raton, FL.
4. Gill, R. K. and Christakos, S., (1993) Vitamin D-dependent calcium binding protein, calbindin-D L: regulation of gene expression. In: Berdanier, C. D. and Hargrove, J. L. (ed). *Nutrition and gene expression* CRC Press, Boca Raton, FL.
5. Anderson, K. E., Conney, A. H., Kappas, A. (1982) Nutritional influences on chemical biotransformations in humans. *Nutr. Rev.* **40**: 161–171.
6. Kappas, A., Anderson, K. E., Conney, A. H., Alvares, A. P. (1976) Influence of dietary protein and carbohydrate on antipyrine and theophylline metabolism in man. *Clin. Pharm. Ther.* **20**: 643–53.
7. Sinha, R., Rothman, N., Brown, E. D., Mark, S. D., Hoover, R. N., Caporas, N. E., *et al.* (1994) Pan-fried meat containing high levels of heterocyclic aromatic amines but low levels of polycyclic aromatic hydrocarbons induces cytochrome P450 1A2 activity in humans. *Cancer Res.* **54**: 6154–9.
8. Fiorio, R., Bronzetti, G. (1995) Diallyl sulfide inhibits the induction of HPRT-deficient mutants in Chinese hamster V79 cells treated with dimethylnitrosamine in the presence of S9 of rats induced with acetone. *Environ. Mol. Mutagen.* **25**: 344–6.
9. Brady, J. F., Wang, M. H., Hong, J. Y. *et al.* (1991) Modulation of rat hepatic microsomal mono-oxygenase enzymes and cytotoxicity by diallyl sulfide. *Toxicol. Appl. Pharm.* **108**: 342–54.
10. Strickland P., Groopman, J. D., (1995) Biomarkers for assessing environmental exposure to carcinogens in the diet. *Am. J. Clin. Nutr.* **61** (Suppl 3): 710S–20S.
11. Butler, M. A., Lang N. P., Young, J. F., *et al.* (1992) Determination of CYP1A2 and NAT2 phenotypes in human populations by analysis of caffeine urinary metabolites. *Pharmacogenetics.* **2**: 116–27.
12. Ames, B. N. (1983) Dietary carcinogens and anticarcinogens. *Science* **221**: 1256–64.
13. Ames, B. N. (1995) The causes and prevention of cancer. *Proc. Natl. Acad. Sci. USA* **92**: 5258–65.
14. Wakabayashi, K., Sugimura T., Nagao, M. (1991) Mutagens in food. In: Li, A. P., Heflich, R. H., (ed.). *Genetic toxicology.* CRC Press, Boca Raton, FL 303–38.
15. Aguilar, F., Harris, C. C., Sun, T., Hollstein, M., and Cerutti, P., (1994) Geographic variation of p53 mutational profile in non-malignant human liver. *Science* **264**: 1317–19.
16. Cerutti, P., Hussain, P., Pourzand, C., and Aguilar, F. (1994) Mutagenesis of the H-ras proto-oncogene and the p53 tumor suppressor gene. *Cancer Res.* **54 (Suppl 7)**: 1934S–38S.
17. Lininsky, W. and Shubik, P. (1964) Benzo[a]pyrene and other polynuclear hydrocarbons in charcoal-broiled meat. *Science.* **145**: 53–5.
18. Fazio, T., and Howard, J. W. (1983) Polycyclic aromatic hydrocarbons in foods. In: Bjorseth, A., (ed.). *Handbook of polycyclic aromatic hydrocarbons.* Vol. 1. Marcell Dekker, New York. 461–505.
19. Yamamoto T., Tsuji, K., Kosuge, T., Okamoto, T., Shudo, K., Takeda, K. *et al.* (1978) Isolation and structure determination of mutagenic substances in L-glutamic acid pyrolysate. *Proc. Jpn. Acad.* **54**: 248–50.

20. Felton, J. S. and Knize, M. G. (1991) Occurrence, identification, and bacterial mutagenicity of heterocyclic amines in cooked food. *Mutat. Res.* **259**: 205–17.
21. Hasegawa, R., Tanaka, H. Tamano, S., Shirai, T., Nagao, M. Sugimura, T. *et al.* (1994) Synergistic enhancement of small and large intestinal carcinogenesis by combined treatment of rats with five heterocyclic amines in a medium-term multi-organ bioassay. *Carcinogenesis.* **15**: 2567–73.
22. Potter, J. D. and McMichael, A. J. (1986) Diet and cancer of the colon and rectum: a case-control study. *J. Nat. Cancer Inst.* **76**: 557–69.
23. Willett, W. (1989) The search for the causes of breast and colon cancer. *Nature.* **338**: 389–94.
24. Ames, B. N., Profet, M. and Gold, L. S. (1990) Dietary pesticides (99.99% all natural). *Proc. Natl. Acad. Sci. USA* **87**: 7777–81.
25. Sunderman, F. W. Jr (1986) Carcinogenicity and mutagenicity of some metals and their compounds. In: O'Neill, I. K., Schuller, P. and Fishbein, L .(ed.). *Environmental carcinogens. Selected methods of analysis. Vol. 8: Some metals: As, Be, Cd, Cr, Ni, Pb, Se, Zn.* IARC Scientific Publications, No. 71, International Agency for Research on Cancer, Lyon, France. 17–43.
26. Branda, R. F., Albertini, R. J. (1995) Effect of dietary components on hprt mutant frequencies in human T-lymphocytes. *Mutat. Res.* **346**: 121–7.
27. Anderson D., Yu, T. W., Phillips, B. J., Schmezer, P. (1994) The effect of various anti-oxidants and other modifying agents on oxygen-radical-generated DNA damage in human lymphocytes in the COMET assay. *Mutat. Res.* **307**: 261–71.
28. Weindruch, R. (1996) Caloric restriction and ageing. *Sci. Am.* **274**: 32.
29. Pfohl-Leszkowicz, A., Grosse, Y., Carriere, V., Cugnenc, P.-H., Berger, A., Carnot, F. *et al.* (1995) High levels of DNA adducts in human colon are associated with colorectal cancer. *Cancer res.* **55**: 5611–16.
30. Pearce, N., de Sanjose, S., Boffetta, P., Kogevinas, M., Saracci, R., Savitz, D. (1995) Limitations of biomarkers of exposure in cancer epidemiology. *Epidemiology.* **6**:190–4.
31. Shankel, D. M. (1991) Antimutagens. In: Li, A. P. and Heflich, R. H. (ed.). *Genetic toxicology.* CRC Press, Boca Raton, FL. 339–57.
32. De Flora, S., Zanacchi, P., Izzotti, A. and Hayatsu, H. (1991) Mechanisms of food-borne inhibitors of genotoxicity relevant to cancer prevention. In: Hayatsu, H. (ed.). *Mutagens in food: detection and Prevention.* CRC Press, Boca Raton, FL. 158–80.
33. Hayatsu, H., Negishi, T., and Arimoto, S. (1993) Dietary inhibitors against mutagenesis and carcinogenesis. In: Bronzetti, G., Hayatsu, H., De Flora, S., Waters, M. D., and Shankel, D. M. (ed.). *Antimutagenesis and anticarcinogenesis mechanisms III.* Plenum Press, New York. 387–418.
34. Kohlmeier, L., Simonsen, N., Mottus, K. (1995) Dietary modifiers of carcinogenesis. *Environ. Hlth. Persp.* **103**: 177–84.
35. Hood, L. (1988) Biotechnology and medicine of the future. *J. Am .Med. Assoc.* **259**: 1837–44.
36. Guengerich, F. P. (1994) Catalytic selectivity of human cytochrome P450 enzymes: relevance to drug metabolism and toxicity. *Toxicol. Lett.* **77**: 133–8.
37. Guengerich, F. P. (1995) Influence of nutrients and other dietary materials on cytochrome P450 enzymes. *Am. J. Clin. Nutr.* **61** (Suppl 3): 651S–8S.
38. Guengerich, F. P., Shimada, T., Yun, T-H., Yamazaki, H., Raney, K. D., Thier, R., *et al.* (1994) Interactions of ingested food, beverage, and tobacco components involving human cytochrome P450 1A2, 2A6, 2E1, and 3A4 enzymes. *Environ. Hlth. Persp.* **102** (Suppl 9): 49–53.
39. Lang, N. P., Butler, M. A., Massengill, J., Lawson, M., Stottos, R. C., Hauser-Jensen, M., *et al.* (1994) Rapid metabolic phenotypes for acetyltransferase and cytochrome P450 1A2 and putative exposure to food-borne heterocyclic amines increases the risk for colorectal cancer or polyps. *Cancer Epid. Biomarkers Prevention.* **3**: 675–82.

40. Vineis, P., and Martone, T., (1995) Genetic–environmental interactions and low level exposure to carcinogens. *Epidemiology* **6**: 455–7.
41. Vineis, P., Bartisch, H., Caporaso, N., Harrington, A. M., Kadlubar, F. F., Landi, M. T., *et al.* (1994) Genetically based N-acetyltransferase metabolic polymorphism and low-level environmental exposure to carcinogens. *Nature* **369**: 154–6.
42. Bell, D. A., Badawi, A. F., Lang, N. P., Ilett, K. F., Kadlubar, F. F. and Hirvonen, A. (1995) Polymorphism in the N-acetyltransferase 1 (NAT1) polyadenylation signal: association of NAT1*10 allele with higher N-acetylation activity in bladder and colon tissue. *Cancer Res.* **55**: 5226–9.
43. Bell, D. A., Stephens, E. A., Castranio, T., Umbach, D. M., Watson, M., Deakin, M. *et al.* (1995) Polyadenylation polymorphism in the acetyltransferase 1 gene (NAT1) increases risk of colorectal cancer. *Cancer Res.* **55**: 3537–42.
44. Badawi, A. F., Hirvonen, A., Bell, D. A., Lang, N. P. and Kadlubar, F. F. (1995) Role of aromatic amine acetyltransferase, NAT1 and NAT2, in carcinogen-DNA adduct formation in the human urinary bladder. *Cancer Res.* **55**: 5230–7.
45. Hwang, S-J., Beaty, T. H., Liang, K.–L., Coresh, J. and Khoury, M. J. (1994) Minimum sample size estimation to detect gene–environment interaction in case-control designs. *Am. J. Epid.* **140**: 1029–37.
46. Slattery, M. L., O'Brien, E., and Mori, M. (1995) Disease heterogeneity: does it impact our ability to detect dietary associations with breast cancer? *Nutr. Cancer* **24**: 213–20.
47. Piegorsch, W. W., Weinberg, C. R., and Taylor, J. A. (1994) Non-hierarchical logistic models and case-only designs for assessing susceptibility in population-based case-control studies. *Stat. Med.* **13**: 153–62.
48. Cole, T. J. (1991) Sampling, study size, and power. In: Margetts, B. M. and Nelson, M. (ed.). *Design concepts in nutritional epidemiology.* 1st edn. Oxford University Press, Oxford. 53–78.
49. Morgenstern, H. and Thomas, D. (1993) Principles of study design in environmental epidemiology. *Environ. Hlth. Perspect.* **101** (Suppl 4): 23–38.
50. Weinberg, C. R. (1993) Toward a clearer definition of confounding. *Am. J. Epid* .**137**: 1–8.
51. Upfal, M., Divine, G., and Siemiatycki, J. (1995) Design issues in studies of radon and lung cancer: implications of the joint effect of smoking and radon. *Environ. Hlth. Perspect.* **103**: 58–63.
52. Tamai, S., Sugimura, H., Caporaso, N. E., Resau, J. H., Trump, B. F., Weston, A., *et al.* (1990) Restriction fragment length polymorphism analysis of the L-*myc* gene locus in a case-control study of lung cancer. *Int. J. Cancer* **46**: 411–15.
53. Breitner, J. C. S., Murphy, E. A. and Woodbury, M. A. (1991) Case-control studies of environmental influences in diseases with genetic determinants, with an application to Alzheimer's disease. *Am. J. Epid.* **133**: 246–56
54. Khoury, M. R. and Beatty, T. H. (1994) Applications of the case-control method in genetic epidemiology. *Epid. Rev.* **16**: 134–50.
55. Wei, Q., Matanowski, G. M. and Grossman, L. (1994) DNA repair and susceptibility to basal cell carcinoma: a case-control study. *Am. J. Epid.* **140**: 598–607.
56. Breslow, N. and Day, N. (1980) *Statistical methods in cancer research. I. The analysis of case-control studies.* Vol. 32. IARC Scientific Publications, Lyon, France.
57. Weinberg, C. R. and Sandler, D. P. (1991) Randomized recruitment in case-control studies. *Am. J. Epid.* **134**: 421–32.
58. Weinberg, C. R. and Wacholder, S. (1993) Prospective analysis of case-control data under general multiplicative–intercept risk models. *Biometrika.* **80**: 461–5.
59. Piegorsch, W. W. (1994) Statistical models for genetic susceptibility in toxicological and epidemiological investigations. *Environ. Hlth. Perspect.* **102** (Suppl. 1): 77–82.
60. Breslow, N. E. and Storer, B. E. (1985) General relative risk functions for case-control studies. *Am. J. Epid.* **122**: 149–62.

61. Kleinbaum, D. G., Kupper, L. L. and Morgenstern, H. (1982) *Epidemiologic research: principles and quantitative methods*. Lifetime Learning Publications, Belmont, California.

62. Gardner, M. J. and Munford, A. G. (1980) The combined effect of two factors on disease in a case-control study. *Appl. Stat.* **29**: 276–81.

63. Piegorsch, W. W. and Taylor, J. A. (1992) Statistical methods for assessing environmental effects on human genetic disorders. *Environmetrics*. **3**: 503–18.

64. Wald, A. (1943) Tests of statistical hypotheses concerning several parameters when the number of observations is large. *Trans. Am. Math. Soc.* **54**: 426–82.

65. Greenland, S. (1983) Tests for interaction in epidemiologic studies: a review and a study of power. *Stat. Med.* **2**: 243–51.

66. Schlesselman, J. J. (1974) Sample size requirements in cohort and case-control studies of disease. *Am. J. Epid.* **99**: 381–4.

67. Rao, B. R. (1986) Joint distribution of simultaneous exposures to several carcinogens in a case-control study: sample size determination. *Comm. Stat. – Theory and Methods*. **15**: 3035–65.

68. Dupont, W. D. and Plummer, M. (1990) Power and sample size calculations: a review and computer program. *Controlled Clin. Trials*. **11**: 116–28.

69. Smith, P. and Day, N. E. (1984) The design of case-control studies: the influence of confounding and interaction effects. *Int. J. Epid.* **13**: 356–65.

70. Begg, C. B. and Zhang, Z.-F. (1994) Statistical analysis of molecular epidemiology studies employing case-series. *Cancer Epid., Biomarkers and Prevention*. **3**: 173–5.

71. Lawrence, C. and Greenwald, P. (1977) Epidemiologic screening: a method to add efficiency to epidemiologic research. *Am. J. Epid.* **105**: 575–81.

72. Burr, M. L. (1991) Cohort studies. In: Margetts, B. M. and Nelson, M. (ed.). *Design concepts in nutritional epidemiology*. 1st edn. Oxford University Press, Oxford. 369–84.

73. Kupper, L. L., McMichael, A. J. and Spirtas, R. (1975) A hybrid epidemiologic study design useful in estimating relative risk. *J. Am. Stat. Assoc.* **70**: 524–8.

74. Prentice, R. L. (1986) A case-cohort design for epidemiologic cohort studies and disease prevention trials. *Biometrika*. **73**: 1–11.

75. Margetts, B. M. and Rouse, I. L. (1991) Experimental studies. In: Margetts, B. M. and Nelson, M. (ed.). *Design concepts in nutritional epidemiology*. 1st edn. Oxford University Press, Oxford. 385–408.

76. Breslow, N. and Day, N. (1987) *Statistical methods in cancer research. II. The analysis of cohort studies*. Vol. 82. IARC Scientific Publications, Lyon, France.

77. Kaaks, R., Riboli, E. and van Staveren, W. (1995) Sample size requirements for calibration studies of dietary intake measurements in prospective cohort investigations. *Am. J. Epid.* **142**: 557–66.

78. Yanagawa, T. (1979) Designing case-control studies. *Environ. Hlth. Perspect.* **32**: 143–56.

79. Lubin, J. H. and Gail, M. H (1990) On power and sample size for studying features of the relative odds of disease. *Am. J. Epid.* **131**: 552–66.

80. Clayton, E. W., Steinberg, K. K., Khoury, M J., Thomson, E., Andrews, L., Kahn, M. J. E., *et al.* (1995) Informed consent for genetic research on stored tissue samples. *J. Am. Med. Assoc.* **274**: 178–92.

Part C   The design of nutritional epidemiological studies

12. Ecological studies

Janet E. Hiller and Anthony J. McMichael

12.1 Introduction

When epidemiologists use the term 'ecological' it does not refer to the environmental context in which living organisms exist but to a research study design in which the focus is on characteristics of population groups rather than their individual members. In ecological studies of the association between nutrition and disease, population or group indices of dietary intake or nutritional status are related to population or group indices of health status. The unit of analysis is not an individual but a group defined by time (calendar period, birth cohort), geography (country, province, or city), or by socio–demographic characteristics (e.g. ethnicity, religion, or socio–economic status). In nutritional epidemiology, ecological studies have predominantly examined geographic relationships of indices of dietary intake or nutritional status and health. An important example is the early series of ecological observations suggesting the importance of blood cholesterol and dietary fats in the aetiology of coronary heart disease[1] and showing the association between plasma cholesterol, dietary intake of saturated fats, and coronary heart disease rates.

Ecological studies are frequently the first stage in constructing an epidemiological picture of the differential distribution of diseases among people with different risk profiles. Variation in disease risk between different categories of persons can indicate differences in genetic composition, differences in environmental exposures, differences in both genes and environment, or interaction between the two. Ecological studies of migrant populations have been widely used to partition causation between genetic and environmental factors. These comparisons usually take advantage of routinely collected data and are therefore considered relatively inexpensive.

Similar techniques can be used to investigate correlations over time. For instance, the age–standardized mortality rate from coronary heart disease, which has decreased in the United States since the mid-1960s, has been linked to the increase in the per capita alcohol consumption over the same period (Fig. 12.1).[2]

Even more information may be obtained by simultaneously examining variations in both space and time, as did Dwyer and Hetzel[3] in their examination of time trends in coronary heart disease mortality in three countries in relation to changes in major risk factors.

Ecological analyses are only of value when the groups or communities being compared are relatively heterogeneous in their mean levels of exposure to dietary factors. For this reason, they have been used most extensively for between-country rather than within-country comparisons. For example, although extensive maps, indicating

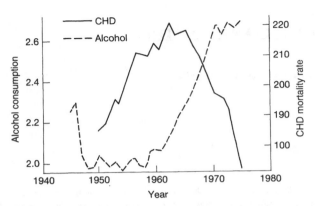

Fig. 12.1 Time trends in the age-standardized coronary heart disease (CHD) mortality rate (per 10^5 population) and per capita alcohol consumption (gal/yr), US, 1945–1975. (Source: Kuller *et al.*[2])

regional differences in disease incidence[4], are available for the United States, regional variations in most components of dietary intake in that country are limited. It has been estimated that 90% of adults in the United States eat between 30% and 44% of their calories as fat, while, worldwide, 90% of adults eat between 11% and 42% of their calories as fat.[5]

The People's Republic of China offers an opportunity for the application of ecological techniques in the examination of the association between diet, other aspects of lifestyle, and disease because there are wide variations in disease rates from one region to another, accompanying substantial differences in culture, behaviour and lifestyle. This between-regional heterogeneity was the rationale behind a large, ecological study in China in which disease rate patterns between regions were correlated with dietary and lifestyle data collected in those same regions.[6]

The ecological approach is limited as a source of causal inference because of the inability to determine whether the index of dietary intake of interest is actually associated with health status at the level of the individual. The 'ecological fallacy' is a term applied to errors that may result from making inferences about exposure–effect relationships at the level of individuals on the basis of relationships observed at the group level.[7] The use of a summary measure of exposure for each group being compared overlooks the actual heterogeneity in exposure levels among the individual members of a group.

Ecological studies frequently provide a useful first look at relationships. When used in a frankly exploratory context (for example, the study by Armstrong and Doll[8] on international variations in cancer incidence and mortality), they may suggest new hypotheses worthy of further study. They are also useful for preliminary appraisal of newly-proposed hypotheses.

Further, they are frequently the only research method of value in the investigation of the association between various aspects of diet and disease risk, either because exposure data are not available at the individual level (for example, fluoride in drinking water), or because within-population variations in exposure may be insufficient to cause detectable within-population variations in disease risk.[9]

Population-level studies have highlighted gaps in our understanding of the causes of coronary heart disease. The French 'paradox', in which coronary heart disease mortality in these communities is lower than would be predicted from well-documented risk factors, suggests that another hitherto unsuspected dietary factor is important.[10] Conversely, ecological studies can be used to expand and support the conclusions drawn from individual-level investigations, for example, the European Prospective Investigation into Cancer and Nutrition (EPIC)[11], in which a series of cohort studies is being undertaken focusing on diet and cancer. The within-community comparisons will rely on individual level data while the between-community comparisons, which will be able to investigate the effects of a wider range of nutritional intakes, will be more ecological in approach.

Well-designed ecological studies such as EPIC frequently collect data on non-dietary confounders – information that typically is not available in opportunistic ecological studies. An example of research designed to collect group-level data, rather than relying on existing data sources, is the series of studies sponsored by the International Agency for Research on Cancer (WHO) comparing fibre consumption in populations with differences in colorectal cancer incidence. In these Scandinavian-based studies, faecal chemistry, bacteria, and bulk were examined as well as estimated average population intakes of dietary fibre (Fig. 12.2).[12]

Ecological measures have been used to complement individual-level data in the development of multi-level models to describe the combined effects of social factors and individual behaviours on health and disease.[13] This methodological development creates opportunities for nutritional epidemiologists to develop explanatory models on an individual level that utilize community-level data. As nutrition is strongly influenced

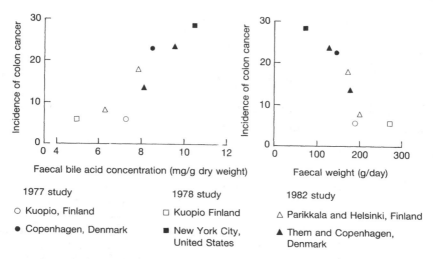

Fig. 12.2 The relationship between faecal bile acid concentration and faecal weight and the incidence of colon cancer in three studies, made in 1977, 1978, and 1982. (Source: Muir[12])

by cultural forces as well as individual opportunity and choice, multi-level analysis will encourage the stronger integration of ecological techniques and individual-level study designs.

12.2   Indices of dietary intake

12.2.1   Average consumption

Estimates of average individual intake can be made from pre-existing (usually commercially-oriented) data or from population survey data collected *de novo* (Table 12.1).[14]

National food supply or food 'disappearance statistics'

The Food and Agricultural Organization (FAO) publishes food balance sheets for 146 countries[15] which estimates the average amount of food available per person on a daily basis. These food 'disappearance' statistics are calculated by estimating the quantity of food produced in a given country, added to the quantity of food imported, and subtracting the food exported, lost in storage, fed to animals, or used for non-dietary purposes. The resulting figure is converted to an estimate of per capita consumption by dividing by the total population. These data tend to reflect food availability patterns rather than actual dietary intake and they are, therefore, a reflection of food wastage as well as of food consumption.

Validation studies comparing estimates of dietary intake from aggregate data with estimates derived from survey data can improve the quality of ecological measures of

Table 12.1   Estimates of per capita consumption.

Parts of the food chain surveyed	Type of data published	Scope and limitation of survey data
National food supply	Food balance data collected by agricultulre ministries, collated by FAO	Allows for home production, imports and exports, changing food stocks
Market distribution	Industrial data	Limited to specific sectors
Household budget	Economic statistics	Limited to financial outlay of whole households on food: costs do not relate to nutritional value of purchases
Household consumption	Household food survey	Often fails to allow for food eaten elsewhere; food waste assumed
Individual nutrition	Individual food and nutrition intake	Numerous methods available of varying reliability

From James *et al. Healthy nutrition.*[14]

average dietary intake. The validity of the measures of subtypes of fatty acids derived from FAO data has been assessed in a study comparing the mean intakes of these same subtypes derived from individual dietary surveys.[16] Although absolute quantities of fatty acid intake varied with age, measures of intake expressed as a per cent of total energy intake were less likely to vary. This relative measure may be more useful in ecological studies than absolute measures as it adjusts for the over-estimation of food inherent in the use of food disappearance data. Such a measure of population dietary intake that is assumed to be invariant with age and gender can be used as an effect modifier or confounder in cross-cultural comparisons of patterns of disease.[17]

National governmental agencies tend to collate similar data, and make similar estimates of per capita food 'disappearance'. Such surveys provide crude estimates of average national consumption; there is seldom sufficient information to estimate consumption for subgroups, such as people of a given age or gender or socio-economic group. The use of these crude estimates of nutritional intake is a frequent source of error in taking an ecological approach to nutritional epidemiology.

National food 'consumption' statistics have proved useful in preliminary examinations of hypotheses. Dwyer and Hetzel[3] used these types of data in their examination of time trends in ischaemic heart disease mortality and its major risk factors in Australia, the United Kingdom, and the USA. They inferred that the absence of a decline in mortality in the 1970s in the United Kingdom – in contrast with the marked declines in Australia and the USA – reflected the lack of change in national indicators of a number of risk factors, including per capita consumption of dietary fat based on national food disappearance data. Between-country comparisons that include both rich and poor nations may, however, be subject to biases in the quality of data collected at national levels, in which case the calculation of adjusted measures of intake and validation studies assume greater importance.

Household or population survey data

National population surveys have been used to collect more detailed dietary information on subgroups of the population. Presuming appropriate sampling techniques have been used, these data are then extrapolated to the general population. In Australia, detailed 24-hour dietary data have been collected on samples of the population, as part of cross-sectional studies of changes in risk factors for coronary heart disease undertaken by the National Heart Foundation.[18] It has been argued that 24-hour recalls are only suitable for ecological studies, such as those being described in this chapter, and not for individual-based investigations of the association between disease and diet. The wide daily variation in an individual's diet (especially in micronutrients) renders a 24-hour recall more subject to error in estimating that individual's intake than an instrument based on usual consumption of foods.[19] On the other hand, 24-hour dietary data may provide a reasonable estimate of the diet of a given population, enabling comparisons to be made with other populations. Dietary intake data from different countries can be collected by food frequency questionnaires, weighed inventories, diet histories, 24-hour recall, two-day recall, household food surveys, and other methods (see Chapter 6). Combining or comparing data derived using very different collection methods adds an additional source of error.

Frequently, data derived from household food surveys are available only on a household basis and are not analysed by age or gender categories[20], limiting their usefulness in examining associations with age- or gender-specific disease rates. The validity of models for estimating within household distribution is now being assessed (Section 6.4.1). Recent data available from a study of diet and nutrition in British adults however, does provide age and gender-specific data derived from 7-day weighed intakes, albeit on a much smaller number of individuals.[21]

On other occasions, small-area data collected on individuals (e.g. dietary histories from a sample of the population in a given town) are presumed to typify intake in the area or region as a whole. These data are often collected in the form of household food inventories in which food intake for a given time period is estimated by trained field workers who visit the participating households. Average per capita intake is calculated by dividing the total household intake by the number of individual family members. Inferences are then drawn about the effect of regional differences in dietary intake on regional differences in indices of health status.

When analysing the health status of different subgroups in the population, indirect methods of estimating per capita consumption derived from aggregate data for the population as a whole must be interpreted with caution. In particular, associations between age- or gender-specific disease rates and per capita dietary consumption (for example, examining the correlation between national death rates from breast cancer in women and per capita consumption of dietary fat) presume that dietary patterns are relatively constant in all population subgroups. However, population-based dietary information is seldom published in a disaggregated form that would enable the calculation of average dietary intake in these specific population subgroups. The United States Health and Nutrition Survey (HANES) is an exception, as intake can be estimated for various age-, gender-, and ethnic-group-specific populations.

In-depth surveys of population subgroups

Ecological analyses of cross-cultural variations in mortality have used detailed nutritional analysis of the diets of small samples of individuals from those countries. For example, in an ecological analysis of the Seven Countries Study, which originally was designed to investigate associations between diet and cardiovascular disease, dietary recall data and laboratory analysis of average food intake were used to derive estimates of the average intake of anti-oxidant vitamins in each of the communities studies. These measures of average intake were correlated with mortality from lung, stomach, and colorectal cancer among the 16 cohorts of the study. Thus detailed dietary data were derived from small subsets of the populations included in the mortality analysis.[22]

12.2.2   National indirect indicators of consumption

In the absence of direct measures of dietary consumption, various indirect markers have been used. For example, sales or tax records have been used to estimate per capita consumption of alcohol. Such an indicator was used to examine the relationship of laryngeal cancer mortality time trends to those of alcohol consumption in the UK and Australia (Fig. 12.3).[23] This method may either underestimate true intake because

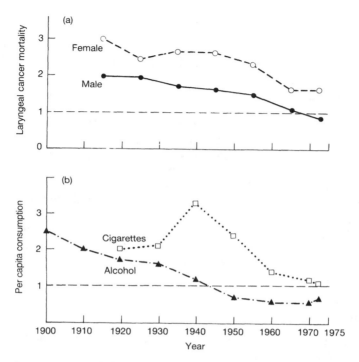

Fig. 12.3 Time trends in ratios of British versus Australian age-standardized laryngeal cancer mortality, by gender; and of British versus Australian consumption of alcohol and cigarettes. (Source: McMichael[23])

estimates of consumption do not include illegally purchased alcohol, exempt beverages, and home-brew, or it may overestimate intake by not accounting for wastage. However, if this type of unmeasured alcohol intake is a relatively constant proportion of all alcohol intake between the compared populations or time periods, then variations in the population marker of consumption may be a reliable indicator of changes in average individual consumption. It does not take into account variations in extremes of consumption which may be associated with particular diseases (e.g. cirrhosis of the liver).

In the absence of population data on diet, proxy indicators of intake including anthropometric measures of body mass index, weight-for-height and height-for-weight indices have been used in a study undertaken in the Congo to determine the population prevalence of stunting and wasting – indices of overall under-nutrition.[24]

Another example of an indirect indicator of consumption is that of applying estimates from a source population to some derivative (presumably representative) subpopulation. Typically, this method is used in migrant studies in which the diet in the country of birth is used as an indicator of likely diet in the host country.[25] Caution is needed in such an analysis because of the lack of information about post-migration secular trends in patterns of dietary behaviour.

12.2.3 Community-level indirect indicators of exposure

Community-level indicators of nutritional intake have been developed as part of community trials (Chapter 16). For example, grocery shop shelf space has been used to estimate changes in individual diets following the introduction of community nutrition programs.[26] This measure is used to make an inference about the dietary intake of those individuals using the grocery shops. This approach has also been used to indicate usual diet in remote Aboriginal communities in Australia where the local food store provides the majority of food consumed in that community.

Recent theoretical work on ecological studies, however, highlights that community level measures of the social environment in which individuals live may reflect combinations of effects that are not apparent when individuals are measured separately.[27] Examples of this effect, outside nutritional epidemiology, are provided by the work of Humphreys and Carr-Hill[28] who demonstrated that the poverty level of a community in which an individual lives has an effect on morbidity separate from the actual poverty level of that individual; and by the work of Koopman and others on infectious diseases, in which the disease risk for individuals is dependent on the disease risk for other individuals in their community.[29]

12.2.4 'Macroscopic generalization'

Occasionally, statements are made about dietary patterns in populations, based on observations of subgroups that have not been specifically sampled for the purpose. Thus, generalizations about dietary intake in the population are global statements not founded in sampling procedures. A well-known instance of this reasoning is the work of Burkitt and Trowell.[30] Stimulated by the large differences in disease profiles between eastern African and Western populations, they made casual observations about the traditional African diet replete with high-fibre, unprocessed foods; they presumed that this diet typified that of all non-urbanized Africans. They then inferred that dietary fibre was the crucial factor protecting African populations from the prevalent chronic diseases of Western countries, where fibre formed a much less significant component of the typical diet (limitations discussed further in Section 12.7). Similar global statements have been made about emerging chronic disease risks in Asia and South America, based on limited information about changes in dietary intake over time.[31]

12.2.5 Average food/soil concentrations of micronutrients

The intake of various micronutrients may be inferred from known deficiencies or excesses in the food or soil of a particular region. This estimate of intake is particularly appropriate when most food sources for a region are local. In the event of substantial importation of food from outside the local area, estimates of dietary intake derived from food or soil concentrations are likely to be misleading.

For example, in China, ecological analyses have demonstrated that areas with low soil levels of molybdenum (and low nitrate uptake) have higher rates of oesophageal cancer.[32] In addition, molybdenum levels analysed in hair samples were low in the high risk regions. Soil supplementation programmes in areas of China at high risk have been noted to increase the molybdenum level of vegetables and decrease their nitrate levels.[33] Thus, these analyses have correlated disease rates with the soil and food deficiencies and have also been able to demonstrate that changes in molybdenum content of locally grown foodstuffs occurred with supplementation programmes.

Concentrations of micronutrients can be influenced by changes in production processes. Changes in flour milling procedures during World War II increased the amount of fibre in flour.[34] This change correlated with reduced mortality from colon cancer in affected countries some 15 years after this dietary change (although the confounding effect of other wartime dietary changes was not excluded in the analysis).

The concentration of trace elements in drinking water has been linked with cardio-vascular disease rates in ecological studies that are between- and within-country. The analysis of the effect of drinking water quality on health is one that lends itself to ecological studies. In most communities, it is unlikely that drinking water to individual households would be supplied from a variety of sources (unlike London in the days of John Snow). Thus, any potential effect would need to be estimated by comparisons among communities with different water sources. In a British study[35] both water contents and disease rates were estimated at the town level. Some socio–economic and environmental measures were also available for the same unit of analysis and therefore could be used in multivariable analyses to adjust for confounding.

12.2.6   Average food/water concentrations of toxins

Variation in the amount of toxins in the local diet can be correlated with variations in disease occurrence in a group of communities. Again, such an analysis is only valuable in communities that do not consume foodstuffs that are grown elsewhere in any significant quantity. The motor-neurone disease, lytico, that occurs commonly in Guam, has been associated with the consumption of the cycad, a palm-like plant that is the source of edible starch.[36] These plants contain a non-protein amino acid (BMAA) that has been found to cause a motor-neurone disease among monkeys that resembles the Guam disorder.

Investigations of dietary causes of liver cancer have correlated the aflatoxin contamination of peanuts with liver cancer rates in east Africa.[37] More extensive research of the role of aflatoxin in liver cancer in the aforementioned large-scale Chinese ecological study on diet and disease[6] was able to examine the prevalence of hepatitis B infection in the same communities in which liver cancer rates and aflatoxin exposure were determined. In fact, chronic HBV infection was determined to be of far greater importance than aflatoxin – highlighting the importance of considering the potential effect of confounding variables when interpreting the findings of ecological studies.

There have been limited investigations of the consequences of heavy metal contamination of soils and their uptake into vegetables and grasses and hence into the food chain. This issue may become of increasing importance in vulnerable populations with poor nutritional status.[38]

12.2.7 Biological indices of dietary intake or nutritional status

In the face of scepticism about the validity and reliability of dietary survey data, developments in molecular epidemiology offer opportunities to use biomarkers of exposure[39] that reflect both intake and metabolism.[40] As disease rates presumably reflect environmental exposures in the past, the biological specimen will have maximum validity if it is an indicator of past consumption. Unfortunately, few available biomarkers both persist over time and reflect the total intake of the nutrient other than those that are fat soluble or those that are stored in hair or nails. Despite these limitations, the analysis of blood[41], urine[42,43], faeces[44,45,12], toe-nail clippings[46], saliva[47], and breast-milk[48], has provided useful information about presumed dietary intake of a range of foods and toxins. In particular, these biological specimens appear to provide useful measures of micronutrient intake.[49]

Since some disturbances of biological indices may reflect an aspect of the disease process itself, and not merely the causal pathway, ecological studies have an advantage over case-control studies in the way in which biological indices can be interpreted. In cases with disease, an abnormal profile of biological indices may reflect disease-induced metabolic derangements, or an abnormal exposure history. Even cohort studies of disease with long and unknown latent periods may be subject to the same limitation. In ecological studies, using samples of predominantly healthy persons, no such ambiguity exists.

Some biological indices are particularly suited for ecological studies rather than for individual-level studies. For example, serum vitamin A concentration is not an accurate measure of an individual's nutritional status. In populations, however, the frequency of very low or very high serum concentrations of vitamin A is a useful measure of the average nutritional status of that community.[48]

12.2.8 Collection and analytical methods

The determination of mean values for indicators of dietary intake could theoretically involve the handling and analysis of many separate food samples or biological specimens from a particular geographic region. A less expensive approach is to use pooled samples to derive estimates of intake for each geographic region. This approach necessarily forfeits information about the underlying distribution among individual study subjects, and precludes calculation of standard deviations and standard errors. It also assumes that the pooled mean reflects the averages of the individual values of the specimens contributing to the pool.

The large Chinese ecological study[6] used pooled biological samples, instead of individual samples, to derive estimates of nutrient intake for given communes. This approach increased the size of the biological sample, enabling the investigation of a wider range of indices, and provided a substantial cost-saving (again permitting the investigation of more markers). Instead of analysing fifty individual samples to get an estimate for a given commune, far fewer analyses were necessary. Blood and urine specimens were combined into either gender-specific pools or age-gender-specific pools for each commune and then analysed.

Validation assays were conducted on a random subsample of 150 individual specimens, which were then placed into six pools of 25 specimens. The results of these assays indicated good agreement between the mean of the individual assays and the value derived from analysis of the pooled specimens.

An additional disadvantage is incurred if there is a non-linear association between the dietary component being estimated and disease risk. In such circumstances, pooled estimates of intake would not correlate with disease rates and the true association would be obscured. A further problem occurs if the intention is to use a standardized value (e.g. urine metabolite from casual specimens expressed per mg creatinine). Differences between groups may be obscured if there is large variation in the concentration of the standard between individual specimens (i.e. the denominator) which is not taken into account; an approach to the solution to this problems is given by Nelson et al.[50]

Calibration studies can be used to enhance the quality of the exposure data used in ecological research. Biases in population level analyses can be corrected by using detailed dietary intake data collected on individual members of the populations being compared or biomarkers assessed in subgroups.[51]

12.3 Indices of health status

12.3.1 Routine measures of mortality and morbidity

Some of these measures have been alluded to in the section on indices of nutritional status. The measures of mortality or morbidity most frequently used in ecological studies include international, national, and small-area data[51] usually available through World Health Organization publications[52] or from special reports from national governments.[53] Age- and gender-specific disease rates or summary statistics (adjusted for age and, less frequently, gender) such as summary mortality rates or standardized mortality ratios can be used. These data have the advantage of routine availability, compatibility, and comprehensiveness, but are usually compiled only for the largest geographic unit, i.e. individual countries. International differences in mortality registration, diagnosis of cause of death, and survival may influence the interpretation of these data. Within-country comparisons must rely on national and local data sources, which may not collect the required information on a routine basis. However, in addition to mortality data, various measures of morbidity typically exist within developed countries for a variety of disorders such as cancer incidence and national estimates of decayed, missing, and filled teeth (DMFT) (Fig 12.4).[54] Accurate measures of disease incidence are not universally available, thus mortality data frequently are used as a proxy measure of disease risk. The development of accurate small area health statistics, as has occurred in the UK and Australia, facilitates within-country comparisons of both mortality and morbidity.[55,56]

12.3.2 Biological indices as (presumptive) disease-mediating processes

Biological specimens such as blood, urine, or faeces can be used as markers of stages in the disease process, or as direct measures of the presence of disease (for example, in

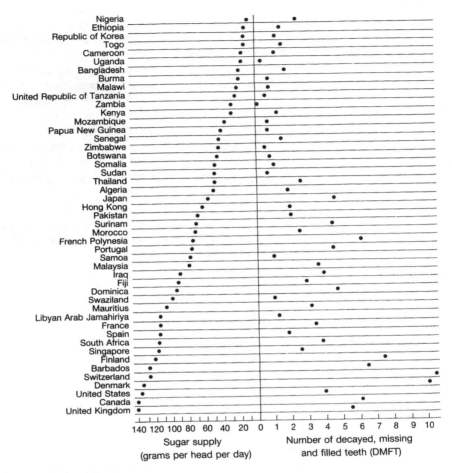

Fig. 12.4 Prevalence of dental decay, expressed as decayed, missing, and filled teeth (DMFT) in children aged 12 years, and per capita daily sugar supply in 47 countries. (Source: Sreebny[54])

diabetes). Such indices are not available routinely but must be collected as part of a special population survey. Data collected on representative subsamples of the population are presumed to be indicative of general associations.

Blood   A more direct measure of disease-mediating mechanisms has been provided in studies of the effect of marine oil ingestion on haemostasis in Eskimos, a group with a low death rate from coronary heart disease despite a high intake of animal fats.[57]

Faeces   IARC has completed two studies of regional variation in diet and faecal measures (concentration, absolute amounts, etc.) of primary and secondary bile acids as indicators of stages in the genesis of colon cancer.[44,45] These studies indicate a limitation of the ecological approach. Although bile acid concentrations varied between areas with high and low incidence of colon cancer, the researchers were unable to identify definitively the dietary components that contributed to these variations in bile acids.

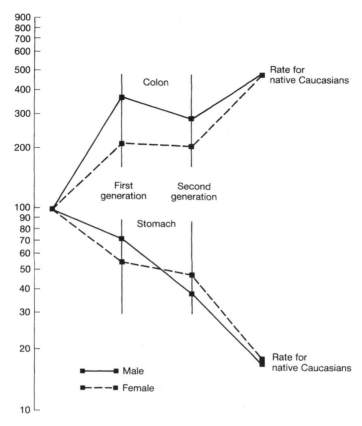

Fig. 12.5 Mortality from cancer of the stomach and colon in Japanese immigrants to the United States. (Source: Wynder *et al.*[61])

The final unravelling of the causal pathway may rely on research techniques better able to control for the various non-dietary factors that affect colon cancer risk.

Other Various other *ad hoc* methods of assessing the biomedical status of compared groups have been used. The tools of metabolic epidemiology can refine diet–disease associations being examined in ecological studies, for example by correlating the presence of DNA-adducts in urine with liver cancer rates.[58]

12.4 Populations or groups studied

12.4.1 Migrants

Changes in disease patterns among migrant populations away from those of their country of origin and towards that in the host country, have provided opportunities for the exploration of the relative effect of genetic predisposition and environmental exposures on disease. National per capita dietary consumption data derived from FAO data can be used to infer usual diet in the host country and in the migrants' countries of origin. These dietary data can then be compared with disease rates experienced by the various migrant groups in the host country. In the analysis of gastrointestinal cancer mortality among recent European migrants to Australia[25], migrants from countries with rates of stomach cancer that differed from the Australian rates, initially had correspondingly different rates from those in the Australian-born population. However, with increased duration of residence in Australia, and presumably, concomitant acculturation in dietary pattern, the disease patterns increasingly reflected those experienced by the native Australian population.

More definitive studies of the effect of acculturation and passage of time on diet in migrant populations have provided direct evidence of the gradual cultural adaptation to dietary patterns of the host population. Such studies have occurred in Australia amongst Italian[59] and Greek migrants[60] and in the United States where first-, second-, and third-generation Japanese migrants have been compared with Japanese in Japan and the rest of the citizens of the United States. The number of generations of residence in the United States is used as a proxy for change in diet from a traditional low fat Japanese diet to an American pattern of food consumption. Comparisons between cancer sites of the generations taken for a migrant group to assume the disease profile of the host population may provide clues to carcinogenic processes (Fig. 12.5). For example, colon cancer rates in migrant groups rapidly assume the pattern of the host population; stomach cancer rates take a little longer; and breast cancer rates take one to two generations to assume a new pattern, thereby indicating different effects on the initiation and promotion stages of carcinogenesis.[61]

Migrant studies recently supported by the International Agency for Research on Cancer have investigated the effects of Jewish immigration to Israel, in which people migrated from many different countries of origin, and the effects of Italian emigration to a range of host countries.

12.4.2 Religious groups

There have been many ecological studies of Seventh-Day Adventists, who frequently follow a lacto-ovovegetarian diet. When their cancer mortality is compared with mortality data for the general population there are indications of reduced risk for colon cancer and equivocal results for breast cancer.[62,63] Vegetarian English nuns have similarly provided a unique social group for the investigation of the effect of dietary restrictions on disease risk.[64] Limited conclusions can be drawn from many of these studies as religious groups frequently are distinctive in behaviours other than their diets.

Ecological analyses of disease patterns among religious groups may even suggest covert patterns of social behaviour. For example, in analysing the high rates of oral cancer in Iran, which cannot be explained by reported alcohol and tobacco consumption (as they have been in studies of many other populations), undercover illicit alcohol consumption may be considered.

12.4.3 Groups with distinct behaviour

Other sub-populations with distinctive dietary patterns have been investigated to determine whether these patterns are associated with similarly distinctive disease patterns. Observations on Eskimo populations have revealed relatively low rates of coronary heart disease, despite the consumption of diets high in fat and cholesterol which are presumed to increase the risk of this disease. The habitual consumption of large quantities of cold-water fish with long-chain polyunsaturated fatty acids of the omega-3 type, was presumed to be responsible, in part, for these low rates. The effect of this diet on thrombosis has been inferred by an examination of bleeding times in Eskimos and in Danish populations that have a different diet.[57] Eskimos were noted to have longer bleeding times.

12.4.4 Groups in cultural transition

Omran coined the term 'epidemiologic transition' to describe the changes, over time, in patterns of disease and health in different cultures.[65] In general, societies move from famine and pestilence, through an era during which infectious disease has the greatest impact on mortality, to a stage when degenerative or chronic diseases are the greatest health problems. Recent work has noted a subsequent pattern, particularly in some industrialized countries, characterized by behavioural change[31] leading to increased intake of fruits, vegetables, and complex carbohydrates and decreased intake of refined foods and dietary fats.

Westernization has frequently been accompanied by dramatic increases in the rates of non-insulin dependent diabetes mellitus (NIDDM) and other chronic disease.[66,67] In his early epidemiological observations on diabetes among the Pima Indians, West noted that diabetes, which had been uncommon before 1940 when most American Indians had been slender, became much more common as these populations became obese.[68] Zimmet and his colleagues have documented the effect of Westernization with its concomitant changes in diet, obesity levels, and physical exercise on various groups of Pacific Islanders who now have some of the highest rates of NIDDM in the world.[69,70] These studies highlight the value of ecological studies in studying phenomena that influence entire communities such as a shared genetic propensity. Individual-level studies in these communities would highlight the triggering effect of obesity rather than the genetic predisposition.

Although the effect on disease of the cultural impact of Westernization has been most widely documented among aboriginal peoples and in developing countries, a similar pattern has been noted in Japan. The incidence of disease associated (on an ecological basis) with high fat diets (cancers of the colon, pancreas, breast, prostate, ovaries, and endometrium, and coronary heart disease) is increasing in Japan as the traditional low fat diet undergoes increasing Westernization.[71]

12.4.5 Groups in social upheaval

Ecological studies have been used to examine the association between nutritional status and widespread social change that is known to affect dietary patterns. For example, following the Third World debt crisis of the 1980s, structural adjustment programmes have been introduced in developing countries at the behest of the World Bank and the International Monetary Fund. The impact of these programmes on measures of

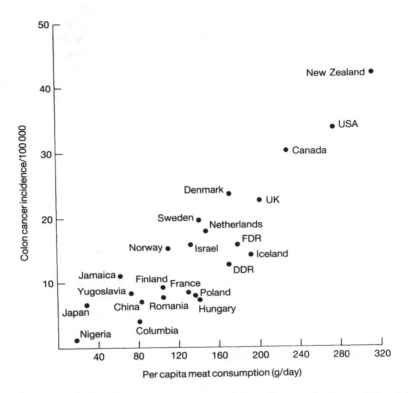

Fig. 12.6 Relationship between meat consumption in various countries and the risk in those countries of developing cancer of the colon. (Source: Peto[47])

population health[72] and the nutritional status of populations[24] has been documented. The effect of the social upheaval of war has been monitored by regular anthropometric surveys of the Bosnian population to allow the United Nations to determine population groups to target for relief work.[40]

12.4.6 Sub-populations displaying sharp cultural or behavioural differences

An ecological study examining possible explanations for the higher incidence of childhood coeliac disease in Sweden compared with Denmark, neighbouring countries with similar health care systems and ethnicity, highlighted differences in infant feeding practices as an explanation for the different pattern in incidence rates. Wheat flour, which has a high gluten content, is introduced at an earlier age and in greater quantities in Sweden.[73] This study demonstrates the advantages of ecological studies in examining the effect of different dietary patterns between groups that are similar in many respects other than dietary differences.

12.5 Techniques in examining relationships

12.5.1 Disease mapping, simple regression, and correlations

Exploratory analysis of geographic patterns of disease may use mapping procedures to compare disease rates between regions and countries. These maps can be displayed along with pictorial representations or scattergrams depicting international differences in nutrient intake (Fig. 12.6). The impressions conveyed by such maps require further investigation using more sophisticated techniques. Calculation of correlation coefficients between disease rates and regional indicators of dietary consumption[8] may be the next stage. These types of data indicate that there are systematic population-based patterns of association between diet and disease. Until recently ecological analyses have relied on such relatively simply statistical methods or correlation analysis.

Analytical issues arise in deciding whether it is appropriate to weight each area by its relative size. In addition, as contiguous areas are often similar in a variety of ways, and assumptions in a regression analysis of independent error terms are unlikely to be correct[35,74], statistical techniques have been developed to deal with autocorrelation.[75,76,77]

The simpler correlation analyses of ecological data can be refined by statistical methods designed to adjust for intercorrelations between indicators of dietary intake and other social indicators and amongst the range of dietary factors. Partial correlation coefficients[8] and stepwise regression techniques[78] have been used to examine the association between national age-adjusted cancer incidence and mortality rates and a variety of dietary and environmental variables (e.g. rainfall, population density, alcohol consumption) while adjusting for potential confounding variables. The stepwise multiple regression procedure was also used by Pocock[35] because it gives adjusted regression coefficients and provides evidence for the relative importance of each of the items included in the model.

The use of correlation techniques in ecological studies has been criticized.[7,79] If the populations being compared are selected because they are heterogeneous with respect to an independent variable (for example, dietary fat), correlation coefficients tend to be inflated because these coefficients are dependent on the relative dispersion of the independent and dependent variables. The variance of the independent variable will be increased relative to the disease or outcome variable, thereby increasing the size of the correlation coefficient.

12.5.2 Time-lagging

Time-lagging techniques are valuable in the analysis of ecological data. In examining associations between diet and patterns of chronic disease morbidity and mortality where latent and induction periods are known to be important, these time-lagging techniques may disclose the time of maximal aetiological influence of the dietary exposure. Rose used time-lagging techniques in an analysis of the association between blood cholesterol and coronary heart disease rates.[80] Data from seven countries on serum cholesterol levels recorded during 1958 and 1964, on men aged 40–59, were related to national mortality from coronary heart disease in the same age cohorts at 5-year intervals for a 15 year period. The correlations between serum cholesterol at baseline and coronary heart.disease mortality rates increased with time reaching a peak of 0.96 after 15 years.

Skog's analysis of the association between per capita alcohol consumption and liver cirrhosis mortality, highlighted a major limitation to correlation analysis of the association between dietary intake and disease rates.[81] Individuals' risk of dying from cirrhosis of the liver in a given year, is a reflection of their drinking history, not merely their alcohol consumption in the last year of life. Similarly, between- and within-country ecological analyses relating alcohol consumption to cirrhosis mortality rates, frequently display a time lag between the period of peak consumption and the time of peak mortality rates. When the regression equation is modified by the addition of a lag parameter, differential weightings are providing to exposures according to their proximity to the year of death or incidence of disease. This method is particularly appropriate when the median latency between exposure and diagnosis is known and can be used in the time-lagged analysis. If the latency is unknown or has wide variability between individuals, time-lagging introduces an additional source of error rather than improving accuracy. In addition, time-lagging presumes a stable population; the estimates of exposure and the subsequent measures of disease refer to the same or similar individuals. Both immigration and emigration can substantially alter the underlying population.

Time-lagging will acquire a greater role in the analysis of ecological studies as public health nutrition moves to an awareness of the long-term consequences of nutritional deficiencies and excesses.[82,83]

12.5.3 Cohort analysis

Government policy, or some other major social change, may affect the dietary intake for particular areas resulting in a sudden change in diet for the population. The effect of that change can be examined by investigating disease rates prior to the change and disease rates in population cohorts following the change. For instance, birth cohort-based analysis of changes in age-specific oesophageal cancer rates in Australia highlighted a decline in risk from cohort to cohort commencing around the turn of the century with a recent increase in rates at younger ages.[84] Graphs of time trends in per capita consumption of alcohol in beer, wine, and spirits for 1900–1975 suggested that the drop in alcohol consumption (especially of spirits consumption) in the first third of this century was associated with the changing pattern of oesophageal cancer rates in successive cohorts. The prevalence of low birthweight, the percentage of wasting among children less than one year of age, and the prevalence of chronic energy deficiency among mothers in Brazzaville increased from 1986 to 1991 following the introduction of a structural adjustment programme supported by the International Monetary Fund.[24]

12.5.4 Adjusting for confounders

Ecological analyses have been criticized because they can lead to spurious and often curious associations, especially in simple correlation studies. Analysis of the effect of confounding variables in ecological studies is not possible at the individual level, creating an additional source of error. This complication has been documented in studies of water hardness and cardiovascular disease, in which disease rates are not only associated with soft water, but with three other well-documented risk factors for cardiovascular disease – smoking, blood pressure, and serum cholesterol.[53] Certainly, it has been claimed that associations between dietary fat, or total calories, and chronic diseases associated with economic development, are confounded by other indicators of gross national product. Is the putative association between national diet and national disease rates merely a consequence of an association between some other factor affected by socio–economic development and the disease in question? Adjustment for confounding variables has been a problem in the analysis of ecological data because these data were often not available nor easily measured on a geographical basis.[35]

The problem of confounding is not insurmountable as statistical developments have demonstrated the feasibility of combining routinely collected, aggregate-level, adjusted (usually for age and gender) disease rates with detailed data on exposures and confounding factors collected on subsets of each population group being compared.[85]

In the analysis of liver cirrhosis death rates by Qiao et al.[86], partial correlation coefficients for a variety of dietary constituents and disease rates have been adjusted for alcohol consumption because data were available on a per capita basis for all dietary constituents examined. Unfortunately, data on confounding factors are not always available covering the same geographic units included in the ecological analysis.

In the absence of small-area data on the distribution of confounding variables, researchers have used proxy measures that are available. In an ecological analysis of arsenic in drinking water and vascular disease mortality in 30 counties in the United States[87], smoking was considered to be a potential confounder. As smoking-related causes of death were not available at the county level, the researchers used the relative risks of smoking-related causes of death as age-adjusted proxy measures for smoking. An adjustment for socio–economic differences has used data on the percentages of households without amenities as an indicator of both hygiene and of social class.[88] The observed positive association between potato and sugar consumption and acute appendicitis rates was reduced after controlling for the percentage of households without a bath in each of the 90 areas of England, Wales, Scotland, and Eire. The inverse relationship between vegetable consumption (other than potatoes) and appendicitis was also weakened following the adjustment, via partial correlations, for social class. However, the partial correlation of −0.41 remained a strong indication of an inverse association between diet and appendicitis.

Other creative adjustment methods may be available. Dobson[89] examined trends in cardiovascular risk factors in Australia, determined from serial risk factor prevalence surveys, to determine their possible contribution to mortality declines. Proportional hazards models, derived from data from the Framingham study in the United States, were used as a source of coefficients to examine the contributions of average changes in risk factors among groups on group death rates. Beta coefficients were thus derived from longitudinal data collected on North American individuals and applied to changes in average cholesterol levels, systolic blood pressure, and cigarette smoking in Australia. Age- and gender-specific grouped data risk factor levels were available. This analytical method enabled the examination of the effect of each of these risk factors after adjusting for the other two in the equation.

Large-scale ecological studies that have been conducted in the 1980s and 1990s have been designed to collect data on the distribution of confounding variables in the communities being compared directly.[6]

12.5.5 Multi-level analysis

This technique (described in section 12.1) incorporates individual-level and ecological data in the same model. Although it has not yet been used in nutritional epidemiology except in the evaluation of community trials of nutritional interventions, it offers considerable opportunities to reduce the bias of less sophisticated approaches to the analysis of ecological data in making inferences about determinants of individual behaviour.

12.6 Criteria of 'proof' in ecological associations between diet and disease

The criteria for legitimizing the drawing of causal inferences are no different in ecological studies than in other epidemiological investigations, although emphases may differ. Particular attention should be paid to the biological plausibility of associations identified from ecological studies and the overall coherence of data, given the possibility of identifying associations that are nonsensical. For example, the ecological examination of the protective role of non-starch polysaccharides in large bowel cancer is limited by difficulties in obtaining the appropriate dietary information. However, the coherence of the strong inverse association observed with basic science research lends credibility to the findings.[90]

The specificity of association is a criterion that can be readily tested. Is the association specific to the dietary component of interest and the disease of interest, or is there a variety of unconnected associations that may reflect the quality of data rather than true associations? An ecological analysis of the association between Alzheimer's disease and aluminium in drinking water determined that there was no association with another neurological disorder, epilepsy, although the risk for Alzheimer's disease in areas with higher aluminium concentration was 1.5 times the risk in low concentration areas.[91]

The calculation of correlation and regression coefficients, and the use of time series analysis to test co-variation, incorporate the notion of the dose–response criterion.

Temporal relationships can be evaluated by investigating disease rates following changes in exposures. For example, the association between dental decay and fluoridation can be documented by examining indicators of dental health prior and subsequent to the introduction of a fluoridation programme.

12.7 Limitations

Beyond the logical problem of the ecological fallacy, there are methodological difficulties in ecological studies, particularly when used to draw inferences at the level of the individual. Confounding is a particular problem in ecological studies of diet and diseases associated with industrialization (Section 12.5.4). Studies conducted within a country can usually control for some of the socio–economic factors associated with level of development, such as standard of medical care, quality of recording, and exposure to non-dietary risk factors.

Between-country comparisons may be restricted by the absence of comparable data, usually on dietary intake, although cause of death may also be subject to international differences in data quality. On the other hand, within-country comparisons (e.g. between Francophone and Flemish areas of Belgium) that may not suffer from lack of compatibility of data, may yet be restricted by the limited size of the population in each region and the consequent instability in rates, as well as by homogeneity of exposures within the country as a whole.

Where there is marked individual variation in the dietary component of interest within each geographical region (i.e. heterogeneity of exposure), summary exposure measures (e.g. average consumption data) may have such large, but unknown, error terms associated with them that correlations with disease rates would be rendered useless. As a corollary to that limitation, there is a presumption that within a region of interest there are no systematic differences in dietary exposure between sub-regions. For instance, if only one county within a given region experiences unusual dietary intake patterns and disease rates, then this association may either be obscured, or else erroneous conclusions may be drawn about the region as a whole, i.e. a type of 'ecological fallacy' would occur. As with other types of epidemiological studies, inferences are limited by the details and quality of the data.

In addition, some reports of ecological associations between chronic diseases and dietary indices have disregarded the long preclinical induction periods inherent in these diseases[74] and have examined correlations between contemporaneous indicators of dietary patterns and disease rates. Unless some time lag analysis is used, there must be an assumption that current consumption patterns reflect past consumption. This assumption will be flawed when the exposure to the dietary factors being investigated has changed dramatically over time.[31]

The population unit being used for analysis of morbidity or mortality is often inappropriate for the analysis of exposure to diet. In addition, one must ensure that the same geographical boundaries are used for all analyses. Mortality and incidence data may be available for different age, race, and gender groupings while dietary data may only be available for much larger aggregates.

Interactions between a variety of dietary exposures and a disease outcome or between diet and other exposure factors and disease cannot be assessed in ecological studies because data are not available about joint probabilities of exposure at the level of the individual.

12.8   When are ecological studies the method of choice?

Ecological studies are ideal for examining newly-proposed hypotheses. They have been particularly useful in situations where it is possible subsequently to study causal relationships at an individual level. An analysis of the relationship between dietary factors and liver cirrhosis death rates indicated a potential protective effect of calcium[86] that had not been documented previously.

Ecological studies are invaluable when intake (or outcome) data are unavailable on an individual level. Despite the oft-stated proviso that ecological analyses can only generate hypotheses that should be tested subsequently using more rigorous observational or experimental methods[79], it should be borne in mind that the ecological approach is frequently the only one available for the examination of hypotheses when exposure cannot be defined meaningfully on an individual level. For example, the association between the cumulative prevalence of dental decay in children aged 12 and sugar intake, can be readily documented using FAO data on per capita daily sucrose utilization in 47 countries. It may not be possible (or at least practicable) to measure individual sugar intake because estimates should be based on total dietary intake, including processed foods, although data may not be available for individual items.

In addition, ecological studies may be more appropriate when there is great variability at the individual level in the measure of exposure (regression dilution bias). The collection and analysis of individual food records is difficult, may not reflect habitual intake, and cannot measure individual variability in the metabolic response to a given diet. Because of the innate (and/or acquired) variability in individual response to diet intake, the dietary risk factors for some diseases may be more evident for groups/populations than for individuals. The relationship between dietary salt and blood pressure is widely considered to provide an example of this important issue. The correlation between salt and blood pressure on an individual level may be further attenuated by the homogeneity of exposure among individuals within a given population. The ecological data are not easily dismissed given their strength and their concordance with experimental data. The INTERSALT Study, which examined this relationship in 52 populations in 32 different countries, analysed data with individuals as units of analysis and with communities as units of analysis and thus, within the same study, were able to examine the relationship between sodium, potassium, and blood

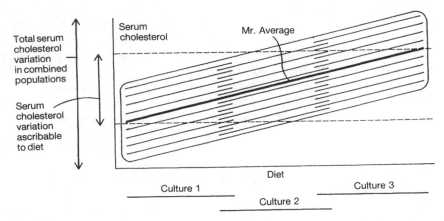

Fig. 12.7 A schematic representation of the variation of serum cholesterol ascribable to diet across three communities representing different cultures. (Source: Fraser[95])

pressure using the strengths and weaknesses of both levels of analysis.[92] Ecological analysis of these data were enhanced by the availability of information on confounding factors such as age, gender, BMI, and alcohol consumption on the same units of measurement as the blood pressure data (see Section 12.5.4). The availability of data on exposure, outcome, and confounders on the same population groups enhances the quality of ecological analyses. Such analysis of cross-sectional data however, is limited by the inability to time-lag.

Ecological studies are also valuable in the investigation of associations between dietary exposure and disease when, within a given population, there is insufficient heterogeneity in exposure experience. This issue has been debated at length in interpretations of the contradictory findings on the association between dietary fat and breast cancer risk in ecological and individual-level studies, be they case-control or cohort in design (which, it should be noted, may also suffer from an inability to collect dietary data at the critical period in determining breast cancer risk for a given individual).[9,93,94]

Instruments assessing dietary intake on an individual level are subject to measurement error (as are instruments measuring population levels of dietary intake). Narrow gradient of exposure combined with the inherent limitations of measuring instruments reduce the power of cohort and case-control studies to detect an increase in risk. Fraser's illustration[95] (Fig. 12.7) of the limited variation in serum cholesterol levels within cultures demonstrates this phenomenon. Ecological studies on the other hand, that use average measures of intake, or blood nutrient analyses based on large numbers of individuals, are less likely to be affected by the attenuation of effect estimate that would be found in individual-level studies.

Thus, ecological studies may be invaluable not only for investigating diseases where there is no *a priori* method for measuring exposure on an individual level (and are therefore seen as the method of second choice) but may be the method of choice even when exposure can be measured at an individual level.

A revival of interest in ecological studies has reflected a need for epidemiology to examine patterns of disease and health at a population level and to appreciate that at least some determinants of these patterns, particularly the social, cultural, economic, and environmental, cannot be measured at the level of the individual.[96] Recent theoretical work has challenged the entire discipline to re-adjust its focus to examine community- and population-level determinants of disease risk.[27] It is argued that study designs that incorporate ecological elements are the only ones that can examine these contextual factors.[97]

Acknowledgements
Thanks to Liddy Griffith and Wendy Keeves for their assistance with searching the literature.

References

1. McGill, H. C. Jr. (ed.). (1968) *Geographic pathology of atherosclerosis.* Williams and Williams, Baltimore.
2. Kuller, L. H., LaPorte, R. E. and Weinberg, G. B. (1977) The decline in ischemic heart disease mortality: environmental and social variables. In: Havlik, R.J. and Feinleib, M. (ed.). *Proceedings of the conference on the decline in coronary heart disease mortality.* DHEW Pub. No. (NIH) 79–1610 Washington, DC. Government Printing Office, Washington DC. 312–339. (Figure 6, p334)
3. Dwyer, T. and Hetzel, B. S. (1980) a comparison of trends of coronary heart disease mortality in Australia, USA, and England and Wales with reference to three major risk factors–hypertension, cigarette smoking and diet. *Int. J. Epid.* 9: 67–71.
4. Blot, W. J. and Fraumeni, J. F. Jr. (1982) Geographic epidemiology in the United States. In: Schottenfeld, D. and Fraumeni J. F. Jr. (ed.) *Cancer epidemiology and prevention.* W. B. Saunders, Philadelphia.
5. Wynder, E. L. and Hebert, J. R. (1987) Homogeneity in nutritional exposure: an impediment in cancer epidemiology. *J. Natl. Cancer Inst.* 79: 605–7.
6. Chen, J., Campbell, T. C., Junyao, L. and Peto, R. (1990) *Diet, lifestyle, and mortality in China: a study of the characteristics of 65 Chinese counties.* Oxford University Press, Oxford.
7. Morgenstern, H. (1982) Uses of ecologic analysis in epidemiologic research. *Am. J. Public Hlth.* 72: 1336–44.
8. Armstrong, B. and Doll, R. (1975) Environmental factors and cancer incidence and mortality in different countries, with special reference to dietary practices. *Int. J. Cancer* 15: 617–31.
9. Prentice, R. L., Kakar, F., Hursting, S., Sheppard, L., Klein, R. and Kushi, L. H. (1988) Aspects of the rationale for the Women's Health Trial. *J. Natl. Cancer Inst.* 80: 802–14.
10. Renaud, S. and de Lorgeril, M. (1992) Wine, alcohol, platelets, and the French paradox for coronary heart disease. *Lancet.* 339: 1523–6.
11. Riboli, E. (1992) Nutrition and cancer: background and rationale of the European prospective investigation into cancer and nutrition (EPIC). *Ann. Oncol.* 3: 789–91.
12. Muir, C. S. and James, P. (1982) Diet and large bowel cancer in Denmark and Finland: report of the Second IARC International Collaborative Study. *Nutr. Cancer.* 4: 1–79.
13. Von Korff, M., Koepsell, T., Curry, S. and Diehr, P. (1992) Multi-level analysis in epidemiologic research on health behaviours and outcomes. *Am. J. Epid.* 135: 1077–82.
14. James, W. P. T., Ferro-Luzzi, A., Isaksson, B. and Szostak, W. B. (1988) Healthy nutrition: preventing nutrition-related diseases in Europe. WHO Regional Publications, European Series, No. 24. WHO Regional Office for Europe, Copenhagen.
15. Food and Agriculture Organization of the United Nations. (1994) FAO quarterly bulletin of statistics 7: nos. 2/3/4. FAO, United Nations, Rome.
16. Sasaki, S. and Kesteloot, H. (1992) Value of Food and Agriculture Organization data on food balance sheets as a data source for dietary fat intake in epidemiologic studies. *Am. J. Clin. Nutr.* 56: 716–23.
17. Kesteloot, H., Sasaki, S., Verbeke, G. and Joossens, J. V. (1994) Cancer mortality and age: relationship with dietary fat. *Nutr. Cancer.* 22: 85–98.
18. Calvert, G. D., English, R., Wahlquest, M. L. (1987) Changing eating patterns in Australia. In: Wahlquest, M., King, R. W. F., McNeil, J. J. and Sewell, R. (ed.). *Food and health issues and directions.* John Libbey and Company Ltd., London.
19. Beaton, G. H., Milner, J., Corey, P., McGuire, V., Cousins, M., Stewart, E., *et al.* (1979) Sources of variance in 24-hour dietary recall data: implications for nutrition study design and interpretation. *Am. J. Clin. Nutr.* 179: 2546–59.
20. Ministry of Agriculture, Fisheries and Food. (1994) *Household food consumption and expenditure survey*, 1992. HMSO, London.

21. Gregory J., Foster, K., Tyler, H. and Wiseman, M.(1990) *The dietary and nutritional survey of British adults.* HMSO, London.

22. Ocké, M. C., Kromhout, D., Menotti, A., Aravanis, C., Blackburn, H., Buzina, R., *et al.* (1995) Average intake of anti-oxidant (pro)vitamins and subsequent cancer mortality in the 16 cohorts of the seven countries study. *Int. J. Cancer* **61**: 480–4.

23. McMichael, A. J. (1978) Increases in laryngeal cancer in Britain and Australia in relation to alcohol and tobacco consumption trends. *Lancet.* **i**: 1244–7.

24. Cornu, A., Massamba, J. P., Traissac, P., Simondon, F., Villeneuve, P. and Delpeuch, F. (1995) Nutritional change and economic crisis in an urban Congolese community. *Int. J. Epid.* **24**: 155–64.

25. McMichael, A. J., McCall, M. G., Hartshorne, J. M. and Woodings, T. L. (1980) Patterns of gastrointestinal cancer in European migrants to Australia: the role of dietary change. *Int. J. Cancer.* **25**: 431–7.

26. Cheadle, A., Psaty B., Curry S., Wagner, E., Diehr, P., Koepsell, T., *et al.* (1993) Can measures of the grocery store environment be used to track community-level dietary change? *Prev. Med.* **222**: 361–72.

27. Schwartz, S. (1994) The fallacy of the ecological fallacy: the potential misuse of a concept and the consequences. *Am. J. Public Hlth.* **84**: 819–24.

28. Humphreys, K. and Carr-Hill, R. (1991) Area variations in health outcomes: artefact or ecology? *Int. J. Epid.* **20**: 251–7.

29. Koopman, J. S. and Longini, I. M (1994) The ecological effects of individual exposures and nonlinear disease dynamics in populations. *Am. J. Public Hlth.* **84**: 836–42.

30. Burkitt, D. P. and Trowell, H. C. (ed.). (1975) *Refined carbohydrate foods and disease. Some implications of dietary fibre.* Academic Press, London.

31. Popkin, B. M (1994) The nutrition transition in low-income countries: an emerging crisis. *Nutr. Rev.* **52**: 285–98.

32. Yang, C. S. (1980) Research on oesophageal cancer in China: a review. *Cancer Res.* **40**: 2633–44.

33. Luo, X. M., Wei, H. J., Hu, G. G., Shang, A. L., Liu, Y. Y., Lu, S. M., *et al.* (1981) Molybdenum and oesophageal cancer in China. *Fed. Proc.* **40**: 928. [abstract 3962].

34. Powles, J. W. and Williams, D. R. R. (1984) Trends in bowel cancer in selected countries in relation to wartime changes in flour milling. *Nutr. Cancer.* **6**: 40–8.

35. Pocock, S. J., Cook, D. G. and Shaper, A. G. (1982) Analysing geographic variation in cardiovascular mortality: methods and results. *J. Roy. Statist. Soc. Ser. A.* **145**: 313–41.

36. Lancet. (1987) [editorial]. A poison tree. *Lancet.* **2**: 947—8.

37. Linsell, C. A. and Peers, F. U. (1977) Field studies on liver cell cancer. In: Hiatt, H. H., Watson, J. D. and Winston, J. A. (ed.). *Origins of human cancer, book A.* Cold Spring Harbor Laboratory, New York.

38. Thornton, I. (1994) Heavy metal contamination from historical mining and smelting and the food chain: a global perspective. In: Wahlqvist, M., Truswell, A. S., Smith, R. and Nestel, P. J. (ed.). *Nutrition in a sustainable environment.* Proceedings of the XVth International Congress of Nutrition, Smith-Gordon, London. 44–7.

39. Kohlmeier, L. (1995) Future of dietary exposure assessment. *Am. J. Clin. Nutr.* **61**: 702S–9S.

40. James, W. P. T. and Ralph, A. (1994) Matching nutrition knowledge to nutritional needs. In: Wahlqvist, M., Truswell, A. S., Smith, R. and Nestel, P. J. (ed.). *Nutrition in a sustainable environment.* Proceedings of the XVth International Congress of Nutrition, Smith-Gordon, London. 73–86.

41. Marmot, M. G., Syme, S. L., Kagan, A., Kato, I. I., Cohen, J. B. and Belskly, J. (1975) Epidemiologic studies of coronary heart disease and stroke in Japanese men living in Japan, Hawaii, and California: prevalence of coronary and hypertensive heart disease and associated risk factors. *Am. J. Epid.* **102**: 514–25.

42. Gleibermann, L. (1973) Blood pressure and dietary salt in human populations. *Ecol. Food and Nutr.* **2**: 143–50.

43. Elliott, P. and Stamler, R. (1988) Manual of operations for 'INTERSALT', an international cooperative study on the relation of sodium and potassium to blood pressure. *Controlled Clin. Trials.* **9**: 1S–118S.

44. Jensen, O. M., MacLennan, R. and Wahrendorf, J. (1982) Diet, bowel function, fecal characteristics, and large bowel cancer in Denmark and Finland. *Nutr. Cancer.* **4**: 5–19.

45. International Agency for Research on Cancer, Intestinal Microecology Group. (1977) Dietary fibre, transit time, faecal bacteria, steroids, and colon cancer in two Scandinavian populations. *Lancet.* **ii**: 207–11.

46. Morris, J. S., Stampfer, M. J. and Willett, W. (1983) Toenails as an indicator of dietary selenium. *Biol. Trace Elem. Res.* **5**: 529–37.

47. Peto, R. (1986) Cancer around the world: evidence of avoidability. In: Hallgren, B., Levin, O. and Rossner, S. (ed.). *Diet and prevention of coronary heart disease and cancer.* Fourth International Berzilius Symposium sponsored by the Swedish Society of Medicine. Raven Press, New York.

48. Udomkesmalee-Wasantwisut, E. (1994) Newer approaches to the assessment of vitamin A status. In: Wahlqvist, M., Truswell, A. S., Smith, R. and Nestel, P. J. (ed.). *Nutrition in a sustainable environment.* Proceedings of the XVth International Congress of Nutrition, Smith-Gordon, London. 266–9.

49. Hetzel, B. S. and Baghurst, K. I. (ed.). (1981) The assessment of the nutritional status of the individual and the community. *Transactions of the Menzies Foundation.* **3**.

50. Nelson, M., Quayle, A. and Phillips, D. W. (1987). Iodine intake and excretion in two British towns: aspects of questionnaire validation. *Hum. Nutr.: Appl. Nutr.* **41A**: 187–92.

51. Clayton, D. (1994) Measurement error: effects and remedies in nutritional epidemiology. *Proc. Nutr. Soc.* **53**: 37–42.

52. WHO (1995) *World health statistics annual, 1994.* WHO, Geneva.

53. Pocock, S. J., Shaper, A. G., Powell, P. and Packham, R. F. (1985) The British Regional Heart Study: cardiovascular disease and water quality. In: Thornton, I. (ed.). *Proceedings of the first international symposium on geochemistry and health.* Science Reviews, Middlegender. 141–57.

54. Sreebny, L. M. (1982) Sugar availability, sugar consumption and dental caries. *Community Dent. Oral Epid.* **10**: 1–7.

55. Social Health Atlas Project. (1990) *A social health atlas of South Australia.* South Australian Health Commission, Adelaide.

56. Elliott, P., Westlake, A. J., Hills, M, Kleinschmidt, I., Rodrigues, L., McGale, P., *et al.* (1992) The small area health statistics unit: a national facility for investigating health around point sources of environmental pollution in the United Kingdom. *J. Epid. Comm. Hlth.* **46**: 345–9.

57. Dyerberg, J. and Jorgensen, K. A. (1982) Marine oils and thrombogenesis. *Prog. Lipid Res.* **21**: 255–69.

58. Autrup, H. and Wakhisi, J. (1988) Detection of exposure to aflatoxin in an African population. In: Bartsch, H., Hemminki, K. and O'Neill, I. K. (ed.). *Methods for detecting DNA damaging agents in humans: applications in cancer epidemiology and prevention.* IARC Scientific Publications No. 89. International Agency for Research on Cancer, Lyons. 63–6.

59. Hopkins, S., Margetts, B. M., Cohen, J. and Armstrong B. K. (1980) Dietary change among Italians and Australians in Perth. *Comm. Hlth. Stud.* **4**: 67–75.

60. Powles, J., Ktenas, D. and Sutherland, C. (1986) *Food habits in southern European migrants: a case study of migrants from the Greek Island of Levkada.* Department of Social and Preventive Medicine, Monash Medical School, Prahran.

61. Wynder, E. L., McCoy, G. D., Reddy, B. S., Cohen, L., Hill, P., Spingarn, N. E., *et al.* (1981) Nutrition and metabolic epidemiology of cancers of the oral cavity, oesophagus, colon,

breast, prostate and stomach. In: Newel, G. R. and Ellison, N. M. (ed.). *Nutrition and cancer: etiology and treatment.* Raven Press, New York. 11–48.

62. Phillips, R. L. (1975) Role of lifestyle and dietary habits in risk of cancer among Seventh-Day Adventists. *Cancer Res.* **35**: 3513—22.

63. Phillips, R. L., Garfinkel, L., Kuzma, J. W., Beeson, W. L., Lodz, T. and Brin, B. (1980) Mortality among Californian Seventh-Day Adventists for selected cancer sites. *J. Natl. Cancer Inst.* **65**: 1097–107.

64. Kinlen, L. J. (1982) Meat and fat consumption and cancer mortality: A study of strict religious orders in Britain. *Lancet.* **i**: 946–9.

65. Omran, A. R. (1971) The epidemiologic transition: a theory of the epidemiology of population change. *Milbank Mem. Fund Q.* **49**: 509–37.

66. Young, T. K. (1988) Are subarctic Indians undergoing the epidemiologic transition? *Soc. Sci. Med.* **26**: 659–71.

67. Schooneveldt, M., Songer, T., Zimmet, P. and Thoma, K. (1988) Changing mortality patterns in Nauruans: an example of epidemiological transition. *J. Epid. Comm. Hlth.* **42**: 89–95.

68. West, K. M (1974) Diabetes in American Indians and other native populations in the New World. *Diabetes.* **23**: 841–55.

69. Zimmet, P. Z. (1979) Epidemiology of diabetes and its macrovascular manifestations in Pacific populations: the medical effects of social progress. *Diabetes Care* **2**: 144–53.

70. Zimmet, P. Z. (1987) Diabetes and other non-communicable disease in Paradise – the evolutionary and genetic connection. *Med. J. Aust.* **146**: 457–8.

71. Hirayama, T. (1979) Diet and Cancer. *Nutr. Cancer.* **1**: 67–81.

72. Pearce, N., Matos, E., Koivusalo, M. and Wing S. (1994) Industrialization and health. In: Pearce, N. (ed.). *Occupational cancer in developing countries.* IARC Scientific Publications No. 129. International Agency for Research on Cancer, Lyons. 7–22.

73. Weile, B., Cavell, B., Nivenius, K. and Krasilnikoff, P. A. (1995) Striking differences in the incidence of childhood celiac disease between Denmark and Sweden: a plausible explanation. *J. Pediatr. Gastroenterol.* **21**: 64–8.

74. Stavraky, K. M. (1976) The role of ecologic analysis in studies of the etiology of disease: a discussion with reference to large bowel cancer. *J. Chron. Dis.* **29**: 435–44.

75. Morgenstern, H. (1995) Ecologic studies in epidemiology: concepts, principles, and methods. *Annu. Rev. Publ. Hlth.* **16**: 61–81.

76. Cook, D. G. and Pocock, S. J. (1983) Multiple regressions in geographical mortality studies, with allowance for spatially correlated errors. *Biometrics.* **39**: 361–71.

77. Clayton, D. G., Bernadinelli, L. and Montomoli, C. (1993) Spatial correlation in ecological analysis. *Int. J. Epid.* **22**: 1193–202.

78. Yanai, H., Inaba, Y., Takgagi, H. and Yamamoto, S. (1979) Multivariate analysis of cancer mortalities for selected sites in 24 countries. *Environ. Health Perspect.* **32**: 83–101.

79. Piantadosi, S., Byar, D. P. and Green, S. B. (1988) The ecological fallacy. *Am. J. Epid.* **127**: 893–904.

80. Rose, G. (1982) Incubation period of coronary heart disease. *Br. Med. J.* **284**: 1600–1.

81. Skog O.-J. (1980) Liver cirrhosis epidemiology: some methodological problems. *Br. J. Addict.* **75**: 227–43.

82. Scrimshaw, N. S. (1995) The new paradigm of public health nutrition. *Am. J. Publ. Hlth.* **85**: 622–4.

83. Barker, D. J. P. (1992) *Foetal and infant origins of adult disease.* British Medical Journal, London.

84. McMichael, A. J. (1979) Alimentary tract cancer in Australia in relation to diet and alcohol. *Nutr. Cancer* **1**: 82–9.

85. Prentice R. L. and Sheppard, L. (1995) Aggregate data studies of disease risk factors. *Biometrika.* **82**: 113–25.

86. Qiao, Z-K., Halliday, M. L., Coates, R. A. and Rankin, J. G. (1988) Relationship between liver cirrhosis death rate and nutritional factors in 38 countries. *Int. J. Epid.* **17**: 414–18.
87. Engel, R. and Smith, A. H. (1994) Arsenic in drinking water and mortality from vascular disease: an ecologic analysis in 30 counties in the United States. *Arch. Environ. Hlth.* **49**: 418–27.
88. Barker, D. J. P. and Morris, J. (1988) Acute appendicitis, bathrooms, and diet in Britain and Ireland. *Br. Med. J.* **296**: 953–5.
89. Dobson, A. J. (1987) Trends in cardiovascular risk factors in Australia, 1966–1983. Evidence from prevalence surveys. *Comm. Hlth. Stud.* **11**: 2–14.
90. Cassidy, A., Bingham, S. A. and Cummings, J. H. (1994) Starch intake and colorectal cancer risk: an international comparison. *Br. J. Cancer.* **69**: 937–42.
91. Martyn, C. N., Barker, D. J. P., Osmond, C., Harries, E. C., Edwardson, J. A. and Lacey, R. E. (1989) Geographical relation between Alzheimer's disease and aluminium in drinking water. *Lancet.* **1** : 59–62.
92. Stamler, J., Rose, G., Elliott, P., Dyer, A., Marmot, M., Kesteloot, H., *et al.* (1991) Findings of the International Cooperative INTERSALT Study. *Hypertension.* **17** (Suppl. I): I9–I15.
93. Willett, W. C., Stampfer, M. J., Colditz, G. A., Rosner, B. A., Hennekens, C. H. and Speizer, F. E. (1987) Dietary fat and the risk of breast cancer. *N. Engl. J. Med.* **316**: 22–8.
94. Geenwald, P. (1988) Issues raised by the Women's Health Trial *J. Natl. Cancer Inst.* **80**: 788–90.
95. Fraser, G. E. (1986) *Preventive cardiology.* Oxford University Press, Oxford. 71.
96. McMichael, A. J. (1995) The health of persons, populations, and planets: epidemiology comes full circle. *Epidemiology.* **6**: 633–6.
97. Susser, M. (1994) The logic in ecological: I. The logic of analysis *Am. J. Publ. Hlth.* **84**: 825–9.

13. Cross-sectional studies

Janet E. Cade

13.1 Introduction

To find out about the food and nutrient intake of any community, the first place to start would be by reviewing existing data. These data could include: previously published research, routine data such as mortality and morbidity statistics, market prices, rainfall, anthropometry, etc. This type of data may be of limited application to specific populations. It may not be related to the population of interest; it may be inaccurate, biased, and out of date. The next step could be to carry out a rapid assessment[1,2] of the population to give a preliminary understanding of the situation. This may be done by conducting focus group discussions, key informant interviews, or direct observations. Rapid assessment methods can provide useful qualitative information, but are not usually statistically rigorous and so biased results may be obtained. If a more objective measure were required, the next stage would be to conduct a cross-sectional survey.

13.2 Definition of a cross-sectional survey

A cross-sectional survey is a type of observational or descriptive study, where the researcher has no control over the exposure of interest (e.g. diet). It involves identifying a defined population at a particular point in time and measuring a range of variables on an individual basis which can include past and current dietary intake. These data may then be explored in relation to the presence or absence of disease or other health related outcome. However, since the data represent a snapshot of information about the population at one point in time, it is not possible to determine whether the exposure and the outcome are causally related. Cross-sectional surveys are also known as prevalence surveys, since they can be used to estimate the *prevalence* of disease in a population[3], that is, the number of cases in the population at a particular point in time expressed as a rate.

Example:

Data on 4302 children, aged 0–6 years, from rural India, were analysed to study the prevalence of vitamin A deficiency and the efficacy of vitamin A in preventing xerophthalmia co-existing with malnutrition. The prevalence of xerophthalmia was higher in the normal and mild to moderately malnourished children, and lowest in the severely malnourished children (graded by weight for age) (Fig. 13.1).[4] Since the data

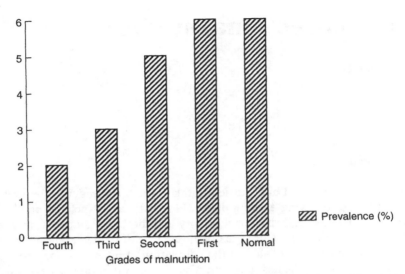

Fig. 13.1 Prevalence of xerophthalmia in 0–6 year-old children by their nutritional status (IAP classification). (Source: Gopaldas *et al.*[4])

are cross-sectional it is not clear which is cause and which is effect. That is, it may be that children who are malnourished are more likely to have a reasonable level of vitamin A due to reduced tissue requirements, or that children without xerophthalmia are more likely to become malnourished than children with xerophthalmia due to, for example, increased physical activity because of better eyesight. One other possibility is that the mortality rate is higher in children with severe malnutrition and vitamin A deficiency, so that this group is more likely to have already died, and so not be available for inclusion in the study.

13.3   Uses of cross-sectional studies

1. *Prevalence surveys*: These studies are commonly used to describe the burden of disease in the community and its distribution. These are known as prevalence surveys. For rare conditions, the sample size required may be very large. In the study by Gopaldas *et al.*[4] described above, vitamin A deficiency was rather common, signs of deficiency were seen in about 10% of children. Another study in the area to confirm the prevalence to within ±0.5% would require a sample size of about 160 children.[5] However, a similar study of children in the UK would require a much larger sample size since vitamin A deficiency is very rare.

2. *Describe population characteristics*: They are also commonly used to describe population characteristics, often in terms of person (who?) and place (where?). The British National Diet and Nutrition Surveys are examples of cross-sectional studies which are used to describe various age groups in the population in terms of food and

nutrient intake and a range of other personal and lifestyle characteristics. The results of a survey of 2197 adults were published in 1990[6] and preschool children in 1995.[7]

Figure 13.2 shows the percentage of energy coming from the main food groups for men by region. There is little variation between regions in the sources of energy. Men in Scotland and northern England were consuming rather more of their energy from beverages, including alcohol, and they were consuming less energy from cereal products than those in the central and southern regions. Descriptive cross-sectional studies can also be used to study local samples, and might be published in health authority annual reports.

3. *Migrant studies*: Some migrant studies may fall into the classification of cross-sectional studies. These studies give clues as to the association between genetic background and environmental exposures on the risk of disease. For example, one study looked at coronary risk factors in a randomly selected group of 247 migrants, from the Indian subcontinent of Punjabi origin, living in West London, and compared them with 117 siblings living in the Punjab in India.[8] The West London group had greater BMI, systolic blood pressure, serum cholesterol, apolipoprotein B, fasting blood glucose, and lower high-density lipoprotein cholesterol than their siblings in the Punjab. Differences in outcomes between places may be due to differences in the environment or in the people who live in each place. A study of the prevalence (percentage) of coronary heart disease among men of Japanese ancestry living in Japan, Honolulu, and the San

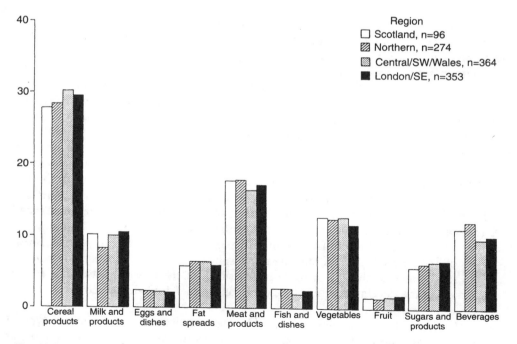

Fig. 13.2 Men: percentage of energy from main food groups by region. (Source: Gregory *et al.*[6])

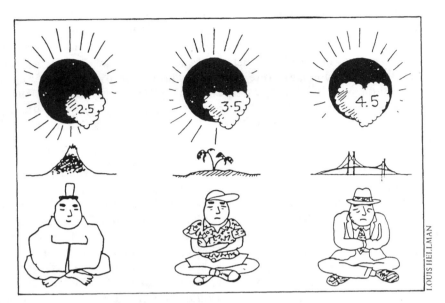

Fig. 13.3 Prevalence (percentage) of coronary heart disease (as indicated by Q waves in electro-cardiogram) among men of Japanese ancestry living in Japan (left), Honolulu (centre), and San Francsico Bay area (right). (Source: Marmot and Davey-Smith.[9])

Francisco Bay area showed the highest rates among those who had migrated to the United States. It was concluded that these changes must be due to differences in environment or lifestyle, such as dietary changes (Fig. 13.3).[9]

Examination of disease rates in people who migrate can help to unravel the relative importance of the genetic susceptibility and environment. In general, those who migrate to the United Kingdom have disease rates which are intermediate between the rates in the country of origin and rates in the new host country. If migrants keep the same rates of disease as in the country of origin then this would suggest that either (i) the pattern of disease was genetically determined; (ii) they do not change their lifestyle; or (iii) that early environmental influences persist. If, however, the migrants change their disease rate to that of the new country, this suggests a role for the environment in the new country.[10] A cross-sectional study of risk factors for hypertension and diabetes in different black populations has found that rates of hypertension are highest in African-Caribbeans living in Manchester compared with rates in Jamaica and Cameroon, the lowest rates being in the rural Cameroonian population (Cruickshank, unpublished). Levels of obesity are highest in Manchester, despite dietary fat intakes being lower than in the rural Cameroonians.[11] In order to see which of the factors measured are most important in the development of diabetes, a follow-up study will be needed.

4. *KAP studies*: KAP (knowledge, attitudes, and practice) studies are also a type of cross-sectional study. These studies are purely descriptive and help to build up a better understanding of the behaviour of the population, without necessarily relating this to

any disease or health outcome. For example, a cross-sectional survey of 400 subjects systematically sampled from electoral registers in Southampton aimed to explore knowledge of dietary fat and its relationship to coronary heart disease.[12] Overall knowledge levels were found to be high. There were, however, some specific gaps in knowledge concerning the polyunsaturated fat content of fish; the fat content of butter, margarine, and low-fat spreads; and the relationship of dietary cholesterol and saturated fat to plasma cholesterol and heart disease.

5. *Management tool*: Health service managers and planners may make use of cross-sectional surveys to assess utilization and effectiveness of services. A study of the determinants of nutritional status in south-west Uganda found that children living in households more than four miles from a health unit had worse nutritional status than those living nearer.[13] This information could be used to help plan outreach services. The study of vitamin A deficiency by Gopaldas in India[4] found that the ability of vitamin A prophylaxis to prevent xerophthalmia was greatest in severely malnourished or normal children.

6. *Development of hypotheses*: Hypotheses on the causes of disease may be developed using data from cross-sectional surveys. The diets of 2340 middle-aged men and women living in three English towns were recorded using a one-day food record. Consumption of fat and the other main nutrients was lowest in the northern industrial town, which had the highest death rates from ischaemic heart disease. The findings suggested that differences in diet in middle age were not likely to be a major cause of differences in adult mortality.[14] This work has added support to other findings that the explanation for these differences in adult mortality rates may lie more in the nutrition and development of children.[15] These results have encouraged further work in the area of infant and neonatal origins of adult onset disease.

13.4 Limitations of cross-sectional studies

The main disadvantage of this type of study is that since the exposure and disease/outcome are measured at the same time it is not possible to say which is cause and which effect. For example, a reanalysis of the National Diet and Nutrition Survey of British Adults showed that people who were eating a high fat diet were also more likely to be obese than those eating a low fat diet.[16] From this study which measured food intake and body mass index at the same time, it is not possible to say whether the high fat intake is a cause of obesity or whether people who are obese tend to eat a high fat diet. To test the hypothesis that high dietary fat intakes cause obesity, a different type of study, such as a cohort study, would have to be conducted. This would take a group of people before they had become obese (the outcome) and measure their fat intake (the exposure), then follow them up over a period of time to see whether those who became obese were more or less likely to be eating a high fat diet (see Chapter 14).

Confounding factors may not be equally distributed between the groups being compared and this unequal distribution may lead to bias and subsequent misinterpretation. A confounding factor is a variable which is related both to the exposure (diet) and the outcome (disease). Age, gender and ethnicity are often confounders. The impact of known individual confounders may be removed by appropriate sampling (such as studying only women) or stratifying by the confounder at the analysis stage. If numbers for any one level of the confounder are small – for example, in a study of the determinants of anaemia, out of 400 subjects only five men were found to be anaemic – it will be difficult to adjust adequately for gender differences. It is almost always the case that there will be residual confounding (related to variables measured poorly or not at all). The effect this may have on the results needs to be considered.

Cross-sectional studies may measure current diet in a group of people with a disease. Current diet may be altered by the presence of disease. In this case the outcome is having an influence on the exposure variable. A cross-sectional study which looked at diet in groups of Asian and European patients with non-insulin dependent diabetes found that the percentage of fat in the diets of the Asian patients was 46%, and in the Europeans, 42%.[17] No conclusions could be drawn from these results about any previous diet leading up to the development of diabetes, since it is likely that the dietary intake of the subjects has changed due to the development of the condition. Current exposure is not equivalent to past exposure because diet may change over time even when subjects are not affected by disease (see Section 6.12).

A further limitation of cross-sectional studies may be due to errors in recall of the exposure and possibly also outcome (see Section 6.9.5). A cross-sectional study of 284 middle-aged and elderly women studied the effects of recalled historical milk consumption on current bone mineral density at the hip and spine. The results showed that milk consumption up to age 25 years was a significant independent predictor of bone mineral density in a multiple linear regression analysis adjusting for a range of other factors.[18] It was concluded that frequent milk consumption before age 25 favourably influenced hip bone mass. However, since the recall period was a long time, 50 years for the 74-year-old women, it could equally well be concluded that good memory makes strong bones or vice versa![19]

Prevalence (incidence × duration) studies may be affected by Neyman's bias. This occurs where subjects are not included in the prevalence measure because they have died early from the disease or the symptoms have gone. For example, it was possible that the results found in the study looking at vitamin A deficiency in relation to malnutrition were due to Neyman's bias. This study found that the most severely malnourished were least likely to be deficient in vitamin A. One reason for this may be that those who were deficient in vitamin A had already died and so were not available to be included in the study.[4]

13.5 Design of cross-sectional surveys

As with any other type of epidemiological study, cross-sectional studies need to be carefully designed. The problem to be studied must be clearly described and a thorough literature review undertaken before starting the data collection. Specific objectives need to be formulated. The information has to be collected and data collection techniques need to be decided. Sampling is a particularly important issue to ensure that the objectives can be met in the most efficient way. For example, to study risk factors for a rare condition it may be better to sample from a high risk population such as i.v. drug users in a study of HIV infection. The sample should be representative of the population to be studied, if not it may be biased in some way and the results could not be generalized to the population as a whole. For example, a study of the association between caffeine consumption and indigestion, palpitations, and other symptoms was studied cross-sectionally in a group of *volunteers*. A multiple logistic regression analysis showed a weak positive association between caffeine consumption and palpitations.[20] These results can not be extrapolated to the general population. People who volunteered for the study may be those who drink a lot of coffee and have symptoms.[21]

Fieldwork needs planning. Who is available to collect the data? Do they need training? If more than one interviewer is to collect the data then it is necessary to assess between-observer variation. This may be done by getting each interviewer to take measurements on the same subjects. If this is not done a systematic difference in results may occur and results will need presenting by each interviewer separately. Figure 13.4 shows results from the three towns study. One interviewer (JC) had collected data in each site along with one local interviewer per site. Interviewer JC had consistently slightly higher results than the results from each of the local interviewers.

The collation, coding, and entry of data need planning. It is also useful to have at the outset a clear idea of the tables of results to be presented, in order to ensure that the right data are being collected in the right way. If ethical approval is required, time should be allowed for this and it should be obtained before data collection begins.

A pilot study is essential to test the proposed methods and make any alterations as necessary. A pilot study was conducted before the main data collection phase of the three towns study.[22] This involved testing the acceptability of a 1-day food diary describing food in terms of household measures and comparing this to weighed

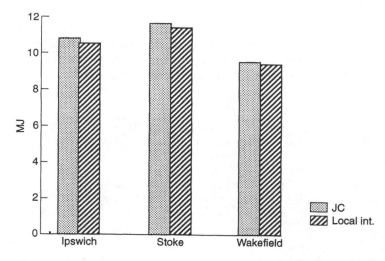

Fig. 13.4   Energy intake for men by interviewer (JC vs. Local) – three towns study.
(Source: Cade *et al.*[14])

amounts of the same foods in a sample of 22 adults. It was found that men were less able than women to describe their portion sizes accurately. The method was adapted so that the food diary included a ruled edge along the bottom of each page and the interviewer used 2-D food models to help in the description of portion sizes. Further pilot work in 33 additional subjects, using the new food diary, showed that subjects were better able to describe portion sizes with the changes made.

Steps to be taken in the design of a cross-sectional study are summarized in Fig. 13.5. These also include ensuring an adequate budget and planning appropriate presentation of the results.

13.6   Dietary assessment in cross-sectional studies

Different dietary assessment techniques have been discussed in detail earlier in this book. They are not all appropriate for use in cross-sectional studies. Some important characteristics are summarized in Box 13.1. Particularly relevant to the cross-sectional study is the ability of the method to assess individual intake, and it should not require long-term follow up or repeat measures. Methods which assess diet at the community level such as food balance sheet data or food sales data are not suitable for cross-sectional studies, but will be appropriate for ecological studies (see Chapter 12). Individual methods which assess actual or usual intake can be used for cross-sectional studies. The weighed intake used to be thought of as the gold standard. It has been used in the National Diet and Nutrition Survey of British Adults (NDNS).[6] The method used in the NDNS records current intake for one week. It is a time-consuming and expensive method, requiring a high degree of cooperation from subjects. Some subjects may not be used to food weighing scales and may be unwilling or unable to use them. The method itself may lead to changes in dietary patterns, or the subject may consume an untypical diet for the recording week. The NDNS had a response rate of 70% to the study. There appeared to be a considerable amount of under-reporting using the weighed intake method. A comparison of calculated basal metabolic rates (BMR) to energy intakes (EI) found that 30% of men and 47% of women in the sample had reported BMR:EI ratio of less than 1.2. Habitual intakes of this level are unlikely to meet requirements.

Box 13.1   Some characteristics of dietary assessment methods for cross-sectional studies.

- Measures an individual's intake at one point in time
- Does not require long-term follow up or repeat measures
- Valid
- Reproducible
- Suitable for aim of study
- Cost within study budget

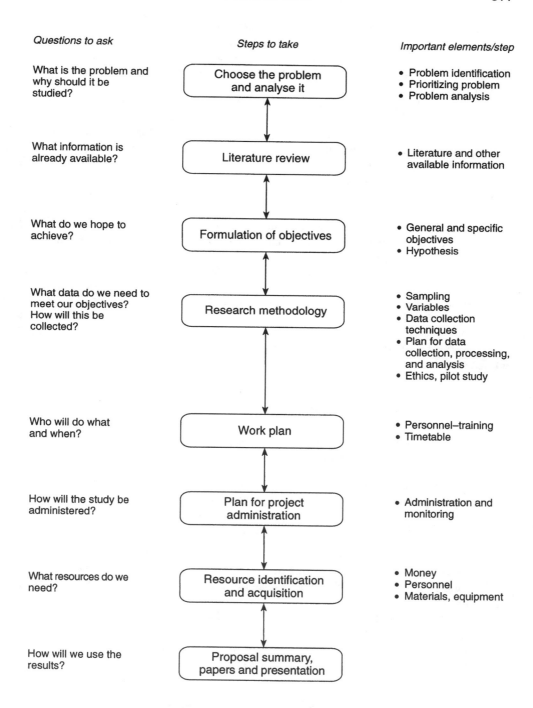

Questions to ask

What is the problem and why should it be studied?

What information is already available?

What do we hope to achieve?

What data do we need to meet our objectives? How will this be collected?

Who will do what and when?

How will the study be administered?

What resources do we need?

How will we use the results?

Steps to take

Choose the problem and analyse it

Literature review

Formulation of objectives

Research methodology

Work plan

Plan for project administration

Resource identification and acquisition

Proposal summary, papers and presentation

Important elements/step

- Problem identification
- Prioritizing problem
- Problem analysis

- Literature and other available information

- General and specific objectives
- Hypothesis

- Sampling
- Variables
- Data collection techniques
- Plan for data collection, processing, and analysis
- Ethics, pilot study

- Personnel–training
- Timetable

- Administration and monitoring

- Money
- Personnel
- Materials, equipment

Fig. 13.5 Steps in the design of a cross-sectional study. (Modified from Varkevisser *et al.*[23])

Food records using descriptions in household measures have been used in cross-sectional studies.[14] The method is less disruptive for the subject than the weighed intake. There may be a problem, however, in converting descriptions to portion weights. Recent work has been done to develop food photographs which may aid description of portion sizes.[24]

The recall method attempts to quantify diet over a defined period in the past, usually 24 hours. Subjects cannot alter their food habits, but invention or omission is possible. This method relies on memory and so may not be suitable for all in the population such as the young or very old. People may also tend to remember and report information which is socially acceptable.

The most commonly used dietary assessment method which attempts to measure *usual* intake is the food frequency questionnaire (FFQ). Like the recall it depends on memory and so may lead to reporting errors. The method may be simple to use and can be done by non-technical personnel. Some versions may be administered postally and completed by the subject alone. This is particularly useful if subjects are spread out in location or a large sample size is to be used. It is preferable to develop a new FFQ for each study and undertake appropriate validation (see Chapter 8), since a questionnaire designed for use in one population group may not be appropriate for use in another population. For example, a questionnaire designed for use by female vegetarians may not be suitable for completion by male students. Researchers should be careful not to misuse FFQs in this way. The development of a FFQ may be time consuming, but once developed, administration and analysis of the data is much quicker than for the other methods.

13.7 Deciding which dietary assessment method to choose

A number of questions may be asked before deciding which of the dietary assessment methods is most appropriate for a study.

1. What is already known about the population?
   - Very little – a more detailed method may be required such as a weighed intake or food record
   - Some information – a FFQ may be developed

2. What are the objectives of the study?
   - Detailed food and nutrient intake required – use a weighed intake or measured food diary; some FFQs may be suitable (portion size information may be required)
   - Food intake patterns of interest – a recall, FFQ, or food checklist
   - Meal patterns – recall, food list, food diary, weighed intake
   - Food knowledge and attitudes – consider using focus group discussions, semi-structured questionnaires, or interviews

3. Who are the subjects?
   - Literate – weighed intake, food records may be appropriate
   - Illiterate – recall, interviewer administered FFQ

- Motivated – weighed intake
- Less motivated or short of time – recall, FFQ

4. What resources are available?
   - Finance limited – an FFQ or recall methods may be cheaper, or use published/routine data
   - Personnel limited/inexperienced – FFQ

5. What is the level of cooperation required of the subjects?
   - Weighed intake and food record methods require a high degree of cooperation
   - FFQ and recall methods require less cooperation

6. Statistical issues
   - Consider how many days of intake need to be recorded by weighing or food record. In population studies it is most efficient to maximize the sample size and minimize the number of recording days per individual
   - All methods should be validated in a subsample against an alternative measure of diet with independent errors, such as a biomarker.

13.8 Analysis of cross-sectional studies

Analysis of any study requires a logical progression through a series of checks and tests. Many of these procedures will also be appropriate for analysis of other study types. Where possible, analysis should be planned, with the help of a statistician, prior to data collection, to avoid 'dredging' of data.

Before starting any formal analysis the data should be checked for any errors and outliers. Obvious errors should be corrected. The records of outliers should be examined, subjects should not be excluded just because they are at the top or the bottom of the distribution.

The data should be explored graphically, e.g., plot the frequency distributions of various nutrients. For example, Fig. 13.6 shows the frequency distributions for energy and alcohol intakes for 55 vegetarian women who had completed a 7-day weighed intake (Cade, unpublished). The energy intake has a fairly normal distribution; however, the distribution of alcohol intake is very skewed. Almost half of the sample did not consume any alcohol at all. The normality of the distribution should be checked; this may be done statistically, for example, using the Kolmogorov-Smirnov Goodness of Fit Test. This matches the distribution of the study data to a normal distribution curve, giving a K-S statistic and a 2-tailed P-value. If the distribution is not normal, the data should be transformed (see Chapter 3), or non-parametric tests should be used. Alcohol usually has a very skewed distribution, and so cannot be successfully transformed, due to the number of people who drink no alcohol at all and the presence of a few very heavy drinkers.

Standard descriptive statistics can then be used: measures of location such as the mean, median, quartiles, and mode; measures of dispersion or variability such as the range, the interquartile range, and the standard deviation; and measures of precision such as the standard error and confidence intervals. Prevalence rates can also be calculated, such as the prevalence of smoking in the sample.

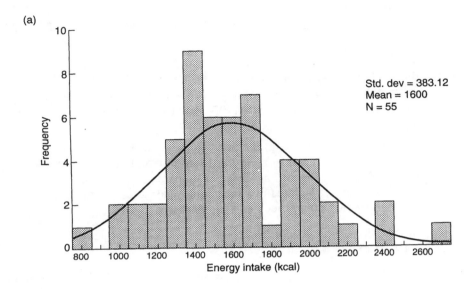

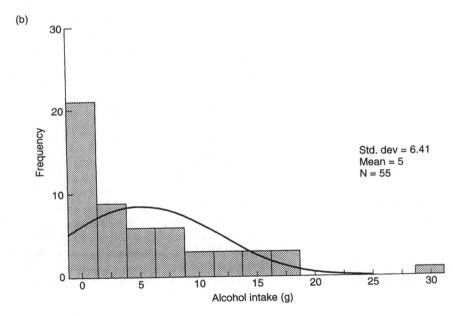

Fig. 13.6 Frequency distribution for energy and alcohol from 7-day weighed records in vegetarian women. (Source: Cade, unpublished.)

Associations can be explored using correlation and regression for continuous variables. However, it is important to remember that a correlation between two variables shows that they are associated and does not necessarily imply a cause and effect relationship. Means can be compared using t-tests or analysis of variance (ANOVA). More complex multivariate analysis can be carried out such as multiple and logistic regression, to investigate how a dependent variable is related to more than one explanatory variable. The study of milk consumption and bone mineral density in women[18] presents results in various ways. For example, the mean bone mineral density (g/cm^2) of the hip for women who, up to age 25, consumed less than one glass of milk per week was 0.84; women who consumed less than one glass of milk per day had a mean density of 0.86; and women who consumed one glass of milk or more per day had a density of 0.90. These means were then adjusted for possible confounding factors of age and body mass index (BMI) and compared using ANOVA. The unadjusted P value for the relationship between milk intake up to age 25 and hip bone density was 0.023. After adjusting for age and BMI, the P value had risen to 0.039, suggesting that there was some effect of age and BMI on the relationship. A multiple linear regression analysis was then carried out controlling for age, BMI, menopausal status, smoking, hormone replacement therapy, oral contraceptive use, physical activity, and years since menopause. Milk consumption before age 25 years remained a small but significant predictor of bone mineral density at all sites, accounting for 1.5–2.0% of the variance in current spine and hip bone mineral density.

13.9 Concluding remarks

Cross-sectional studies are one of the first epidemiological methods to be used in studying associations between diet and disease. The data represent a snapshot of the population at one point in time; therefore it is not possible to determine cause and effect from these studies. These studies are commonly used to describe population characteristics and may provide ideas for further research.

References

1. Scrimshaw, S. C. M. and Hurtado, E. (1987) *Rapid assessment procedures for nutrition and primary health care.* UCLA Latin American Centre Publications, Los Angeles.
2. Scrimshaw, N. S. and Gleason, G. R. (ed.). (1992) *RAP (Rapid Assessment Procedures)* INFDC, Boston.
3. Last, J. M. (1988) *A dictionary of epidemiology.* 2nd edn. Oxford University Press, Oxford.
4. Gopaldas, T., Gujral, S. and Abbi, R. (1993) Prevalence of xerophthalmia and efficacy of vitamin A prophylaxis in preventing xerophthalmia co-existing with malnutrition in rural Indian children. *J. Trop. Paed.* 39: 205–8.
5. Kirkwood, B. R. (1988) *Essentials of medical statistics.* Blackwell Scientific Publications, Oxford.
6. Gregory, J., Foster, K., Tyler, K. and Wiseman, M. (1990) *The Dietary and Nutritional Survey of British Adults.* HMSO, London.
7. Gregory, J., Collins, D., Davies, P., Hughes, J. and Clarke, P. (1995) *National diet and nutrition survey: children aged 1.5 to 4.5 years.* Vol 1. HMSO, London.

8. Bhatnagar, D., Anand, I. S., Durrington, P. N., Patel, D. J., Wander, G. S., Mackness, M. I., *et al.* (1995) Coronary risk factors in people from the Indian subcontinent living in West London and their siblings in India. *Lancet.* **345**: 405–9.

9. Marmot M. G. and Davey-Smith, G. (1989) Why are the Japanese living longer? *Br. Med. J.* **299**: 1547–51.

10. Marmot, M. G. (1989) General approaches to migrant studies: the relation between disease, social class and ethnic origin. In: Cruickshank, J. K. and Beevers, D. G. (ed.). *Ethnic factors in health and disease.* Wright, Oxford.

11. Sharma, S., Cade, J., Jackson, M., Mbanya, J. C., Chungong, S., Forrester, T., *et al.* (1996) Cross-cultural assessment of diet in three population samples of African origin from Cameroon, Jamaica and Caribbean migrants to the UK: method development. *Eur. J. Clin. Nutr.* **50**: 479–86.

12. Tate, J. and Cade, J. (1990) Public knowledge of dietary fat and coronary heart disease. *Hlth. Educ. J.* **49**: 32–5.

13. Vella, V., Tomkins, A., Nviku, J. and Marshall, T. (1995) Determinants of nutritional status in south-west Uganda. *J. Trop. Paed.* **41**: 89–95.

14. Cade, J. E., Barker, D. J. P., Margetts, B. M. and Morris, J. A. (1988) Diet and inequalities in health in three English towns. *Br. Med. J.* **296**:1359–62.

15. Barker, D. J. P. and Osmond, C. (1986) Infant mortality, childhood nutrition and ischaemic heart disease in England and Wales. *Lancet.* **i**: 1077–81.

16. Macdiarmid, J. I., Cade, J. E. and Blundell, J. E. High and low fat consumers, their macronutrient intake and body mass index: further analysis of the National Diet and Nutrition Survey of British Adults *Eur. J. Clin. Nutr.* **50**: 505–12.

17. Peterson, D. B., Fisher, K., Carter, R. D. and Mann, J. I. (1994) Fatty acid composition of erythrocytes and plasma triglyceride and cardiovascular risk in Asian diabetic patients. *Lancet.* **343**: 1528–30.

18. Murphy, S., Khaw, K–T., May, H. and Compston, J. E. (1994) Milk consumption and bone mineral density in middle-aged and elderly women. *Br. Med. J.* **308**: 939–41.

19. Seppa, K. (1994) Bone density and milk. [letter.] *Br. Med. J.* **308**: 1566.

20. Shirlow, M. J. and Mathers, C. D. (1985) A study of caffeine consumption and symptoms: indigestion, palpitations, tremor, headache and insomnia. *Int. J. Epid.* **14**: 239–48.

21. Abramson J. H. (1988) *Making sense of data.* Oxford University Press, Oxford.

22. Cade, J. E. (1988) Are diet records using household measures comparable to weighed intakes? *J. Hum. Nutr. Dietet.* **1**: 171–8.

23. Varkevisser, C. M., Pathmanathan, I. and Brownlee, A. (1991) *Health systems research training series.* Vol 2, pt 1. IDRC, Canada.

24. Nelson, M., Atkinson, M., Darbyshire, S., (1994) Food photography 1. The perception of food portion size from photographs. *Br. J. Nutr.* **72**: 649–3.

14. Cohort studies

Michael L. Burr

14.1 General considerations

A cohort was a tenth part of a Roman legion and contained 300–600 men who marched together. The word has been adopted by epidemiologists to refer to a group of persons, identified at one point in time, who march off together into the future under the watchful eye of an investigator. The essence of a cohort study is that a group of persons is defined, certain characteristics about each individual are recorded, and they are then followed up in such a way that new events (such as disease and death) or other changes in their characteristics are detected. These new events and changes can then be related to the original observations in order to discover what aspects of the initial status of the subjects predict their subsequent experience.

There are two main types of cohort study. The more usual type is conducted prospectively, so that baseline information is collected when subjects enter the study and they are followed up over its duration. Sometimes, however, a 'historical cohort' is identified with reference to some point in the past (e.g. all the patients who attended a diabetic clinic five years ago) and followed up to see what has happened to the people in the meantime. This approach is possible only where adequate records exist; it has the advantage that the effects of a long period of time can be observed during a relatively short period of study.

The principal use of the cohort study is in the elucidation of aetiology. If we suspect that nutrition affects health in some way, we can assess the nutritional status of a group of people (by recording heights and weights, dietary intakes, or biochemical measurements), follow them up, and see whether their disease experience is related to their initial status. Another use is in studying the natural history of a disease, and how this is modified by treatment. Here the investigator defines a group of persons with a given disease, taking care to obtain a group that represents all patients with the disease, usually at the point of diagnosis. The patients are then followed up to investigate the course of the disease, e.g. in what proportion does the disease remit, and can its remission or advance be linked with anything in the patients' condition at the start?

There are important reasons for preferring the cohort type of study to the case-control approach. Firstly, it enables the investigator to obtain accurate information about the individuals before the onset of the disease being investigated. This is particularly important in dietary enquiries, because diet is liable to change over time and it is unrealistic to expect people to remember their dietary pattern of several years ago. The difficulty is even greater when the disease in question is likely to affect the subject's diet. For example, if we want to know whether diet affects the risk of gastro-intestinal cancer, we are interested in the diet taken before the disease arose. A case-control design requires us to ask patients (and controls) about the diet they took some years ago. But the disease itself has probably affected their eating habits, and they may find it difficult to remember what they used to eat before their diet changed. A cohort design obviates this difficulty, in that the diet is recorded before the subject acquire the condition. Secondly, information obtained prospectively is not only more accurate but is also less open to bias than that obtained retrospectively, when the outcome is known. Thirdly, the cohort design allows us to detect unexpected effects of the initial factors, whereas a case-control analysis is restricted to the selected condition. A good cohort study provides a database that can be used afterwards to test hypotheses that were not thought of when it was set up. Fourthly, the findings show the strength of an association in public health terms, so that the 'population attributable risk' can be calculated (i.e. the degree to which the factor in question is responsible for the amount of the disease in the population).

The disadvantages of the cohort study are inherent in its design. Prospective aetiological studies are inevitably large, long, and expensive, even for the more common diseases, and not usually feasible for less common diseases. It may happen that the subjects alter their eating habits, either spontaneously or as a result of changes in dietary fashion, to such an extent that the original observations are irrelevant. Other disadvantages are the difficulties of tracing all the subjects, unforeseen changes in the personnel involved in the study, and the ultimate hazard that the hypothesis being tested becomes superseded, so that the investigator finds that the wrong baseline information has been recorded.

Occasionally, a 'nested' design is used, combining the cohort and case-control approaches. If a large cohort is being followed up, and a sample of every member's serum as been stored, a case-control analysis can be made within the cohort at a later date. Persons who acquire a given disease are identified, and controls (usually two or three per case) are selected from the cohort, each control being matched with a case in respect of age and gender. The sera of cases and controls are extracted and appropriate biochemical analyses are made. The sensitivity of the comparison is not much less than it would be if the specimens from all the subjects were used, and the expense of the analysis is greatly reduced. The advantages of the cohort methods are thus retained, together with the greater efficiency of the case-control design.

14.2 Practical issues

The design of a cohort study will, of course, depend on the hypothesis under investigation, but certain general principles apply in all cases. It is wise to obtain expert statistical advice at the planning stage so as to ensure that the study is likely to be large and long enough but not greatly in excess of the requirements. Calculations of size and duration will be based on the expected numbers of endpoints in the study (see Chapter 3 and appendix 14.1). The cohort itself is then defined, e.g. all babies born in a given hospital between certain dates; a random sample of 300 persons aged 65–74 years registered with general practitioners in a certain town; all the residents in homes for the elderly in a certain area. Permission is obtained from the consultant, general practitioners, and other appropriate authorities for their patients to be involved. Suitable forms are designed on which information can be collected and coded for easy computerization. Alternatively, portable computers can be obtained and programs designed to permit direct data entry. It is wise to conduct a short pilot study to test the procedures that will be used in the survey. The information is collected by the person who interviewed the subject, so that ambiguities and obvious errors can be dealt with while memories are fresh. It is frustrating to find, months (or years) later, that the data cannot be used because of some omission that could easily have been rectified at the time.

If the cohort is to be followed up for several years, it is inevitable that some of the subjects will change their diet, so that the initial information no longer applies. Insofar as such changes occur as a consequence of alterations in the subjects' state of health, it is the previous diet that the investigators are usually interested in, and the cohort rather than the case-control design will have been chosen precisely to obtain information about it. But some of the changes in diet will occur for other reasons, and the investigator may wish to know to what extent the original data characterize the subjects during the whole period in question. It may not be feasible for the entire cohort to be re-examined periodically, but information can be obtained from a sub-sample and will provide some estimate of the stability of the original measurements in the group being studied.

Follow-up needs careful planning. It may be the intention to acquire information during the whole of the follow-up period (e.g. about illnesses experienced during the next two years). Contact will then have to be made with the subject periodically, either by visiting or by telephone. If day-to-day information is required (e.g. on infant feeding methods) a diary may be used. In some studies the intention is to review the cohort at some time in the future rather than continuously. The problem then arises that some of the subjects will have moved or died, and information may not be easily obtained, particularly in a free-living population. Plans should be made at the start of the study about how the subjects will be traced. Persons who are 'lost to follow-up' are almost certainly different from the rest in several important respects, and if they are at all numerous some serious biases may arise. If the follow-up extends over several years it may be very difficult to trace persons who moved soon after they entered the study.

Various techniques can be used, and the successful investigator has to acquire skills similar to those of private detective agencies. The cardinal rule is to anticipate the difficulties that will undoubtedly arise. It may be advisable to have periodic contact with all the subjects (say at annual intervals), by telephone or reply-paid cards, simply in order to detect those who have left the area. Someone who moved recently is much easier to find than someone who moved several years ago, whose neighbours may have lost the information or moved themselves. Telephone directories and electoral registers are helpful in locating people whose whereabouts are approximately but not exactly known. If the study is hospital-based, the subjects' hospital numbers should be recorded. The next of kin is routinely recorded in hospital notes and may assist in finding people. If the subjects' National Health Service numbers are obtained at the start, the NHS records can be flagged by the Central Register so that deaths (with causes) are notified automatically to the investigators. Another way of minimizing the difficulties of finding subjects is to select them from certain occupations whose members are particularly easy to trace. Medical practitioners are all registered with the General Medical Council and listed in the Medical Registry; their names also appear in the Medical Directory. Civil Servants can be traced through their pension arrangements. Several long-term cohort studies have utilized these opportunities by enlisting subjects from these or similar occupational groups. The main drawback of these groups is that they do not entirely represent the population at large, but are drawn from specific social classes. Furthermore, people who are employed or who volunteer always tend to be healthier than others of their age-group (the 'healthy worker' and 'health volunteer' effects). In consequence, such cohorts are likely to have fewer deaths and disease events over a given period, so that the cohort may need to be larger. Furthermore, the results may not apply exactly to the wider population – for example, associations occurring in a largely non-smoking cohort may be different in smokers.

Other potential difficulties should be anticipated as far as possible. If the intention is to look for changes in biochemical variates (e.g. serum cholesterol), the study should be discussed with the biochemist at the start so as to avoid a change in laboratory methodology, which will invalidate comparisons. Changes in staff or collaborators may be more difficult to foresee and can have a disastrous effect if the newcomer does not have the same degree of interest or commitment as the person with whom the study was set up. If the final measurements (e.g. of blood pressure) are to be made by someone other than the person who made the initial measurements, attention should be paid to standardization and comparability. It may also be desirable for the person recording the final measurements or endpoints to be unaware of the initial data, so as to avoid bias.

A few examples will be given of cohort studies in different age groups to illustrate the use of this approach.

14.3 Infancy and childhood

Infancy provides perhaps the best possible opportunity for cohort studies. A cohort of babies can easily be defined in terms of place and time of birth. Some information (e.g. regarding birthweight and initial mode of feeding) is collected routinely and can be supplemented with other details as required. The duration of such studies can in principle be extended indefinitely; even the longevity of the original investigators need not be a limitation! Large national birth cohorts have been set up in which all the children born during a single week (or a random sample of them) were identified and followed up. The National Survey of Health and Development[1], the National Child Development Study[2], and the Child Health and Education Study[3] were based on children born in Britain during one week in 1946, 1958, and 1970, respectively, and have yielded much useful information. Nutritional aspects of these studies include longitudinal data on height and weight, and the relationship between mode of feeding in infancy with the subsequent development of various diseases.

Localized studies allow these issues to be looked at more frequently and in greater detail to see what nutritional and other factors affect development, for example, one cohort study monitored the growth of about a thousand babies in two South Wales towns up to the age of five years.[4]

Length (or height), weight, head circumference, and skinfold thickness were measured six times up to one year and at six-monthly intervals thereafter. It was found that those whose birth weight was less than 2500g tended to be substantially smaller than the other children at the age of five, when growth in head circumference was a year behind that of the others, while height and weight were 25 and 40 weeks behind, respectively. The majority of children 'tracked' along their growth centiles, more than 80% remaining in the same or an adjacent fifth during the whole period of the study. Children in the different social classes tended to diverge after the age of two years, height and head circumference increasing more rapidly in those from the upper social classes than in the others. Another cohort study examined the relationship between feeding method in pre-term infants and intelligence at age 7½–8 years.[5] It was found that the children who received breast milk had, on average, significantly higher intelligence quotients than the other children, even when allowance was made for mothers' education and social class. This study illustrates the difficulty of allowing for confounding variables in cohort studies; it is possible that the babies given breast milk had on average a better genetic endowment or a more stimulating environment than those who were not. The investigators attempted to allow for such factors, but it is impossible to be sure that they were entirely successful.

If there are records of a population of babies who were born many years ago, the opportunity arises for a historical cohort to be defined and followed up to the present time. A series of such studies has been conducted by Barker and colleagues.[6] Records have been preserved of babies born in Hertfordshire between 1911 and 1930 who were weighed at birth and at one year of age. The population was followed up in the 1980s, to see which subjects had died and of what diseases. The death rate from coronary heart disease fell steeply with increasing weight at one year, and to a lesser extent with increasing birthweight; deaths from non-circulatory conditions did not show these trends. Some of the men from this cohort who still lived in the area were traced and interviewed. Their mean systolic blood pressure fell with increasing birthweight, while plasma fibrinogen (a major predictor of coronary heart disease) was inversely related to weight at one year. Other factors that were negatively associated with weight at one year included prevalence of impaired glucose tolerance and of chronic obstructive airways disease. It is clear that early influences have long-term predictive effects. It is difficult to rule out potential confounding variables (e.g. long-acting adverse environmental factors or genetic influences), but a good case has been made for an aetiological effect of factors acting in early life on diseases occurring in middle age.

14.4 Adults

Cohort studies in adults have been very useful in elucidating the role of diet in the causation of disease. Nutrition is a major determinant of health, so it is obviously important to investigate its influence on morbidity and mortality. Everybody eats food, but not necessarily the same food, so there are ample opportunities for comparing the effects of different dietary habits within the same population.

Ischaemic heart disease (IHD) is a good example of a relationship between diet and health, and has been investigated in this way. Table 14.1 summarizes nine cohort

Table 14.1 Some cohort studies of dietary factors associated with IHD incidence or mortality.

Study	Dietary methods	No. subjects	Dietary factors		
			Positively associated	Negatively associated	Not associated
Framingham[7]	24-h recall	859		Energy Alcohol	Fat Sugar
Honolulu[7]	24-h recall	8006	Fat	Energy Alcohol	Sugar
Ireland–Boston[8]	Food frequency	1001	Fat	?Fibre Vegetables	Energy Sugar
London[9]	Weighed intakes	337		Fibre Energy	Fat Sugar
Puerto Rico[7]	24-h recall	9150	Fat	Energy Alcohol	Sugar
Rancho Bernardo[10]	24-h recall	859		Fibre	Fat Energy Alcohol
Seven Countries[11]	Weighed intakes (subsample)	12770	Fat		Sugar
Western Electric[12,13]	Detailed history	1900	Fat score	Fish	
Zutphen[14,15]	Detailed history	871		Energy Fish	Fat

studies that have reported associations between diet and heart disease.[7-15] These studies showed considerable differences in methodology and analysis, and this summary of their findings is somewhat over-simplified. The various dietary methods have different degrees of reliability, which, together with the wide range of numbers and the variety of countries, presumably explain the differences between the results. Thus, it is not entirely surprising that the same dietary factors do not emerge as important in every study. But some consistent features may be seen: no factor had a significant positive association in one study and a significant negative association in another; fat showed positive associations in several studies (although in the Puerto Rico study the association was with polyunsaturated rather than saturated fat); energy, fibre, and alcohol showed negative associations; while sugar was not associated with IHD in any study. The interpretation of these findings illustrates some of the weaknesses of observational cohort studies. Most studies rely on dietary recall, which is particularly unreliable for people whose food is prepared for them: for example, many married men often have only a vague idea of what their wives give them to eat, or even what they ate yesterday. If a precise account is obtained about intake over a short period of time (e.g. using weighed intake records), it may not represent habitual intake.

A more profound issue concerns the interpretation of the associations that were reported. To what extent is an association likely to be causal, or could it be the result of confounding with some other dietary or non-dietary factor? In several of these studies, fibre has emerged as apparently protective. Is this because it is actually protective, or is the relationship attributable to a tendency for people to take a high fibre diet as part of a healthy lifestyle, other aspects of which may be more important? The inverse relationship between IHD and energy intake presumably reflects a protective effect of exercise, although in some individuals inability to take exercise is a consequence (rather than a cause) of heart disease and related illnesses. The cohort design enables information about pre-existent illness to be recorded at the start, so that the analysis can be confined to persons who were then apparently healthy. A further refinement is to exclude persons who die or acquire IHD in the first year or two after entering the study. Fat intake (as a percentage of total energy) is an adverse factor in several studies; to some extent it is confounded with other 'non-healthy' habits, such as smoking and lack of exercise. These difficulties of interpretation all arise because people who choose a diet high in fibre and low in fat are likely to differ from other people, and only a controlled trial can distinguish clearly between causal and non-causal associations.

Some cohort studies have examined one or two specific dietary factors rather than a wide range of foods. Intakes of coffee, tea, and alcohol are more easily described and likely to be fairly constant for any individual, so that drinking habits are sometimes available when other dietary information is absent. Coffee consumption has been positively related to IHD in some prospective studies, while a moderate intake of alcohol seems to confer protection.

Cohort studies have yielded useful information about nutritional factors in relation to other common diseases. The Framingham study indicated a protective effect of fruit and vegetables against stroke.[16] Breast cancer has been positively associated with alcohol intake[17] and negatively with vitamin A.[18] In the Prospective Basel Study, plasma anti-oxidants (carotene and vitamins A, C, and E) were measured in 2974 Swiss men; in the following 12 years, lung cancer was associated with initially low plasma carotene and stomach cancer with low vitamin C and lipid-adjusted vitamin A levels.[19]

14.5 The elderly

There are several reasons for expecting cohort studies to be particularly easy and fruitful in the elderly. Old people tend to have fairly definite likes and dislikes so that the diet of an old person is likely to be more uniform (and therefore more easily characterized) than that of a younger person. Nutritional deficiency is more common in old age than at other periods of life, yet many elderly people eat very well. The dietary variation between individuals is therefore large in comparison with the variation within individuals. Furthermore, morbidity and mortality are very high in the elderly, so more endpoints will occur per person–year of follow-up than at younger ages.

Several nutritional cohort studies have been conducted in the elderly. The subjects' initial condition has been recorded in terms of body mass index, dietary intake, and various biochemical indices. For example, a sample of 830 persons over the age of 65 years was selected from general practitioners' lists in one area and stratified so as to provide relatively more over the age of 75 years.[20] Height, weight, plasma and leucocyte ascorbate concentration, and other variables were measured, and the subjects were followed up and reweighed eight years later. There was a tendency for initial ascorbic acid status to be inversely related to mortality, but it is not entirely clear how this should be interpreted. It may be that vitamin C deficiency is a common cause of ill-health in the elderly, so that a low vitamin C status results in a greater risk of death. Alternatively, the causal relationship may be in the opposite direction: old people who are in poor health for any reason are likely to have some impairment of appetite (and perhaps of their metabolism), such that their intakes and blood levels of various nutrients will be low and vitamin C happened to be the nutrient that was monitored in this study. A third possibility is that a low vitamin C intake tends to accompany other adverse factors, such as low socio–economic status, without necessarily being the main causal link between poverty and ill-health.

The Zutphen Elderly Study examined the intake of anti-oxidant flavinoids of 805 men aged 65 to 84 years.[21] The habitual consumption of relevant foods was estimated by means of a cross-check detailed dietary history, and the flavinoid content of representative samples of these foods was measured biochemically. In the following five years the risk of death from IHD (adjusted for age and other risk factors) was significantly and inversely related to flavinoid intake. The major source of flavinoids was tea, followed by onions, apples, and other vegetables and fruits. These results support other evidence pointing to a protective effect of dietary anti-oxidants against IHD.

The confounding effect of differential ageing is particularly important in old age, and is well illustrated by the paradoxical finding that obesity is a favourable prognostic index in the elderly.[20] Over the age of 65, people tend on average to lose weight as they grow older; this was noticed by Shakespeare in his description of the seven ages of man (As You Like It, Act II, scene 8); the fifth age is 'the justice, in fair and round belly', while the sixth age is 'the lean and slipper'd pantaloon, . . . his youthful hose well sav'd, a world too wide for his shrunk shank' (i.e. his old trousers are now too big for him). But not everybody ages at the same rate. Some enter Shakespeare's sixth age ahead of their contemporaries; they tend to be leaner and to die earlier, while those who are biologically young for their chronological age are on average fatter and less likely to die in the next few years. But it does not necessarily follow that thin old people would live longer if they managed to put on weight.

14.6   Concluding remarks

Cohort studies allow more rigorous testing of aetiological hypotheses than other observational studies. They also provide unique information about the natural history of disease. Their disadvantages firstly concern feasibility, because they tend to be large, long, and suitable only for the study of common diseases. Secondly, they share other weaknesses of the observational approach, in that subjects who choose to eat one type of diet probably differ from people who eat a different diet in other ways that could affect their risk of disease. This confounding is particularly important when the nutritional variables are likely to be associated with particular lifestyles or the initial state of health and senescence of the subjects. Insofar as it is not possible to conduct long-term, randomized controlled trails of dietary changes in free-living populations, cohort studies provide the best available evidence of aetiology.

Appendix I: Checklist for planning a cohort study

1. Purpose of the study
(a) What hypotheses will the study examine?
(b) What other specific questions will it address?

2. Value of the study
(a) If the hypotheses are confirmed, will we be any better off (e.g. in our ability to understand disease or treat patients)?
(b) If the hypotheses are not confirmed, will other scientists be interested?

3. Definition of the cohort
(a) Is the cohort to be identified retrospectively or prospectively?
(b) What are the inclusion criteria (age, gender, area of residence, etc.)?
(c) What exclusion criteria apply (e.g. presence of certain diseases, residence in institutions)?
(d) If the cohort is recruited over a period of time, at what point do the subjects have to meet the age and other criteria (e.g. at the start of the study, or when the subjects are seen)?
(e) Are there any ambiguities in the way the criteria are defined or recorded?
(f) Will the cohort comprise a total population defined as above, or will it be a sample of the population, and, if so, how will the sample be selected (e.g. randomly or by volunteering)?

4. Numbers
(a) How large will the cohort be and how has its size been calculated (expected differences, statistical power, etc.)?
(b) What allowances have been made for non-response and migration of subjects?

5. Recruitment of the subjects
(a) How will the subjects be identified?
(b) How accurate and up-to-date is the sampling?
(c) Over what period will recruitment continue?
(d) Can we foresee any biases arising during recruitment (e.g. from selective identification or response of subjects)?

6. Baseline data
(a) What data are to be collected at baseline (including potential aetiological factors and possible confounders)?
(b) What checks could be conducted on reproducibility, validity, comprehensibility of questionnaires, etc., so that the findings will be accepted as true?
(c) How soon can the data be checked, coded, and computerized so as to allow early detection and correction of errors and omissions?
(d) If blood is taken, should specimens of serum/plasma be kept deep-frozen for future analysis in case further hypotheses are suggested?

7. Tracing of subjects
(a) How will the subjects be traced and when?
(b) What secondary methods of tracing are available for subjects who cannot be traced by the primary methods?
(c) What biases are likely to arise from incomplete tracing?

8. Collection of follow-up data
(a) After what interval(s) will follow-up data be collected?
(b) What information will be required (repeat baseline data, outcome events, new tests)?
(c) What checks should be made on the quality of the data to be collected (e.g. reproducibility, validity, comparability with the baseline data)?
(d) Can we ensure that the outcome events are recorded 'blind' with regard to the initial observations?
(e) If some subjects are not available (e.g. through migration or refusal), is there any useful information that we can obtain about them?

9. Analysis of data
(a) Is a statistician (preferably the person who will undertake the analysis) involved in the design of the study?
(b) What analyses of the data will be performed?

10. General considerations
(a) What ethical issues arise (e.g. concerning explanation and information given to subjects; signed consent forms for tests and follow-up procedures)?
(b) What issues of professional etiquette must be considered (e.g. whose permission needs to be obtained; who should be informed as a courtesy)?
(c) If the data collection could disclose abnormalities in the subjects (e.g. a high serum cholesterol), what is our criterion of abnormality and what do we do when we find it?
(d) What are the costs of the study and what personnel will be required?
(e) Is this the best time to start the study, or would it be better to wait (e.g. until the relevant technology has improved)?
(f) Should the methodology of the study be made comparable to that of any other study (e.g. by using similar questionnaires)?
(g) What experts should be consulted to increase the likelihood that the findings will be accepted as conclusive?
(h) Is somebody keeping a list of all the people we promise to inform about the conclusions of the study?

Appendix II: Analysis of cohort studies

Clive Osmond

Cohort studies may be classified according to both the type of data that are collected at baseline and the nature of the eventual outcome measure. The combination determines the appropriate strategy for analysis. Below we consider four common combinations, mention the usual method of analysis, and give an example of each.

Design 1

Measurements are made on individuals. The outcome is the time to an event. The time may be censored (that is, the event is known not to have occurred up to the time specified). The usual method of analysis is by the Cox proportional hazards model.[22,23,24] The effect size is measured by the hazard ratio, rather similar to a relative risk.

Example
Gale *et al.*[25] studied 730 elderly men and women who had completed a 7-day dietary record in 1973. They followed up the cohort for 20 years, noting when subjects died from stroke or other causes. Allowing for age, gender, and known cardiovascular risk factors, those who were in the highest third of vitamin C intake had a relative risk of 0.5 for stroke (95% confidence interval 0.3–0.8) compared with those in the lowest third. A similar gradient in risk was present for plasma ascorbic acid concentrations.

Design 2

Measurements are made on individuals. The outcome is a notionally continuous measurement. The usual method of analysis is by multiple linear regression and analysis of covariance.[26] The effect size is measured by the regression coefficient. This assesses the change in the outcome variable for a unit change in a predictor variable. Thus when a predictor variable is binary the regression coefficient describes the contrast between two groups.

Example
Lucas *et al.*[27] studied 502 pre-term babies who were randomized to receive one of two different diets during their early weeks – mature donor breast milk or pre-term formula. At age 18 months the survivors were given mental development assessments. A development score with mean close to 100 (standard deviation about 20) was obtained from each child. Regression adjustment was made for gender, gestational age, and social class. No clear difference in mental development was found between the two feeding groups.

Design 3

Measurements are made on individuals. The outcome is a binary 'yes/no' variable. The usual method of analysis is by multiple logistic regression.[28] The effect size is measured by the regression coefficient, and this can be transformed into an odds ratio.

Example

Richardson and Baird[29] studied the milk intake and calcium supplement use of a cohort of 9291 pregnant women in California. 268 women experienced pre-eclampsia, the 'yes/no' outcome variable in the study. Allowing for possible confounders such as number of previous pregnancies and body mass index, the odds ratio for pre-eclampsia was 1.9 (95% confidence interval 1.2–2.9) in those who drank less than one glass of milk a day relative to those who drank two glasses of milk a day. The odds ratio was also higher (1.8; 95% CI 1.1–3.0) in those who drank four or more glasses a day, again using as the comparison group the two glass drinkers. The authors interpreted the association of low levels of milk consumption with pre-eclampsia as consistent with data on calcium and hypertension. The association of high milk consumption with pre-eclampsia was unexpected. The authors suggested that it needed to be replicated.

Design 4

Comparisons are made at a group level. The outcome is a survival time (possibly censored). This is known at the individual level. Thus rates can be calculated for the groups.

Age and gender standardization of rates is necessary. The analysis can be with an internal comparison group, when Poisson rates models are useful.[23,24] An external comparison group, often implied by the use of national cause-specific mortality rates, leads to standardized mortality ratios as the measures of effect size.[23,24] These are often scaled so that 100 corresponds to the rates in the external standard population.

Example

Thorogood et al.[30] studied 6115 members of the United Kingdom Vegetarian Society and 5015 of their meat-eating friends and relatives. The subjects were followed up for 12 years. Standardized mortality ratios (England and Wales = 100) for ischaemic heart disease were 51 (95% confidence interval 38–66) for the meat-eaters and 28 (20–38) for the vegetarians. Figures for all cancer were 80 (64–98) and 50 (39–62) for meat-eaters and vegetarians, respectively.

More complicated designs

If repeated measurements are made on members of the cohort on different occasions, then it is inefficient merely to average the data and incorrect to regard all the observations as statistically independent. More appropriate models are needed[31], and it will almost certainly be necessary to seek statistical support. Indeed even the simpler designs carry their own subtleties, making it wise to work routinely in collaboration with a statistician.

Table 14.2 Summary of methods of analysis for 4 cohort study designs.

	Design 1	2	3	4
Meaasurements are made on	individuals	individuals	individuals	groups
Outcome variable	time to an event	continuous measurement	yes/no variable	time to an event; rate
Method of analysis	Cox proportional hazards model	Multiple linear regression; anlaysis of covariance	Multiple logistic regression	Standardisation; Poisson rates model
Measure of size of effect	Hazard ratio (cf relative risk)	Regression coefficient	Odds ratio	Standardised rate ratio

References

1. Atkins, E., Cherry, N. M., Douglas, J. W. B., Kiernan, K. E. and Wadsworth, M. E. J. (1981) The 1946 British Birth Survey: an account of the origins, progress and results of the National Survey of Health and Development. In: Mednick, S. A. and Baert, A. E. (ed.). *An empirical basis for primary prevention: prospective longitudinal research in Europe.* Oxford University Press, Oxford. 25–30.

2. Fogelman, K. and Wedge, P. (1981) The National Child Development Study. In: Mednick, S. A. and Baert, A. E. (ed.). In: *An empirical basis for primary prevention: prospective longitudinal research in Europe.* Oxford University Press, Oxford. 30–43.

3. Taylor, B., Wadsworth, M. E. J. and Butler, N. R. (1983) Teenage mothering, admission to hospital, and accidents during the first five years. *Arch. Dis. Child.* **58**: 6–11.

4. Elwood, P. C., Sweetnam, P. M., Gray, O. P., Davies, D. P. and Wood, P. D. P. (1987) Growth of children from 0–5 years: with special reference to mother's smoking in pregnancy. *Ann. Hum. Biol.* **14**: 543–57.

5. Lucas, A., Morley, R., Cole, T. J., Lister, G., Leeson-Payne, C. (1992) Breast milk and subsequent intelligence quotient in children born pre-term. *Lancet.* **339**: 261–4.

6. Barker, D. J. P., Martyn, C. N. (1992) The maternal and fetal origins of cardiovascular disease. *J. Epid. Comm. Hlth.* **46**: 8–11.

7. Gordon, T., Kagan, A., Garcia-Palmieri, M., Kannel, W. B., Zurkel, W. J., Tillotson, J., et al. (1981) Diet and its relation to coronary heart disease and death in three populations. *Circulation.* **63**: 500–15.

8. Kushi, L. H., Lew, R. A., Stare, F. J., Ellison, C. R., El Lozy, M., Bourke, G., et al. (1985) Diet and 20-year mortality from coronary heart disease: the Ireland–Boston diet–heart study. *N. Engl. J. Med.* **312**: 811–18.

9. Morris, J. N., Marr, J. W. and Clayton, D. G. (1977) Diet and heart: a postscript. *Br. Med. J.* **2**: 1307–14.

10. Khaw, K. T. and Barrett-Connor, E. (1987) Dietary fibre and reduced ischaemic heart disease mortality rates in men and women: a 12-year prospective study. *Am. J. Epid.* **126**: 1093–102.

11. Keys (1987) *Seven countries: a multivariate analysis of death and coronary heart disease.* Harvard University Press, Cambridge, Massachusetts.

12. Shekelle, R. B., Shryock, A. M., Paul, O., Lepper, M., Stamler, J., Liu, S., et al. (1981) Diet, serum cholesterol, and death from coronary heart disease. *N. Engl. J. Med.* **304**: 65–70.

13. Shekelle, R. B., Missell, L. V., Oglesby, P., Shryock, A. M. and Stamler, J. (1985) Fish consumption and mortality from coronary heart disease. *N. Engl. J. Med.* **313**: 820.

14. Kromhout, D., Bosschieter, B. and Coulander, C. de Le (1982) Dietary fibre and 10-year mortality from coronary heart disease, cancer and all causes: the Zutphen study. *Lancet.* **ii**: 518–22.

15. Kromhout, D., Bosschieter, B. and Coulander, C. de Le (1985) The inverse relation between fish consumption and 20-year mortality from coronary heart disease. *N. Engl. J. Med.* **312**: 1205–9.

16. Gillman, M. W., Cupples, L. A., Gagnon, D., Posner, B. M., Ellison, R. C., Castelli, W. P., et al. (1995) Protective effect of fruits and vegetables on development of stroke in men. *J. Am. Med. Assoc.* **273**: 1113–17.

17. Friedenreich, C. M., Howe, G. R., Miller, A. B. and Jain, M. G. (1993) A cohort study of alcohol consumption and risk of breast cancer. *Am. J. Epid.* **137**: 512–20.

18. Hunter, D. J., Manson, J. E., Colditz, G. A., Stampfer, M. J., Rosner, B., Hennekens, C. H., et al. (1993) A prospective study of the intake of vitamins C, E, and A and the risk of breast cancer. *N. Engl. J. Med.* **329**: 234–40.

19. Stähelin, H. B., Gey, F. J., Eicholzer, M., Lüdin, E., Bernasconi, F., Thurneysen, J., *et al.* (1991) Plasma anti-oxidant vitamins and subsequent cancer mortality in the 12-year follow-up of the Prospective Basel Study. *Am. J. Epid.* **133**: 766–75.

20. Burr, M. L., Lennings, C. I. and Milbank, J. E. (1982) The prognostic significance of weight and vitamin C status in the elderly. *Age Ageing* **11**: 249–55.

21. Hertog, M. G. L., Feskens, E. J. M., Hollman, P. C. H, Katan, M. B. and Kromhout, D. (1993) Dietary anti-oxidant flavinoids and risk of coronary heart disease: the Zutphen Elderly Study. *Lancet.* **342**: 1007–11.

22. Cox, D. R. (1972) Regressions models and life tables (with discussion). *J. Roy. Stat. Soc.,* Series B. **34**: 187–220.

23. Breslow, N. E. and Day, N. E. (1987) *Statistical methods in cancer research.* Vol. II. *The design and analysis of cohort studies.* International Agency for Research on Cancer, Lyon.

24. Clayton, D. and Hills, M. (1993) *Statistical models in epidemiology.* Oxford University Press, Oxford.

25. Gale, C. R., Martyn, C. N., Winter, P. D. and Cooper, C. (1995) Vitamin C and risk of death from stroke and coronary heart disease in a cohort of elderly people. *Br. Med. J.* **310**: 1563–6.

26. Altman, D. G. (1991) *Practical statistics for medical research.* Chapman and Hall, London.

27. Lucas, A., Morely, R., Cole, T. J. and Gore, S. M. (1994) A randomised multicentre study of human milk versus formula and later development in pre-term infants. *Arch. Dis. Child.* **70**: F141–6.

28. Breslow, N. E. and Day, N. E. (1980) *Statistical methods in cancer research.* Vol. I. *The analysis of case-control studies.* International Agency for Research on Cancer, Lyon.

29. Richardson, B. E. and Baird, D. D. (1995) A study of milk and calcium supplement intake and subsequent pre-eclampsia in a cohort of pregnant women. *Am. J. Epid.* **141**: 667–73.

30. Thorogood, M., Mann, J., Appleby P. and McPherson, K. (1994) Risk of death from cancer and ischaemic heart disease in meat and non-meat eaters. *Br. Med. J.* **308**: 1667–71.

31. Diggle, P. J., Liang, K-Y. and Zeger, S. L. (1994) *Analysis of longitudinal data.* Oxford University Press, Oxford.

15. Case-control studies

Hazel Inskip and David Coggon

15.1 Introduction

In a case-control or case-referent study, patients with a disease (cases) are compared with controls who do not have the disease. The prevalence of past exposure to known or suspected risk factors is measured in each group, and from this the relative risk associated with each factor can be estimated.

Case-control studies are usually quicker and cheaper than cohort studies, but difficulties arise in the choice of appropriate controls and in the unbiased ascertainment of exposure. By definition, exposure must be established retrospectively, and this poses problems in nutritional studies, especially when a disease has a long pre-clinical phase and the effects of diet are only manifest after a corresponding latent interval. Nevertheless, useful information has been obtained from nutritional case-control studies. For example, studies of stomach cancer have consistently shown a protective effect of fresh fruit and salad vegetables, thus pointing to possible preventive strategies.

The theory of the case-control technique has in the past been confused by its incomplete symmetry with the cohort method. Ideally, in a cohort study, controls should be similar to exposed subjects in all ways other than their exposure to the risk factors under investigation. This has led to the erroneous recommendation that in a case-control study, controls should be similar to cases in all respects other than their disease status. If carried to the extreme, the outcome of such a policy would be to ensure that the exposure pattern of cases and controls was identical, and no study would ever produce a positive result!

The case-control design is better understood if it is regarded as an efficient method of retrospective sampling within a (usually theoretical) cohort study. A weakness of the cohort method, particularly in the investigation of rare diseases, is that information about exposure must be collected for a large number of subjects who do not go on to develop the disease. The imbalance between the number of cases and non-cases in a cohort study is statistically inefficient. A case-control study attempts to overcome this weakness by measuring exposure in only a sample of non-cases.

There is no simple algorithm which can be followed when planning a case-control study. The important features of the method are discussed below under a series of headings, but the order in which these aspects are considered in the design of a particular investigation will depend upon individual circumstances.

15.2 Study population and selection of cases

Ideally, an investigator who is planning a case-control study should first formulate the questions that are to be asked in the study, and then select the best population in which to address those questions. The study population must be large enough and have a high enough incidence of disease to provide a sufficient number of cases over the course of the investigation. Furthermore, within the study population there should be adequate diversity of exposure to the risk factors under examination. If everyone in the study population eats a similar diet, then it will be difficult to identify and evaluate nutritional causes of disease. This is particularly so when (as is usual in retrospective studies) dietary habits can only be crudely assessed, since random errors in the measurement of exposure tend to obscure associations with disease (see Chapter 4).

In practice, the choice of a study population is often constrained by operational requirements. For example, the investigator may only have resources to conduct the study in the area where he/she normally works. In these circumstances it is still important to assess the suitability of the study population at the planning stage. If the population is too small or too uniformly exposed to the risk factors of interest, then it may be better not to waste time on the study.

Occasionally the study population is the starting point of an investigation, and the choice of risk factors for examination is decided secondarily. The trigger to such an investigation might be an unexplained focus of disease. For example, the observation of high rates of stomach cancer in South Louisiana prompted a case-control study to look for a possible dietary explanation.[1] This is a reasonable approach, but it will not be successful if the dietary factor underlying the local excess of disease affects all members of the population uniformly (e.g. the quality of a town's water supply).

Some case-control studies have exploited special circumstances leading to an unusually heterogeneous diet within a population. In Greece, a gradual trend from a traditional Mediterranean diet to the consumption of Western-style foods produced distinctive variation in eating habits. Manousos and colleagues took advantage of this situation to examine the role of diet in the causation of diverticular disease.[2] The associations that they found with high consumption of meat and low consumption of vegetables would have been much less easily demonstrated in a population with more uniform dietary habits.

In the simplest situation the study population is explicitly defined (e.g. all male residents of a town with year of birth 1911–30), and the cases comprise all members of the study population in whom the disease is newly diagnosed (according to specified criteria) during a defined study period. The cases might be identified from hospital or general practice records or perhaps from a cancer registry. Fatal or prevalent cases of disease are sometimes used as an alternative to incident cases because they are easier to ascertain or more numerous. If so, however, associations must be interpreted with care, since they may reflect an effect not on the rate of occurrence of the disease, but on survival after the disease has developed. For example, an association between mortality from lung cancer and low levels of serum beta-carotene might occur not because the vitamin inhibits the development of the disease, but because it is associated with a higher cure rate or longer survival once a tumour is present.

Even when incident cases are used, interpretation may be complicated if the disease is not diagnosed uniformly throughout the study population. In a case-control study of acute appendicitis it would be reasonable to take as cases all members of the study population admitted to hospital as an emergency with histologically confirmed inflammation of the appendix. Acute appendicitis produces severe symptoms that almost always lead to hospital admission and operation. In contrast, diagnosis of uncomplicated duodenal ulcer does not automatically follow the development of disease. Some patients will be asymptomatic or insufficiently concerned about their symptoms to consult a doctor. Some doctors will treat dyspeptic symptoms without attempting to diagnose the specific underlying cause. If the influences that determine the recognition of duodenal ulcer were related in some way to diet (e.g. if stoical individuals tended to eat differently from those who readily complain to a doctor), then spurious associations might arise in a case-control study based on newly diagnosed patients. One way of overcoming this difficulty would be to set up an *ad hoc* surveillance programme within the study population to ensure that cases were ascertained by uniform criteria. Alternatively, it might be acceptable to use the cases that come to diagnosis through the normal channels, but to make allowance for the ensuing biases when interpreting the findings of the study.

Another consideration in the selection of cases is the specificity of the diagnosis. Any advantage from the larger number of cases that can be obtained with a broader definition of disease must be weighed against the loss of sensitivity that will result if an association applies to only a sub-category of the diagnosis under examination. If, for example, a vitamin protects against squamous carcinoma of the bronchus but not against other histological types, the effect will tend to be obscured in an analysis based on all lung cancers combined. If there is no clear *a priori* indication that an association is limited to a specific diagnostic sub-category, it may be better to use a broader definition but at the same time to collect more detailed diagnostic information. Insofar as numbers allow, analyses can then be carried out on subsets of cases to test whether the strength of association varies for different diagnostic sub-categories. For example, in a study to examine the effect of chilli pepper consumption on gastric cancer, there was an indication that the relationship was stronger for intestinal-type than for diffuse-type gastric cancer.[3]

If the number of cases occurring within a study population is too large to be studied, it is quite acceptable to sample within the case group. Ideally, such sampling should be random, but it is often easier to use a non-random sampling method e.g. including only those patients who are admitted to hospital on specified days of the week. Usually this type of systematic sampling creates no problems, but the investigator should always consider the scope for bias if a non-random sampling method is employed.

So far it has been assumed that cases will come from a clearly delineated study population, but in practice this is often not so. A physician might wish to study newly diagnosed patients that present in his or her clinic, but the clinic may not receive all the cases that occur within the catchment population of the hospital. Some patients may be seen by colleagues working in the same or related specialities. Furthermore, the catchment population of the hospital may not be clearly defined. Patients living at the periphery of the catchment area may sometimes be referred to a different centre. In this situation one option might be to seek collaboration from the colleagues who are also seeing cases, and at the same time to restrict attention to cases resident in an area immediately around the hospital from which referral to other centres would be unlikely. Such an approach may facilitate the choice of a control group (see below), but it is not essential that the study population be explicitly defined. If the cases do not come from an explicitly defined population, it is still helpful to think in terms of a theoretical study population in which individuals are each represented to the extent that they would be likely to be included as cases should they develop the disease under investigation. The arguments for using incident rather than prevalent or fatal cases, and the considerations regarding diagnostic specificity, remain unaltered.

Whether defined or theoretical, the study population can be thought of as a cohort that is followed for a finite period – the time over which the cases are diagnosed. The controls provide an estimate of exposure patterns in the members of this cohort who are at risk of becoming cases during the period of follow-up. Risk estimates then correspond to those which would be obtained if information about exposure were available for the complete cohort.

15.3   Ascertainment of exposure

Exposure must be measured both to risk factors of interest and also to factors which might confound their association with the disease under study. If the disease has a long pre-clinical phase, the relevant exposures may have occurred many years before diagnosis, and in nutritional studies this can pose particular difficulties. Most studies rely on recalled dietary histories, but research has shown that people have difficulty in remembering past dietary practices, and that answers to questions about previous diet are strongly influenced by current eating habits.[4] This will lead to error if the diet has changed, and particularly if cases and controls have altered their diet to a different extent. Changes in dietary practice are quite likely in diseases such as cancer or renal failure which affect the appetite, and also where symptoms are aggravated or relieved by certain foods. Patients with gallstones may avoid fatty foods because they cause discomfort, and patients with duodenal ulcer may increase their consumption of milk in order to relieve dyspepsia. In some diseases, dietary manipulation may form part of the treatment. For example, in a case-control study of renal stones it was difficult to obtain reliable measures of pre-morbid fluid intake because most patients with renal colic had been advised to increase their fluid consumption when they first presented to hospital.[5]

Sometimes it is helpful to ask subjects whether they are aware of having altered their diet, although information of this type can usually be only loosely quantified. Another approach has been to identify cases before their disease becomes symptomatic. For example, the relation of breast cancer to diet has been examined in patients diagnosed at screening clinics, and dietary risk factors for stomach cancer have been sought by comparing subjects with intestinal metaplasia of the stomach (a precursor of carcinoma) and controls. However, this strategy can only be employed when the disease has a pre-clinical phase that can be detected by cheap and ethically acceptable methods.

A common method of measuring diet in case-control studies is by a simple food frequency questionnaire or by a food frequency questionnaire with some estimate of portion size. However, where the diet is relatively constant and unaffected by the presence of the disease (e.g. in a study of early asymptomatic breast cancer detected by screening) it may be possible to use other techniques such as 24-hour dietary recall, or a prospective food diary. If the study hypothesis concerns a specific nutrient, it may not be necessary to make a complete dietary assessment. In a study of fractured neck of femur in which calcium was the main nutrient of interest, intake of the mineral was estimated from the consumption of six key foods – milk, bread, cheese, puddings, cakes, and biscuits.[6] This was possible using a relatively simple questionnaire, the validity of which was assessed by comparison with duplicate portion analysis and a 7-day weighed record.[7]

Increasingly, case-control studies are using biochemical measures of nutrition (see Chapter 7). For example, in a study to examine the relation between micronutrients and childhood cancer, levels of a variety of nutrients including retinol, beta-carotene, alpha-tocopherol, zinc, and vitamins A and E were assayed in the blood.[8] Again, there is an assumption that the variable measured has not changed as a consequence of the disease process. A particular advantage of biochemical measures is that they sometimes allow an assessment of long-term nutritional status. For example, levels of selenium in toenail clippings may reflect chronic dietary intake[9] (see Chapter 7).

A confounding factor is associated with the risk factor under study and independently influences the risk of developing the disease. It may give rise to a spurious association when in fact the risk factor is not a cause of the disease, or it may mask a true causal association. Many non-dietary causes of disease, such as smoking habits, physical activity, personal hygiene, and exposure to infection, are associated with diet and have the potential to confound its effects. A good example is the association between pancreatic cancer and coffee-drinking which has been demonstrated in several case-control studies, but is thought to be due, at least in part, to a confounding effect of smoking.[10] In addition, one dietary variable may confound the effects of another. Interpretation of dietary associations in case-control studies requires that potential confounders be reliably measured. (Errors in the measurement of confounders may mean that their effects are not fully controlled.) However, the impact of a confounder will be large only if it is strongly associated both with the disease and also with the dietary risk factor of interest.

15.4   Selection of controls

The choice of a suitable control group is one of the most difficult aspects of case-control design. The aim is that controls should give a reliable estimate of exposure to risk factors and confounders among members of the defined or theoretical study population who are at risk of becoming cases during the period of study. This objective leads to two requirements:

1. The exposure of controls should be representative of that in members of the study population who are at risk of becoming cases.
2. The exposure of controls should be ascertainable with the same accuracy as for cases. (Ideally, exposure would be measured with complete accuracy in all subjects. In

practice this ideal is rarely attainable, but if the distribution of measurement errors is similar for cases and control, the effect will tend to be conservative. It may mask a true association, but it will not give rise to spurious associations – see Chapter 4.)

It is in trying to reconcile these two requirements that problems are encountered. Two types of control are commonly used.

15.4.1 Patients with other diseases

Patients with other diseases are frequently a convenient sources of controls, especially in hospital-based studies. They have the advantage that ascertainment of exposure can often be made comparable to that for cases. One of the dangers in studies based on recalled data is that, because of a natural interest in trying to find out why they have become ill, cases are more motivated to remember past exposures than controls. However, if the controls are also ill, they too will be seeking an explanation for their disease. It may be possible to blind subjects to the exact purpose of the study so that controls are not aware that their illness is not of prime interest. Furthermore, in studies which collect information at interview, it may be feasible to blind the interviewer as to whether he or she is dealing with a case or control, and so eliminate the possibility that, deliberately or subconsciously, questions are addressed differently to cases and controls. Another advantage of using other patients as controls in hospital-based studies is that control diagnoses can be chosen so that their catchment population is similar to that for cases. This is helpful where the boundaries of the catchment area of the hospital are ill-defined.

The main weakness of using patients with other diseases as controls is that their exposure may not be representative of that in members of the study population who are at risk of becoming cases. For example, controls with peptic ulcer or diabetes would be unlikely to have diets typical of those in the general population. It is of course open to the investigator to exclude from the control group diseases which have known dietary associations, but the possibility of unrecognized bias remains. The effect of such unsuspected biases is potentially greatest when all the controls have the same disease. For this reason, when using patients with other diseases as controls, it is better to include a range of control diagnoses.

15.4.2 Subjects selected from the general population

Various methods have been used to select controls from the general population. Some studies have used a predetermined algorithm to choose controls living in the same street or neighbourhood as cases; in Britain and Scandinavia population registers derived from censuses or health services records are often taken as a sampling frame; and in countries such as the United States where almost everyone has a telephone, controls can be obtained by random digit dialling.

In general, the exposures of controls selected in these ways are likely to be more representative of those in the population at risk of becoming cases, although biases may occur if there is a poor response rate from controls. (The exposure patterns of non-responders are often different from those of subjects who agree to take part in surveys.)

The main problem with community controls lies in the ascertainment of exposure, since subjects selected from the general population will usually be less motivated than cases to put time and effort into helping with a study. Where such recall bias is a concern, its magnitude can sometimes be gauged by including dummy questions about variables which the investigator thinks are unlikely to be related to the disease under study. However, this technique does not eliminate the bias.

Usually there is no perfect control group, and the choice of controls must be a compromise. Three general rules are worth bearing in mind:

1. Controls should always come from the study population, i.e. they should be people who would have become cases had they developed the disease during the period of study.
2. Where possible the method used to ascertain exposure should be similar for cases and controls. For example, if controls are to be interviewed at home, it is better if cases are also interviewed at home.
3. If information is to be obtained at interview or by physical examination (e.g. measurement of height, weight, skinfold thickness), this should, where possible, be carried out blind to the case/control status of the subject. Similarly, laboratory analyses should be performed without knowledge of whether specimens come from cases or controls. If it is not practical to keep an interviewer or examiner blind to a subject's status, then it is an advantage to keep him or her unaware of the exact purpose of the study. Subconscious biases in the method of questioning or examination are then less likely.

Having fixed on a control group, the investigator should try to assess the likely magnitude and direction of any resultant bias, and take that bias into account when interpreting the findings. Interpretation may sometimes be easier if two control groups are used such that any biases are likely to be in opposite directions (perhaps one comprising patients with other diseases and one from the general community). The true relative risk can then be expected to lie somewhere between the estimates obtained with each set of controls.

15.4.3 Matching

In many case-control studies, controls are chosen to match the cases in one or more ways. The matching may be on an individual basis (e.g. each case is paired with a control of the same age and gender) or in groups (e.g. controls are chosen to include similar proportions of current, ex-and non-smokers to the case group). Matching is used in case-control studies for three reasons:

1. To permit allowance for confounders which are complex or difficult to define, e.g. by comparing within identical twin case/control pairs it is possible to allow for ill-defined genetic confounders.
2. To make allowance for confounders statistically more efficient. Efficient analysis requires that there be a similar ratio of cases to controls at each level of exposure to the confounding variable.

3. To reduce biases in the ascertainment of exposure, e.g. if some cases are deceased, it may still be possible to elicit useful dietary histories from their spouses. However, such information is unlikely to be as accurate or complete as would be obtained from the subjects themselves. To make the collection of information for cases and controls comparable, deceased cases could be matched with deceased controls.

Unlike in a cohort study, matching in a case-control study does not in itself eliminate the effects of a confounder. On the contrary, if the factor matched is associated with the exposure under study but is not itself a risk factor for the disease, then confounding may be introduced where none was previously present. (In the extreme, matching on a variable that correlated perfectly with exposure would eliminate all differences between cases and controls, even when exposure was a genuine cause of the disease.) Thus, when matching is employed in the design of a case-control study, it is essential to allow for the matching in the analysis. Matching for a variable which is associated with the exposure under study but not with the disease is statistically inefficient (in effect it removes some of the variation in exposure within the study population), and should if possible be avoided. Matching for a variable associated with the disease but not with the exposure does not compromise statistical efficiency in the same way, but should only be carried out when there is good reason (e.g. matching on vital status to make collection of information about cases and controls more comparable).

Once a variable has been matched it cannot be examined as an independent risk factor in the analysis (although it is still possible to explore whether it modifies the effect of other risk factors). Also, matching on more than two or three variables can become very time-consuming and expensive – especially if effort is required to establish whether a potential control fulfils the matching criteria, and a high proportion end up being rejected because they do not meet the requirements. Matching is therefore usually limited to age and gender (which are almost always potential confounders) and perhaps one other variable.

A matched set in which exposure data are missing for all of the cases or all of the controls contributes nothing to the analysis. Any information about the exposure which has been collected for members of such a set is thus wasted. Insofar as such redundancy is more likely to occur with the smaller sets that are formed by individual matching, it may be preferable to employ group matching where feasible. For example, in relation to age it may be better to group match within five-year age bands rather than individually match to within two years of age.

When matching is employed, the exposures of controls should be representative of those at-risk members of the study population within each matching stratum.

15.4.4   Controls who are lost from the study

One common source of concern in the design of case-control studies is controls who are lost from the study because they cannot be contacted or refuse to participate. Is it permissible to replace lost controls? Clearly, if drop-outs have different exposure to risk factors from participants, their loss will introduce bias. However, replacing lost controls does not increase the bias, and may in some circumstances be advantageous. For example, when cases and controls are individually matched in pairs, failure to replace a lost control will lead to any information about the corresponding case being wasted.

15.4.5 Controls who go on to become cases

Another area of concern is the control who goes on to develop the disease. In a three-year study of incident cases of myocardial infarction with controls selected from the general population, what should happen if a control chosen in the first year proceeds to become a case in year three? Understanding of this problem becomes clearer if the case-control study is viewed in the context of the cohort within which it samples. If the entire cohort were studied, subjects who developed the disease would contribute person–years at risk up to the time at which they became cases. Thus, in the case-control study it is quite legitimate that a control should contribute information about the exposure of persons at risk even though he subsequently goes on to become a case. Statistical calculations become more complicated, however, if some subjects appear in the analysis as both cases and controls, and it may be simpler to discard controls who later become cases. In practice the event is usually so rare that it makes little difference whether they are included or excluded.

15.5 Nested case-control studies

The case-control approach has been presented as a method of efficient sampling within a theoretical cohort study. Occasionally, however, case-control investigations are 'nested' within real cohort studies. For example, a study looking at the relation of colon cancer to vitamin D metabolite levels, drew cases and controls from within a cohort of 20 305 people from whom blood specimens had been taken 10–17 years earlier and stored in appropriate conditions. The assays were only performed on the samples which had been taken from the 57 people who subsequently developed colon cancer (the cases) and from two matched controls for each case. Thus, only 171 assays were performed out of the 20 305 that would have been required had this been a full cohort study, resulting in a considerable saving of resources.[11]

The principles of the design of nested studies are the same as for any case-control investigation. Controls chosen for a particular case should be members of the cohort who were themselves at risk of becoming cases at the time the case was diagnosed.

15.6 Study size and statistical power

When designing a case-control study it is important to include sufficient individuals to give a reasonable chance of detecting relative risks of interest. In other words, the study must have adequate statistical power. The power will not only depend on the numbers of cases and controls but also on the distribution of the exposure of interest in the population at risk of becoming cases, and the relative risk of disease that the study aims to detect. Issues of statistical power and study size are discussed in Chapter 3 along with the formulae for calculating the numbers of cases and controls required.

Where the aim of the study is to establish whether an association exists (i.e. whether the relative risk is different from one), and there is no constraint on the availability of cases and controls, the optimal ratio of controls to cases is 1:1. However, in some studies only a limited number of cases is available for study, or information can be obtained more cheaply and easily for controls than for cases. In these circumstances it may be better to have more than one control per case. There is, however, a law of diminishing returns, and little is gained by having more than four controls per case. (see Fig. 15.1). Normally, a ratio of controls to cases greater than 4:1 would only be used if additional controls were very readily available. In a matched case-control study it is not necessary to have the same ratio of controls to cases in all matched sets or strata. Modern analytical techniques easily deal with a variable ratio.

It is worth noting that the sample size for an unmatched study can be obtained easily from the computer package 'Epi Info' which is in the public domain and can be freely copied.[12] Sample size is based upon formulae given by Fleiss[13], the method being described in the Epi Info manual.[12] As with most formulae for calculating study size, no allowance is made for confounders, so the numbers given must be considered as a lower limit. Epi Info does not provide estimates of sample size when matching is to be used, but in practice the numbers for an unmatched study without considering confounders can be used as an adequate approximation (see Chapter 3).

15.7 Analysis and interpretation

The main measure of association commonly derived from case-control studies is the odds ratio (OR). In most circumstances the odds ratio approximates closely to the relative risk.

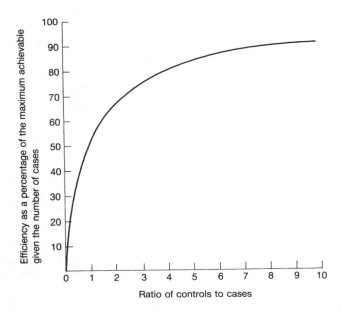

Fig. 15.1 Relation between statistical efficiency and ratio of controls to cases.

15.7.1 Analysis of unmatched studies

In an unmatched study with dichotomous exposure distributed between cases and controls as in Table 15.1, the odds ratio is estimated by the cross-product ad/bc. Approximate 95% confidence limits for this estimate are given by the formula:

$$\exp\left\{\ln\left(\frac{ad}{bc}\right) \pm 1.96\sqrt{\frac{1}{a}+\frac{1}{b}+\frac{1}{c}+\frac{1}{d}}\right\} \tag{15.1}$$

The statistical significance of the association is assessed by the chi-squared test. The computer package Epi Info[12] can be used for the analysis of this type of data, whether presented as individual records or in the form of a summary 2×2 table as in Table 15.1.

As an example, consider the results of the study on chilli pepper consumption and gastric cancer in Mexico mentioned in Section 15.2.[3] The main study results are presented in Table 15.2 from which it can be seen that chilli pepper consumption is quite strongly associated with gastric cancer in Mexico. Such an analysis, however, takes no account of the amount of chilli pepper consumed. The study participants were asked to rate their level of consumption into one of four categories – non, low, medium, or high. By considering the numbers in each consumption category against the 'none' category, odds ratios for low, medium, and high consumption were found to be 4.2, 4.6, and 18.3 respectively. It is possible to test the trend in these odds ratios, and this too can be performed in Epi Info, giving a chi-squared value of 62.1 (p<0.01) indicating a strong trend. Finding a trend gives extra weight to the association as, if chilli pepper is a cause of gastric cancer, then we might expect those who eat it most to be at the greatest risk.

Table 15.1 Distribution of exposure in unmatched case-control studies.

	Cases	Controls
Exposed	a	b
Unexposed	c	d

Table 15.2 Chilli pepper consumption and gastric cancer in Mexico

Chilli pepper	Cases	Controls
Yes	211	607
No	9	145

Odds ratio = 5.6, 95% confidence interval 2.7–12.0

The methods of analysis discussed so far take no account of confounding factors, such as age and gender. This can be done by analysing the data within each age and gender group (and within levels of other confounders where appropriate). A pooled estimate of the odds ratio can be obtained which is adjusted for the effects of the confounders. This method is known as a stratified analysis. However, another method known as logistic regression is now more often used to take account of confounding. Again, it gives estimated odds ratios and their associated confidence intervals that are adjusted for the confounders. Such methods can also deal with exposure variables which have more than two levels or are continuous in nature. Interpretation does not require complete understanding of the underlying mathematics, but the epidemiologist should at least be aware of any biological assumptions that are inherent in the analytical model. For example, in a standard logistic regression analysis there is an assumption that when risk factors are present in combination, their odds ratios multiply. The investigator must decide whether this supposition is justified. It is possible to test for interactions (which indicate that the odds ratios do not multiply) within the statistical model, but a final decision as to its acceptability will rest also on an understanding of the biological mechanisms which are thought to underlie the relevant associations. If two risk factors act at different stages in a carcinogenic sequence then their effects might be expected to multiply. If they both act in the same way at the same stage, then an additive effect would perhaps be more likely and different analytical methods might be appropriate.

15.7.2   Matched studies

Matched studies require a completely different form of analysis to take account of the difference in the design. In the situation in which there is one control for each case the standard presentation of the data is as in Table 15.3. Note that each cell of the table gives a number of case-control pairs rather than the number of individuals as in Table 15.1. The odds ratio is simply calculated as the ratio s/t and an approximate 95% confidence interval is given by:

$$\exp\left\{ \ln\left(\frac{s}{t}\right) \pm 1.96 \sqrt{\frac{s+t}{st}} \right\} \tag{15.2}$$

Statistical significance is assessed by McNemar's test which is described in many epidemiological texts.[14–16] Epi Info can handle data from matched pairs, but only if records are available for each individual. Information cannot be entered in the form of a summary 2×2 table as in Table 15.3. An example of a matched study, given in Table 15.4, is taken from a study to examine risk factors for *Cryptosporidium* diarrhoea in children in Guinea Bissau.[17] This indicates that the storage of cooked food for later use increases the risk of diarrhoea more than two-fold.

More complex statistical techniques are needed to analyse exposures at various levels; to take account of confounding variables other than those for which matching was performed; and to consider interactions (both with the matched variables and with other exposures or potential confounders). Also, many studies use matched sets with control:case ratios other than one, which makes analysis more complex. The standard

Table 15.3 Distribution of exposure in matched case-control studies.

	Control exposed	Control unexposed
Case exposed	r	s
Case unexposed	t	u

Table 15.4 Storage of cooked food and risk of *cryptosporidium* diarrhoea.[17]

		Control	
		Stored cooked food	Did not store cooked food
Case	Stored cooked food	35	39
	Did not store cooked food	18	33

Odds ratio = 39/18 = 2.2, 95% confidence interval 1.3–4.2.

form of analysis for individually matched studies uses conditional logistic regression which, though still providing estimates of odds ratios and requiring the same consideration in the interpretation of the results, is not to be confused with (unconditional) logistic regression as applied in unmatched studies. In the study of diarrhoea described above, use of conditional logistic regression to adjust for a variety of other confounders reduced the odds ratio associated with storage of cooked food to 1.8, although this was still significantly raised.

Although unconditional logistic regression can be performed by many standard statistical packages such as SPSS[18] and SAS[19], only a few packages such as EGRET[20] and STATA[21] provide standard routines for both types of logistic regression. For further information on the analysis of case-control studies readers should consult specialized texts such as those by Schlesselman[14], Rothman[15], and Breslow and Day[16].

15.7.3   Interpreting an association as a causal relationship

It is important that interpretation of the statistical analysis takes into account the possibility of biases in the study method and of unrecognized confounders. Measurement error is a special problem in all dietary studies and can produce substantial bias (see Chapter 4). Furthermore, case-control studies based on dietary histories are at particular risk of recall bias.

Assessment of whether an observed association is likely to be directly causal and not the result of unrecognized confounding depends upon several considerations:

1. The size of the relative risk. In general, higher relative risks are less likely to be explained by unknown confounders. The confounding exposure would have to carry an even higher risk, and as such one might expect it to be recognizable.
2. The presence of a dose-response relation. The observation of a higher risk in subjects with a greater exposure to the risk factor favours a direct causal relationship.
3. The existence of plausible biological mechanisms which might explain a causal relationship.

15.7.4 Attributable risk per cent

In a case-control study the ratio of diseased to disease-free individuals is set up by the investigator and it is impossible to obtain estimates of absolute risk or the risk difference (attributable risk) between the exposed and the unexposed. However, it is possible to estimate the attributable risk per cent associated with a risk factor in exposed subjects. This is a measure of the proportion of cases in the exposed population that can be attributed to the risk factor (assuming that the effect of the risk factor is not confounded). The formula for calculating attributable risk per cent is:

$$\frac{OR - 1}{OR} \times 100 \tag{15.3}$$

Thus, in the chilli pepper and gastric cancer example (see Table 15.2), the attributable risk per cent is $((5.6-1)/5.6) \times 100 = 82$, which suggests that 82% of gastric cancer cases in chilli pepper-eaters might be avoided if they stopped eating chillies (assuming that the association between chilli pepper and gastric cancer is not explained by unknown confounders or a result of bias).

15.7.5 Population attributable risk per cent

Population attributable risk per cent (also known as attributable fraction or aetiologic fraction[22]) provides a useful measure for public health purposes. It indicates the reduction in disease in the whole population that might be achieved by eliminating a risk factor. It can be estimated from a case-control study if information about the prevalence of exposure in the population is available. Provided that the disease is not too common, such estimates can be obtained by considering the proportion of controls who are exposed (as, if the percentage of diseased individuals is small in the population, cases have little impact on the overall proportion of exposed individuals). Then the population attributable risk per cent can be obtained as follows:

$$\frac{p(OR - 1)}{1 + p(OR - 1)} \times 100 \tag{15.4}$$

where p is the estimated prevalence of exposure in the population.

In the chilli pepper example, the proportion of controls who ate chilli pepper was $607/752 = 0.81$ and so the population attributable risk per cent is estimated as:

$$\frac{0.81(5.6 - 1)}{1 + 0.81(5.6 - 1)} \times 100 = 79$$

which suggests that gastric cancer burden in Mexico City might be reduced by 79% if everyone stopped eating chillies. Note that this value is lower than the attributable risk per cent, as we are now considering the effect in the whole population rather than in just those who eat chilli peppers.

References

1. Correa, P., Fontham, E., Pickle, L. W., *et al.* (1985) Dietary determinants of gastric cancer in South Louisiana inhabitants. *J. Nat. Cancer Inst.* **75**: 645–54.
2. Manousos, O., Day, N. E., Tzonou, A., Kapetanakis, A., Polychronopoulou, A., Trichopoulos, D. (1985) Diet and other factors in the aetiology of diverticulosis: an epidemiological study in Greece. *Gut.* **26**: 544–9.
3. López-Carrillo, L., Avila, M. H., Dubrow, R. (1994) Chili pepper consumption and gastric cancer in Mexico: a case-control study. *Am. J. Epid.* **139**: 263–71.
4. Wu, M. L., Whittemore, A. S., Jung, D. L. (1988) Errors in reported dietary intakes: II. Long-term recall. *Am. J. Epid* **128**: 1137–45.
5. Power, C., Barker, D. J. P., Nelson, M., Winter, P. D. (1984) Diet and renal stones: a case-control study. *Br. J. Urol.* **56**: 456–9.
6. Cooper, C., Barker, D. J. P., Wickham, C. (1988) Physical activity, muscle strength, and calcium intake in fracture of the proximal femur. *Br. Med. J.* **297**: 1443–6.
7. Nelson, M., Hague, G. F., Cooper, C., Bunker, V. W. (1988) Calcium intake in the elderly: validation of a dietary questionnaire. *J. Hum. Nutr. Dietet.* **1**: 115–27.
8. Malvy, D.J.-M., Burtschy, B., Arnaud, J., Sommelet, D., Leverger, G., Dostalova, L., *et al.* (1993) Serum beta-carotene and anti-oxidant micronutrients in children with cancer. *Int. J. Epid.* **22**: 761–71.
9. Morris, J. Stampfer, M. J., Willett, W. (1983) Dietary selenium in humans. Toenails as an indicator. *Biol. Trace Element Res.* **5**: 529–37.
10. La Vecchia, C., Liati, P., Decarli, A., Negri, E., Franceschi, S. (1987) Coffee consumption and risk of pancreatic cancer. *Int. J. Cancer.* **40**: 309–13.
11. Braun, M. M., Helzlsouer, K. J., Hollis, B. W., Comstock, G. W. (1995) Colon cancer and serum vitamin D metabolite levels 10–17 years prior to diagnosis. *Am. J. Epid.* **142**: 608–11.
12. Dean, A. G., Dean, J. A., Coulombier, D., Brendel, K. A., Smith, D. C., Burton, A. H., *et al.* (1994) *Epi Info, Version 6: a word-processing, database, and statistics program for epidemiology on microcomputers.* Centers for Disease Control and Prevention, Atlanta, Georgia.
13. Fleiss, J. L. (1981) *Statistical methods for rates and proportions.* John Wiley and Sons. New York.
14. Schlesselman, J. J. (1982) *Case-control studies: design, conduct, analysis.* Oxford University Press, Oxford.
15. Rothman, K. J. (1986) *Modern epidemiology.* Little, Brown and Co., Boston.
16. Breslow, N. E. and Day, N. E. (1980) *Statistical methods in cancer research.* International Agency for Research on Cancer, Lyon.
17. Mølbak, K., Aaby, P., Højlyng, N., da Silva, A. P. J. (1994) Risk factors for *Cryptosporidium* diarrhoea in early childhood: a case-control study from Guinea Bissua, West Africa. *Am. J. Epid.* **139**: 734–40.
18. Norušis, M.J./SPSS, Inc. (1993) *SPSS for Windows. Advanced statistics.* Release 6.0. SPSS Inc., Chicago.
19. SAS Institute, Inc. (1988) SAS *Language guide for personal computers* Release 6.03 edn. SAS Institute Inc., Cary, NC.

20. Statistics and Epidemiology Research Corporation. *EGRET* (email: egret@sercnw.com). Statistics and Epidemiology Research Corporation, Seattle, Washington.
21. StataCorp. (1995) *Stata statistical software*. Release 4.0. Stata Corporation, College Station, Texas.
22. Last, J. M. (ed.). (1988) *A dictionary of epidemiology*. 2nd edn. Oxford University Press. Oxford.

16. Experimental studies: clinical trials, field trials, community trials, and intervention studies

Barrie M. Margetts and Ian L. Rouse

Experimental studies differ from observational studies described reported in previous chapters in that they set out to alter, rather than simply to observe, the exposure of interest. There are many different approaches used in experimental studies, from very tightly controlled laboratory experiments to large scale community intervention programmes. In broad terms, experimental studies either focus on assessing change at the level of the individual or the group. The distinctions between these approaches will be covered in more detail later in this chapter. The most important aspect of experimental studies, no matter what study group is used, is to ensure that the allocation of the study group to the different treatments/interventions/exposures under investigation is done randomly. Apart from the way in which subjects are randomly allocated by the investigator, the principles of experimental design are very similar to those that apply to cohort studies. As in all scientific investigations, having a clear understanding of what research question the study seeks to address is essential. The development of the research protocol will then focus primarily on how to measure the effect of an exposure on an outcome with due consideration of the effects that other factors (potential confounders as well as factors related to the efficacy of the delivery of the intervention) have on the observed relationship. This chapter will present the basic principles essential to the design and analysis of experimental studies. As with other chapters in this book the primary objective here is to provide an overview of issues relevant to the design of experiments in human nutrition.

16.1 Historical introduction

Experimentation has been the method used to discover cause and effect for as long as humans have existed. Others have reviewed this literature in detail and it is beyond the scope of this chapter to repeat the detail of those historical accounts. Lind and Louis are two notable workers who used experimentation to attempt objectively to assess the effect of a treatment on a disease. In 1753, Lind (quoted in Carpenter[1]) described an experiment in which 12 sailors with scurvy were put on the same standardized diets, and then allocated to one of six treatment groups for 14 days. Those receiving oranges and lemons were much improved after six days. While Lind may have subsequently misinterpreted his findings, his study must be considered one of the first controlled clinical trials. It was some eighty years later, in 1834, that Louis (quoted in Pocock[2]) articulated further guidance to follow regarding study design. These included consideration of the number of subjects required to show benefit of one treatment over another; the need to observe disease progress accurately in treated and controlled groups; the need to define precisely disease state before the experiment; and the importance of observing deviations from intended treatments. While there were some advances in experimental designs during the nineteenth and early twentieth centuries, the first randomized controlled trials were not undertaken until the later 1940s by the Medical Research Council. These were trials of steptomycin in the treatment of pulmonary tuberculosis (1948)[3] and antihistamines for the treatment of the common cold (1950).[4] This latter study was a double-blind, placebo-controlled trial.

In 1950 Cochran and Cox published an important textbook on experimental designs.[5] While drawing largely from agricultural experiments, this book clearly and simply described the major statistical consideration relevant for experimental studies. Bradford-Hill was also an important force in making the design of clinical trials more rigorous.[6] In his book *Principles of medical statistics* he has a lengthy chapter on clinical trials which is still very relevant today. Truelove, in 1959, summarized the current thinking on experimental design where he clearly described the essential elements of a therapeutic trial as follows[7]:

1. The trial should be planned so that decisive answers can be given to one or more important questions.
2. Patients should be selected for inclusion in the trial before it is known into which group they will go. After admission to the trial, patients should be allocated at random to one or other treatment group.
3. Systematic and pertinent observations should be made on patients so that relevant data are available for analysis at the conclusion of the trial.
4. When possible, trials should be so arranged that neither the physician nor the patient knows which treatment is being used – the so-called double-blind system.

From the early 1950s there has been a rapid expansion of the use of experimental studies in human nutrition. In Section 16.3 we will expand on some of the points so clearly stated by Truelove in 1959 and still very relevant today.

16.2 Definitions of experimental studies

The terminology used to describe the different types of experimental studies is at times confusing. Table 16.1 summarizes the range of terms used. In broad terms there are two major types of experimental study: those where the unit of measurement and exposure is the individual, and those where the unit of measurement and exposure is the population. Individual-based experimental studies are sometimes sub-divided on the basis of the level of the outcome as clinical trials (or therapeutic, secondary, or tertiary prevention trials) where the subjects have a defined clinical state; and field trials (primary prevention trials) where the subjects do not have any defined level of outcome which may be classified as disease. In addition, a third group of individual-based studies are called intervention studies, which we will call field intervention studies, where the

Table 16.1 Summary of terminology used to define different types of experimental studies.

Unit of measurement	Description	Selection of subjects in relation to exposure and outcome
Whole communities/ populations		
	Community trials – Community intervention studies	Whole towns and villages without regard to exposure or outcome (unless initial screening removes clinically diagnosed subjects at baseline)
Individuals		
	Clinical trials – Therapeutic trials – Secondary or tertiary prevention trials	Selected on basis of outcome; may have additional exclusion criteria
	Field trials – Primary prevention trials	Usually no selection, healthy volunteers, with range of exposures and levels of the outcome variable (for continuously distributed measures e.g. blood pressure)
	Field intervention studies	Usually no selection, but clinically diagnosed outcomes may be excluded at baseline

individuals who have the outcome of interest above a certain level at baseline are excluded (e.g. in a trial of vitamin A supplementation children with xerophthalmia are excluded).

Experimental studies in whole populations (communities) are usually referred to as community trials or community intervention studies. Some distinction can be drawn between community trials and community intervention studies. As commonly used, the term community trial focuses on mass education campaigns aimed at changing people's knowledge and attitudes (see Table 16.3 for examples). For community intervention studies, the exposure is usually given to subjects (for example, in the form of supplements, food fortification, or injections) or involves some manipulation of the environment to control access to the exposure of interest (for example, by vector control to reduce malaria, pit latrines for clean water), or to reduce work load and/or to increase disposable income. These community intervention studies have also been characterised as:

(1) explicitly nutritional
   (a) nutrition oriented food programmes; (b) feeding programmes; (c) weaning foods; (d) fortification; (e) nutrition education;

(2) implicitly nutritional
   (a) health related, e.g. immunization, sanitation; (b) economic, e.g. income generation or substitution; (c) labour-saving, e.g. cereal mills;
(3) integrated
   combinations of (1) and (2) above.[8]

Both field and community intervention studies tend to be more complex and less tightly
controlled; they may be conducted without the participants even knowing they are
involved in a study. Some community intervention studies have rather naively assumed
that increasing the supply of food will automatically reduce malnutrition; unless there is
absolutely no doubt about the intervention leading only to a positive change in health,
the effect of pragmatic interventions still need to be compared to control centres who
have not had the intervention.

The term *experimental studies* will be used when a topic is relevant to all types of
study designs. Another way of considering experimental studies is presented in Table
16.2. Here the emphasis is on whether the study seeks to measure effectiveness or
efficacy; do the researchers want to know whether changing the exposure leads to a
change under strictly controlled conditions or under the conditions that apply in the
'real world'. Testing a question under 'real world' conditions asks whether there are
practical, social, and cultural factors which affect the take-up of the treatment/
intervention being offered. This is the question which needs to be asked in a public
health setting; these studies are often called intervention (both field and community)
studies as outlined above. In clinical and field trials the question being asked is: can
changing the exposure lead to change in the outcome; is it effective? These effectiveness
studies may be more helpful in exploring causal mechanisms.

Table 16.2 Comparison between clinical trials and intervention studies.

	Clinical or field trials	Community or field intervention studies
Outcome	Measures exposure and outcome under controlled conditions	Measures exposure and outcome under less well controlled conditions
	Measures effectiveness	Measures efficacy
Question answered	Does the treatment work in theory (is it theoretically feasible) without consideration of the practical constraints imposed in the 'real world'	Does the treatment work in practice under day-to-day conditions which apply in the 'real world'
Major objective	Explores causal mechanisms	Assesses factors which affect implementation

Tables 16.3(a) and (b) Examples of different study designs. (Selected list of examples are presented to illustrate different design principles in different types of studies.)

(a) Community trials-whole community

Author	Study name/location	Intervention	Outcome measures
Fortmann et al. 1995[9]	Stanford Five-City project/USA	Two treatment cities (6-year community-wide multifactor education programmes targeted to specific groups)/ two control cities; one city for outcome data only; *assignment not random*	Total morbidity (and changes in risk factors) and mortality data; four cross-sectional surveys in independent samples; four repeated surveys in a cohort of selected subjects; baseline data collected
Murray 1995[10]	Minnesotta Heart Health programme/USA	Three pairs of communities selected, each with one education and one comparison site; intervention-advocated hypertension prevention and control, healthy eating, non-smoking, and regular physical activity, operated at the individual, group, and community level using mass media, health professionals; communities matched; *assignment not random*	Vital statistics monitored; periodic cross-sectional surveys in up to 500 subjects; cohort surveys in baseline samples
Paradis et al. 1995[26]	Coeur en santé St-Henri/ Canada	Two communities (low income urban) matched on size, location, language, level of education, income and CHD mortality: five-year multifactor (39) interventions (low fat diet, non-smoking, physical activity, cholesterol, and blood pressure control); 18–65 years, emphasis mainly on women. For earch targeted behaviour intervention in each of the five axes of the Ottawa Charter for Health Promotion (strengthen community action, create supportive environments, build public health policy, develop personal skills, reorient health services). *No detail on basis of assignment*	Long-term mortality and morbidity: baseline characteristics monitored in subset from two communities

Table 16.3 (*cont.*)

(b) Clinical trials

Author	Study name/location	Subjects	Intervention	Exposure measure	Outcome measure
Education					
Wood *et al.* 1994[27]	Family Heart Study/UK	In 26 general practices in 13 towns across UK; 12 472: men (7460) and their partners (5012) aged 40–59 years	Randomized control trial; intervention practice and internal control within the practice and an external control from another practice; a nurse-led lifestyle intervention programme (client centred counselling, subject given their risk score; personally negotiated lifestyle change) for one year	No dietary assessment	Pairs compared for difference in total coronary risk score, blood pressure, blood cholesterol and glucose, smoking
Muir *et al.* 1994[28]	Oxcheck/UK	In 5 general practices in Bedfordshire; 5803 subjects aged 35–64; attended for health check	Effect of health check in 1989 and 1992 compared with health check only in 1992; intervention – counsel patients about risk factors; ascertained views on change; negotiated priorities and targets	Validated dietary score	Serum cholesterol, BMI, blood pressure, smoking

Nutrient supplementation

Albanes et al. 1995[29]	ATBC Cancer Prevention Study/ Finland	29 133 male cigarette smokers aged 50–69 years	2*2 factorial design: 20 mg beta-carotene, 50 mg alpha-tocopherol; both or placebo daily for 5–8 years	Check on capsule compliance	5–8 year mortality from various cancers
MacLennan et al. 1995[30]	Australia	424 patients at colonoscopy	306 subjects at 48 months follow-up; RCT double-blind, placebo controlled; fat 25% dietary energy, 25 g wheat bran and 20 mg β-carotene (seven groups and one control)	No dietary assessment	Total new adenomas; risk of large adenomas
Bostock et al. 1995[31]	USA	193 sporadic adenoma patients	RCT double blind placebo: 64 on 1 g calcium, 63 on 2 g calcium and 66 on placebo for six months	No dietary assessment	Rectal biopsy; cell proliferation (labelling index)
Blot et al. 1993[32]	China	455 males aged 40–60 years	5 years; factorial design with combinations of micronutrients and minerals compared with placebo	Plasma measures	Incidence and mortality
Hennekens et al. 1996[33]	US Physicians	22 071 males, aged 40–84 years (11% current smokers, 39% ex-smokers)	Randomized double blind, placebo controlled; β-carotene for 12 years	Plasma measures (subset taken without prior warning in three geographic areas)	Reports of malignant neoplasms, CVD, or death
Dibley et al. 1996[34]	Indonesia	1036 children aged 6–47 months in 43 villages in Central Java	Randomized (fixed geographic pattern), placebo controlled; vitamin A (different doses in children under 12 months) + vitamin E compared with vitamin E alone; 2 years	Serum retinol	Acute respiratory and diarrhoeal illness

The outcomes studied in experimental research cover the whole range of measures discussed elsewhere in this book; these could include changes in knowledge, attitudes, or behaviour (such as eating patterns). The outcome variable may be changed in a continuously distributed variable such as blood pressure or serum cholesterol or blood glucose, or changes in incidence or mortality from specific diseases or risk factors such as obesity, low birth weight babies, or hypertension (all derived from continuous variables). The outcome may be measured in individuals (clinical trials) or groups/populations (community intervention trials). Table 16.3 summarizes the design of a selection of different experimental studies.

Irrespective of the disease state or outcome measure being investigated, all subjects or groups should be measured in the same way, and allocation to treatment (exposure) groups should not be influenced by the disease state or level of the outcome measure (unless randomization to groups is blocked in some way, see Section 16.3.2) of the subjects or groups in the study. All eligible subjects or groups should be randomly allocated to treatments.

Although the specific statistical methods used and the interpretation of results from community trials may differ from other types of experimental studies, the basic principles remain that change in outcome in the treatment group must be compared to any change in outcome measures which may have occurred in the control group. It is not appropriate to measure a 'statistically significant' reduction in an outcome measure in the treatment group and ignore any change that may have occurred independently of treatment in control groups. Whatever the type of study, the main objective is to explore an exposure–outcome (cause–effect) relationship free from bias.

16.3   General considerations in experimental studies

There are a number of general principles that are relevant to all experimental studies. These include:

(1) selection of the study population;
(2) allocation of treatment regimes;
(3) length of observation;
(4) observer effects;
(5) participant effects;
(6) compliance;
(7) ascertainment of exposure and outcome;
(8) statistical power;
(9) analysis and interpretation.

The key points are summarized for clinical and community trials in Table 16.4.

16.3.1   Selection of study population

In Chapter 1, considerable discussion was devoted to the issues of internal and external validity. In all studies, the aim is to design a study so that it is free from bias and internally valid. The internal validity of the study will be compromised if subjects do not comply with the intervention, or are lost to follow-up (same concern as expressed in cohort studies). For short-term, tightly controlled metabolic studies, compliance and loss to follow-up are less likely to be a problem. In a larger, less tightly controlled intervention trial which requires a longer follow-up to assess the desired effect, poor compliance and loss to follow-up may be crucial. In clinical trials, volunteers are usually recruited who are not necessarily representative of the general population; here the main concern is to demonstrate whether a change in exposure leads to a change in an outcome (effectiveness). In community intervention studies, the aim is to assess whether the intervention works at a practical level (efficacy), and some notion of the representativeness of the study sample is important in order to be able to generalize the results.

For clinical trials where a therapeutic agent or procedure is to be tested, consideration may need to be given as to admission criteria. These criteria may include certain demands for exclusion and inclusion, and may primarily be intended for pragmatic and ethical purposes. The restriction of subjects to be included in the study may also relate to the underlying hypothesis being tested; for example, the effect of changing the exposure may differ at different levels of the exposure and the researcher may only be interested in the effects in those with either a high or low intake.

In a clinical trial the investigator may want to specify suitable clinical indications for treatment. (It is not ethical to withhold a treatment which is mandatory or to give a treatment which is likely to be harmful.) It is not appropriate under any circumstances to allocate subjects within the study sample, however that sample is derived, into treatments in a way that results in the treatment groups not being equivalent in clinical state and exposure to other variables.

Apart from the issues already raised there may be other pragmatic issues relating to sample selection. If the aim is to determine the effect of a treatment on an outcome, it may be important to consider whether the selected subjects can complete the study and provide complete and reliable information. If an intervention is to last several years it is important to have a sample which is geographically stable, and therefore likely to have a lower loss to follow-up. This pragmatic choice of study population limits the generalizability but is likely to give a more internally valid result.

In a community trial the selection of towns may be influenced by the treatment to be tested. If the treatment is a general media campaign it will be necessary for the treatment and comparison communities to be sufficiently discrete as to minimize exposure of the control community to the treatment. For example, it may be important to check whether there are relatives living in treatment and control communities who may share information or swap treatments. The selection of such towns may also be influenced by other pragmatic issues, such as ease of access to the town by the investigators or support from local community leaders in staging the research. Irrespective of these pragmatic issues, the towns should be randomly allocated to treatment group and monitored at baseline and followed-up in the same way.

16.3.2   Allocation of treatment regimes

Irrespective of how the study sample is selected, once selected, the optimal way of assigning subjects to treatment and comparison (control) groups is by randomization.

Table 16.4 Comparison of general considerations/contrasts in design for studies in individuals and communities.

	Study group	
	Individuals	Communities
Study population	Exposure and outcome measured and linked at the level of the individual	Exposure and outcome not linked at the level of the individual; individuals receive exposure in the form of, for example, radio or TV health messages, or immunization or vitamin supplements, malaria control programmes to water supplies; in some studies subsets of individuals are measured
Selection of study population	Relevant to study question, and who will be able to comply and not be lost to follow-up; representativeness less important than compliance; exclusion rules may be applied	Representative communities, main concern is to avoid overlap of treatment/exposure between communities, consider geographic/linguistic spread and contact between communities
Allocation of treatment regime	Randomly; matched/blocked as required; comparison group essential; may be placebo or other treatment	Randomly; matched/blocked as required; comparison group essential (secular trends)
Length of observation	Vary from minutes to weeks to months to years depending on question; observation period needs to be long enough for the effect to occur if it is going to; often have a run-in period to get subjects used to the protocol	Usually takes years; observation period needs to be long enough for the effect to occur if it is going to
Observer effects	Ideally, observer taking measurements and involved in giving treatment is blinded as to treatment allocation	Blinded
Participant effects	Ideally, subjects are blinded as to the true nature of study	Blinded
Compliance	The extent to which subjects receive the treatment should be measured objectively; the need to measure compliance depends on the way treatment is given; the measured degree of compliance needs to be considered in the analysis	The extent of the effects of non-compliance varies depending on the intervention from minimal (where subjects given capsules or injections) to a great deal (nutrition education advice to change knowledge, attitudes and behaviour); needs to be considered in analysis and interpretation

Ascertainment of exposure	May not be needed in a feeding study; if a dietary treatment in free-living subjects needs to measure habitual diet at baseline and change in diet during intervention accurately (weighed record plus biological markers of treatment and treatment effects on causal pathway); depends on within person variability and accuracy of methods used	Depends on intervention; sometimes in subsets of individuals when intervention is advice or information; where injection given sometimes blood samples taken to measure changes in levels
Ascertainment of outcome	Outcome measure needs to be measured at baseline and after treatment with required accuracy to observe biologically relevant change; consider within- and between-person variability and accuracy of measuring instruments; outcome may also be measured using mortality data; loss to follow-up may be an issue for longer studies	Outcome measured using routine statistics, for example, morbidity or mortality data before and after intervention in intervention and control communities; subsets analysed; loss to follow-up
Study size/statistical power	Number of subjects required depends on effect expected and accuracy of methods used to measure effect; can be from a few subjects to several hundreds; power altered by study design, but determined by number in treatment group, thus a parallel design with a treatment and control group is less powerful for the same number of subjects than crossover design where all subjects receive the treatment and the control regime	The unit of study is the number of communities studied, not the number of subjects within each community; matching and increasing contacts increases power
Analysis	The true measure of effect is the difference in the change from baseline in the treatment compared with the control group; the above effect should also be assessed taking into account the effects of potential confounding factors; use analysis of variance to test for interaction between treatment, outcome and other factors; also use multiple regression analysis	The difference in the change from baseline in the intervention compared with control group
Interpretation	Consider the effects of chance, bias, and confounding	Consider possible biases: the effects of non-compliance; loss to follow-up of sections of the population with different risk; differences in completeness of ascertainment of outcome, and deaths from competing causes

Random assignment implies that individuals or communities are allocated randomly to each study group and that allocation of subjects to a group is independent of the allocation of other subjects. In a community trial randomization occurs at the level of the community; subjects within a community are not randomly assigned to treatment or control group. However, for practical reasons the two largest community trials in the US[9,10] did not fully randomly allocate towns, and this may undermine the confidence with which the results of these studies are judged.

The purpose of randomization is to ensure that differences between treatment and control groups or towns/populations in potential confounders and levels of other important variables arise by chance alone. Tables of random numbers (and computer programs) are available for the randomization of subjects.

The random allocation of subjects to groups also ensures that neither the observers nor the individual participating in the study can influence, by way of personal judgement or prejudice, who is allocated to receive which treatment. If the observer controls the allocation of subjects to treatment group, there is the strong possibility of bias occurring. Whether consciously or subconsciously, it is possible that the observer may allocate into the treatment group all those people more likely to comply.

Where the study sample is small and a factor is known to be an important determinant of the outcome, it is common to block on that factor to ensure that differences between treatment groups for levels of that factor do not occur by chance. For example, subjects are often blocked on age and gender to ensure that groups are balanced for these factors. Within a block, the allocation to a treatment or control group is still random. For large trials, it is not usually necessary to block, as it is possible in the analysis to consider the treatment–outcome effect in subcategories of the factor of interest. While the effect of these blocking factors could be considered in the analysis, if the experiment is small and the chance variation large, it may be difficult to adjust for these effects in the analysis.

Some studies make use of historical controls as a comparison group. For example, a new treatment may have been developed to the extent that it is considered unethical to withhold it from any subjects. In this situation, how subjects responded to past treatments can be used. There are, however, considerable limitations in this approach. It may be very difficult using historical controls to ensure that conditions other than the treatment of interest are comparable for the treatment and control periods.

It is also possible to use exclusion criteria and matching to take account of the effects of other factors. If, for example, smokers behave differently from non-smokers and this difference is believed to influence the way treatment affects outcome, it may be advisable to restrict the study to non-smokers (or smokers) only, or to block on smoking status if this is feasible.

While it may be ideal for subjects to be similar in their exposure variables prior to a study, unless a particular exposure level is a contraindication for the participation in the study, the subject should be included and randomly allocated to a treatment group. It is not acceptable to allocate all the sickest children to a treatment and to allocate the less sick children to a control regime. This bias in subject allocation may lead to either a falsely optimistic or falsely pessimistic outcome. If it is considered unethical to withhold treatment the trial should not begin, or should be carried out on the basis of the comparison of two treatments (current practice versus new treatment). If there is no doubt about the benefit of the new treatment or intervention, then there is no need for a study.

16.3.3 Length of observation

An experiment should be just long enough to allow the effect of exposure change to result in the hypothesized change in outcome. In deciding on the length of the study the investigator must have an idea as to the mechanism of action of the proposed treatment and thereby some idea as to how long it should take to affect the various steps in the pathway (whether related to change in knowledge, attitudes, or behaviour). The outcome of interest will affect the length of observation. If the aim is to assess the acute effects of food on, for example, catecholamines or glucose metabolism, the study may only last a few hours. For studies of diet and serum cholesterol or blood pressure the study may need to last weeks. For endpoints such as death the length of observation will need to be longer, perhaps many years.

It is clear that a careful consideration of the length of observation is dependent on the hypothesis being investigated. For short-term clinical trials, it may be important to consider whether the short-term changes being assessed are representative of what may occur when the diet is adopted over a longer period of time. The length of observation may also be influenced by statistical power considerations which have already been discussed in Chapter 3 and will be discussed further later in this chapter.

For the study to be worthwhile there must be sufficient events (outcomes), and the longer the observation in a large-scale trial, the more events will occur and therefore the greater the statistical power of the study. For longer-term studies, the effects of secular trends in the underlying rates of the outcome measure being studied need to be considered.

It may also be advisable to establish some rules whereby it would be permissible to extend the period of observation of a study in order to increase the number of endpoints and thereby its statistical validity. On the other hand, where a very substantial effect of a treatment emerges early in a clinical trial, it may be unnecessary, or even unethical, to continue the trial. If the treatment (or lack of treatment in the control group) appears to be resulting in an increased rate of disease, it may also be advisable to stop the trial. Where it may be considered likely that either of the above situations could occur, there should be clearly defined stopping rules incorporated into the study design. For more details about the implementation of stopping rules in clinical trials, readers are referred to other texts.[11–12]

16.3.4 Observer effects

It is possible that if the observer knows to which group a subject has been allocated, they may encourage or in some way alter the behaviour of the subject in the treatment group *differently* from a subject in a control group. If a subject knows they are in a treatment group, they may comply differently than if they are in a control group. It is therefore desirable that both the observer and the participants are blinded as to the participants' treatment group. Prior to the commencement of the study, all personnel involved in the study must be carefully trained to ensure uniformity in the administration of the protocol. The instruments, be they for measuring height, weight, or blood pressure; biochemical assay methods; dietary questionnaires; or any other source of ascertainment of information about the study, subjects must be carefully piloted to ensure that they measure what was intended and also that they measure it in a way that gives reliable information.

In a multi-centre trial, it may not be possible for the same observer to make all the measurements. If different observers are involved, careful consideration needs to be given as to the effect this may have on the consistency of results between centres. If one observer measures blood pressure in one centre and another measures it in another centre and the centres produce different effects, it may not be possible to determine whether the effect was due to the different observers or due to a real difference between the centres. If this type of problem can be thought of in the design stage, it may be better to consider an observer-independent means of measuring the variable of interest. If this is not possible, it will be necessary to have a standardized comparison of the differences between observers which should occur in the training/pilot phase of the study. It is also important that a subset of subjects in each community have repeat measures taken by an observer from another centre. By doing this it may be possible to establish the potential effect that observer differences may have on the outcome. Where possible, analyses should be controlled by one coordinating centre. For example, if blood or urine or other tissue samples are being collected, they should be analysed in one centre or at least in centres with identical analytical and standardization procedures.

When any measurements are being made or data are being collected by interview, the observer should be blind as to the treatment or intervention group of that subject. This will ensure that any effect of the observer on the measurement will be random. It may be difficult for all those in the research team to be blinded as to the nature of the intervention, but as far as possible any field worker collecting information from subjects should not also be the person giving advice or information to the subjects as part of the intervention. As well as a clear and standardized research protocol and procedures manual, there should be strict quality control procedures throughout. It is important to have a measure of the size of the likely intra-observer variation. This should also be established prior to the commencement of the study. An assessment of intra-observer variation should also, where appropriate, be undertaken during the study.

16.3.5 Participant effects

The aim is to standardize the conditions under which the experiment is conducted so that the response of the participant to the intervention can be attributed to the treatment. Subjects in any study will have some notion of what the intervention should be doing to them, and this may alter their response; as long as subjects do not know what intervention they are getting it is likely that the effect of subjects guessing the intervention will be randomly distributed between study groups, and therefore will have no effect on the interpretation of the results.

To be a participant in the trial a person must be recruited and give free and informed consent to participate. They should be aware of the general nature of the research and aware of what they will be expected to do, and have done to them. The provision of adequate information about the study for the participants is important to improve subject compliance. The exact detail given to the participants needs to be balanced with the requirement that as far as possible the subjects be blinded as to the treatment allocation. For some trials this is relatively simple, where, for example, one drug is given compared to another or to a placebo. For dietary interventions this is much more difficult and it is likely that the subject will know the treatment group. This may affect their response to the treatment. In community trials, subjects will probably not be asked if they agree to being involved in the study, and may not even know that they are in a study. Here the researcher must be sure that the treatment is ethical and not likely to harm the members of the community.

The way a subject passes through the research protocol should be carefully standardized. Any violation of the protocol should be noted. For example, if a subject is scheduled to have their blood pressure measured in the morning, they should always have their blood pressure measured at the same time. In practice this is not always possible and when it does not occur it should be noted. Subjects should be given clear and consistent instructions for the completion of dietary records and questionnaires. If they are to provide urine or blood samples, they should be given clear, written instructions about what they need to do, for example, whether to fast the night before or, for a urine sample, how long the urine collection is for and when it is to stop and start.

We have already said that allocation to treatment groups should be random. This should ensure that other variables likely to influence outcome are randomly distributed. However, it is still important to measure these potentially important variables. While it is not appropriate to analyse for statistically significant differences between these variables at the baseline measurement (because of randomization any differences which occur will be by chance anyway), it is appropriate to assess how these variables change during the study and to assess how these changes (and baseline levels) may have affected the treatment–effect relationship. These variables need to be measured with sufficient precision for their effect to be properly considered. As mentioned repeatedly elsewhere, measurement error in potential confounders is just as important as in the exposure and outcome measures.

The way information is collected needs to take account of the within-subject variability. Just as repeat measures give an idea of observer effects, they also give an indication of subject variability. In a clinical trial the aim is to characterize the individual, and measurements need to be precise enough to achieve this. The prime concern must be the internal validity – that all aspects about subject participation in the study are comparable and that deviation from this ideal can be documented. In a community trial, participants may not even know they are participating in a study; if they do, then the same issues as mentioned for clinical trials need to be considered.

16.3.6 Compliance

Much of what we have already said with respect to participant effects relates to compliance. Deviation from the protocol needs to be documented in all subjects, not just those on the treatment. It may be that a comparison or control group alters their behaviour so as to make them more like the treatment group in their exposure status. Perhaps more commonly, participants will forget or deliberately fail to take drugs, or, if they have been placed on a dietary regime, they may occasionally 'break-out' and deviate from the protocol.

Measurement of compliance is essential in any clinical (dietary) trial. The study must be designed so that all variables of importance can be measured during the trial with sufficient precision to give a sensitive and specific (valid) indication of the level of each variable. In many situations the observer is reliant upon the participant honestly reporting whether they have deviated from the protocol. Where possible, an independent measure of compliance should be used. For example, measuring changes in the levels of fatty acids in serum, red blood cells, or a fat biopsy enables the researcher to assess the compliance with dietary advice to alter fat intake.[13] If a dietary intervention aims to increase fibre intake, it may be possible to include in the fibre diet a marker which can subsequently be measured in faecal samples. The level in the faecal sample may give an indication of the amount of fibre supplement eaten. From our experience it is helpful to tell participants that we are checking their compliance by taking blood or urine samples.

It may be more difficult to measure individual compliance in a community trial, but by random sampling of subjects within each study community, it should be possible to measure at least whether subjects are aware of the community intervention and whether it has had any effect on their knowledge, attitudes, behaviour, or levels of some outcome variables. It may be reasonable to assume in a community trial that compliance will be similar in all centres and that it is therefore not necessary to select a random sample of subjects within the community. The efficiency of the treatment as measured by changes in community rates of disease may be adequate. Not measuring change in levels of the exposure which was supposed to be changed in the study may lead to a false impression of the effect of the exposure on the outcome (either positive or negative).

The use of a run-in or familiarization period may improve compliance. It gives the subjects time to adjust to the rigours of the study protocol. However, the diet being fed during this period should not have any effect on the outcome measure. In theory it should be similar to the subject's usual diet. If the trial is for a therapeutic agent, the run-in period should only use a placebo or usual care treatment. The run-in period should be before randomization, so that any drop-outs which occur during this period do not affect the internal validity of the study.

There are situations where it may not be possible or appropriate to have a run-in period. For example, where the experiment is assessing the effect of treatment following an acute event such as angina or myocardial infarction, or where the effect of different oral rehydration therapy on survival in an acutely malnourished child is being assessed.

16.3.7 Ascertainment of exposure and outcome

The aim of an experiment is to assess the effect of a defined change in exposure on the outcome of interest. To assess whether the change in exposure has affected the outcome requires that some measure of each can be obtained to confirm the changes. The measure required will vary depending on the method of changing the exposure, the outcome, and the study design. In clinical trials where subjects are fed, there is no need to ask subjects to measure their intake. For studies where subjects are given advice as to how to change their diet, a measure of compliance with this advice is required; this will usually require an accurate assessment of an individual's intake. Some studies will use biological measures to assess change in exposure, but caution must be exercised in assuming that biological markers relate directly to dietary intake for any nutrient of interest.

Irrespective of the measures required to assess exposure and outcome, the protocol should be administered in the same way in all subjects or groups included; it is not acceptable to use different measures of exposure and outcome in intervention and control groups.

Ascertainment of exposure

If an accurate measure of dietary intake is required, and the only choice is to elicit this information from the subject, then the considerations outlined in Chapter 6 must be considered. If diet is measured poorly, it may be impossible to detect the desired change in exposure which the study has sought, and the study may wrongly conclude that the subject's diet did not change significantly as a result of the intervention.

Studies aimed at achieving dietary change by giving people dietary advice, but without measuring diet, and where the advice has not lead to statistically significant change in the outcome measure, are open to the criticism that the reason the advice did not lead to change in the outcome measure was because the advice did not achieve the desired change in diet (as well as concerns about statistical power and length of follow-up). For studies aiming to change people's behaviour by changing people's knowledge, there is a need to consider the complex series of steps involved in going from knowledge to attitudes to behaviour. There is good evidence that knowing what to eat does not always lead people to eating that food. More recently, intervention studies seeking to change behaviours by dietary advice have measured psychological factors related to the subjects' readiness to change (transtheoretical models of behaviour in general[14], and in relation to change in fat intake[15]) and taken this into account when exploring the outcome measure.

Because of the limitations of assessing dietary intakes by subject-based recording methods, alternative methods of assessing intake have been sought. Biochemical markers of intake are discussed in more detail in Chapter 7. While the actual variability of the marker may be much smaller than for a dietary intake measure, the relevance of these markers must be considered. There is little point in precisely measuring, for example, a blood or urinary constituent that is not involved in or affected by the exposure of interest.

Potentially important confounding factors should also be measured during the study; the effects of measurement error or misclassification need to be considered when selecting the method for measuring the confounding factor. Measurement error in confounders is as important as it is in the exposure measure of interest.

Ascertainment of outcomes

Outcomes in experimental studies are measured in the same way as in a cohort study. The outcome measures may be routinely collected data sources (death certificates or hospital activity/medical records), may be collected by the participants themselves (by completion of a questionnaire), or may be collected by the investigator (by personal interviewer or medical examination). The outcome of the study is dependent on the completeness and validity of the information obtained. Where routinely collected data are to be used to measure outcome, it must be possible to ascertain for all subjects whether they have died or been admitted to hospital. It may be relatively simple to determine vital status and obtain a death certificate where there is a central registry of deaths. It may be much more difficult to obtain complete hospital admission data in the absence of a suitable computerized system.

If the investigator finds that a subject has died or had an event of interest (in a hospital or elsewhere), they are then reliant upon the accurate ascertainment (usually by some other person) of the cause of death or clinical details related to the hospital admission. For an outcome measure such as, for example, fractured neck of femur, which is not likely to be recorded on a death certificate as an underlying cause of death, under-ascertainment of outcome will occur if the death certificate is the only source of information about outcome. Even for common causes of death, the detail written on a death certificate may not accurately reflect the major underlying disease process that resulted in the death. If hospital records are to be used, the investigator must be sure that all relevant hospitals to which the study subjects may be admitted are checked for any admissions. Where general practitioners' records are to be used, the investigator must also be assured that subjects only attend that practice and that if an illness occurs they go to the same practitioner. The more subjects and information lost to follow-up, the more likely that a biased result will occur.

Where outcome measures are obtained either by self-report or observer measurement, it is essential that information is obtained in the same way for all subjects. Any under-ascertainment of outcome will effect the validity of the study. Observer blindness will reduce the risk of ascertainment bias and will also ensure that follow-up procedures to obtain outcome will not be influenced differentially in treatment groups. It is also essential that the measure of outcome is precise enough to categorize subjects correctly.

There is no substitute, in designing an experiment with accurate ascertainment of outcome, to having a clear understanding of the biological process under investigation and the potential errors associated with the outcome measure.

16.3.8   Statistical power/sample size

The aim is always to have a study with sufficient participants or groups to ensure that the result obtained is likely, to the best of your knowledge, to be a statistically viable one. This has been discussed in detail in Chapter 3. Before the study commences an estimate of its statistical power is required. To estimate the statistical power for clinical trials, the investigator needs to be able to estimate the likely random errors in the measurements being used and the number of events or changes in an outcome measure to be expected. The investigator also needs to specify the acceptable level of statistical significance and confidence.

It may be that on the basis of the power calculations the study can not be undertaken with the population and finance available. It is wasteful, and in some cases unethical, to commence a study that is never going to produce a statistically and biologically meaningful result.

The statistical power of community trials relates to the number of communities, not the number of individuals, in each group. The power of community trials can be increased by matching intervention and control centres, stratifying on a baseline variable which is strongly related to the outcome, and also by increasing the number of times a community is observed.[10,16]

16.4 Analysis and interpretation

The analyses to be undertaken need to be specified before the study commences. This will ensure both that there are sufficient subjects available in subsets of the sample and that the data are collected in a way that is appropriate for the required analysis. In general, the correct estimate of the effect of the intervention will be the difference in the change from baseline in the intervention compared with the control group, irrespective of the exposure or outcome measure. The statistical significance can be expressed using the 95% confidence interval around the mean difference. In clinical trials, with data collected at the level of the individual, the change from baseline can be measured for each subject and the average change assessed for all subjects.

For community trials the analysis will be of the change in the population incidence or mortality. Community trials often sample subsets of the population in which change in the underlying factors can be estimated, although some caution is required in interpreting the results of these subsets because of the potential effects of sampling and information bias. Murray[10] has recently pointed out that observations on persons within clusters, such as communities, tend to be correlated.

The effects of other factors on the difference in the change between intervention and control groups can be assessed by multiple regression analysis.

It is recommended that some form of graphical presentation of the data are made (for example, see Fig 16.1); this gives a more intuitive feel for the relationship under investigation than a simple level of statistical significance derived from a regression analysis.

Where measuring the outcome of interest (e.g. blood pressure) may itself influence the measure, and may therefore be considered as an intervention in its own right, some researchers have argued that it is not appropriate to make this measurement at baseline. In this situation, the analysis simply measures the difference between groups in the outcome at the end of the study, and assumes that because of randomization baseline differences will not affect the final differences seen. Some caution should be exercised in adopting this approach, which seems attractive and efficient. From our experience, if things can go wrong in research they do, and not having any information about subjects at the beginning of a study may make interpretation difficult. If the baseline measure is measured in all groups, the observed effect of the treatment will be independent of the effect of the baseline measurement, although the overall effect may be attenuated. We believe that, unless there are well argued circumstances, baseline measures should be included in all studies.

There are two major approaches to the consideration of the subjects in the analysis of the data for clinical trials. One view is that once subjects have been randomly allocated to treatment groups they should be included in the analysis irrespective of whether their

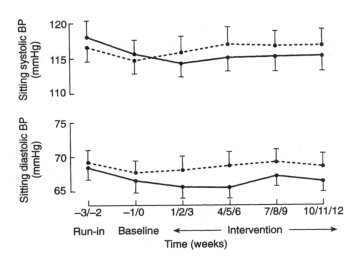

Fig. 16.1 Sitting systolic and diastolic BP in the meat (●————●) and non-meat (●- - - -●) groups (*n*=25 in each group) at different periods during the trial. Results are means with bars representing SEM. (Source: Prescott *et al.*[25])

compliance was good or bad or whether they dropped out or not. This is sometimes referred to as analysing on an 'intention to treat' basis. Excluding subjects who have 'measured' compliance below a certain level is arbitrary and may give optimistically positive results. Since it is not possible to measure compliance perfectly accurately, the decision to exclude those whose compliance measure is below a certain level may give misleading results.

A second view would argue that if the aim of the study was simply to demonstrate that a treatment can effect an outcome, then it may be acceptable to use a restricted subset (on the basis of compliance) of the data. If this approach is taken, consideration must be given to the effect that breaking the balanced group allocation may have on any comparisons. It may be that those who comply sufficiently well to be included are either different in other important characteristics from those not adequately complying and/or the distribution of those characteristics may be different in treatment and control groups.

If the objective of the research is to see whether the offering of the treatment affects outcome, then all subjects must be included in the analysis, irrespective of compliance scores. This latter question is more relevant to public health issues, where the investigator wants to know whether the treatment works in the community. For more detailed consideration on statistical analysis readers are referred to other texts.[5,17–21]

16.5 Designs used in experimental studies

A basic premise for all experimental studies is that the effect of any treatment on an outcome must be compared with the effect of a control treatment on outcome.

Uncontrolled studies of any design are very difficult to interpret. Without a control group being studied in the same way and over the same period, it is difficult to estimate the effects that regression to the mean, familiarization, seasonality in response, and the effects that other unknown factors may have on outcome. For example, in trials measuring blood pressure as the outcome, it is very common to see blood pressures falling in all groups throughout the study; without a control group it would be impossible to separate out the effect of this treatment from the general 'familiarization' effect. In both the Stanford Five Town Study and the Minnesota Heart Health Program, there were secular trends both in the exposure and the outcome measures; without control communities, the real magnitude of the effect of the intervention would have included the secular trend plus the effect of the intervention.[9,10]

Broadly, there are two approaches used in allocating treatment and control regimes: either parallel or crossover. A parallel design is where subjects receive only one treatment and the change in outcome response in one group of subjects (receiving treatment of interest) is compared with that in another group of subjects receiving a different (or control) treatment. In a crossover design each subject receives both (all) treatments in a randomized order with suitable gaps between treatments (wash-out) and outcomes/response is compared within subjects.[22]

In a factorial experimental design, the effects of a number of different factors can be investigated at the same time. The basic design may be parallel or crossover. The treatments are formed by all possible combinations that can be formed from the different factors. For example, Burr and colleagues assessed the effects of both a high fibre diet and a high fish oil diet on recurrence of infarction. Subjects were firstly randomly assigned to receive either the high fibre diet or control diet and then within these groupings they were randomly assigned to receive either the fish oil or the control diet. The advantage of this approach is that the investigator can assess the effect of the interaction between treatments as well as whether one treatment may be more effective than another treatment. If treatments are considered to be acting independently, a factorial design is effectively a number of independent experiments that are being conducted at the same time; it is therefore a cost-effective approach. It may, however, be considerably more difficult for the researcher to keep control of the study and generally factorial designs are limited to only two factors.

An advantage of the crossover design over the parallel design is that subject characteristics are approximately constant for both treatment groups (exposure categories) and it is therefore possible to separate out the effect of the treatment from those which may be due to the individual. This is not the case in parallel studies where subjects do not receive all treatments. Another advantage of a crossover design is that, as all subjects receive the treatment under investigation, the statistical power of the study is greater than in a parallel study of equivalent size, where only a proportion of the subjects receive the treatment under investigation.

A crossover design may be suitable for a single-dose treatment of a micronutrient, but may not be suitable where the treatment is given continuously throughout the treatment period. The latter is most often the case in feeding studies. Single dose studies tend to be used more in pharmacological trials and testing the effects of different drugs in the same patient, with, for example, asthma, where the condition is relatively stable over time and may be the optimal design. Where the condition being studied is likely to vary over time a parallel design is likely to give results which will be easier to interpret.

The most important issues to consider in choosing between a parallel and a crossover design is whether there is likely to be any carry-over or period effects in a cross-over study.[23,24]

In a crossover design, the effect of the first or earlier treatment may carry over into the following period and hence influence the outcome measure during that period. For a two period design it means that the response in period two may be affected by the treatment given in period one. The response in period two will be a combination of the effect of the second treatment and an additional residual effect of treatment in the first period. Some investigators use a wash-out period between treatments to minimize this carry over effect; this assumes that the diet eaten in the wash-out period reverts to the baseline diet and is consumed for long enough to return the outcome measure to baseline. This may only be likely to occur for studies which assess the acute effects of feeding different diets on, for example, blood glucose levels. It is hard to imagine many dietary based experiments aimed at assessing the effects of changing people's diets on risk factors such as lipids or blood pressure, or longer-term measures such as morbidity or mortality, where a crossover design would be free from the potential effects of carry over. Senn has recently argued that it is virtually impossible to be sure that carry over effects are not present.[23]

Balaam has suggested optimal designs which can be used to assess the effects of carry over, without the use of a wash-out period[24]: these include groups of subjects with all combinations of treatments and in different periods. For example, in a two treatment design (A or B) subjects are randomly allocated to one of four groups: AA, BB, AB, BA. The responses in each group are then compared.

For long-term trials, the outcome measure may alter during the study. Disease status may progress, regress, or have a cyclical pattern of response. If the subjects have been randomly allocated to groups (or blocked on disease state if disease state is considered important), these period effects are not likely to lead to a systematically biased outcome. It may be that overall response is different in latter periods where disease may have progressed.

Where it is not known what carry over effects exist, and where it is not feasible (time and money, subject compliance) to use the more complex designs required to assess its likely effect, it is advisable to use a parallel design.

16.6 Systematic reviews of clinical trials – the role of meta-analysis

Over the last few years there has been a massive collaborative effort to bring together all the randomized controlled trial data from all over the world. The Cochrane Collaboration has enabled researchers to do meta-analysis of pooled data from many different studies. These pooled analyses provide pooled estimates of effect with much smaller confidence intervals and provide more reliable estimates of the likely effect. Some caution is required in the use of meta-analysis, particularly to ensure that all relevant studies have been included (no publication bias), that it is appropriate to pool data from different studies, and that the correct statistical methods are used. See Chapter 1 for more details.

16.7 Concluding remarks

A properly controlled randomized experiment offers the best test of causality. If properly conducted it is less likely to give a biased estimate of the effect of an exposure on an outcome. Experiments are, however, not free from the problems of non-experimental studies. Measurement error and the effects of confounding variables may still affect the outcome.

A clearly defined aim for the research is essential and establishes the structure for the research protocol. The question being asked in the experiment needs to be clear, and exposure and outcome need to be able to be measured with precision and freedom from the effects of other variables. The design used needs to be appropriate to the research question and population under study. For clinical and field trials, all subjects, once included in the study, should be observed and followed-up in exactly the same way. Poor compliance, subjects dropping out, and incomplete ascertainment of outcome seriously affect the validity of the study. There should be sufficient subjects, observed for an adequate period of time, included in the study to allow appropriate analyses to be conducted.

For community trials or community intervention studies, which are often aimed at addressing more pragmatic questions related to efficacy of the intervention, there is the same need to pay close attention to the design of the study. Recent experience suggests that the major difficulty in starting a community trial may be the ability to predict the secular trend which is going to occur in the study population, and thereby weaken the power of the study to detect change in outcomes.

References

1. Carpenter, K. (1986) *The history of scurvy and vitamin C.* Cambridge University Press, Cambridge.
2. Pocock, S. J. (1983) *Clinical trials: a practical approach.* Wiley, New York.
3. Medical Research Council. (1948) Streptomycin treatment of pulmonary tuberculosis. *Br. Med. J.* 2: 769–82.
4. Medical Research Council. (1950) Clinical trials of antihistamine drugs in the prevention and treatment of the common cold. *Br. Med. J.* 2: 425–9.
5. Cochran, W. G., Cox, G. M. (1957) *Experimental designs.* 2nd edn. John Wiley & Sons, New York.
6. Bradford-Hill, A. (1971) *Principles of medical statistics.* 9th edn. The Lancet Ltd, London.
7. Truelove, J. C. (1959) Follow-up studies. In: Witts, L. J. (ed.). *Medical surveys and clinical trials.* Oxford University Press, Oxford. 91–104.
8. Geissler, C. (1995) Nutrition intervention. In: Ulijaszek, S. J. (ed.). *Health intervention in less developed countries.* Oxford University Press, Oxford. 23–48.

9. Fortmann, S. P., Flora, J. A., Winkleby, M. A., *et al.* (1995) Community intervention trials: reflections on the Stanford Five-City Project experience. *Am. J. Epid.* **142**: 576–86.

10. Murray, D. M. (1995) Design and analysis of community trials: lessons from the Minnesota Heart Health Program. *Am. J. Epid.* **142**: 569–72.

11. Whitehead, J. (1983) *The design and analysis of sequential clinical trials.* Horwood, Chichester.

12. Armitage. P., Berry, G. (1994) *Statistical methods in medical research.* 3rd edn. Blackwell Scientific Publications, Oxford.

13. Margetts, B. M., Beilin, L. J., Armstrong, B. K., *et al.* (1985) Blood pressure and dietary polyunsaturated and saturated fats: a controlled trial. *Clin. Sci.* **69**: 165–75.

14. Prochaska, J. O., DiClemente, C. C. (1982) Transtheoretical theory: toward a more integrative model of change. *Psychother: Theory, Res. Practice.* **19**: 276–88.

15. Lamb, R., Joshi, S. (1996) The stage model and processes of change in dietary fat reduction. *J. Hum. Nutr. Dietet.* **9**: 43–53.

16. Donner, A., Klar, N. (1996) Statistical considerations in the design and analysis of community trials. *Clin. Epid.* **49**: 435–9.

17. Meinert, C. L. (1986) *Clinical Trials. Design, conduct, and analysis.* Oxford University Press, Oxford.

18. Norman, G. R. (1989) Issues in the use of change scores in randomized trials. *J. Clin. Epid.* **42**: 1097–105.

19. Peto, R., Pike, M. G., Armitage, P., *et al.* (1976) Design and analysis of randomized clinical trials requiring prolonged observations of each patient. I. Introduction and design. *Br. J. Cancer.* **34**: 585–612.

20. Peto, R., Pike, M. G., Armitage, P. *et al.* (1977) Design and analysis of randomized clinical trials requiring prolonged observations of each patient. II. Analysis and examples. *Br. J. Cancer.* **35**: 1–39.

21. Louis, T. A., Lavori, P. W., Bailar, J. C., Polansky, M. (1984) Crossover and self-controlled designs in clinical research. *N. Engl. J. Med.* **310**: 24–31.

22. Jones, B., Kenward, M. G. (1989) *Design and analysis of cross-over trials.* Chapman and Hall, London.

23. Senn, S. (1993) *Cross-over trials in clinical research.* John Wiley and Sons, Chichester.

24. Balaam, L. N. (1968) A two-period design and t^2 experimental units. *Biometrics.* **24**: 61–73.

25. Prescott, S. L., Jenner, D. A., Beilin, L. J., Margetts, B. M., Vandongen, R. A. (1988) Randomized controlled trial of the effect on blood pressure of dietary non-meat protein versus meat protein in normotensive omnivores. *Clin. Sci.* **73**: 665–72.

26. Paradis, G., O'Loughlin, J., Elliott, M., *et al.* (1995) Coeur en Santé St-Henri – a heart health promotion programe in a low income, low education neighbourhood in Montreal, Canada: theoretical model and early field experience. *J. Epid. Comm. Hlth.* **49**: 503–12.

27. Wood, D. A., Kinmonth, A. L., Davies, G. A. *et al.* (1994) Randomized controlled trial evaluating cardiovascular screening and intervention in general practice: principal results of British Family Heart Study. *Br. Med. J.* **308**: 313–20.

28. Muir, J., Mant, D., Jones, L., Yudkin, P. (1994) Effectiveness of health checks conducted by nurses in primary care: results of the OXCHECK study after one year. *Br. Med. J.* **308**: 308–12.

29. Albanes, D., Heinonen, O. P., Huttunen, J. K., *et al.* (1995) Effects of alpha-tocopherol and beta-carotene supplements on cancer incidence in the Alpha-Tocopherol Beta-Carotene Cancer Prevention Study. *Am. J. Clin. Nutr.* **62**: 1427S–1430S.

30. MacLennan, R., Macrae, F., Bain, C., *et al.* (1995) Randomized trial of intake of fat, fiber, and beta-carotene to prevent colorectal adenomas. *J. Nat. Cancer Inst.* **87**: 1760–6.

31. Bostick, R. M., Fosdick, L., Wood, J. R., *et al.* (1995) Calcium and colorectal epithelial cell proliferation in sporadic adenoma patients: a randomized, double-blinded, placebo-controlled clinical trial. *J. Nat. Cancer Inst.* **87**:1307–15.

32. Blot, W. J., Li, J. Y., Taylor, P. R., *et al.* (1993) Nutrition intervention trial in Lianxian, China: supplementation with specific vitamin/mineral combinations, cancer incidence, and disease specific mortality in the general population. *J. Nat. Cancer Inst.* **85**: 1483–92.

33. Hennekens, C. H., Buring, J. E., Manson, J. E., *et al.* (1996) Lack of effect of long-term supplementation with beta-carotene on the incidence of malignant neoplasms and cardiovascular disease. *N. Engl. J. Med.* **334**: 1145–9.

34. Dibley, M. J., Sadjimin, T., Kjolhede, C. L., Moulton, L. H. (1996) Vitamin A supplementation fails to reduce incidence of acute respiratory illness and diarrhoea in preschool-age Indonesian children. *J. Nutr.* **126**: 434–42.

Index